The Assessment of
Child and Adolescent Personality

The Assessment of
Child and Adolescent Personality

Edited by

Howard M. Knoff
THE UNIVERSITY OF SOUTH FLORIDA

THE GUILFORD PRESS
New York   *London*

To Cindy—for always

© 1986 The Guilford Press
A Division of Guilford Publications, Inc.

PRINTED IN THE UNITED STATES OF AMERICA
Last digit is print number: 9 8 7 6 5

Library of Congress Cataloging-in-Publication Data
Main entry under title:

The Assessment of child and adolescent personality.

   Includes bibliographies and index.
   1. Personality assessment of children.   2. Personality
assessment of youth.   I. Knoff, Howard M.   [DNLM:
1. Personality Assessment—in adolescence.
2. Personality Assessment—in infancy & childhood.
3. Personality Development.   WS 105.5.P3 A846]
RJ503.7.P47A87   1986   155.4   85–30585
ISBN 0-89862-668-4

Contributors

David C. Boersma, PhD. Center for Forensic Psychiatry, Ann Arbor, Michigan

Carol A. Boliek, MA. School Psychology Program, University of Northern Colorado, Greeley, Colorado

Marla R. Brassard, PhD. Department of Educational Psychology, University of Georgia, Athens, Georgia

Douglas T. Brown, PhD. Department of Psychology, James Madison University, Harrisonburg, Virginia

Jack A. Cummings, PhD. Department of Counseling and Educational Psychology, Indiana University, Bloomington, Indiana

Stephen T. DeMers, EdD. Department of Educational and Counseling Psychology, University of Kentucky, Lexington, Kentucky

James Garbarino, PhD. Erikson Institute for Advanced Study in Child Development, Chicago, Illinois

Darrell H. Hart, PhD. Educational Support Systems, Inc., Salt Lake City, Utah

Stephen Hooper, PhD. Department of Psychiatry, Vanderbilt University School of Medicine, Nashville, Tennessee

Allen E. Ivey, EdD. Counseling and School Psychology Program, University of Massachusetts, Amherst, Massachusetts

Shagufa Kapadia, MA. Department of Individual and Family Studies, The Pennsylvania State University, University Park, Pennsylvania

Harold R. Keller, PhD. Department of Psychology and School of Education, Syracuse University, Syracuse, New York

Rex B. Kline, PhD. Department of Psychology, University of Saskatchewan, Saskatoon, Saskatchewan, Canada

Howard M. Knoff, PhD. Department of Psychological and Social Foundations of Education, University of South Florida, Tampa, Florida

David Lachar, PhD. Institute of Behavioral Medicine, Good Samaritan Medical Center, Phoenix, Arizona

Roy P. Martin, PhD. Department of Educational Psychology, University of Georgia, Athens, Georgia

Ena Vazquez Nuttall, PhD. Counseling and School Psychology Program, University of Massachusetts, Amherst, Massachusetts

John E. Obrzut, PhD. Department of Educational Psychology, University of Arizona, Tucson, Arizona

H. Thompson Prout, PhD. School Psychology Program, State University of New York at Albany, Albany, New York

Jeffrey Snow, PhD. Department of Counseling and Educational Psychology, University of Missouri, Columbia, Missouri

Irving B. Weiner, PhD. Office of Academic Affairs, Fairleigh Dickinson University, Rutherford, New Jersey

Foreword

The field of personality assessment of children is alive and well, as this fine collection by Howard Knoff amply attests. Presenting a much broader scope than traditional personality assessment texts, this book offers the reader discussions of both projective and objective techniques. While the text has a strong school focus, those interested in clinical approaches will not be disappointed. Likewise, its behavioral emphasis does not slight psychodynamic approaches.

In its attempt to provide a comprehensive picture of this field, *The Assessment of Child and Adolescent Personality* leaves almost no stone unturned. Topics include theoretical, legal, and practical issues involved in assessment; interviewing techniques; the Rorschach and thematic approaches; projective drawings; sentence completion techniques; the Personality Inventory for Children; rating scales; behavioral observation approaches; family assessment; ecological assessment; actuarial and automated assessment approaches; report writing; and intervention strategies.

The wisdom of many specialists can be found in *The Assessment of Child and Adolescent Personality*, and readers will find a wealth of invaluable information about how tests and other assessment procedures are used in schools and clinics. The book also is an excellent source for obtaining references for further study. The volume fills a void in the field and is a welcome addition to the assessment literature. It should prove to be a valuable guide to students and practitioners in the field of clinical child psychology and school psychology.

Jerome M. Sattler
San Diego State University

Preface

The field of personality assessment has long been focused on adults and their emotional and adjustment difficulties. This is not surprising given the history and development of specific personality theories and theorists, and the post–World War II history of clinical psychology. Clearly, this adult focus has resulted in a great number of effective personality assessment approaches, tools, and techniques. However, many of these approaches, initially geared to adult populations and concerns, have been adapted for use or simply used with children and adolescents. In view of the clinical differences which exist between childhood and adult personality development—typical and atypical—many of these approaches are misplaced in the child or adolescent's personality assessment battery.

This book is testimony to the need for personality assessment approaches that are conceptualized, developed, and standardized specifically for the developmental periods of childhood and adolescence. Personality assessment has and must continue to become specific to the various subsets of individuals across the lifespan. Clearly, childhood and adolescence is one such subset—one, within the field of personality assessment which, in many ways, is just emerging. Hopefully, from this emergence, the entire field of personality will be expanded and enriched.

Among the newest (and perhaps oldest) concepts discussed in this book are reciprocal determinism; multitrait, multisetting, multimethod assessment; ecological assessment and evaluation; and multimodal therapy and intervention. Also included are the newest and most updated assessments in the behavior rating scale, projective technique, objective inventory, and family and ecological approach areas. Many of these have been developed specifically for children and adolescents; some are still aspiring to that goal. All of these developments are integrated into a comprehensive, problem-solving process of personality assessment for children and adolescents. Using the steps of problem identification to problem analysis to intervention to evaluation, personality assessment is presented as a broad process where each step is contingent upon the preceding step and where intervention is inextricably tied to problem identification and analysis. This process, additionally, forms an heuristic model which can guide further research and improvements. All of this is accomplished in the book's four parts.

In Part I, the conceptual and theoretical models of disturbance are discussed along with the classification systems which currently exist in the mental health field; the various legal and ethical issues relevant to personality assessment are reviewed; and a conceptual and pragmatic problem-solving process of assessment with children and adolescents is presented.

In Part II, the various personality assessment approaches are discussed: diagnostic interviewing, the Rorschach, the Thematic approaches, projective drawing and sentence completion techniques; the Personality Inventory for Children; behavior rating scales and behavioral observation approaches; and family and ecological assessments. Each of these chapters addresses the assessment process in both school and clinic or agency settings, and each chapter presents one or more case studies demonstrating the specific technique and its clinical usefulness. Part II concludes with a review of the current status of automated/actuarial assessment in the field.

In Part III, the assessment to intervention process is described. Here, the topics include the personality assessment report and the post-assessment/feedback conference, a conceptual and clinical approach to intervention with disturbed and disturbing children and adolescents, and the place of consultation within the comprehensive assessment and intervention process.

Part IV concludes the book with a summarization of its major conceptual and pragmatic points, and a discussion of future needs in the field.

This book has been written for two related audiences: first, graduate students in the mental health fields who need a comprehensive resource to guide their personality assessment processes with children and adolescent clients—from their first academic courses in this area through their clinical practice or internship experiences; and, second, experienced mental health practitioners who wish a comprehensive, updated review of the literature across the multitude of assessment approaches, as well as a review of the newest techniques in the field. The projected "mental health" audience includes clinical, counseling, and school psychologists, psychiatrists or other medical specialists, clinical or psychiatric social workers, mental health and family counselors, psychiatric or other related nursing professions, and other licensible mental health professionals. Clearly, however, any individual who uses the approaches described in this book should use them within the bounds of their expertise and experience and their ethical and moral principles.

When undertaking a book of this magnitude, there is an enormous participating and supporting cast. Initially, I would like to thank all of my colleague/authors who worked painstakingly and professionally to produce chapters of exceedingly high quality and usefulness. They are all experts in this field, and their contributions are much appreciated. Many thanks are due to Tom Prout, who encouraged me to write this particular book first and who has been an excellent professional and personal role model, and to my colleagues at the State University of New York at Albany where much of this book was written. To Mirabel Gray, the word processing "Wang Wizard" at SUNY–Albany's School of Education, I can not give enough thanks. She stuck through this production from beginning to end, lending her technical and personal support, scanning these hundreds of pages with precision and dedication.

In many ways, a book's quality is also a function of its editorial support system. I have been fortunate to work with many superb professionals at The Guilford Press. Many thanks go to Seymour Weingarten, Editor-in-Chief who supported this project from its beginning; Sharon Panulla, production editor extraordinaire; Russell Till, who provided expert production services; and to the entire staff at The Guilford Press.

Finally, to my wife Cindy: for the untold hours that I wasn't there, for all my nights until 3:00 a.m., for the pressure and the anxiety of deadlines—both real and imagined, for all her love and support . . . this is for you.

Howard M. Knoff

Contents

3. A Conceptual Model and Pragmatic Approach toward Personality Assessment Referrals

57

Howard M. Knoff

II. Personality Assessment Approaches and Techniques with Children and Adolescents

4. The Diagnostic Interview Process

105

Ena Vazquez Nuttall and Allen E. Ivey

5. Assessing Children and Adolescents with the Rorschach

141

Irving B. Weiner

6. Thematic Approaches to Personality Assessment with Children and Adolescents

173

John E. Obrzut and Carol A. Boliek

7. *Projective Drawings*   199

Jack A. Cummings

8. *The Sentence Completion Techniques*   245

Darrell H. Hart

9. *The Personality Inventory for Children: Approaches to Actuarial Interpretation in Clinic and School Settings*   273

David Lachar, Rex B. Kline, and David C. Boersma

10. *Behavior Rating Scale Approaches to Personality Assessment in Children and Adolescents*   309

Roy P. Martin, Stephen Hooper, and Jeffrey Snow

11. *Behavioral Observation Approaches to Personality Assessment*   353

Harold R. Keller

12. *Family Assessment Approaches and Procedures*   399

Marla R. Brassard

13. *Ecological Assessment Procedures*   451

James Garbarino and Shagufa Kapadia

IV. *Summation and Integration*

I
Theories, Issues, and Procedures in Personality Assessment

Before choosing a personality assessment battery to evaluate a referred child or adolescent, it is important to have a comprehensive understanding of the theories, issues, and conceptual models underlying the entire process. These components form the foundation which guides personality assessment—both its planning and its evaluation. This section of the book reviews relevant conceptual, theoretical, and empirical research and writing in the field to create this foundation. In Chapter 1, the theories of disturbed and disturbing behavior are discussed; the classification systems currently utilized in mental health and educational settings to specify different types of atypical behaviors and affects are reviewed; and important professional and ethical issues which arise when children and adolescents are referred and assessed are considered. In Chapter 2, the important legislative mandates and legal decisions related to assessment in general and personality assessment in particular are discussed. Finally, in Chapter 3, there is a presentation of conceptual and pragmatic approaches toward assessment. The former approach is an integration of the theoretical models of disturbance across a problem-solving process; the latter approach is a "hands-on" process which considers the research literature, ultimately suggesting a practical, efficacious assessment routine.

1

Identifying and Classifying Children and Adolescents Referred for Personality Assessment: Theories, Systems, and Issues

Howard M. Knoff

In a sense, children and adolescents' personalities and social–emotional statuses are constantly, formally and informally, being evaluated by parents, educators, mental health professionals, and community "others" (e.g., community and religious leaders, peers, adult acquaintances). Anchoring these evaluations is, minimally, a general sense of expected or typical behavior from a societal, cultural, developmental, and/or legal perspective. Sound personality development and competent social–emotional interactions are important to a child or adolescent's physiological, cognitive, academic, and vocational maturation or progress. Certainly, the relationship between positive self-concept and general interpersonal adjustment has been well discussed (Rogers, 1961, 1980) and demonstrated, for example, in the achievement and school performance domains (e.g., Bandura, 1969; Knoff, 1983; Taylor, Winne, & Marx, 1975). Personality assessment, then, initially is based on an understanding of normative expectations and typical personality development across the life span. Further, personality assessment provides the baseline and ongoing evaluation data that demonstrate the integral relationship between social–emotional status and all facets of human activity.

Formal personality assessment by a mental health practitioner (a school, counseling, or clinical psychologist, psychiatrist, social worker, guidance counselor, psychiatric nurse) often occurs when a child or adolescent's behavior problems, interactions, or ecological situation become so significantly disruptive that mental health intervention appears warranted. Thus, while personality assessment can be proactive and commonplace (as when used to evaluate positive interpersonal adjustment), it is most often used for referred individuals with significant behavioral or emotional disorders or disruptions. Formal personality assessment involves a number of diverse perspectives, approaches, and techniques which help to identify and characterize the referred individuals' social–emotional status and their attitudes, behaviors, and reactions to specific and recent or general and long-existing situations or environments. With children and adolescents, personality

Howard M. Knoff. Department of Psychological and Social Foundations of Education, School Psychology Program, University of South Florida, Tampa, Florida.

3

assessment occurs most often in a school or community mental health (private or public) setting.

While mental health practitioners investigate and explore personality assessment referrals, they need to explore why the referral has occurred, what their theoretical notions of an "appropriate" referral include, and how they feel about potentially describing or classifying the referred individual. These concerns directly involve perspectives that influence referral decisions, theoretical models of disturbed behavior, and classification systems that categorize atypical developmental and social–emotional behavior, respectively. These will be discussed below, all from the focus of personality assessment.

Perspectives That Influence Referral Decisions

The decision to refer a child or adolescent to a mental health practitioner is ultimately the parent or guardian's unless, for extenuating circumstances, a social service agency or court-ordered caretaker has the authority to take that step. These circumstances aside, the referral may be initiated individually by the parents or as suggested by a significant other who feels and convinces the parents that the referral is necessary. At times, the "referred" child is the "significant other" who initiates the (self-)referral which ultimately requires the parents' approval and cooperation.

When a referral for personality assessment and intervention occurs, the practitioner should immediately clarify how the referral decision was reached and why his or her help is being sought. Often, the referral is the result of a perceived discrepancy between the referred child's behaviors, attitudes, or interpersonal interactions in some situation or environment and some more optimal level desired and defined by the referral source. The basis of the discrepancy may come from one or more perspectives which conceptually define acceptable versus unacceptable behavior.

The Sociocultural Perspective

The sociocultural perspective represents the most pervasive influence on a child's present and emerging behavior because it shapes the normative values, ideologies, attitudes, and behaviors of countries, communities, families, and individuals who interact with the child. One's sociocultural environment includes those socioeconomic, racial, religious, national, geographic, or idiosyncratic characteristics which create group or community identities and mores. These identities and the behaviors that operationalize community standards represent the "norm" of typical, acceptable behavior.

While dramatically powerful, the sociocultural environment is surprisingly malleable and ever changing. For example, one generation's emphasis on individual and differentiated sex roles (e.g., in the 1950s) may later become obsolete to the next generation's insistence on more androgenous and shared sexual roles and responsibilities (e.g., in the 1980s). These changes, therefore, demonstrate that a culture's concept of "acceptable" behavior and attitude is also constantly changing. Practitioners considering referrals for personality assessment, then, must be particularly sensitive to these changes and to current sociocultural perspectives of "normality."

From this perspective, a child or adolescent might be referred when he or she manifests behaviors or attitudes that represent unacceptable societal standards. For example, the child who destroys property and shows no remorse or strides toward behavioral change, by most community standards, would be appropriately referred. However, some children might be referred when manifesting acceptable, contemporary behavior which, nonetheless, is considered unacceptable given the referral source's sociocultural background or upbringing. An example of this anachronistic situation might involve an immigrant parent's struggle with an "Americanized" adolescent's behavior and attitudes toward responsibility. While both types of referrals might require mental health attention, the practitioner's analysis and understanding of the specific sociocultural variables and interactions should facilitate the best assessment and therapeutic choices and directions.

To summarize, the sociocultural environment creates a broad community consensus on acceptable behavior which becomes a norm or standard for comparison. Some children or adolescents may be referred for personality assessment because they differ from this norm. The mental health practitioner must consider both the sociocultural norm and the referred child's behavior to decide if a discrepancy indeed does exist, and then if the apparent discrepancy is disruptive to the child's overall psychological and developmental growth and future.

The Community Subgroup Perspective

Sometimes a specific dominant community subgroup can define its own norms for "typical" and "acceptable" behavior that may differ from the broader sociocultural norms. This may occur when the community subgroup is well defined or organized, is relatively homogeneous in its interactions with children and adolescents, and/or is able to significantly influence these norms and behaviors in a pervasive perhaps day-to-day way. These subgroups might include small sociocultural subgroups within a community as well as educational, medical, legal or governmental, mental health, or community recreational subgroups. A sociocultural subgroup might be the affluent, upper class suburbanites that live on one side of a community's train tracks, or the subgroup that comprises the "Italian North End" of a large urban community. Given their individual definitions of expected behavior, then, a subgroup may identify a child for a personality assessment referral when he or she substantially differs from the subgroup's norms. For example, a child who significantly and/or persistently breaks a district's disciplinary code might prompt a referral based purely on past experience with such students within this educational domain. Similarly, the judicial system might order psychological assessment for certain types of infractions at certain ages (e.g., firesetting by a delinquent youth) given its experience with such adjudications and their recidivism rates.

Referrals, therefore, from a community subgroup must be analyzed and understood from the subgroup's perspective, ecology, and environmental conditions. A child might be considered inappropriate or disruptive within one subgroup and be accepted or acceptable in another. The practitioner should acknowledge potential subgroup differences and explore the broad implications of a child's unacceptable behavior in one setting, yet that behavior's acceptance in all other settings. On the other hand, a referral from one subgroup's perspective might substantiate other subgroups' reactions and impressions of an individual and prompt more pervasive, comprehensive communication and calls for personality assessment. The referring community subgroup, therefore, might be reacting to a sample of a child's behavior compared to their specific norms, or might be seeing problem behaviors which exist across many subgroups and which should be evaluated through personality assessment. Hopefully, the practitioner can assess the referral across different subgroup perspectives. This maximizes the validity of the referral and minimizes the potential for specific subgroup bias.

The Setting-Specific Perspective

Often within the community subgroups are individual settings and people who have their own ecological and personal norms of acceptable and unacceptable behavior. In spite of the sociocultural and subgroup norms, these personal norms may result, for example, from experiences within single settings with children at one chronological or developmental age level. Thus, these norms may arise without the benefit of a larger environmental and life-span context, a limitation that may be unrecognized by the individual and that may require a conscious effort to minimize (e.g., through continuing education or by taking time to observe children of other ages or in various settings).

A referral from the setting-specific perspective often occurs when a child manifests behaviors that are discrepant to a significant degree from certain setting and individual norms. For example, the former junior high school classroom teacher forced to teach first grade due to declining enrollments might refer a first-grade child for personality assessment because he or she is unable to socially interact or express important social needs. This referral may refect the teacher's setting-specific perspectives and may be inappropriate if he or she is using past junior high school socialization criteria to evaluate this first-grader's behavior and to rationalize the personality assessment referral. Or, two parents might express setting-specific concerns about a child's nightmares and specific fears because their other children never exhibited such behavioral reactions at the same age, despite the fact that such occurrences are not unusual for most children at that specific age.

Once again, the mental health practitioner must explore and understand these setting and person-specific perspectives of typical or acceptable behavior in order to fully address any referral's concerns. This process always entails some reality testing with the referral source to determine the true extent of the discrepancy between actual and desired behavior and generally involves some determination of the pervasiveness and severity of the referred behavior to the child, his or her surroundings, and his or her future development. Ultimately, this comparison of the referred behavior to a broader mental health context requires the practitioner to determine the validity of the referral, a decision which certainly implicates his or her *own* comprehensive attitudes and beliefs of what constitutes acceptable versus unacceptable behavior.

This entire discussion focuses on the reality that different elements of society, whether they involve sociocultural, community subgroup, or setting-specific perspectives, consider different values, behaviors, and attitudes as acceptable or unacceptable. While there is often an "unwritten" definition or consensus of typical behavior at any one point in time in any one culture or community, any specific referral must be assessed individually for its appropriateness; that is, the practitioner should not accept the assumption that often underlies the referral process: If the referral source finds a need to make a referral, there certainly must be a significant problem that must be as stated by that source. The practitioner must be willing to make the difficult decision of rejecting an inappropriate referral. Such rejections can help the referral source to reassess his or her perspective of the referred child and his or her attitudes toward what is typical versus atypical behavior. Ultimately, these reassessments can change societal perspectives; indeed Szasz's notions (1961) of the myth of mental illness and Ryan's notions (1976) of "blaming the victim" have had wide-reaching effects.

To conclude, while the sociocultural, community subgroup, and setting-specific perspectives of acceptable behavior have been discussed separately, they are actually interdependent and unavoidably correlated. A definition of normality depends on all three perspectives along with the practitioner's knowledge of typical psychological development and mental health theory, experience, and application. At times, the mental health practitioner is unable to determine how acceptable a referred child's behavior is until after a complete personality assessment. Thus, while some referrals are rejected as inappropriate, others will require assessment to determine the absence of any significant problems. Normality, therefore, despite these three perspectives and a practitioner's experience and expertise, is not always immediately evident. Nonetheless, the practitioner is wise to consider often the question of "what is typical" and to explore the many domains that help with its answer.

Personality Assessment and the Theoretical Models of Disturbed Behavior

While there are cultural and community perspectives of typical and atypical behavior, there are also theoretical models that define and explain disturbed behavior. Personality assessment often is guided by these theoretical definitions, and in many cases, assessment results help to validate the theoretical notions of psychological disturbance and help to operationalize the definitions themselves. Currently, there are eight major theoretical models of disturbed behavior: the neurobiological, psychoanalytic, humanistic, cognitive-developmental, behavioral, psychoeducational, interactionalist, and ecological models. While some theories do share various elements or ideas and while some referred behaviors can be explained satisfactorily with two or more (or a combination of) theories, the eight models will be discussed in detail separately. These discussions will first define the model's definition and explanation of disturbed behavior and then discuss the model in the context of personality assessment.

The Neurobiological Model

The neurobiological model assumes that disturbed behavior occurs because of some genetic, chromosomal, biochemical, neurological, or physiological malfunction or damage which directly or indirectly influences the individual's social-emotional control. While early discussions considered the neurobiological–behavioral interaction as unidirectional (neurobiological dysfunctions cause disturbed behavior), the field now recognizes the interaction between these two conditions; that is, a neurobiological condition may not occur unless some environmental, behavioral, or stressful condition occurs triggering the biological reaction which then triggers the disturbed social–emotional reaction. Thus, the child or adolescent may be neurobiologically predisposed, but the environmental stress is necessary to make that predisposition a reality. Technically, this is called the *diathesis-stress* notion, and it has been used to explain why both identical twins do not become schizophrenic when one twin is schizophrenic (Thomas, 1979; Wicks-Nelson & Israel, 1984).

Despite the neurobiological–behavioral interaction, neurobiological conditions have been shown to cause directly some atypical social–emotional reactions. For example, the Lesch–Nyhan syndrome, a genetic/chromosomal disorder which occurs only in males because it is sex-limited to the *X* chromosome, causes unusual motor development, mental retardation, and extreme self-mutilation during childhood. Caused by a defective gene, this disorder usually results in death before adulthood is reached. Feingold (1975) has hypothesized a biochemical explanation of hyperactivity which identifies a child's allergic reaction to certain food additives as the cause. While some have criticized his methodology, some studies using the "Feingold diet" have resulted in decreases in children's hyperactive behavior (Connors, Goyette, Southwick, Lees, & Andrulonis, 1976; Swanson & Kinsbourne, 1980). Similarly, Crook (1980) has discussed the effects of allergies to such common foods as milk, sugar, eggs, and chocolate on children's learning capabilities and behavior.

From a neurological perspective, pre- and postnatal traumas are definitely related to significant disruptions in children's cognitive, learning, and behavioral development. Significant brain damage from anoxia at birth is directly related to later developmental deficits as are deficits due to maternal alcohol and drug involvement during pregnancy (Liebert & Wicks-Nelson, 1981). This, actual physiological or structural damage to a child's brain and neurological processing pathways can explain some skill deficits and behavioral impairments (Bower, 1969).

Pragmatically, the neurobiological model can provide insights or explanations for some disturbed behaviors, but comprehensive personality assessment and intervention often requires other models for support and thoroughness. When this model is used exclusively, the practitioner and especially the referral source could fall into the "medical model" trap that all neurobiological and other dysfunctions can be "cured" through some operation or pharmaceutical intervention. Such cures are rare, and even when they are available, they often do not address the comprehensiveness of a behavioral or personality-related problem which often extends beyond the referred child to families, school personnel, and other significant individuals. For example, while Ritalin and other drug interventions can change the hyperactive child's attention span and impulse control, this may not help him to learn any better or more efficiently (Barkley, 1979). Thus, the intervention may change elements of the referred problem, yet leave the comprehensive difficulty unchanged.

With respect to personality assessment, the neurobiological model does not advocate any specific approaches. Certainly a medical doctor would find reliable observations in various settings useful, and he or she might question psychosomatic influences in some cases. Yet, someone using this model would not routinely request personality assessment unless the syndrome of interest medically called for such measures. Within school or community agencies that use multidisciplinary approaches to service delivery, the mental health practitioner will hopefully consider formal personality assessment when appropriate, even if a neurobiological model appears to be the most dominant explanation given a specific referral. Only with a comprehensive assessment can the full implications of the neurobiological–behavioral interaction be realized.

The Psychoanalytic Model

The psychoanalytic model has its roots in Freudian theory, expanding through the psychologies of the neo-Freudians and ego psychologists, including Anna Freud. This model views disturbed behavior as a manifestation of underlying or unconscious conflicts or forces which cannot be resolved by the rationality of the ego, the individual's decision-making and reality-testing psychological structure. According to Freud, these conflicts will generally arise from the id, which is the impulsive, pleasure-seeking personality structure needing immediate gratification, or from the superego, the standard-setting conscience of the personality which sometimes becomes too self-critical and rigid, expecting too high a level of moral behavior. While the ego usually is able to deal with "reality anxiety" (those fears of real dangers in the environment), the ego is not successfully mediating "neurotic anxiety" (the fear that id-driven instincts, for example, of a sexual or aggressive nature, will get out of control) or "moral anxiety" (the fear that the superego's moral expectations will paralyze personality development through, for example, guilt feelings) when these anxieties become debilitating. Here, debilitation involves (*a*) the individual's need to use defense mechanisms that involuntarily compensate for anxiety by creating adjustment patterns which are somewhat socially acceptable, yet restrictive to any further personality development, or (*b*) a total breakdown of the ego structure such that psychosis and loss of touch with reality results.

Other important characteristics of the psychoanalytic model include its developmental and deterministic nature. According to Freud, children develop through five psychosexual stages (oral, anal, phallic, latency, and genital), each with specific conflicts to resolve and specific bodily zones which they depend on for gratification. For example, the oral stage involves a child's mouth as the primary source of satisfaction and consists of two stages (oral–passive and oral–aggressive) describing two styles of gratification a child may adopt and maintain as a long-standing personality style. If the developmental conflict is not resolved at a particular stage, the child may become "fixated" at that stage, and the anxiety and characteristics of the conflict and stage may dominate the personality style and inhibit further personality development.

To summarize briefly, according to this model, a child's disturbed behavior can be analyzed to identify three possible types of anxiety, the presence of defense mechanisms (e.g., repression, denial, projection, displacement), and the stage where the child has become fixated. Disturbed behavior indicates that psychosexual and personality development has not progressed typically and that the ego is dealing with more conflict and "psychic energy" than can reasonably be handled. Psychoanalytic theory does not assume that the individual is aware of any significant conflicts; personality assessment using psychoanalytic methods is necessary to uncover these conflicts.

Given the often unconscious nature of a disturbed child's conflicts, psychoanalytic personality assessment is directed at his or her latent and symbolic content and manifestations. Freud often used hypnosis, free association, dream analysis, symbolic interpretation, and "Freudian slips" to assess an individual's difficulties. More recently, projective techniques have been used because their symbolic content is thought to uncover significant themes, conflicts, or issues that are related to a referred disturbance. Actually, it is the psychoanalytic interpretation of most projective techniques rather than their theoretical foundations or construct developments that makes them, or any other assessment procedure, "psychoanalytic." Certainly a behavioral observation or objective personality inventory (e.g., the Personality Inventory for Children) could be interpreted behaviorally, psychoanalytically, or from another theoretical perspective. The most critical point, however, is that this model does regard personality assessment as a necessary component of a problem analysis process which then sug ests intervention directions.

The Humanistic Model

The humanistic model actually spends more time discussing the characteristics and variables necessary for an individual to be fulfilled or "self-actualized" than the conditions that result in a disturbed child or adolescent. Further, this model is more geared to adult disturbance, given the writings of Rogers (1961) and Maslow (1968), than to difficulties in school-aged children and adolescents. Nonetheless, the humanistic model does describe a pattern of psychological development that explains disturbed behavior from its perspective.

During infancy and early childhood, the individual's primary psychological goal is to develop a sense of self, a sense of self-esteem, and a sense of a desired self or "ideal-self." Through a developmental process that depends on interactions with the environment (primarily the nuclear family), the child develops a sense of reality versus make-believe, a need for positive external- and self-regard, a recognition that some positive regard is conditional or contingency based, and finally an awareness of an unconditional positive regard that exists above any conditional levels. Unconditional positive regard occurs when the child feels loved and respected regardless of individual behaviors which significant others may not appreciate or accept at a specific point in time. These unacceptable behaviors and the external or internal feedback defining them as unacceptable can create feelings of "incongruence" or conflict for the child. Without this sense of unconditional positive regard, these conflicts can decrease the child's personality development and potentially create disturbed behavior.

According to this model, disturbed behavior occurs when incongruence between a child's self and ideal-self is so significant that the potential for ongoing actualization is paralyzed. The discrepancy is minimized by the individual through "perceptual distortion," a process of distorting reality so that it coincides with the desired ideal self, or through "denial," a process of avoiding the discrepancy by ignoring those realities that create it. These "defense mechanisms" exist as a series of self-protective attitudes and behaviors that distort reality and arrest ongoing personality development. Ultimately, the disturbance reaches a level of significant anxiety which disrupts the child's daily routine, increases negative self-concept feelings and perceptions, and threatens his or her reality testing and orientation. Humanists do not describe what specific behaviors would be considered disturbed; this, they believe, is related to the individual and his or her developmental history.

Because of their concern with normal child through adult personality development, the humanists do not emphasize personality assessment for the purpose of defining or analyzing disturbed or aberrant behavior. It is assumed that through the nondirective counseling process, the individual will not only discover his or her significant problems and issues, but also structure him- or herself toward positive reflection and change. Thus, observation primarily during counseling is the predominant "assessment" technique. At times, the Q-sort (Rogers, 1961), a task measuring the individual's perceptions of self versus ideal-self, might be used to assess the discrepancy between those two states. Finally, some structured assessment and therapeutic approaches, such as play therapy, are used to analyze a child's and family's interdependent dynamics, although again the interpretation perspective (e.g., humanistic vs. behavioral vs. psychoanalytic) is more telling than the technique itself.

The Cognitive-Developmental Model

The cognitive-developmental model is specifically based on the work of Jean Piaget and is generally based on the child and adolescent psychology literatures which provide baselines of age-expected personality and behavioral characteristics. This model analyzes the potential impacts of atypical development (e.g., in the physiological, perceptual, learning, socialization, or psychoeducational areas) on a referred child's age-expected versus problem behavior. The theoretical basis of the model, however, emphasizes the importance of cognition and cognitive processes such as memory, perception, language, problem solving, and abstract thinking (Van Evra, 1983). While the other developmental areas support the child's cognitive development, Piaget and advocates of this model suggest that cognitive development and status determine the child's perceptions and interpretations of his or her world and influence his or her interactions with the environment.

The cognitive–developmental model is founded upon a stage perspective of development; that is, the child moves from one developmental stage to the next (i.e., from the sensory-motor to preoperational to concrete to formal operations stages) as the child's ability to perform specific cognitive processes and skills are cognitively possible and actually exhibited. Ultimately, all behavior is guided by the skills ascribed to a child's cognitive stage (or status) and his or her understanding and representation of the environment and its significant people and components. Behavioral change as well as new learning and cognitive development occur as children organize or evaluate the information in their environments and adapt to novel situations. This is accomplished through assimilation processes (fitting these new situations into existing conceptualizations or behavior patterns) or accommodation processes (adopting and/or creating new conceptualizations to fit in situations that cannot be explained by existing schema or conceptualizations). Supporting these processes are, for example, the individual's capacity for selective attention, information processing, motivated thinking, and generalization across settings and individuals (Baldwin, 1969; Kohlberg, 1969).

Disturbed behavior, according to this model, occurs when a child's cognitive functions fail to properly influence appropriate age- and setting-specific behavior. This "failure" may occur because (a) the child has missed or something has interfered with opportunities to develop the cognitive structures, perceptions, and interpretations of self and environment that guide appropriate behaviors and behavioral responses; (b) the child cannot express or inhibits appropriate behavioral reactions even though he or she has the necessary cognitive structures; and (c) the expected behaviors require cognitive structures that differ from the structures assumed to be necessary and experientially nurtured by, for example, teachers or parents (Elkind, 1976; Flavell, 1977). While the cognitive–developmental model frequently has been used to explain child or adolescent disturbances such as hyperactivity, inadequate impulse control, poor problem solving, depression, and

the developmental problems associated with cognitive deficits (e.g., mental retardation or learning disabilities), other more pervasive disorders such as schizophrenia or anxiety disorders could be understood and addressed using it.

The cognitive-developmental model is so focused on cognition that "personality" assessment is a derivative of cognitive assessment and not a distinct conceptual or actual activity. Because the model is concerned with a child's cognitive
stage, skills, and status and how they relate to behavior and personality, norm-
and criterion-referenced assessments are often used to infer and analyze those
underlying structures or internal processes that are responsible for the child's current (inappropriate) behavior and/or thinking. Using this model's developmental
perspective, a practitioner would also compare a child's current social–emotional
status with age norms that represent typical behavioral and other expectations.
This comparison would identify the range and severity of the disturbed behavior,
place it within the development stage or age where it would be expected or considered appropriate, and suggest the next highest developmental stage or behavior
that would be expected through maturation and/or intervention. As with other
models, personality assessment permitting these developmental comparisons
would still be conceptualized within the cognitive framework that guides the entire model's theoretical beliefs and assumptions.

The Behavioral Model

The behavioral model originated with the work of Watson and Raynor (1920),
matured with Skinner (1938, 1953), and now has fully expanded into many different perspectives of behavior and learning. Behavioral advocates believe that
disturbed behavior results from inappropriate conditioned responses; reinforcement patterns, schedules, and contingencies; modeling and social learning; and/or
cognitive beliefs and thinking (Kauffman, 1981; Nelson, 1981; Ross, 1980; Wicks-
Nelson & Israel, 1984). These inappropriate behavior and learning situations relate
to the classical conditioning, operant conditioning, social learning theory, and
cognitive–behavioral paradigms, respectively.

Disturbed behavior, explained within a classical conditioning paradigm, is
evident when a stimulus (the conditioned stimulus, CS) that does not originally
elicit an inappropriate behavior or response (the unconditioned response, UCR)
becomes paired with a separate stimulus (the unconditioned stimulus, UCS) that
does elicit an inappropriate response (the unconditioned response, UCR) such that
the CS eventually does elicit the inappropriate response (the conditioned response,
CR) even when presented alone. For example, a child may exhibit behaviors that
appear to be "school phobic" when further analysis reveals that it is really a fear
(CR) of the school bus (UCS), which previously had skidded and stopped short
of another car, thus creating a fear-provoking situation (UCR) that had later
become paired with the process of leaving the house to go to the bus stop (CS).
The conditioning process is dependent minimally on the pairing process between
the two stimuli and on the number of paired trials necessary to make the CS–CR
connection. Sometimes the conditioning process is not as evident because generalization from the original conditioned stimulus has occurred, resulting in a
larger class of stimuli which elicit the behavioral response (e.g., the fear coming
as the child thinks about getting out of bed to get ready for school).

Operant conditioning theory states that behavior is a function of antecedent
stimulus conditions and consequence response conditions, all of which are ob-

servable in the environment. Simplistically, behavior occurs when antecedent conditions (e.g., the child's attention span, a quiet setting, a prepared teacher, previous learning) facilitate a response which is then reinforced (positively, aversively, or punitively; immediately or after a predetermined number of responses or amount of time). Disturbed or inappropriate behavior occurs when environmental conditions support its manifestation and when the behavior is reinforced in such a way that it becomes learned and entrenched in the child's behavioral repertoire. For example, an adolescent may make an inappropriate remark in class (stimulus) because he perceives a teacher with a weak disciplinary style (environmental condition) and because he gets immediate attention and approval from his peers who laugh and support his behavior (reinforcement). This inappropriate behavior becomes stronger or more resistant to extinction when the teacher punishes the behavior inconsistently and when the adolescent's peers continue to laugh periodically even though asked to refrain by the teacher.

Social learning theory proponents (Bandura, 1977) believe that behavior can be learned by directly modeling a specific task or behavior or by vicariously observing the consequences (positive or negative) that occur when someone else models that behavior. A number of psychological processes are considered necessary for successful direct modeling: attention to the task, retention, motoric reproduction, and the motivation to perform the task. For successful vicarious modeling, factors like the child's identification with the model (age, sex, socioeconomic status), the behavior and situation presented, and the reinforcements and reinforcement contingencies used appear critical. Disturbed behavior within this paradigm occurs when a child has observed and directly models inappropriate behaviors or has generalized multiple observations of different inappropriate behaviors into more complex patterns of disturbed behavior. Disturbed behavior generally involves a disinhibition of behavior, that is, a removal of behavioral control. For example, after observing a group of peers enjoying the aggressive antics of "The Three Stooges," a child might imitate those behaviors at school in a seemingly out-of-context (for the teacher) way. The teacher's negative response to those behaviors hopefully cues the child in to the inappropriateness of that type of aggressiveness and social interaction.

The cognitive-behavioral paradigm expands the notion of behavior to include thoughts, imagery, information processing, and the intrapersonal aspects of attention and problem solving. It is assumed that behind every behavior are cognitive processes which help to create, direct, and support the behavior. Cognitive-behavioral practitioners consider disturbed behavior to reflect improper problem solving, incorrect self-statements or cognitive beliefs, and/or inadequate internal impulse (or other) controls. Meichenbaum (1979), for example, has demonstrated that children can learn greater cognitive–behavioral impulse control by using self-instructions to both monitor their behavior and decrease the behavior that occurs "before they think about it."

The behavioral model does not discriminate between personality assessment and any other type of assessment. A referred problem is behaviorally identified and defined; it is then analyzed by quantifying and observing its occurrence in specific environments along with relevant environmental variables and interactions, and the analysis eventually leads to an intervention paradigm consistent with the collected data. Overt or cognitive behaviors are considered manifestations of one's personality; the behavioral model does not use symbolic interpretation or assume that a behavior represents a symptom of some more pervasive, underlying disorder. Behavior rating scales are also used to generate behavioral descriptions and empirical and statistical methodologies which classify behaviors as typical or atypical in frequency, duration, and/or intensity across specific age levels. Thus, the behavioral model does assess personality by investigating clearly specified behaviors and the interactions of person, environmental, and behavioral characteristics.

The Psychoeducational Model

The psychoeducational model (Fagen, 1979; Long, Morse, & Newman, 1980; Morse, 1975) integrates a psychiatric view that disturbed behavior is caused by conflicts both within the child and due to relationships and stresses in the child's environment, and an educational view that the academic achievement process and its (self-perceived) success is important to the child's well-being, facilitating self-concept, social–emotional growth, and positive interpersonal change. Within this model, the interaction between a child's thoughts and feelings and his or her experience in the educational or academic setting is paramount. For example, it is likely that a child's negative self-concept can affect school learning and success and just as likely that academic failure can initiate the negative self-concept feelings. The psychoeducational model accepts the presence of the disturbed behavior regardless of its "chicken or egg" origination, identifies the child's academic and affective strengths and weaknesses, and begins to create an environment which facilitates both educational and social–emotional support and developmental progress.

In a sense, the psychoeducational model is very individualistic and child oriented in its view of disturbed behavior. Any psychological and educational perspective that helps to identify and clarify a child's unique disturbed behavior and to suggest remedial directions toward resolving the difficulties is considered. Further, the child's disturbance is not described with a "classic" textbook description, classification, or label, nor compared to other children who manifested similar problems. Each child's difficulties are assumed to be unique and, as such, are analyzed individually and addressed with specifically tailored interventions.

Interventions, within the psychoeducational model, occur in the educational setting and may involve changes in the interactions between a child and teacher, a child and the curriculum, a child and the organizational atmosphere and format of the classroom, and/or a child and him- or herself. The ultimate goal of this model is to create a supportive environment, an empathetic and trusting relationship between a child and his or her teacher, greater self-awareness and self-acceptance on the part of the child, and changes toward more positive coping and problem-solving styles resulting in increased feelings of success. Given its individualization, "success" becomes a relative term. While attending to a class lecture for 20 minutes without incident might be success for one child, it may be a regression toward another child's original, preintervention status.

Within the psychoeducational model, personality assessment is an integrated procedure within a broader holistic assessment process, and it is always occurring. As the model encourages the enlistment of any potentially useful assessment (or intervention) approach, the assessment approach will be varied and individualized to the child's specific problems or concerns. Further, as intervention is accomplished within a "therapeutic milieu or environment" and as some crises are used to teach specific coping or adaptation skills, some assessments may actually become interventions and some interventions may later be considered assessments.

Thus, the psychoeducational model does believe in personality assessment, yet the assessment tends to be geared to the individual child and is often accomplished in the environment where and when the actual disturbed behavior occurs.

The Interactionalist Model

Actually, the interactionalist model is not a formal unified "model" explaining personality disturbances, but is more of a theoretical perspective using the works of Rudolf Dreikurs and William Glasser. This perspective, which primarily addresses discipline problems or "disturbing" (rather than "disturbed") behaviors, exists along a conceptual spectrum between the humanistic and the behavioral models; that is, the interactionalist model believes that disturbing children should be forced to take responsibility for their inappropriate behavior and that significant adults need to create the learning and social–emotional atmosphere which supports this goal. This differs from the humanistic model, which assumes that children will actualize their behavior given a maturing, unconditionally positive environment with little direct teaching or adult intervention, and the behavioral model, which emphasizes direct adult control and environmental manipulation in order to facilitate learning and behavioral change (Wolfgang & Glickman, 1980).

Dreikurs' beliefs concerning childhood disturbances emanate from Alfred Adler's social theory of personality. Both theorists believe that all people want to belong to one or more social groupings and want to be accepted by others within those groups. A child's disturbing behavior, therefore, is motivated by a need for social recognition and is orderly, purposeful, and goal directed. Dreikurs identifies four subconscious goals that motivate inappropriate behavior: (a) attention getting, (b) power and control, (c) revenge, and (d) helplessness or inadequacy. Because these goals can be identified consciously for the child and because the behavior is within the child's control, Dreikurs advocates methods that make the child aware of the logical and natural consequences of inappropriate behavior and, thus, encourage independent change (Dreikurs, Grunwald, & Pepper, 1982).

Glasser's "reality therapy" (1975) also adheres to a socially oriented perspective that people must learn to adjust and interact successfully in environments where others also exist. Children, for example, have social–emotional needs that they can fulfill, but not if they significantly infringe upon others' needs and rights (to also develop and progress). Glasser especially emphasizes that children must recognize their responsibility for all their actions and that they must acknowledge their appropriate and inappropriate behavior. Further, when they are inappropriate, children must accept the consequences and commit themselves toward change and responsible action.

The interactionalist model, as seen above, is very child oriented, yet it evaluates a child's disturbance in the context of his or her social stature, needs, and desires in a particular environment or situation. Thus, the interaction between the person and the environment is critical even though the analysis and intervention focus is on the child and his or her need to acknowledge and change inappropriate, disturbing behaviors. Neither Dreikurs nor Glasser advocate specific types of personality assessment measures, procedures, or techniques. They do suggest that a directed process of observing, interviewing, and interacting with the disturbing child while applying their theoretical perspectives should satisfactorily analyze most problems. Certainly more formal personality assessment, within the context of this model, to fully clarify a problem could not be rejected.

The Ecological Model

The ecological model (Hobbs, 1966, 1975; Knoff, 1983; Rhodes, 1967, 1970; Swap, 1978) goes beyond the psychoeducational and interactional models by considering the effects of all possible environments and interactions, not just the school environment and child–educational interaction, on disturbed behavior. In fact, disturbed behavior is not considered solely the child's problem, according to this model; it is considered a function of the entire environment or ecological system. Thus, disturbed behavior occurs when significant environmental, familial, interpersonal, or intrapersonal stresses create a dysfunctional ecological system.

The disturbed ecological system of a disturbed child is identified from a composite system organized into four subsystems which contain specific components that may be interacting with and around the child. The composite ecological system (see Figure 1-1) is made up of (*a*) the microsystem consisting of people, characteristics, or organizational units of the environment where the referred behavior or issues are most evident or where elements exist that most influence the referred behavior/issues; (*b*) the exosystem consisting of people, characteristics, or organizational units which are external to the microsystem, yet still interface and influence the referred behavior/issues; (*c*) the macrosystem comprising societal expectations and values which may have caused the referred behavior/issues to be identified initially and which indirectly guide the objectives of the change process; and (*d*) the mesosystem symbolically acknowledging the inter-

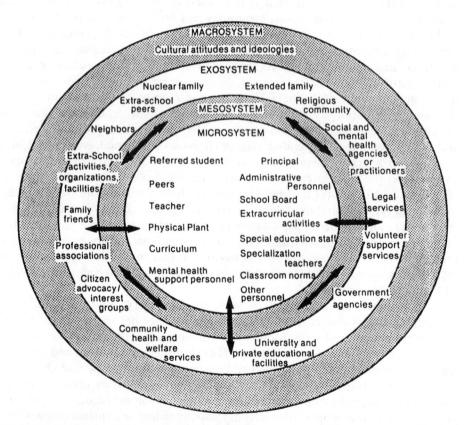

Figure 1-1. The Ecomap, adapted from Bronfenbrenner's ecological system model, showing possible environmental systems.

dependent interactions among components of the other three subsystems (Bronfenbrenner, 1979; Prieto & Rutherford, 1977). An ecological analysis involving a disturbed child can focus on the child in the context of the school, family, or community setting, but it cannot ignore components outside of the specified setting which, nonetheless, may be creating or supporting the disturbed behavior. For example, the presence of a new sibling at home must be considered within an ecological analysis when a child's classroom behavior suddenly deteriorates exactly when the birth has occurred.

Given the systemic perspective of the ecological model, the disturbed system is analyzed not only for its significantly stressful interactions, but also for potential resources and past successes. The model assumes that each ecological system is using its own resources efficiently and effectively when it is functioning well, and that it must depend on its own resources to effect change, compromise, and resolution when the system is in crisis. These resources are often identified through systematic observation and analysis of the system, and they sometimes involve individuals or environments which are available to the system but not currently being utilized. For example, the family in crisis may take the advice of a close friend and go to a community mental health center for counseling, something that was always available but not considered until suggested or motivated by the crisis.

The ecological model does acknowledge the importance of personality assessment, and this assessment involves any theoretical perspective or pragmatic measure that will facilitate a comprehensive understanding of the unique ecological system of concern. Personality assessment here differs somewhat because the focus is on systemic interactions. Thus, the assessment may include many individuals, including the originally referred child, as well as some organizational structures—such as a school's curriculum, a community's social services system, or a society's attitudes toward certain individual behaviors or life circumstances. The ecological model encompasses a comprehensive analysis of person, environmental, organizational, and behavioral interactions, which may include the use of any techniques inherent in the models discussed above. The overriding assessment concern is, however, to understand the entire system and to identify ways for the system to apply its resources toward adjustment and problem resolution.

Classification Systems That Categorize Disturbed Behavior

While the theoretical models comprise different perspectives which explain and analyze disturbed behavior, classification systems attempt to categorize this behavior in standard and consistent ways. The ultimate goals of a classification system are to provide reliable and valid definitions and procedures within a categorization process and to develop a system that has some clinical relevance and utility in service delivery. Definitions or categories must be clearly specified such that there is no confusion as to what they represent or to what a described behavior, condition, or environmental situation refers. Well-operationalized categories often greatly enhance interrater reliability because practitioner assumptions, (mis)interpretations, and "classification" errors are minimized. The categories must also be valid; that is, they should describe disturbances that can be clearly discriminated from one another. Other aspects of validity include predictive validity and concurrent validity. Predictive validity is the ability of a category to

suggest future behavior or prognosis for a child or adolescent and to suggest interventions that, based on previous experience with similarly classified individuals,
have high probabilities of success. Concurrent validity is the ability to use a
correlated category to suggest additional characteristics that may be present in
a classified individual which are related to but not specifically defined within the
initial classifying category (Wicks-Nelson & Israel, 1984).

Personal attitudes toward a classification system's clinical relevance and
utility directly influence its use by the practitioner. Every existing classification
system has individual strengths and weaknesses; overall, the practitioner must
decide if the strengths outweigh the weaknesses. Further, the practitioner must
determine if his or her notion or construct of "disturbance" is exemplified in the
classification system and if the system's use improves the quality of problem identification, problem analysis, intervention, and product or process evaluation. Also
important to clinical utility, the practitioner must consider the impact of being
classified or labeled under a particular classification system on the child or adolescent. If classification improves communication and agreement about the child's
difficulties, yet creates biases among the intervention staff which actually decrease
their commitment to and attitudes about success, then how useful is the classification process and system? This is obviously an individualistic, situation-specific
question, yet it should highlight the potential differences between a classification
system's use in theory versus its use in actual practice. Practitioners need to
evaluate the classification systems that they use in both educational and community settings and be sensitive to their potential child-, staff-, and systems-
oriented impacts.

Four types or approaches to classification will be reviewed below: the educational approach, DSM-III, the GAP, and the empirical approach. Historically, most
early classification systems evaluated only adults' disturbed behavior or emotional
disorders while considering children and adolescents' disorders as "younger" or
"developmentally immature" versions of the adult categories. The DSM-III and
empirically derived classification systems, however, now acknowledge that some
disorders are specific to one age level or developmental status, and that disturbance during childhood does not necessarily lead to analogous disturbances during
adolescence or adulthood. Practitioners should consider the context wherein the
four systems discussed below were developed and in what settings or under what
conditions they will be best used.

Educational Classification: PL 94-142

Public Law 94-142, the Education for All Handicapped Children's Act, was
passed in 1975 and implemented in 1977 to ensure that all school-aged children
with special educational needs receive a free, appropriate, public-funded education in the least restrictive environment. As a legislative approach to classification, the impact of politics and congressional compromise in drafting this law as
well as its on-going legal status and its potential for litigation must be recognized.
Because of this, some PL 94-142 classification definitions noticeably avoid specific
operationalizations and clarity, a weakness which potentially affects the reliability,
validity, and clinical utility of the categories. To be fair, however, PL 94-142 expects all states to write annual service delivery and implementation goals and
reports, and the classification categories can become more specific at the state
or even the individual school district levels.

Within PL 94-142, there are 11 defined handicapping conditions which, between the ages of 3 and 21 years, qualify one for special educational and/or related services: deaf, deaf–blind, hard of hearing, mentally retarded, multihandicapped, orthopedically impaired, other health impaired, seriously emotionally disturbed, specific learning disability, speech impaired, and visually handicapped. While any child or adolescent with any handicapping condition might be administered a personality assessment battery due to disturbed or poor adjustment behavior, issues around the seriously emotionally disturbed definition will be highlighted. Certainly, however, the limitations created by a child's handicap must be considered and controlled for during personality assessment and interpretation. For example, a child's cognitive and intellectual status must always be factored into the assessment process because it may limit the child's ability to understand a technique's directions and to produce scoreable answers, or because the technique assumes or was standardized for a specific cognitive level and its interpretation with other levels would be inappropriate or misleading. In fact, most children or adolescents referred for personality assessment should be individually administered some cognitive or intellectual test to secure an up-to-date ''baseline'' of their skills and status in this area.

The most current definition of seriously emotionally disturbed under PL 94-142 (Section 121a.5) states:

(i) The term means a condition exhibiting one or more of the following characteristics over a long period of time and to a marked extent, which adversely affects educational performance:
(A) An inability to learn which cannot be explained by intellectual, sensory, or health factors;
(B) An inability to build or maintain satisfactory relationships with peers and teachers;
(C) Inappropriate types of behavior or feelings under normal circumstances;
(D) A general pervasive mood of unhappiness or depression; or
(E) A tendency to develop physical symptoms or fears associated with personal or school problems.
(ii) The term includes children who are schizophrenic. The term does not include children who are socially maladjusted unless it is determined that they are seriously emotionally disturbed.

Recent changes, however, have omitted autistic children from this definition, moving it to the other health-impaired category; and potential changes may alter this category's name to ''behaviorally disordered.''

The potential category change to ''behaviorally disordered'' emphasizes some of the weaknesses of this category with respect to its clinical usefulness. First, this is an educationally specific classification system (PL 94-142) and classification category (seriously emotionally disturbed). Because the definition mandates disturbed behavior which affects educational performance, these behaviors will most likely have to be observed in school. Further, disturbed behavior that does not affect school success (e.g., extreme passivity or, despite the definition, ''unhappiness'') may not be identified for intervention. While mental health and not special education intervention might be necessary for the passive or unhappy student, this is not assured by the law, nor is it always practical if a school's mental health practitioner is overrun with PL 94-142 referrals and responsibilities and if administrators restrict the practitioner's role to PL 94-142 duties because his or her position is funded through PL 94-142 money. The change to the behaviorally disordered label, with some additional definitional changes, would emphasize that all children with social–emotional difficulties should receive mental health and/or educational support, that the support should not be tied only to educational progress, and that being "seriously" disturbed (if that can be defined, see below) should not be the criterion. Thus, as it now stands, this category within its classification system is artificially restrictive in its definition. It limits its potential beneficiaries while, parenthetically, forcing them to accept a potentially stigmatizing label in order to receive services.

A second weakness within this category is its general and somewhat vague definition. If not defined more objectively at a state, district, or even individual practitioner level, its reliability and validity could be suspect during the identification and intervention-generating process (Kaufman, Swan, & Wood, 1980; Mealor & Richmond, 1980). For example, what is "a long period of time," "a marked extent," "an inability to learn," "inappropriate feelings," and "normal circumstances?" The subjectivity of this category could result in children being denied services, children being misclassified, or districts manipulating the number of students in classes for emotionally disturbed children by changing the definition's criteria from year to year. While these potential abuses can be balanced by PL 94-142's guarantee of due process, what guides the well-meaning mental health practitioner who wants to best serve his or her clientele? The current definition, at the federal level, needs to be objectively operationalized such that it targets a clearly specified population and such that research into specific interventions for specific types of disorders can be accomplished.

This leads into the third area of weakness. As written, the seriously emotionally disturbed category requires only a "yes or no" identification decision; that is, "yes" this child has special needs in this classification area, or "no" the child does not qualify for these special educational services. As the other three classification systems discussed below will demonstrate, disturbed or disordered behavior is far from homogeneous. Without more subcategory specification, a special education teacher, for example, may not understand the full extent of the child's social–emotional difficulties, may not have the information to educationally and therapeutically plan intervention strategies, and may not have the criteria with which to determine when the child is ready to rejoin the regular education curriculum and/or class. This criticism implies that this category, whatever its designation or label, should be separated into discriminable subcategories—preferably based on behavioral and/or empirical data—such that true individualization of the therapeutic program and intervention can occur. Such a system of subcategories might also facilitate communication between school practitioners and community mental health practitioners if out-of-school services are necessary.

Many of the other categories under PL 94-142's classification system are equally general and subject to potential misuse and abuse. As a system to guide the use and interpretation of personality assessment, PL 94-142 is very weak. Although it focuses on education and educational impact, it still ignores the necessary characteristics that make the classification process reliable, valid, and useful. Hopefully, substantial changes will entirely reorganize PL 94-142's special education categories and definitions to create a more behavioral, empirically based, and heuristic classification system.

Psychiatric Classification: DSM-III
The third revision of the *Diagnostic and Statistical Manual of Mental Disorders* (DSM-III) was published in 1980 by the American Psychiatric Association following the DSM-I (1952) and DSM-II (1968). Compared to its earlier versions,

the DSM-III attempts to describe its various disorders more behaviorally, and it significantly expanded the categories listed specifically as childhood disorders. As a psychiatric classification system, the DSM-III describes specific disorders, the criteria or manifestations characteristic to a disorder, the degree to which these characteristics must be evident, and a minimum length of time that they must be present. According to the Manual, not all criteria must be present to diagnose a specific disorder; usually, a specific subset of the characteristics listed must be present. Given its use in community mental health settings and by insurance companies for third-party payments, the DSM-III will likely continue its dominance, like its predecessors, as the most widely used classification system for child and adolescent disorders. It is not, however, without its weaknesses and critical opponents (e.g., Cantwell, Mattison, Russell, & Will, 1979; Wirt & Lachar, 1981).

The DSM-III classifies individuals along five axes which provide a clinical picture or coding of a specific disorder. Axis I describes the major clinical syndromes (except for the personality and specific developmental disorders coded on Axis II). These are conditions that require therapeutic attention or treatment, yet are not attributable to a mental disorder (e.g., conduct disorders, anxiety disorders, eating disorders), and conditions that involve unspecified, atypical, or deferred diagnoses. As noted above, Axis II codes for personality disorders and specific developmental disorders. Axis III involves physical conditions excluded from the previous two axes (e.g., diabetes or asthma) which, nonetheless, are important for a broad understanding or treatment program for the child or adolescent. These three axes provide the primary diagnostic information which classifies a child or adolescent disorder.

Axes IV and V may be used for either clinical or research purposes and are particularly useful for planning and evaluating treatment programs and/or for predicting treatment effectiveness. Axis IV evaluates the severity of specific "psychological stressors" in the child's life which may affect personality assessment or intervention along a 1 (no apparent psychosocial stressor) to 7 (catastrophic stressor presence) scale. Axis V describes the child's highest level of adaptive functioning during the past year along a 1 (superior adaptive functioning) to 7 (grossly impaired functioning) scale. Both Axes IV and V have a "0" rating category when "no information" or a "not applicable" rating is appropriate.

Generally, the child or adolescent with a significant social–emotional disorder will receive a DSM-III classification which uses all five axes. Exceptions to this rule will occur when the child has a clinical syndrome problem only (where Axis II will not be used) or a specific developmental disorder (where Axis I will be dropped). The DSM-III disorders that are most directly evident during infancy through adolescence (Axes I and II) and descriptions and examples of Axes III, IV, and V are outlined in Table 1-1. Axis I is divided into five categories to describe child or adolescent disorders: intellectual, behavioral, emotional, physical, and developmental. Axis II consists of various developmental or specific learning disorders that are not due to any disorders described or represented in the five categories of Axis I. While Axes I and II outline specific disorders usually evident first in infancy, childhood, or adolescence, other, less age-related categories (e.g., depression) may be used diagnostically to describe a child or adolescent's specific difficulties.

Despite its popularity and/or extensive use, the reliability, validity, and utility of the DSM-III remain to be demonstrated. The DSM-III's reliability (interrater) has been tested only in two field trials prior to its publication, with results indicating acceptable reliability for broad diagnostic classifications, but poor reli-

Table 1-1
DSM-III Classifications That Are Most Directly Applicable to Children and Adolescents[a]

Axis I. Disorders Usually First Evident in Infancy, Childhood, or Adolescence

Mental Retardation:
Mild mental retardation
Moderate mental retardation
Severe mental retardation
Profound mental retardation
Unspecified mental retardation
Attention Deficit Disorder:
with hyperactivity
without hyperactivity
residual type
Conduct Disorder:
undersocialized, aggressive
undersocialized, nonaggressive
socialized, aggressive
socialized, nonaggressive
atypical
Anxiety Disorders of Childhood or Adolescence:
Separation anxiety disorder
Avoidant disorder of childhood or adolescence
Overanxious disorder

Other Disorders of Infancy, Childhood, or Adolescence:
Reactive attachment disorder of infancy
Schizoid disorder of childhood or adolescence
Elective mutism
Oppositional disorder
Identity disorder
Eating Disorders:
Anorexia nervosa
Bulimia
Pica
Rumination disorder of infancy
Atypical eating disorder
Stereotyped Movement Disorders:
Transient tic disorder
Chronic motor tic disorder
Tourette's disorder
Atypical tic disorder
Atypical stereotyped movement disorder

Other Disorders with Physical Manifestations:
Stuttering
Functional enuresis
Functional encopresis
Sleepwalking disorder
Sleep terror disorder
Pervasive Developmental Disorders:
Infantile autism
Childhood onset pervasive developmental disorder
Atypical

Axis II. Specific Developmental Disorders

Developmental reading disorder
Developmental arithmetic disorder
Developmental language disorder

Developmental articulation disorder
Mixed specific developmental disorder
Atypical specific developmental disorder

Axis III. Physical Disorders or Conditions

Axis III permits the clinician to indicate any current physical disorder or condition that is potentially relevant to the understanding or treatment of the individual

Axis IV. Severity of Psychosocial Stressors

Code	Term	Child or Adolescent Examples
1	None	No apparent psychosocial stressor
2	Minimal	Vacation with family
3	Mild	Change in schoolteacher; new school year
4	Moderate	Chronic parental fighting; change to new school; illness of close relative; birth of sibling
5	Severe	Death of peer; divorce of parents; arrest; hospitalization; persistent and harsh parental discipline
6	Extreme	Death of parent or sibling; repeated physical or sexual abuse
7	Catastrophic	Multiple family deaths
0	Unspecified	No information, or not applicable

Axis V. Highest Level of Adaptive Functioning During Past Year

Levels	Child or Adolescent Examples
1. SUPERIOR—Unusually effective functioning in social relations, occupational functioning, and use of leisure time.	A 12-year-old girl gets superior grades in school, is extremely popular among her peers, and excels in many sports. She does all of this with apparent ease and comfort.
2. VERY GOOD—Better than average functioning in social relations, occupational functioning, and use of leisure time.	An adolescent boy gets excellent grades, works part-time, has several close friends, and plays banjo in a jazz band. He admits to some distress in "keeping up with everything."
3. GOOD—No more than slight impairment in either social or occupational functioning.	An 8-year-old boy does well in school, has several friends, but bullies younger children.
4. FAIR—Moderate impairment in either social relations or occupational functioning, or some impairment in both.	A 10-year-old girl does poorly in school, but has adequate peer and family relations.
5. POOR—Marked impairment in either social relations or occupational functioning, or moderate impairment in both.	A 14-year-old boy almost fails in school and has trouble getting along with his peers.
6. VERY POOR—Marked impairment in both social relations and occupational functioning.	A 6-year-old girl needs special help in all subjects and has virtually no peer relationships.
7. GROSSLY IMPAIRED—Gross impairment in virtually all areas of functioning.	A 4-year-boy needs constant restraint to avoid hurting himself and is almost totally lacking in skills.
0. UNSPECIFIED	No information.

Reprinted, with a change in notation, by permission of the publisher from the *Diagnostic and Statistical Manual of Mental Disorders* (3rd ed.) Copyright 1980, American Psychiatric Association.

[a]This table was originally published in Sattler, J. M. (1983). Identifying and classifying disturbed children in the schools: Implications of DSM-III for school psychology. *School Psychology Review, 12*, 386.

ability for specific categorizations. Validity data does not appear to support many DSM-III categories (Rutter & Shaffer, 1980), nor was that validity evident when many of the categories were created (Spitzer & Cantwell, 1980). Finally, the DSM-III's utility appears to have potential given its improvements over previous DSMs, but this can be demonstrated only over time and over consistent documented use. Current weaknesses include its use of adult disorders and descriptions still to classify some childhood disturbances, its use of symptoms and its labeling of symptom clusters, and its lack of a developmental psychology perspective in analyzing child and adolescent disorders (Clarizio & McCoy, 1983).

As noted above, the DSM-III will most likely be used in community mental health settings over public schools or educational settings. Because disturbed or educationally deficient students must be categorized with a PL 94-142 label to receive special education services, the DSM-III classification has few compelling reasons for school mental health practitioner use. However, if community or private mental health services are necessary to supplement school services, a DSM-III classification may be useful for joint practitioner communication and a common reference point. For this reason alone, school practitioners should become conversant in the DSM-III system.

A major criticism of DSM-III from an educational perspective is its inclusion of specific developmental disorders (e.g., reading, arithmetic, language disorders) in a medical–psychiatric classification system (Harris, 1979; Sattler, 1983). Further, the DSM-III criteria for these disorders and the intellectually related Axis I disorders (i.e., mental retardation) are noticeably simplistic and, at times, potentially damaging. For example, DSM-III does not include adaptive behavior assessments as a required part of a mental retardation assessment battery, an omission that ignores common psychoeducational practice (Sattler, 1983). Thus, the school practitioner may need to supplement DSM-III classifications (if used) in these areas with psychoeducational descriptions and analyses, a procedure which may provide the best classification approach of all.

The GAP

The Group for the Advancement of Psychiatry (GAP) proposed an alternative classification system for childhood psychopathology in 1966, with a revision in 1974. A specific strength of this system compared with DSM-III is its attention and sensitivity to developmental variables and characteristics within the social–emotional (and other) domains. Indeed, the GAP specifically includes a "healthy responses" category in its descriptive format. This developmental perspective recognizes that some social–emotional behaviors and reactions are typical at certain age levels (e.g., some fears and nightmares around the ages of 5 to 7), while they are atypical and suggestive of significant disturbance at other ages. This perspective further recognizes that some "atypical" behaviors may be expected and adaptive under certain environmental situations or life circumstances (e.g., the death of a parent), and that children with some psychopathological disturbance still have other individual strengths and resources.

Examples of some psychopathological disorders from the GAP are presented in Table 1-2. The GAP describes criteria for each category of disorders. Reliability, validity, and clinical utility data for this system, however, are not readily available. In fact, the GAP does not appear to have a record of much acceptance

Table 1-2
The GAP Proposed Classification System for
Psychopathological Disorders in Childhood[a]

1. *Healthy Responses*

This category assesses the positive strengths of the child and tries to avoid the diagnosis of healthy states by the exclusion of pathology. The criteria for assessment are the intellectual, social, emotional, personal, adaptive, and psychosocial stage-appropriateness functioning of the child in relation to developmental and situational crises.

Healthy Responses:
   1. Developmental crisis
   2. Situational crisis
   3. Other responses

2. *Reactive Disorders*

This category is based on disorders in which behavior and/or symptoms are the result of situational factors. These disturbances must be of a pathological degree so as to distinguish them from the healthy responses to a situational crisis.

3. *Developmental Deviations*

These are deviations in personality development that may be beyond the range of normal variation in that they occur at a time, in a sequence, or in a degree not expected for a given age level or stage in development.

Developmental Deviations:
   1. Deviations in maturational patterns
   2. Deviations in specific dimensions of development
      a. Motor
      b. Sensory
      c. Speech
      d. Cognitive functions
      e. Social development
      f. Psychosexual
      g. Affective
      h. Integrative
   3. Other developmental deviations

4. *Psychoneurotic Disorders*

These disorders are based on unconscious conflicts over the handling of sexual and aggressive impulses that remain active and unresolved, though removed from awareness by the mechanism of repression. Marked personality disorganization or decompensation, or the gross disturbance of reality testing is not seen. Because of their internalized character, these disorders tend toward chronicity, with a self-perpetuating or repetitive nature. Subcategories are based on specific syndromes.

Psychoneurotic Disorders:
   1. Anxiety type
   2. Phobic type
   3. Conversion type
   4. Dissociative type
   5. Obsessive-compulsive type
   6. Depressive type
   7. Other psychoneurotic disorders

5. *Personality Disorders*

These disorders are characterized by chronic or fixed pathological trends, representing traits that have become ingrained in the personality structure. In most but not all such disorders, these trends or traits are not perceived by the child as a source of intrapsychic distress or anxiety. In making this classification, the total personality picture must be considered and not just the presence of a single behavior or symptom.

Personality Disorders:
   1. Compulsive personality
   2. Hysterical

(continued)

**Table 1-2
(Continued)**

    3. Anxious
    4. Overly dependent
    5. Oppositional
    6. Overly inhibited
    7. Overly independent
    8. Isolated
    9. Mistrustful
  10. Tension-Discharge Disorders:
      a. Impulse-ridden personality
      b. Neurotic personality disorder
  11. Sociosyntonic Personality Disorders:
      a. Sexual deviation
      b. Other personality disorders

6. *Psychotic Disorders*
These disorders are characterized by marked, pervasive deviations from the behavior that is expected for the child's age. They are revealed in severe and continued impairment of emotional relationships with persons, associated with an aloofness and a tendency toward preoccupation with inanimate objects; loss of speech or failure in its development; disturbances in sensory perception; bizarre or stereotyped behavior and motility patterns; marked resistance to change in environment or routine; outbursts of intense and unpredictable panic; absence of a sense of personal identity; and blunted, uneven, or fragmented intellectual development. Major categories are based on the developmental period, with subcategories in each period for the listing of a specific syndrome, if known.
  Psychotic Disorders:
    1. Psychoses of infancy and early childhood
      a. Early infantile autism
      b. Interactional psychotic disorder
      c. Other psychoses of infancy and early childhood
    2. Psychoses of later childhood
      a. Schizophreniform psychotic disorder
      b. Other psychoses of later childhood
    3. Psychoses of adolescence
      a. Acute confusional state
      b. Schizophrenic disorder, adult type
      c. Other psychoses of adolescence

7. *Psychophysiologic Disorders*
These disorders are characterized by a significant interaction between somatic and psychological components. They may be precipitated and perpetuated by psychological or social stimuli of stressful nature. These disorders ordinarily involve those organ systems innervated by the autonomic nervous system.
  Psychophysiologic Disorders:
    1. Skin
    2. Musculoskeletal
    3. Respiratory
    4. Cardiovascular
    5. Hemic and lymphatic
    6. Gastrointestinal
    7. Genitourinary
    8. Endocrine
    9. Of nervous system
  10. Of organs of special sense
  11. Other psychophysiologic disorders

8. *Brain Syndromes*
These disorders are characterized by impairment of orientation, judgment, discrimination, learning, memory, and other cognitive functions, as well as by frequent labile affect. They are basically

(continued)

**Table 1-2
(Continued)**

caused by diffuse impairment of brain tissue function. Personality disturbances of a psychotic, neurotic, or behavioral nature also may be present.
    Brain Syndromes:
        1. Acute
        2. Chronic

9. *Mental Retardation*

10. *Other Disorders*
This category is for disorders that cannot be classified by the above definitions or for disorders we will describe in the future.

ªSource: Adapted by permission from *Group Psychopathological Disorders in Childhood: Theoretical Considerations and a Proposed Classification* (New York: Brunner/Mazel, 1966).

or use by practitioners in either school or community settings. Thus, while the GAP presents an important contrast to the DSM-III, strong statements on its effectiveness in the field are difficult at this time.

Empirical Classification Approaches

With the advent of more sophisticated computer programming and related statistical capabilities, empirical classification systems have become more evident and influential. Using factor analyses, descriptions of disturbed children can be clustered such that first-order (general or broad-band) factors and second-order (specific or narrow-band) factors can be identified and labeled. These descriptions are often chosen from behavior problem checklists which have been normed and standardized with samples of both typical and disturbed children and adolescents. While an individual child's difficulties may be identified with these checklists (see Chapter 10 of this volume), specific factors that are present across a number of checklists may be used to create an empirically based classification system for child and adolescent disorders.

Two of the more common empirically derived classification systems have been reported by Achenbach from his Child Behavior Checklist (1979) and Quay and Peterson from their recently revised Behavior Problem Checklist (1979). Achenbach's Child Behavior Checklist has been used and validated by different observers (e.g., mental health practitioners, teachers, parents) for many different types of disturbed children and adolescents (Achenbach & Edelbrock, 1978). Across almost all the available studies, two consistent broad-band factors characterizing Externalizing or Undercontrolled and Internalizing or Overcontrolled behavior, respectively, have been statistically identified. These two factors delineate hyperactive, delinquent, or aggressive (externalizing) behavioral styles versus depressed, withdrawing, or uncommunicative (internalizing) behavioral styles, respectively (Achenbach, 1982).

At the second-order factor level, 14 possible narrow-band factors were evident, although they did not have the same statistical strength and prevalence across all the research studies. The most pervasive narrow-band factors were labeled Aggressive, Delinquent, Hyperactive, Schizoid, Anxious, Depressed, Social

Withdrawal, and Somatic Complaints. From a classification perspective, these might be considered the most reliable and valid additional categories with which to classify disturbed children and adolescents. Further, the specific rating scale items (behaviors) correlating with each factor could provide the behavioral criteria or characteristics necessary to evaluate the presence of that factor in a child or adolescent. Finally, Edelbrock and Achenbach (1980) noted that these narrow-band factors do differ across age (6–11 and 12–16 years old) and sex; thus, a sensitivity to the developmental nature of some social–emotional disorders is possible with empirically based systems.

Quay and Peterson's recently revised Behavior Problem Checklist (1979) was factor analyzed using four separate samples: children and/or adolescents from two private psychiatric residential facilities (outpatient and inpatient cases), from a private school for children with learning disabilities, and from a community-sponsored school for those with developmental disabilities. The factor analyses resulted in four major factors or scales (Conduct Disorder, Socialized Aggression, Attention Problems-Immaturity, Anxiety-Withdrawal) and two minor scales (Psychotic Behavior, Motor Excess). It is interesting that Quay found evidence in these data for Achenbach's Undercontrolled broad-band factor, but he labeled it Conduct Disorder, and for the Overcontrolled broad-band factor, which he labeled Anxiety-Withdrawal (Wicks-Nelson & Israel, 1984). This demonstrates the need to compare the specific items or behaviors that form the rating scales' major factors, because they may be quite similar despite differences in the factors' names. This also demonstrates the relatively consistent factors generated through factor analytic, empirical approaches, and lends further support for classification systems using these methods.

As a classification system, the factors from the Revised Behavior Problem Checklist may be conceptually grouped into three types of atypical social–emotional patterns: (a) discipline problems (using the Conduct Disorder and Socialized Aggression scales), (b) emotional disturbance problems (using the Psychotic Behavior and Anxiety-Withdrawal scales), and (c) maturation delay problems (using the Attention Problems-Immaturity, Motor Excess, and Anxiety-Withdrawal scales). The Anxiety-Withdrawal scale is included in the latter problem area because it shares 21% of its variance with the Attention Problems-Immaturity Scale. This is a "commonsense" grouping based on the item descriptions from each scale (Quay, 1983). Even without this grouping, the statistical qualities (i.e., reliability and validity) of these factors may make them the best representative categories of disturbed and disturbing behavior available. Indeed, while comparing the Revised Behavior Problem Checklist and the DSM-III, Quay (1983) noted that many DSM-III categories are unaccounted for in the Checklist because their empirical support for existence is so weak.

To summarize, empirical personality assessment approaches statistically correlate and organize individual problem behaviors and descriptions into more unified factors which, despite differences in their labeled names, appear to be somewhat consistent across different behavioral checklists and standardization samples. These factors may be used as categories to organize and classify children and adolescents' disturbed behavior. Or, for more complex disturbances, these classification categories could be combined or profiled together to show their interrelationships and the relative contributions which explain a particular disturbance. Finally, given their behavioral and empirical foundations, these assessment approaches may create the most useful and defensible classification system of those discussed above, a system that may also facilitate the development and application of specific intervention approaches for specific categories or profiles of disturbance.

Issues That Affect the Identification and Classification Process

Having discussed the perspectives influencing referral decisions, different theoretical models of disturbed behavior, and various classification systems that categorize atypical social–emotional behavior, we will now address some specific issues affecting the identification and classification process. These issues include a broad-based perspective of when to consider personality assessment, data on determining the presence of "disturbance," and the effects of labeling.

A Perspective of Personality Assessment Use

Although much of the theoretical discussion in this chapter has emphasized emotionally or behaviorally disturbed children and/or adolescents, this author views behavior along a spectrum from typical behavior to severely disturbed behavior. Within this spectrum are typical behavior patterns and social–emotional states, mild or discipline-related behavioral disturbances, often referred to as "disturbing" rather than "disturbed" behaviors, behavioral disturbances requiring special class placements and/or mental health interventions, especially if they exist in the school setting, and severely disturbed behaviors requiring out-of-school (e.g., institutional) interventions and coordinated community mental health and social services. As noted above, the Quay and Peterson Revised Behavior Problem Checklist (1979) Conduct Disorder and Attention Problems-Immaturity factors might be placed toward the discipline problem end of the spectrum, while the Psychotic Behavior factor would be toward the opposite, severely disturbed end of the spectrum. The Anxiety-Withdrawal, Motor Excess, and Socialized Aggression factors would fall between these diagnostic end points and could suggest discipline, behavioral disturbance, or severely disturbed problems, depending on the specific referred behaviors and their intensity and impact on the referred child and significant others (Knoff, 1985).

Personality assessment is also thought to occur continuously with all children and adolescents. Personality assessment consists of any formal or informal observation, interview, and/or evaluation process involving a child or adolescent's behavior, social–emotional development or progress, or self-concept formation. This is a very broad definition. Thus, a mental health practitioner is assessing personality when he or she is observing the interpersonal interactions of a group of typical students on a playground, and when he or she is completing a behavior rating scale with a parent or teacher who has referred a child for aggressiveness toward peers. This definition is meant to encourage all practitioners to consider every observation or interaction with a child, typical or referred, as part of a sampling process which in total comprises a longitudinal study of the child's personality development. Given this perspective and this definition, personality assessment becomes an everyday activity for the practitioner. Thus, when extensive personality testing with a child becomes necessary, the whole process will hopefully occur in a more normalized context for the practitioner, not a context which identifies the referred child as unusual, requiring a special procedure used only for "special" cases.

Consistent with the idea of continuous personality assessment along a broad behavioral spectrum for all children and adolescents is the notion that the eight theoretical models of disturbance can be applied to explain behavior along the entire spectrum or some specific part of it. Further, any behavior or referred situation may be best explained by a combination of theoretical perspectives; that is, the existence of one dominant theory of disturbed behavior that explains the entire behavioral spectrum is not realistic or expected; rather, an interactional view using a number of theories may be required and necessary. This creates a rather eclectic potential for personality assessment which permits a very broad, nonrestrictive view of behavior and the many conditions and circumstances under which it occurs. This view becomes advantageous to the practitioner who must understand and address a child or adolescent's behavior pragmatically, not theoretically or abstractly.

Agreements and Disagreements on the Presence of "Disturbance"

As noted above, especially for DSM-III, the reliability and validity of a practitioner's diagnostic impressions on the presence or absence of a childhood disturbance is not consistently high. Even among groups of mental health practitioners (e.g., school psychologists) who analyze data from similar case studies, diagnostic agreement is mixed (Clarizio & McCoy, 1983). Stuart (1970) identified four factors that contribute to practitioners' low diagnostic agreement: (a) practitioner variance and error, (b) referred child characteristics and their impact or bias on the diagnostic process, (c) poor classification systems, and (d) differential attention to the child's ecological systems and specific situations and environments.

Practitioner variance involves the different theoretical beliefs, diagnostic biases, expectations, and practices, interpretive strategies and conceptualizations, and technical and evaluative skills that cause two or more practitioners to evaluate the same referral problem in different ways and/or to analyze the same set of data differently. Practitioner error includes gaps in knowledge, skill, experience, or objectivity which cause technical and pragmatic errors to occur; they do not involve professional differences of opinion, interpretation, or procedure. Child characteristics, such as socioeconomic status, race, religion, style of dress, nationality, sex, verbal expressiveness, or presence of a dialect, sometimes contribute to inappropriate, prejudiced referrals and/or to inappropriate assessment procedures and interpretations. These biases unevenly influence practitioners' and significant others' attitudes and beliefs about a child, and they may cause favorable or unfavorable diagnostic impressions and decisions by affecting not necessarily the data, but how the data are interpreted or differentially evaluated. Finally, attention to the referred child's ecology includes understanding the context around the referral situation (e.g., how many people perceive the problem and how powerful they are within the diagnostic team or environment, what resources are available, how many interventions have been previously attempted), as well as understanding the extent to which different practitioners have examined the various home, school, and community interactions, strengths, and potential resources and their effects on diagnostic opinions and eventual intervention programs. Here, practitioners may react differently to organizational pressures and ecological characteristics such that diagnostic disagreements occur.

Diagnostic agreements and disagreements will always exist unless a single theoretical and procedural process is universally accepted and utilized. As this is unlikely, practitioners must be aware of the variables and characteristics causing unnecessary diagnostic variance and, more critically, judgmental errors during the assessment process. Only by minimizing these differences can diagnostic decisions become more consistent and more appropriate for the referred child and those working toward successful problem resolution and intervention planning.

The Effects of Labeling

While many research studies investigating the effects of labeling have focused on educationally as opposed to emotionally or behaviorally handicapped children, the practitioner still should be sensitive to the potential positive and negative implications of labeling. In general, the research results remain inconclusive as to whether labeling is consistently bad or good; the results primarily indicate that labeling is a complex phenomenon with differential influence. For example, some laboratory studies have reported that labels negatively influence teachers' expectations for a student (Ysseldyke & Foster, 1978), yet other studies indicate that labels affect teachers' checklist scores, but not their behavioral observations or grading of academic work (Fogel & Nelson, 1983). With respect to labeled youngsters, MacMillan, Jones, and Aloia (1974) found no evidence of a direct, causal relationship between self-concept and labeling.

Given the current research, practitioners are encouraged to understand how to best use labels and how to best minimize their potential negative effects for specific referred cases. Among the advantages of labels are their ability (*a*) to facilitate professional communication about a specific status or condition that affects a child and about analysis procedures and/or interventions that can successfully resolve or ameliorate the labeled condition (especially when the label is specific, well operationalized or defined, and used consistently among peer professionals); (*b*) to secure services, for example, in the educational domain (through PL 94-142) or in the community (through DSM-III and third-party insurance payments); (*c*) to identify specific groups of individuals who because of their labeled conditions receive greater public attention, services, and support; and (*d*) to encourage further research and innovation because a well-defined population (by virtue of the label) exists, needs mental health support, and therefore will (need to) generate a body of specific knowledge. Among the disadvantages of labels are their potential (*a*) to create prejudice, stereotyping, and negative or incorrect expectations in identified children; (*b*) to lead significant others to ignore a child's unique strengths, weaknesses, and individuality; (*c*) to result in classrooms and/or therapies that are geared to the label and not to the child's specific ecology or manifestations; (*d*) to encourage a "medical model" view that a child "owns" a problem such as a physiological malady or pathology that needs to be "cured"; and (*e*) to create a public record that, if handled inappropriately, results in a loss of confidentiality that affects or biases a child's social, educational, and vocational future (Clarizio & McCoy, 1983; Hallahan & Kauffman, 1982). These advantages and disadvantages coexist whenever labels are considered or used. The practitioner must consider a label's effects throughout the referral and personality assessment process, evaluating their effects to personal and professional practice, to the referred children, and to significant others involved in the referred case.

Summary

There are many theories, systems, and issues involved in the identification and classification of children and adolescents referred for personality assessment. The theories explaining emotional disturbance will be discussed further in Chapter 3 of this volume and integrated into a comprehensive personality assessment, problem-solving process. These theories contribute to the potential understanding of any referred child; no theory should be categorically dismissed. The systems, especially PL 94-142 and DSM-III, are used in the field and, despite their weaknesses, they do influence and sometimes dictate the delivery of services to referred and identified children and adolescents. The practitioner must understand the various systems, evaluate their pragmatic utility, and minimize their potential limitations and abuses. The issues, and certainly this chapter has neither exhausted the issues nor their discussion, must always be in the practitioner's awareness. The practitioner must be sensitive to their influences and implications, maximize their strengths and uses, and minimize their weaknesses and disadvantages.

References

Achenbach, T. M. (1979). The Child Behavior Profile: An empirically based system for assessing children's behavioral problems and competencies. *International Journal of Mental Health, 1*, 24–42.

Achenbach, T. M. (1982). Empirical approaches to the classification of child psychopathology. In J. R. Lachenmeyer & M. S. Gibbs (Eds.), *Psychopathology in children* (pp. 30–52). New York: Gardner Press.

Achenbach, T. M., & Edelbrock, C. S. (1978). The classification of child psychopathology: A review and analysis of empirical efforts. *Psychological Bulletin, 85*, 1275–1301.

American Psychiatric Association. (1952). *Diagnostic and statistical manual of mental disorders* (1st ed.). Washington, DC: Author.

American Psychiatric Association. (1968). *Diagnostic and statistical manual of mental disorders* (2nd ed.). Washington, DC: Author.

American Psychiatric Association. (1980). *Diagnostic and statistical manual of mental disorders* (3rd ed.). Washington, DC: Author.

Baldwin, A. L. (1969). A cognitive theory of socialization. In D. A. Goslin (Ed.), *Handbook of socialization theory and research* (pp. 325–345). Chicago, IL: Rand McNally.

Bandura, A. (1969). *Principles of behavior modification*. New York: Holt, Rinehart, & Winston.

Bandura, A. (1977). *Social learning theory*. Englewood Cliffs, NJ: Prentice-Hall.

Barkley, R. A. (1979). Using stimulant drugs in the classroom. *School Psychology Review, 8*, 412–425.

Bower, E. M. (1969). *The early identification of emotionally handicapped children in school* (2nd ed.). Springfield, IL: C. C Thomas.

Bronfenbrenner, U. (1979). *The ecology of human development*. Cambridge, MA: Harvard University Press.

Cantwell, D., Mattison, R., Russell, A., & Will, L. (1979). A comparison of DSM-II and DSM-III in the diagnosis of childhood psychiatric disorders: Difficulties in use, global comparisons, and conclusions. *Archives of General Psychiatry, 36*, 1227–1228.

Clarizio, H. F., & McCoy, G. F. (1983). *Behavior disorders in children* (3rd ed.). New York: Harper & Row.

Connors, C. K., Goyette, C. H., Southwick, D. A., Lees, J. M., & Andrulonis, P. A. (1976). Food additives and hyperkinesis: A controlled double-blind experiment. *Pediatrics, 58*, 154–166.

Crook, W. G. (1980). Can what a child eats make him dull, stupid, or hyperactive? *Journal of Learning Disabilities, 13*, 281–285.

Dreikurs, R., Grunwald, B. B., & Pepper, F. C. (1982). *Maintaining sanity in the classroom: Classroom management techniques*. New York: Harper & Row.

Edelbrock, C., & Achenbach, T. M. (1980). A typology of child behavior profile patterns: Distribution and correlates for disturbed children aged 6–16. *Journal of Abnormal Child Psychology, 8*, 441–470.

Elkind, D. (1976). Cognitive development and psychopathology: Observations on egocentrism and ego defense. In E. Schopler & R. J. Reichter (Eds.), *Psychopathology and child development* (pp. 167–183). New York: Plenum Press.

Fagen, S. A. (1979). Psychoeducational management and self-control. In D. Cullinan & M. Epstein (Eds.), *Special education for adolescents: Issues and perspectives* (pp. 235–272). Columbus, OH: Charles E. Merrill.

Feingold, B. F. (1975). *Why your child is hyperactive.* New York: Random House.

Flavell, J. H. (1977). *Cognitive development.* Englewood Cliffs, NJ: Prentice-Hall.

Fogel, L. S., & Nelson, R. O. (1983). The effects of special education labels on teachers' behavioral observations, checklist scores, and grading of academic work. *Journal of School Psychology, 21,* 241–252.

Glasser, W. (1975). *Reality therapy: A new approach to psychiatry.* New York: Harper & Row.

Hallahan, D. P., & Kauffman, J. M. (1982). *Exceptional children* (2nd ed.). Englewood Cliffs, NJ: Prentice-Hall.

Harris, S. L. (1979). DSM-III: Its implications for children. *Child Behavior Therapy, 1,* 37–46.

Hobbs, N. (1966). Helping disturbed children: Psychological and ecological strategies. *American Psychologist, 21,* 1105–1115.

Hobbs, N. (1975). *The futures of children.* San Francisco, CA: Jossey-Bass.

Kauffman, J. M. (1981). *Characteristics of children's behavioral disorders* (2nd ed.). Columbus, OH: Charles E. Merrill.

Kaufman, A., Swan, W., & Wood, M. (1980). Do parents, teachers, and psychoeducational evaluators agree in their perceptions of black and white emotionally disturbed children? *Psychology in the Schools, 17,* 185–191.

Knoff, H. M. (1983). Personality assessment in the schools: Issues and procedures for school psychologists. *School Psychology Review, 12,* 391–398.

Knoff, H. M. (1985). Best practices in dealing with discipline referrals. In J. Grimes & A. Thomas (Eds.), *Best practices manual in school psychology* (pp. 251–262). Kent, OH: NASP Publications.

Kohlberg, L. (1969). Stage and sequence: The cognitive-developmental approach to socialization. In D. A. Goslin (Ed.), *Handbook of socialization theory and research* (pp. 347–480). Chicago, IL: Rand McNally.

Liebert, R. M., & Wicks-Nelson, R. (1981). *Developmental psychology.* Englewood Cliffs, NJ: Prentice-Hall.

Long, N. J., Morse, W. C., & Newman, R. G. (Eds.). (1980). *Conflict in the classroom* (2nd ed.). Belmont, CA: Wadsworth Press.

MacMillan, D. L., Jones, R. J., & Aloia, G. F. (1974). The mentally retarded label: A theoretical analysis and review of research. *American Journal of Mental Deficiency, 79,* 241–261.

Maslow, A. (1968). *Toward a psychology of being.* New York: Van Nostrand.

Mealor, D., & Richmond, B. (1980). Adaptive behavior: Teachers and parents disagree. *Exceptional Children, 46,* 386–389.

Meichenbaum, D. H. (1979). Teaching children self-control. In B. B. Lahey & A. F. Kazdin (Eds.), *Advances in clinical child psychology* (Vol. 2, pp. 1–33). New York: Plenum Press.

Morse, W. C. (1975). The education of socially maladjusted and emotionally disturbed children. In W. M. Cruickshank & G. O. Johnson (Eds.), *Education of exceptional children and youth* (3rd ed., pp. 553–612). Englewood Cliffs, NJ: Prentice-Hall.

Nelson, C. M. (1981). Classroom management. In J. M. Kauffman & D. P. Hallahan (Eds.), *Handbook of special education* (pp. 663–687). Englewood Cliffs, NJ: Prentice-Hall.

Prieto, A. G., & Rutherford, R. B. (1977). An ecological assessment technique for behaviorally disordered and learning disabled children. *Journal of Behavioral Disorders, 2,* 169–175.

Quay, H. C. (1983). A dimensional approach to behavior disorder: The Revised Behavior Problem Checklist. *School Psychology Review, 12,* 244–249.

Quay, H. C., & Peterson, D. R. (1979). *Manual for the Behavior Problem Checklist.* Privately printed.

Rhodes, W. C. (1967). The disturbing child: A problem of ecological management. *Exceptional Children, 33,* 637–642.

Rhodes, W. C. (1970). A community participation analysis of emotional disturbance. *Exceptional Children, 36,* 309–314.

Rogers, C. R. (1961). *On becoming a person.* Boston, MA: Houghton-Mifflin.

Rogers, C. R. (1980). *A way of being.* Boston, MA: Houghton-Mifflin.

Ross, A. O. (1980). *Psychological disorders of children* (2nd ed). New York: McGraw-Hill.

Rutter, M., & Shaffer, D. (1980). DSM-III: A step forward or back in terms of the classification of child psychiatric disorders? *Journal of the American Academy of Child Psychiatry, 19,* 371–394.

Ryan, W. (1976). *Blaming the victim*. New York: Vintage Books.

Sattler, J. M. (1983). Identifying and classifying disturbed children in the schools: Implications of DSM-III for school psychology. *School Psychology Review, 12*, 384–390.

Skinner, B. F. (1938). *The behavior of organisms: An experimental analysis*. New York: Appleton-Century-Crofts.

Skinner, B. F. (1953). *Science and human behavior*. New York: Macmillan.

Spitzer, R. L., & Cantwell, D. P. (1980). The DSM-III classification of the psychiatric disorders of infancy, childhood, and adolescence. *Journal of the American Academy of Child Psychiatry, 19*, 356–370.

Stuart, R. (1970). *Trick or treatment—how and when psychotherapy fails*. Urbana, IL: Research Press.

Swanson, J. M., & Kinsbourne, M. (1980). Artificial color and hyperactive behavior. In L. M. Knights & D. J. Bakker (Eds.), *Treatment of hyperactive and learning disordered children* (pp. 131–150). Baltimore, MD: University Park Press.

Swap, S. (1978). The ecological model of emotional disturbance in children: A status report and proposed synthesis. *Behavioral Disorders, 3*, 186–196.

Szasz, T. S. (1961). *The myth of mental illness*. New York: Harper & Row.

Taylor, T. D., Winne, P. H., & Marx, R. W. (1975, April). *Sample specificity of self-concept instruments*. Paper presented at the meeting of the Society for Research in Child Development.

Thomas, R. M. (1979). *Comparing theories of child development*. Belmont, CA: Wadsworth Press.

Van Evra, J. P. (1983). *Psychological disorders of children and adolescents*. Boston, MA: Little, Brown.

Watson, J. B., & Raynor, R. (1920). Conditioned emotional reactions. *Journal of Experimental Psychology, 3*, 1–14.

Wicks-Nelson, R., & Israel, A. C. (1984). *Behavior disorders of childhood*. Englewood Cliffs, NJ: Prentice-Hall.

Wirt, R., & Lachar, D. (1981). The Personality Inventory for Children. In P. McReynolds (Ed.), *Advances in psychological assessment* (Vol. 5). San Francisco, CA: Jossey-Bass.

Wolfgang, C. H., & Glickman, C. D. (1980). *Solving discipline problems*. Boston, MA: Allyn & Bacon.

Ysseldyke, J. E., & Foster, G. G. (1978). Bias in teacher's observations of emotionally disturbed and learning disabled children. *Exceptional Children, 44*, 613–615.

Legal and Ethical Issues in Child and Adolescent Personality Assessment

Stephen T. DeMers

Introduction

Since the introduction of the Binet Intelligence Scale around the turn of the century, the use of psychological assessment procedures in this country has become widespread. Indeed, it is likely that every American citizen has been affected in some way by their results (Haney, 1981). Testing now shapes the process whereby major decisions about people's lives are made in government, hospitals and clinics, industry, and, most certainly, schools and colleges. School children probably are tested more than any other group of people in our society. It has been estimated that over 200 million standardized tests of academic aptitude and achievement, perceptual–motor coordination, personality, and vocational interests are given to children each year (Hopkins & Stanley, 1981). Significantly, this figure does not include the myriad classroom and other nonstandardized assessments also used.

While tests often have positive outcomes, such as college admission, student feedback, and career guidance, they also can serve to label, segregate, track, institutionalize, and deny access to desired goals. As the use of tests for these exclusionary purposes has increased, so has their potential for causing unjustified negative consequences. When those consequences incurred legally recognized injuries, psychological tests and assessment practices began to be examined by the legal system. As a result, there is probably no activity performed by psychologists or other mental health practitioners which is so closely scrutinized by the law (Bersoff, 1981).

This chapter examines the major legal decisions and statutes affecting psychological assessment practices in this country with a particular emphasis on those cases and laws affecting personality assessment of children and adolescents. The chapter begins with a brief, historical review of legal involvement in general psychological assessment practices. Remaining sections describe in more detail

Stephen T. DeMers. Department of Educational and Counseling Psychology, University of Kentucky, Lexington, Kentucky.

cases and statutes of particular relevance to both personality assessment (as opposed to ability testing) and assessment of children and adolescents (as opposed to adults).

Most of the legal activity affecting psychological assessment has occurred in two settings: personnel selection of adults in the workplace and ability testing of children in the public schools (Bersoff, 1982d). Relatively few court cases and legal mandates directly address the issue of personality assessment of young people. Thus, to some extent, this chapter must extrapolate from the decisions involving adults and/or ability testing to identify legal implications for personality assessment with children and adolescents. Specific issues addressed include what constitutes informed consent, invasion of privacy, and the limits of confidentiality when the client is a minor; do clients' legal protections change in the private as opposed to the public service setting; and does the type of credential possessed by a psychologist or mental health practitioner affect the legal rights of the client? Because both the law and personality assessment practices are constantly changing, a final section offers some speculations as to potential sources of conflict and legal action in the future.

A Brief History of Psychological Testing and the Law

Although social, political, and psychological experts have criticized psychological tests throughout their period of increasing popularity (Bersoff, 1973; Black, 1963; Cronbach, 1975; Gross, 1962; Kamin, 1974; Lippman, 1922; Williams, 1970), the courts, legislators, and legal scholars have examined their use only in the past 20 years. The recent increase in legislation and litigation involving testing, however, has caused many behavioral scientists to reexamine and question some long-accepted beliefs. For example, the American Psychological Association (APA) recently devoted an entire issue of the *American Psychologist* (Glaser & Bond, 1981) and a full day at its 1981 convention to testing. Similarly, the National Academy of Sciences established three blue ribbon panels (Heller, Holtzman, & Messick, 1982; Sherman & Robinson, 1982; Wigdor & Garner, 1982) to study testing practices. What are these legal influences that have so dramatically affected the previously unexamined arena of psychological and educational assessment?

Constitutional Safeguards and Assessment Practices

Courts and legislative bodies typically do not interfere in the work of trained experts such as psychologists by defining or insisting on their own notions of appropriate psychological practice. Indeed, to the extent that psychologists administer tests as employees of state agencies such as public schools, the Supreme Court as recently as 1977 warned the courts not to interfere in the operation of the public schools unless basic constitutional safeguards are in danger. Yet, in two decisions that reaffirmed this need for judicial restraint (*Epperson* v. *Arkansas*, 1968; *Ingraham* v. *Wright*, 1977), the Supreme Court also noted the court's obligation to intervene where constitutional values were threatened. Thus, over the past 20 years, the majority of Supreme Court and other federal and lower state court decisions affecting psychological assessment have involved constitutional guidelines. Among these decisions, psychologists (and other mental health practitioners) have been directed to warn potential victims threatened by their clients in psychotherapy, to stop giving IQ tests to minority students being considered for special education and to secure the informed consent of both parents and children before administering a questionnaire about potential drug abuse among students.

Most of the litigation and legislation related to psychological assessment has involved one or both of the following constitutional safeguards: equal protection of the law, and due process of law.

Equal protection of the laws refers to that aspect of the Fourteenth Amendment to the Constitution which forbids a state (including schools and school officials) to treat persons who are similarly situated differently unless there is a justifiable reason. The equal protection clause is relevant to the psychological assessment of children and adolescents mostly as it relates to the assessment practices of psychologists employed by the state, typically public schools and mental health clinics. The equal protection clause comes into play whenever public schools or clinics seek to treat some group or class of people differently, for example, placing handicapped students in special education, placing minority children in inferior neighborhood schools, or providing inferior treatment to minority clients in mental health settings. If such differential treatment results in a disadvantage for a particular group, then the school or clinic must prove that it has an important, and in some cases, a compelling reason for such discrepancies in treatment.

Another constitutional safeguard in the Fourteenth Amendment is the due process clause which prevents the government from denying persons life, liberty, or property without (a) a legitimate reason and (b) providing some meaningful and impartial forum to prevent arbitrary deprivations of those protected interests. The Supreme Court has defined property and liberty interests broadly to include, for example, such assessment-related interests as a child's right to a free public education and the right to be free of any stigmatizing labels (e.g., emotionally disturbed, mentally retarded). Liberty includes not only freedom from involuntary incarceration in a prison or commitment to a mental institution, but also encompasses the right to privacy, personal security, and reputation. Thus, much of what psychologists do—including observing and evaluating students, writing and maintaining confidential reports, and counseling—falls under the right to privacy aspect of the due process clause.

In addition to these constitutional safeguards, there are numerous federal and state statutory protections that may be invoked to challenge the actions of psychologists. State licensing laws for psychologists, including provisions for privileged communication, federal and state laws governing release of confidential information to third parties, and laws prohibiting undue invasion of privacy, are just a few examples. Given the highly serious and sensitive nature of psychologists' primary activities, it is hardly surprising that some courts have viewed their assessment practices as unduly denying some individuals their legally protected rights.

Litigation Related to Ability Testing in Public Schools

The use of psychological assessment in a variety of social and public settings recently has spawned numerous legal actions by plaintiffs claiming harm from such evaluations. To date, the greatest legal activity involving the use of tests has centered around education and employment decisions. This section briefly describes the major court cases addressing the use of psychological assessment in the schools, while a following section describes legal activities related to employment testing. For a more thorough discussion of the legal aspects of ability testing in schools, the reader is referred to Bersoff (1981, 1982b), DeMers and Bersoff (1985), and Reschly (1980).

Before reviewing the legal decisions affecting education, a Supreme Court decision which set the precedent for these cases needs to be mentioned. While not directly investigating the merits of psychological assessment, the Supreme Court declared in a 1969 decision that "students in school as well as out of school are 'persons' under our Constitution. . . . possessed of fundamental rights which the States must respect" (*Tinker* v. *Des Moines Independent Community School District*, 1969, p. 511). The case involved the rights of students to protest the Vietnam War, and the Court not only upheld the student's right to free speech but, for the first time, also explicitly defined minors as "persons" for constitutional purposes. In two subsequent cases (*Goss* v. *Lopez*, 1975; *Wood* v. *Strickland*, 1975), the Court's view of minors as persons possessing constitutional rights was reaffirmed.

Without this precedent and these supporting decisions, legal arguments about school testing practices (or other legal complaints involving minors) might now be burdened to first demonstrate how parent's constitutional rights have been violated, since their children would have no separate legal rights under the law. However, with minors recognized as persons under the law, these decisions led, perhaps inevitably, to increased complaints from students that negative consequences which resulted from some assessment procedures or situations constituted denials of their protected rights. These complaints especially focused on negative consequences which seemed disproportionately to affect certain racial minorities. Such complaints formed the basis for the three cases which most directly challenged the use of psychological assessments in the public schools.

Hobson v. Hansen

The primary issue in *Hobson* v. *Hansen* (1967) was the constitutionality of racial disparities when allocating financial and educational resources in a public school system. However, the court ultimately faced the issue of whether group ability and achievement tests measured black students' innate capacity to learn, because the school system defended its higher proportion of minority students in the lower tracks of their program based on the higher proportion of minority students scoring lower on the standardized tests.

The court decided that classification on the basis of ability was defensible only if such judgments were based on measures that assessed children's capacity to learn (i.e., their innate endowment) and not their present skill levels. The court's underlying rationale was that these skill levels might be lower due to the disadvantages experienced by these minority children, specifically their (families') reduced social and economic opportunities. The court concluded that the assessment devices used by the district did not accurately reflect the students' learning ability, and therefore, the classification of students into tracks based on such tests was unconstitutional. More importantly, the court concluded that since these measures "are standardized on and are relevant to a white middle class group of students, they produce inaccurate and misleading test scores when given to lower class and Negro students . . . " (*Hobson* v. *Hansen*, 1967, p. 514).

Although the decision in *Hobson* focused on group ability and achievement tests only, the court's decision to ban tests used to track minority students, unless they clearly measured these children's innate capacity to learn, demonstrates the stringent criteria that the courts can demand to protect the constitutional rights of minority students. Despite the extensive research on both group and individual ability tests, no psychologist, including Jensen (1980), could show that such tests measure the hereditary endowment of intellect (e.g., Anastasi, 1976; Cleary, Humphreys, Kendrick, & Wesman, 1975; Reynolds, 1982). An important final note specifically mentioned in the *Hobson* decision concerned the inappropriate use of tests standardized with a white middle-class bias to evaluate the ability of non-white, non-middle-class students. This same complaint formed the basis for two subsequent cases involving individual IQ tests.

(Larry) P. v. *Riles*

Perhaps no legal decision has so greatly affected psychological assessment practices as the California suit known as *(Larry) P.* v. *Riles* (1972). The case involved a group of black children in San Francisco who filed suit in 1971 claiming that the state-approved administration of individual intelligence tests had resulted in discrimination and their misplacement in classes for the educably mentally retarded (EMR). The plaintiffs further claimed that they were not mentally retarded; they were so classified only because the IQ tests used to place them were culturally biased. They requested and won a preliminary injunction barring the school system from administering IQ tests to other black children being considered for EMR classes until a full trial could be held.

The legal significance of *(Larry) P.* lay in the plaintiffs' contention that the testing practices of the school system violated the Constitution's equal protection clause, causing a disproportionate and harmful impact on black children. Thus, for the first time, the court was forced to rule on the constitutionality of individual psychological testing when used to place racial minorities in potentially adverse situations. In a case involving two phases, the plaintiffs first sought the preliminary injunction barring the use of IQ tests until a decision was reached, and second, participated in the actual trial.

This trial phase began in late 1977 and involved extensive testimony by nationally known psychologists and other social scientists who had expertise in psychological assessment. Prior to the trial and between the first and second phases of this case, significant and relevant federal legislation (e.g., Education of All Handicapped Children's Act of 1975; Family Educational Rights and Privacy Act of 1974) and other court decisions presented additional obstacles complicating the school system's defense of its assessment practices. These obstacles included provisions that tests be validated for the specific purposes of their use, that no single assessment procedure be used as the main determinant of a placement decision, and that a multidisciplinary team make placement decisions based on a variety of measures and evidence. Significantly, the plaintiffs were allowed to amend their original complaint to include claims that the school system's assessment practices violated these newly passed statutory protections. Thus, the plaintiffs ultimately claimed infringement of both constitutional (i.e., equal protection) and statutory (e.g., The Education of All Handicapped Children's Act of 1974) rights.

The late-1979 decision in *(Larry) P.* consisted of a long and controversial view of the merits of both psychological assessment and special education. The court generally found in favor of the plaintiffs on both constitutional and statutory grounds, and permanently enjoined the defendants (i.e., the school system and the state) from using individual IQ tests to place minority students in classes for the educably mentally retarded. In addition to the profound effect on the practice of school psychology in California, the judge's written decision had two other important effects: (*a*) it became a legal precendent in other jurisdictions, and (*b*) it carried the potential to alter other states' general psychological assessment practices.

The primary focus of the *(Larry) P.* decision was on the requirement that assessment instruments be validated for the specific purposes of their use; that is, the intelligence tests used to assess minorities for special education placements would have to be validated for each minority group. A second aspect of the decision focused on whether the tests themselves discriminated against blacks and other minority groups. The court ultimately decided that the tests did discriminate against black children, since (*a*) the original versions of the individual IQ tests primarily used by the defendants (the Stanford-Binet and Wechsler scales) did not include blacks in their standardization samples, and (*b*) subsequent inclusions of representative proportions of minorities in updated standardizations did not ensure differential validity for minority groups. Finally, the court also emphasized that despite school system regulations requiring a multidisciplinary team to consider a variety of data and pertinent information, the IQ score was often the sole and clearly most important determinant which placed these children in special education.

Although some school psychologists may view the *(Larry) P.* decision as interfering and restrictive to their professional practice, it could aid school psychologists' attempts to convince school administrators that special education placements require thorough and multifaceted assessments, not quick and cursory evaluations with instruments of questionable validity.

PASE v. *Hannon*

Less than a year after the *(Larry) P.* decision, a federal court in Illinois heard a case similar in issues, facts, and even witnesses. The decision, however, was very different. The *PASE* v. *Hannon* (1980) case was brought on behalf of all black children placed in EMR classes in Chicago's public schools. The two named plaintiffs claimed that they were not retarded despite their placement in EMR classes for several years and that blacks generally were overrepresented in these classes. The plaintiffs further asserted that the misclassification resulted from racial bias inherent in the individually administered IQ tests, and that these tests violated the equal protection clause of the Constitution and the same federal statutes at issue in *(Larry) P.* Updated psychological evaluations showed that these plaintiffs were of normal intelligence, but their learning was hampered by remediable disabilities.

The defendants in *PASE* (i.e., the school system), conceding that IQ tests could be slightly biased, asserted that this did not deprive the tests of their utility or their ability to facilitate accurate classification decisions. Ultimately, according to the defendants, their diagnoses of mental retardation were based on a combination of factors, with the IQ score as only one of those factors. They further asserted that if denied the use of this relatively objective measure, the schools would be forced to make decisions on more subjective criteria.

Although the federal judge who presided over *PASE* had the voluminous testimony from *(Larry) P.* available as well as some of the same witnesses, he dismissed most of the expert testimony. Instead, he chose to review the Stanford–Binet and WISC-R (Wechsler) scales himself, question by question, to form his own opinion of the tests' inherent racial bias. This analysis influenced the court's final decision that only a small minority of items on the two scales was sufficiently biased to warrant exclusion. Furthermore, the judge concluded that even if the IQ tests had been biased, that did not prove that the whole assessment process, which included the use of multiple measures and multidisciplinary teams, was biased. In fact, the judge found that fewer children were ultimately labeled retarded than would have been the case had their IQ scores alone been used.

Thus, the *PASE* decision was almost the opposite of the *(Larry) P.* decision despite the similar claims and issues. These conflicting decisions leave school administrators and psychologists uncertain about using IQ tests to evaluate minority children for special education. DeMers and Bersoff (1985) argue that one possible explanation for the opposing decisions involves the Chicago schools' ability to show more compliance with the new federal regulations, that is, that the placement decisions were made by multidisciplinary teams who used more than just the IQ tests. Regardless, the issues debated in these cases suggest that practitioners should evaluate their assessment programs to best prevent potential abuses of minority or other children *before* they occur or are claimed in a lawsuit.

Legal Influences in Employment Testing

Like ability testing in schools, the use of psychological assessment tools to select and evaluate employees has only recently received attention from judges and lawmakers (Johnson, 1976; Lerner, 1978). Two issues seem to have generated this legal interest in employee testing practices: (*a*) concern over the privacy rights of individuals required to complete personality inventories to obtain a job, and (*b*) claims of racial discrimination when ability tests are used to hire and advance employees. The legal protections and mandates resulting from these two issues and the cases discussed below provide background and legal precedents which could be generalized to the use of personality assessment with children and adolescents. For a more extensive discussion of the legal aspects of employment testing per se, the reader should review Bersoff (1981, 1982c), Johnson (1976), and Lerner (1978).

Public criticism and legal scrutiny of psychological testing in the workplace erupted around 1965. During that year, two separate congressional hearings, one in the House of Representatives and one in the Senate, were held in response to growing public sentiment against psychological testing. This sentiment was fueled further by critics such as Black (1963) and Gross (1962, 1965). The spark igniting these extensive congressional activities was a complaint by federal employees that certain government agencies, who required job applicants to complete personality inventories, were invading their privacy. In his opening remarks to the Special House Subcommittee on Invasion of Privacy, Gallagher (1965) described the issue as "the matter of psychological or personality testing of government employees and job applicants by federal agencies" who subject "federal workers . . . to extensive tests on their sex life, family situations, religion, personal habits, childhood and many other matters" (p. 955). Similar concerns were raised by the Senate investigation (Ervin, 1965).

Following the lengthy debate and analysis of these hearings, psychologists were forced to reexamine and reform their questionable assessment practices. For example, professional associations such as the APA ultimately developed and codified strict standards governing the use of psychological assessment tools in government and industry (American Psychological Association, 1970, 1974, 1980). Although the problems uncovered by these initial hearings and the standards adopted by the psychological community are numerous and complex, the basic issues involved the nature of undue invasion of privacy and the use of tests in situations for which they were not validated. Each of these major concerns is discussed in greater detail later in this chapter.

The second arena of legal activity in employment decisions involved the use of psychological tests to select and promote employees. Here, as in the use of ability tests in schools, the legal issues questioned whether psychological tests were racially discriminatory and, thus, violated the constitutional safeguard of equal protection. The landmark decision which established the legal precedent for several subsequent complaints was the case of *Griggs* v. *Duke Power Co.* (1971). Following the passage of the Civil Rights Act of 1964, the Duke Power Co. introduced a series of standardized ability tests to set criteria for advancement to higher levels and better-paying jobs. As black employees at Duke had been openly restricted to the lowest level jobs before the new civil rights legislation, blacks in the suit contended that the new employment tests were instituted to maintain Duke's now illegal discriminatory practices and that they were not related to job performance.

In a unanimous decision, the Supreme Court found for the black employees and, perhaps more importantly, introduced the notion of "job-relatedness" in employment testing. Job-relatedness refers to the Court's position that employers must demonstrate a rational and meaningful connection between test performance and job success and may not employ "broad and general testing devices" with limited ability to "fairly measure the knowledge and skills required by a particular job" (*Griggs* v. *Duke Power Co.*, 1971, p. 433). The Court used guidelines established by the Equal Employment Opportunity Commission (1966) to buttress its argument of job-relatedness, and these guidelines, like the APA test standards, served to reform and regulate employment testing practices. In a variety of subsequent cases involving both private industry (e.g., *Albermale Paper Co.* v. *Moody*, 1975) and government agencies (*Guardian Association of New York City* v. *Civil Service Commission*, 1980; *Teal* v. *State of Connecticut*, 1981; *United States* v. *City of St. Louis*, 1980), the courts have continued to challenge the job-relatedness of various employment testing practices, even where purposeful discrimination is not an issue (Bersoff, 1982a).

Although not directly related to children and adolescents, these legal decisions involving employment testing of adults in the workplace and ability testing in schools set the stage for legislative actions which may directly affect the assessment of children's personality and emotional status. Further, these decisions set legal precedent and reveal the judicial perspective which might prevail should a legal challenge to personality assessment practices arise.

Legislation and Litigation Affecting Personality Assessment with Children and Adolescents

As the brief history of legal interest in psychological assessment suggests, most of the complaints and decisions involving psychological assessment have concerned ability testing in either the school or the workplace. Bersoff (1982d) noted the irony that ability tests, which have survived decades of empirical analysis and validation, have received such harsh judicial review while personality assessment practices, which have many unanswered questions about their psychometric adequacy, have remained virtually unexamined by the law. This discrepancy in legal interest may be explained by the larger pool of potential litigants that is created by the many more children who receive intellectual assessments over personality assessments. One might also argue that complaints of racial discrimination are more serious or grievous than complaints of poor or misleading personality assessment. However, this argument of less serious consequences seems without merit when one considers that a child could be labeled and placed in a class for the emotionally disturbed or placed in the custody of one or another or neither parent, or that any person could be involuntarily committed or found competent to stand trial rather than insane through a personality assessment.

Two other aspects of personality assessment practices may explain the discrepancy in legal scrutiny. Although criticism of the reliability and validity of many popular personality assessment procedures is extensive (Bersoff, 1973; Gross, 1962; Korchin & Schuldberg, 1981; Meehl, 1959; Mischel, 1977), few, if any, critics have suggested that personality assessment procedures systematically discriminate against a particular group, for example, a racial minority or a specific handicapping condition. Thus, the legal basis for much of the litigation involving ability tests (i.e., the equal protection clause) does not apply to personality assessment. Second, except in cases of special education evaluations in public schools and government personnel selection practices, most instances of personality assessment occur in the private offices of licensed professionals who are voluntarily sought out by private citizens. Since these are voluntary assessments from private practitioners, the second major basis for legal action involving ability tests (i.e., the due process clause which protects private citizens from an unfair denial of their rights by a state) is also irrelevant. Thus, the limited legal attention afforded to personality assessment may be explained best by the limited availability of a legal basis for a complaint rather than the psychometric rigor of these assessment procedures.

This does not suggest that personality assessment practices, particularly those affecting children, are immune from legal intervention. In fact, it is likely that a sizable proportion of personality assessments conducted with children and adolescents are administered by state-employed psychologists in public schools, mental health centers, and hospitals. As such publicly employed psychologists are agents of the state in the eyes of the law, constitutional safeguards like equal protection and due process therefore would apply. Moreover, some legal safeguards such as informed consent and the right to privacy could serve as the basis for a legal complaint even in a private practice situation.

The legislation and litigation related to personality assessment of children and adolescents fall into three main categories: test validation, informed consent, and privacy issues. Each of these major categories is addressed below with a discussion of the nature of the law or case in general and its specific relevance to personality assessment with children and adolescents. Also discussed below are any perceived differences in legal culpability or responsibility between practice in a public versus a private setting.

Test Validation Issues

One of the key issues debated in the legal challenges to ability testing in the schools and the workplace involved the appropriate validation of assessment procedures. As noted above, the issue of proper test validation in these legal challenges was raised in the context of a racial discrimination claim. However, the requirement that tests be properly validated could prompt and support other complaints against mental health practitioners, for example, malpractice suits stemming from alleged misdiagnoses. Such legal complaints could be brought against either publicly or privately employed practitioners.

For practitioners (particularly school psychologists) working with school-children suspected of having educational and social–emotional handicaps which potentially involve special education programming, appropriate test validation is required under The Education of All Handicapped Children's Act of 1975 (PL 94-142). Among many other things, PL 94-142 requires that tests be validated for the specific purposes for which they are used, be reliable for the populations being assessed, and be capable of generating appropriate decisions based on their data and results. This law's significance was evident in the *(Larry) P.* case where the court was able to require some fairly rigorous criteria for the intelligence tests used (e.g., differential validity for separate minority groups). Specific to personality assessment with children, few of the diagnostic procedures used by school psychologists to evaluate children for emotionally disturbed classroom placements were normed or even intended to serve such a purpose. Many of these procedures would be difficult to defend simply on the issue of reliability. Further, many of these procedures were developed and normed on adult populations, not with children or adolescents.

In their review of assessment practices in special education, Salvia and Ysseldyke (1981) challenge the technical adequacy of most personality assessment procedures for children:

> Most personality assessment devices have inadequate norms. . . . Many authors of personality measures do not report evidence of reliability of their tests. When reliability data are reported, the reliabilities are generally too low to warrant use of the tests in making important educational decisions about children. . . . Definitions of traits, needs and behaviors assessed by personality measures is not a common practice by test authors. Yet the absence of operational definitions creates a situation in which it is difficult to determine just what a test is designed to measure. (p. 447)

Such harsh criticism of personality assessment devices is hardly rare; similar attacks appear in the literature over the past 30 years (Bersoff, 1973; Breger, 1968; Meehl, 1954; Mischel, 1968). One needs only to go to the most recent edition of *Buros Mental Measurements Yearbook* (Buros, 1978) to see that the question of adequate reliability and validity remains unanswered for many measures of personality (Haney, 1981), especially those purporting to measure personality in young children (Walker, 1973).

Psychologists in private practice, while not directly affected by PL 94-142, have an ethical responsibility to consider the adequacy and appropriateness of their assessment procedures. Principle 8 of the APA's *Ethical Principles of Psychologists* (1981b) states that "In reporting assessment results, psychologists indicate any reservations that exist regarding validity or reliability because of the circumstances of the assessment or the inappropriateness of the norms for the person tested" (p. 637). Since many state psychology licensing laws have adopted the APA ethical principles as standards for their licensed psychologists, even private practitioners may be held legally responsible for using tests of questionable psychometric quality.

The purpose of this chapter is not to debate whether these criticisms of personality assessment practices are justified or warranted. However, with such a long history of extensive criticism by respected sources, the foundation of a legal challenge against the use of some personality assessment devices due to their invalidated applications and unreliable characteristics is certainly available. One recent court case involving school personality assessment practices came close to being the first true legal challenge on the basis of this test validation issue.

Lora v. *Board of Education of the City of New York* (1978) involved a discrimination complaint under the equal protection clause. However, the plaintiffs were not claiming misdiagnosis due to biased ability tests. Rather, this group of minority students had been diagnosed as emotionally disturbed by what they claimed were vague and subjective evaluation criteria and procedures. Specifically, the plaintiffs charged that the school system had placed a disproportionate number of minority students in a special school for disturbed students while nonminority students with similar problems were placed in classes for the emotionally disturbed in regular schools. Plaintiffs further contended that the tests used to evaluate them were biased against minority children, and that this bias caused the disproportionate placements in the more restrictive environments.

Bersoff (1982b) notes that the central issue in this case should have been whether the diagnostic procedures (e.g., the Bender–Gestalt, TAT, and Rorschach) had been validated with minority children to diagnose their emotional disturbances. The court, however, chose to focus on the lack of procedural safeguards afforded the plaintiffs under the due process clause of the Constitution. The court found for the plaintiffs on these grounds, never directly addressing the differential validity of the assessment procedures used. However, as noted above, the potential for future claims based on these procedures' validities or on related grounds remains.

Informed Consent

The second major category of legal and ethical requirements with specific implications for the personality assessment of children and adolescents involves informed consent. In general, informed consent refers to the receipt of specific permission to do something following a complete explanation of the nature, purpose, and potential risks involved. The term includes the receipt of permission from subjects participating in research projects, from patients receiving medical treatment, or from clients (or their parents or guardians) receiving psychological evaluations. The legal requirement for informed consent which most directly affects the personality assessment of children is found in PL 94-142 governing assessment practices in schools. Section 300.504 of PL 94-142 discusses parents' rights regarding the granting of permission to schools to evaluate and place their children in special education. The intent of this section is clearly to increase parents' participation in the educational decision-making process by requiring schools to notify parents before taking certain actions and to obtain consent before engaging in other actions.

Under PL 94-142, informed consent involves three components:

1. Knowledge. Although not required to reveal every detail of an evaluation or placement decision, the law requires school officials or personnel (e.g., school psychologists) to tell parents (*a*) what they intend to do (i.e., conduct a comprehensive evaluation), (*b*) why they intend to do it (i.e., to decide if special education is necessary), and (*c*) how they intend to do it (i.e., with an intellec-

tual, achievement-oriented, or personality assessment battery). Clearly, the latter or "how" aspect of knowledge is the most difficult to accomplish; it involves describing complicated assessment practices in nontechnical language such that the general public can understand it.

2. Voluntariness. Informed consent involves the willful granting of permission in addition to provision of the knowledge specified above. Schools may not secure the written permission of parents through pressure tactics, threats, misrepresentation, or unfair inducement.

3. Competence. Parents must be legally competent to give consent. Most school officials presume the competence of parents even when limited education, mental ability, or social adjustment makes the receipt of informed consent difficult.

Since school systems typically presume parental competence and probably do not often coerce parents into granting consent, the knowledge component of informed consent tends to receive the most attention by both the schools and the courts. As noted above, the description of the evaluation instruments and assessment process is the most difficult aspect of the knowledge domain. School psychologists are required under PL 94-142 to explain the nature and purpose of complicated psychological assessment procedures (including personality assessment devices) in parents' native language and in nontechnical terms. Bersoff (1982b) notes that the law prescribes a description of each evaluation procedure, not merely a list of the names of those tests to be used.

Ethically, all psychologists, not just school psychologists, have similar knowledge expectations placed on them. Principles 6 and 8 of APA's ethical code require that psychologists respect a client's right to know (a) the nature and purpose of any evaluation procedure as well as (b) the results, interpretations, and conclusions drawn from specific assessment techniques. Psychologists are also ethically bound not to misuse assessment results, an ethic which some authors (Martin, 1983) feel eliminates assessment procedures of limited technical adequacy from use. As seen in the previous section on test validation, this interpretation of ethical responsibility could seriously restrict the use of many popular personality assessment procedures. Although the provisions of PL 94-142 do not apply directly to assessments completed outside of the public schools, these provisions do serve as legal precedents and could be viewed (in combination with the ethical responsibilities noted) as defining appropriate professional practice. This perspective could provide clients of psychologists outside of the public schools with a basis for legal complaint when the standards of informed consent are violated.

Thus, psychologists and mental health practitioners would do well to develop a method of communicating the nature and use of personality (and other) assessment instruments to parents. Minimally, parents should be told (a) what tests and procedures their children will be given, (b) each test's purpose and administration methods, and (c) each test's contribution to the relevant placement and/or programming issues. Perhaps in the future, practitioners, like physicians, will be required to inform parents of the potential risks involved for each assessment and the margin of error inherent in each measure. Ethically, psychologists may already be bound to convey the risks and limitations of chosen diagnostic procedures to their clients (Martin, 1983). However, the typical interpretation of the legal requirements under PL 94-142 and the ethical responsibilities of psychologists does not yet require such a comprehensive disclosure to secure informed consent (Bersoff, 1982b; DeMers & Bersoff, 1985).

Invasion of Privacy

The third major category of legal and ethical requirements is a broad and complicated collection of legislation, litigation, and ethical principles that is perhaps best labeled as the right to privacy. While not specifically guaranteed in the Constitution, the right to privacy has been cited as a component of the Fourteenth Amendment's right to liberty, and it has served as a basis for many legal decisions (e.g., *Merriken* v. *Cressman*, 1973). Since the Fourteenth Amendment protects citizens from unnecessary intrusions by a state, the use of some of these legislative and legal decisions is limited to those psychologists (or practitioners) who function as agents of the state. Yet, recent case law and those professional ethics related to privacy issues apply to virtually all psychologists licensed to practice. Thus, this right should be protected by all practicing psychologists. This section is divided into three subsections (i.e., access to assessment records, confidentiality/privileged communication, and privacy as informed consent), each dealing with one aspect of the privacy issue.

Access to Assessment Records

Throughout their histories, many psychological assessment procedures have been shrouded in secrecy to prevent public disclosure. In the past, members of the APA could have been expelled from the Association or suffered other professional sanctions had they violated the Code of Ethics provision (now changed) that limited access to psychological tests and other assessment devices to "persons with professional interests who will safeguard their use" (APA, 1963, p. 59). However, consistent with other consumer-oriented disclosure laws (Robertson, 1980), some federal and state statutes now require greater accessibility of test materials to examinees (and their parents in the case of children).

The first major federal legislation affecting public disclosure of tests and their results was the Family Educational Rights and Privacy Act (FERPA) of 1974. FERPA (and its implementing regulations published in 1976) requires school systems receiving federal support from the Department of Education to allow parents (and emancipated minors) access to records concerning their children. Additionally, this law, also known as the "Buckley Amendment," provides an opportunity for parents to challenge these records. FERPA clearly applies to psychological reports prepared by school psychologists, since these are part of a child's school record.

Developing law also indicates that parents probably have a legal right to review the test protocols themselves (Bersoff, 1982b). Under the Buckley Amendment, test protocols and answers were often withheld from parents under the provision that documents in the sole possession of the maker (e.g., the psychologist) and not accessible or revealed to anyone else are not considered part of a pupil's record. However, to the extent that the information from such tests is revealed to others, that is, it appears in assessment reports and is discussed during placement meetings, then it is arguable that such test protocols are part of the child's record and, therefore, available for inspection. PL 94-142, which included portions of FERPA to describe parents' right to review records of their handicapped children, requires that schools permit parents to inspect and review records that are collected, maintained, and used by the school in its special education decision making. Psychological tests and their results are almost always "used" in this process and, thus, could be considered accessible.

In 1979, two states (namely, New York and California) enacted "truth-in-testing" legislation which requires testing agencies to disclose information about tests and test-takers' performance. The California law requires only that the test-maker supply test subjects with sample questions and explanations of scoring procedures. The New York law is much more stringent, requiring test-makers to reveal not only background and statistical data pertaining to the test, but also the contents of the test itself. In fact, the test-maker is required to file the necessary documents so that a test-taker may request a copy of the test questions, his or her own answers, and the correct answers according to the test developer. The statute was passed despite protests from the Educational Testing Service (ETS) and others who claimed that it would violate test security and necessitate prohibitively expensive revisions of tests after each administration. Despite the lobbying these pieces of legislation caused (indeed, a federal version may be introduced), surprisingly few of the test-makers' dire predictions have occurred. For example, relatively few test-takers have requested disclosure of test materials, and only a modest increase in the cost of taking tests (like the Graduate Record Examination administered by ETS) has resulted due to the need to develop alternate forms of the tests (APA, 1981a).

At the present time, these truth-in-testing laws apply only to large-scale standardized tests used for admissions purposes. However, the legal principles and judicial climate seem clear; the rights of the test-taker over the test-maker are currently favored. Therefore, mental health practitioners' clients may soon have the legal right to demand access to assessment data which influenced important decisions about them (or their children). This right could even become the norm in private practice and community-based settings.

Confidentiality/Privileged Communication

Extending confidentiality to children, separate from their parents or guardians, is also legally risky in the mental health field. While most training programs emphasize those professional and ethical responsibilities and practices which maintain a client's confidence, practitioners who work with children must be aware of the legal limitations of these practices given a child's status as a minor. Except where specifically contradicted in federal or state statutes or specific legal decisions, minors have no rights to privacy separate from their parents. Consequently, practitioners who have acquired information about a child during counseling, testing, or other psychological functions have no right to withhold such information from parents unless the parents have voluntarily waived their right to know as a condition of treatment. But even with a voluntary waiver, the practitioner would have to prove that the conditions of informed consent (i.e., knowledge, voluntariness, and competence) were met when obtaining the waiver should the parents decide to recant their decision.

Besides a waiver, there are other limited circumstances when practitioners may legally withhold information obtained from and about children from their parents. Many states currently have passed statutes which allow mental health practitioners, physicians, and other professionals to withhold such information when it involves potential child abuse, drug use, and requests for information about contraception, although such statutes usually require the professional to inform other parties (e.g., the police, the courts) (Overcast & Sales, 1982). Thus, except for these special situations, confidentiality with minors is perhaps best applied as a joint protection of children and their parents from the release of information to a third party (e.g., the school, the courts, a potential employer), not as a specific protection of information from or about a child from his or her parents.

Practitioners should also consider their legal status and right to extend confidentiality. Many state psychology licensing laws include provisions for "privileged communication" (as confidentiality is legally termed) for those professionals licensed under that act; however, some licensing laws may not provide for this right. In addition, many state boards that regulate psychological practice and licensing may not extend the right to privileged communication to, for example, school psychologists (and others) who function under credentials issued by state departments of education, unless they are also licensed by that board. A few states (e.g., Kentucky, Nebraska) do extend the right of privileged communication to school counselors and psychologists credentialed through their departments of education. It is left to the individual practitioner, however, to determine his or her legal status to claim privileged communication in their own states.

A final limitation to the confidential relationship between practitioners and clients (including children) which may affect personality assessment practices involves the so-called "duty to warn" principle. Demonstrated in a far-reaching California case (*Tarasoff* v. *Regents of the University of California*, 1974), the duty to warn provision permits a court to hold psychologists (and other professionals) liable for damages in cases when they fail to warn targeted individuals who are in danger due to their clients' threats because they choose to maintain client confidentiality. The *Tarasoff* case itself involved a psychologist working with a client in a state university counseling center. The psychologist contacted the campus police after the client threatened the life of his former girlfriend, Tatiana Tarasoff, during a therapy session. The campus police interviewed the client and then released him after deciding that the threat was not serious. The client never returned to therapy, neither the police nor the therapist contacted Ms. Tarasoff to inform her of the client's statements, and 2 months later the client killed Ms. Tarasoff.

The family of Ms. Tarasoff sued the psychologist, his supervisor, and the university for damages in an action ultimately decided by the state supreme court. The court found for the Tarasoffs and not only awarded them damages, but also held that psychologists have a "duty to warn" potential victims of violent threats made by clients, even if the psychologist enjoys the general rights to privileged communication. As Siegel (1979) notes, the court found the Tarasoff case analogous to a physician who, while generally enjoying a confidential relationship with a patient, has the responsibility to warn the public of potential cases of serious communicable diseases.

While the *Tarasoff* decision technically applies only to psychologists in California where the case was brought, it again serves as legal precedent in other jurisdictions. Siegel (1979) suggests that the psychologist in the *Tarasoff* case would have had a better chance for a successful resolution of the conflict had he maintained the client's confidentiality *and* kept him in treatment. The duty to warn principle places the psychologist in the untenable position of choosing whether to defy the law or to ignore professional ethics; the possibility of being sued is present, whichever option is taken. This conflict between legal mandates and ethical principles is hardly new (Bersoff, 1975; Siegel, 1979), but no less disconcerting to the conscientious practitioner.

Many psychologists hoped that the *Tarasoff* decision would be overturned on appeal, thus resolving this conflict between legal and ethical requirements. However, two recent California cases have reaffirmed and strengthened the duty to warn principle. In the cases of *Hedlund* and *Yablonsky* (APA, 1984), the courts stated that therapists must warn "any and all potential victims of possible violence when a person threatens another in therapy'' (p. 1). Although the context of these cases involves a psychotherapeutic relationship, there is little reason to believe that psychologists learning of potentially violent situations during an assessment would be excused by the courts from the duty to warn requirement.

In summary, practitioners must become familiar with the specific statutes in their states. They should investigate their general rights to claim privileged communications and the specific limitations placed on such rights when the client is a minor. Unless otherwise specified by law, parents have a legal right to obtain the information resulting from an assessment of their child. Consequently, practitioners should be careful to inform both the child and the parents of the limits to confidentiality.

Privacy as Informed Consent

The final issue related to privacy and its impact on the psychological assessment of children concerns the legal necessity to obtain informed consent prior to accumulating information about children and/or their families. In the previous section on informed consent, the focus was on the need to inform parents about the nature and limitations of various diagnostic procedures. Here, the focus is on informing parents of the possible invasion of their family's privacy as a consequence of assessing their child. Parents must be informed, since children are legally considered minors and, moreover, are incapable of weighing risks to themselves, making informed and binding decisions, and granting permission for medical or other treatments. Permission for the psychological treatment (including assessment) of children therefore must be secured from a child's parents or legal guardians, and must include a full disclosure of the procedure's potential benefits and/or harmful effects to either the child or the family.

While securing parental permission for testing may constitute informed consent, a classic case suggests that the adequacy and completeness of the disclosure may ultimately determine whether informed consent was fully obtained. The case (*Merriken* v. *Cressman*, 1973) involved a survey of eighth-grade students to determine their potential for drug abuse. A school system hired a private research organization to identify and then treat potential drug abusers. A brief letter sent to all parents to notify them of the program stated only that some diagnostic testing would be part of the program. The letter went on to state that the district would assume parents' cooperation unless notified to the contrary. The survey asked students about themselves, their classmates, the nature of their relationships with their parents (e.g., loving, hostile, strained), and the behavior of their parents in specific situations (e.g., how often they expressed their love to them).

When the mother of one student in the district complained to the school board, the publicity surrounding the complaint resulted in the American Civil Liberties Union entrance into the case on the mother's behalf. Ultimately, the case attempted to permanently enjoin the program, not just to exclude the complainant's child from participation. The federal court found that the program implemented by the school district had invaded the privacy of the family by questioning the child without an adequately informed consent process. Right to privacy becomes an issue in this case because the school system is viewed as a representative of the state which is encroaching on the rights of private citizens.

Although the children were questioned without their agreement or consent, the court found that the *parents'* right to privacy was violated (see Bersoff, 1982d) by survey questions attempting to discover correlates between family life and drug abuse. The court declared that

> the fact that students are juveniles does not in any way invalidate their rights to assert their Constitutional right to privacy. . . . [T]he children are never given the opportunity to consent to invasion of their privacy; only the opportunity to refuse to consent by returning a blank questionnaire. Whether this procedure is Constitutional is questionable, but the Court does not have to face that issue because the facts presented show that the parents could not have . . . given informed consent. . . . (pp. 918–919, 1973)

Thus, the court seems to affirm that minors have a right to privacy, although it never addresses whether they maintain this right independent of their parents. Given this judicial view, it may not be long before practitioners will be required to obtain the child's and the parents' informed consent.

Bersoff (1982b), discussing the implications of this case, notes that a person can certainly waive a constitutional right, but "that such waivers must be shown to be voluntary, knowing, intelligent and done with sufficient awareness of the relevant consequences" (p. 1,065). While the school system's letter in this case obviously failed to meet the legal requirement of informed consent, the question of what constitutes adequate informed consent remains. Would the courts view the typical request for permission to assess a child adequate? If a family crisis has precipitated the request for service, was voluntary permission granted under these circumstances? Would a psychologist in private practice (and thus not an agent of the state) also be expected to obtain informed consent? These are questions that still need to be addressed by the courts or by legislators. In the meantime, however, practitioners doing extensive assessments which include obtaining information from children about their parents and their home life are advised to consider the precedent in *Merriken* v. *Cressman* (1973). Thus, they should make a defensible effort to apprise all parties of the nature, extent, and purpose of the assessment and intervention process that will be employed.

To summarize this section on privacy issues, practitioners working with children need to become familiar with both the legal and ethical constraints involving such issues as access to assessment records, confidentiality, and obtaining informed consent prior to collecting information about private family matters. As noted above, legal and ethical requirements can differ from one another; in fact, they may directly oppose and contradict each other. The privacy issues are further complicated because children, as minors, present special legal problems as to what rights they do and do not possess. Finally, the employment status of the practitioner as either a public servant or private entrepreneur may affect the extent to which certain constitutional protections such as right to privacy apply.

Conclusions and Speculations on Future Legal Involvement in Assessment of Children's Personality

As stated initially, no other activity performed by psychologists has received as much legal scrutiny as psychological assessment. While suits and legislation affecting psychological assessment have a relatively recent beginning, the future will probably bring a steady increase rather than a decrease of legal activity. According to a recent publication from the APA:

> Until very recently, psychologists were somewhat unique among health service professionals in that they were as a group seldom or only occasionally susceptible to malpractice and errors or omissions complaints. That era may be coming to a close now, not so much because psychologists are practicing differently . . . , but because the legal profession is learning how to litigate this type of claim. (p. 3, 1984)

Soon, psychologists, like physicians, may have to pay exhorbitant premiums for liability insurance in light of successful claims against their colleagues. Further, they may need to practice with a constant eye toward avoiding potential lawsuits.

Practitioners who work with children and adolescents are especially likely to see this trend continue for several reasons which are worth repeating here. First, children present special legal challenges because their status as minors complicates the available legal and ethical mandates. Second, many practitioners who work with children are employed in school systems and other public agencies and are therefore viewed by the law as agents of the state. This places additional burdens on them and their organizations to safeguard constitutional protections. Finally, children seen by practitioners are often handicapped or from minority populations. Thus, they receive the benefit of still greater legal protections which may impinge on the practice of psychological assessment.

What specific issues are likely to be challenged in the courts in the near future? Given the public's reaction to the insanity defense in the case of John Hinckley, who attempted to assassinate President Reagan, and the extension of the duty to warn mandate in California, it would seem that the judicial climate is right for a direct legal challenge to the adequacy of personality assessment. This might follow lines similar to the exhaustive scrutiny of IQ tests in the *(Larry) P.* case during the 1970s. Considering the increased role of psychologists and other helping professionals in mediating custody disputes following divorce, the adequacy and dependability of personality assessment used to guide those decisions could also become legally contested, especially given the emotional fervor associated with such decisions. Finally, the increasing availability of computer scoring and report writing programs for a variety of psychological instruments and procedures (including personality assessment devices) is likely to generate controversy, possible abuse, and disputes requiring litigation. This is especially possible given the current absence of any comprehensive ethical guidelines for the appropriate use of computers in psychological assessment.

Given the likelihood of continued legal involvement in issues related to psychological assessment and the distinct possibility that more specific legal scrutiny of personality assessment practices will occur, a comment on the relative merits of this legal interposition in the practice of psychology and mental health services seems warranted. While many practitioners may feel that the intrusion of lawyers and legislators into the mental health domain is unnecessary and purely obstructive to professional practice, a brief review reveals that, for the most part, poor practice often precipitated legal involvement and better practice resulted from the legal decisions. For example, in the case of *(Larry) P.* and *Merriken* v. *Cressman*, potentially dangerous practices such as relying only on IQ tests to place minority children in special education and failing to obtain the parents' informed consent prior to soliciting family-related information were struck down and remediated. Legislative mandates requiring the use of tests consistent with their standardizations and validations and giving parents open access to records maintained on their children in school are some further positive examples.

Some psychologists (Bersoff, 1982a; DeMers & Bersoff, 1985; Overcast & Sales, 1982) see this increase in legal influences as having several potential benefits for psychology in general and the psychological assessment of children in particular. First, it has made the profession of psychology, as well as society in general, more aware of the rights of children and their parents, as well as the special need to protect the rights of minorities and the handicapped. Second, it has alerted psychologists, as well as those who employ them, that they will be held legally responsible for their actions, thereby forcing psychologists to examine their instruments, interpretations, and recommendations. To the extent that such examinations result in better instruments and decisions, then the legal and legislative initiatives have served to improve rather than impede our professional functioning. Finally, these same legal decisions and mandates that guide our professional practice also can serve to protect and support psychologists who are resisting attempts by others (e.g., employers, third-party payers, administrators) to require unethical or illegal practices (*Forest* v. *Ambach*, 1981; Starkman, 1966).

Finally, mental health-related and psychology training programs need to emphasize and practitioners now in practice need to become more familiar with the various legal and ethical constraints on professional functioning. Such increased familiarity will serve to protect practitioners from the increasing attempts to litigate claims against them. More importantly, this should result in better psychological and mental health services to the clients we seek to serve.

References

Albermale Paper Co. v. Moody, 422 U.S. 405 (1975).

American Psychological Association (APA): (1963). *Ethical standards of psychologists*. Washington, DC: Author.

American Psychological Association (APA). (1970). Psychological assessment and public policy. *American Psychologist, 25*, 264–266.

American Psychological Association (APA). (1974). *Standards for educational and psychological tests*. Washington, DC: Author.

American Psychological Association (APA). (1980). *Principles for the validation and use of personnel selection procedures*. Berkeley, CA: Author (Division of Industrial/Organizational Psychology).

American Psychological Association (APA). (1981a). *Committee on tests and assessments: Statement on "truth in testing" legislation*. Washington, DC: Author.

American Psychological Association (APA). (1981b). *Ethical principles of psychologists*. Washington, DC: Author.

American Psychological Association (APA). (1984, August). *Hedlund* and *Yablonsky* decisions expand *Tarasoff* duty to warn burden in California. *Professionally Speaking*, pp. 1–2.

Anastasi, A. (1976). *Psychological testing* (4th ed.). New York: Macmillan.

Bersoff, D. N. (1973). Silk purses into sow's ears: The decline of psychological testing and a suggestion for its redemption. *American Psychologist, 28*, 842–849.

Bersoff, D. N. (1975). Professional ethics and legal responsibilities: On the horns of a dilemma. *Journal of School Psychology, 13*, 359–376.

Bersoff, D. N. (1981). Testing and the law. *American Psychologist, 36*, 1047–1056.

Bersoff, D. N. (1982a). *Larry P.* and *PASE*: Judicial report cards on the validity of individual intelligence testing. In T. Kratochwill (Ed.), *Advances in school psychology*. Vol. 2, pp. 61–95. Hillsdale, NJ: Erlbaum.

Bersoff, D. N. (1982b). The legal regulation of school psychology. In C. Reynolds & T. Gutkin (Eds.), *The handbook of school psychology* (pp. 1043–1074). New York: Wiley.

Bersoff, D. N. (1982c, August). *Regarding psychologists testily: The legal regulation of psychological assessment*. Master lecture presented at the American Psychological Association Convention, Washington, DC.

Bersoff, D. N. (1982d). *Social and legal influences on test development and usuage*. Invited paper presented at the Buros-Nebraska Symposium on Measurement and Testing, Lincoln, NE.

Black, H. (1963). *They shall not pass*. New York: Morrow.

Breger, L. (1968). Psychological testing: Treatment and research implications. *Journal of Consulting and Clinical Psychology, 32*, 176–181.

Buros, O. (Ed.). (1978). *The eighth mental measurements yearbook*. Highland Park, NJ: Gryphon Press.

Civil Rights Act of 1964.

Cleary, A., Humphreys, L., Kendrick, S., & Wesman, A. (1975). Educational uses of tests with disadvantaged students. *American Psychologist, 30*, 15–41.

Cronbach, L. (1975). Five decades of public controversy over mental testing. *American Psychologist, 30*, 1–14.

DeMers, S. T., & Bersoff, D. N. (1985). Legal issues in school psychological practice. In J. Bergan (Ed.), *School psychology in contemporary society: An introduction*. Columbus, OH: Charles E. Merrill.

Education of All Handicapped Children's Act of 1975 (PL 94–142). 20 USC Sec. 401 (Supp. 1975).

Epperson v. Arkansas, 393 U.S. 97 (1968).

Equal Employment Opportunity Commission (1966). *Guidelines on employee selection procedures*. Washington, DC: Author (29 C.F.R. Sec. 1607).

Ervin, S. (1965). Why senate hearings on psychological tests in government? *American Psychologist, 20*, 879–880.

Family Educational Rights and Privacy Act of 1974. 20 U.S.C.A. Sec. 123g with accompanying regulations set down in 45 C.F.R. Part 99.

Forrest v. Ambach, 436 N.Y.S. 2d 119, 107 misc. 2d 920 (Sup. Ct. 1981).

Gallagher, C. E. (1965). Opening remarks. In testimony before House Special Committee on Invasion of Privacy of the Committee on Government Operations. *American Psychologist, 20*, 955–988.

Glaser, R., & Bond, L. (Eds.). (1981). Testing: Concepts, policy, practice, and research. *American Psychologist, 36*, 997–1206.

Goss v. Lopez, 419 U.S. 424 (1975).

Griggs v. Duke Power Co., 401 U.S. 424 (1971).

Gross, M. (1962). *The brain watchers*. New York: Random House.

Gross, M. (1965). Testimony before House Special Sub-Committee on Invasion of Privacy of the Committee on Government Operations. *American Psychologist, 20*, 958–960.

Guardian Association of New York City v. Civil Service Commission, 630 F. 2nd 79 (2d Cir. 1980), *cert. denied*, 452 U.S. 939 (1981).

Haney, W. (1981). Validity, vaudeville, and values. *American Psychologist, 36*, 1021–1024.

Heller, K., Holtzman, W., & Messick, S. (1982). *Placing children in special education: A strategy for equity*. Washington, DC: National Academy Press.

Hobson v. Hansen, 269 F. Supp. 401 (D. D.C. 1967), *aff'r sub nom* Smuck v. Hobson, 408 F.2d 175 (D.C. Cir. 1969).

Hopkins, K., & Stanley, J.C. (1981). *Educational and psychological measurement and evaluation*. Englewood Cliffs, NJ: Prentice-Hall.

Ingraham v. Wright, 430 U.S. 651 (1977).

Jensen, A. (1980). *Bias in mental testing*. New York: Free Press.

Johnson, J. (1976). *Albermale Paper Co. v. Moody*: The aftermath of *Griggs* and the death of employment testing. *Hastings Law Review, 28*, 1239–1262.

Kamin, L. (1974). *The science and politics of IQ*. New York: Wiley.

Korchin, S. J., & Schuldberg, D. (1981). The future of clinical assessment. *American Psychologist, 36*, 1147–1158.

Lerner, B. (1978). *Washington v. Davis*: Quantity, quality, and equality in employment testing. In P. Kurland (Ed.), *Supreme Court Review* (pp. 117–139). Chicago, IL: University of Chicago Press.

Lippman, W. (1922). The abuse of tests. *New Republic, 32*, 297–298.

Lora v. Board of Education of the City of New York, 456 Supp 1211 (E.D.N.Y. 1978). *Vacated and remanded or reworded* 623 F. 2nd 248 or 298 2nd Cir. 1980)

Martin, R. (1983). Ethics column. *School Psychologist, 37*, 10.

Meehl, P. (1954). *Clinical vs. statistical prediction*. Minneapolis: University of Minnesota Press.

Meehl, P. (1959). Some ruminations on the validation of clinical procedures. *Canadian Journal of Psychology, 13*, 102–128.

Merriken v. Cressman, 364 F. Supp. 913 (E.D. Pa. 1973).

Mischel, W. (1968). *Personality and assessment*. New York: Wiley.

Mischel, W. (1977). On the future of personality assessment. *American Psychologist, 32*, 246–254.

Overcast, T. D., & Sales, B. D. (1982). The legal rights of students in the elementary and secondary public schools. In C. Reynolds & T. Gutkin (Eds.), *Handbook of school psychology* (pp. 1075–1100). New York: Wiley.

(Larry) P. v. Riles, 343 F. Supp. 1306 (N.D. Cal. 1972) *aff'r* 502 F.2d 963 (9th Cir. 1974); 495 F. Supp. 926 (N.D. Cal. 1979); *appeal docketed*, No. 80-4027 (9th Cir., Jan. 17, 1980).

PASE v. Hannon, 506 F. Supp. 831 (N.D. Ill. 1980).

Reschly, D. (1980). Psychological evidence in the Larry P. opinion: A case of right problem—wrong solution? *School Psychology Review, 9*, 123–135.

Reynolds, C. (1982). The problem of bias in psychological assessment. In C. Reynolds & T. Gutkin (Eds.), *The handbook of school psychology* (pp. 178–208). New York: Wiley.

Robertson, D. (1980). Examining the examiners: The trend toward truth in testing. *Journal of Law and Education, 9*, 167–199.

Salvia, J., & Ysseldyke, J. (1981). *Assessment in special and remedial education* (2nd ed.). Boston, MA: Houghton-Mifflin.

Sherman, S., & Robinson, N. (Eds.). (1982). *Ability testing of handicapped people: Dilemma for government, science, and the public*. Washington, DC: National Academy Press.

Siegel, M. (1979). Privacy, ethics, and confidentiality. *Professional Psychology, 10*, 249–258.

Starkman, S. (1966). The professional model: Paradox in school psychology. *American Psychologist, 21*, 807–808.

Tarasoff v. Regents of the University of California, 13 C. 3rd 177, 529 P. 2nd 553, Cal Rptr. 129 (1974).

Teal v. Connecticut, 645 F. 2nd 133 (2nd Cir. 1981), *cert. granted* No. 80-2147 (Oct. 5, 1981).

Tinker v. Des Moines Independent Community School District, 393 U.S. 503 (1969).

United States v. City of St. Louis, 616 F. 2nd 350 (8th Cir. 1980). *cert. denied* 452 U.S. 938 (1981).

Walker, D. K. (1973). *Socioemotional measures for preschool and kindergarten children*. San Francisco, CA: Jossey-Bass.

Wigdor, A., & Garner, W. (Eds.). (1982). *Ability testing: Uses, consequences, and controversies*. Washington, DC: National Academy Press.

Williams, R. (1970). Black pride, academic relevance, and individual achievement. *Counseling Psychology, 2*, 18–22.

Wood v. Strickland, 95 S. Ct. 992, 420 U.S. 308 (1975).

A Conceptual Model and Pragmatic Approach toward Personality Assessment Referrals

Howard M. Knoff

There is no single "correct" theoretical or practical approach toward personality assessment referrals and their completions or resolutions. Minimally, the personality assessment process depends on (*a*) the appropriateness of the referral, (*b*) the referral source, (*c*) the theoretical and clinical perspectives of the attending practitioners, (*d*) the characteristics of referred children or adolescents, and the interacting people and environments relevant to these individuals and/or the referred situation, and (*e*) the practitioner's ability to consult with and motivate those participating in the assessment process to demonstrate cooperation and commitment to the referred child, the assessment process, and the importance of change. While practitioners generally develop a personal style and approach of personality assessment based on their experience, they hopefully have a conceptual model of personality development and behavior which guides that approach. This chapter integrates the different theoretical perspectives of disturbed or atypical behavior discussed in Chapter 1 of this volume into a conceptual model structuring the personality assessment of children and adolescents. It also discusses the practical steps, decisions, and assessment procedures necessary to consider and complete a personality assessment referral.

A Conceptual Model of Personality Assessment

Any referral to a practitioner of a child or adolescent who is presenting significant emotional, behavioral, or adjustment difficulties represents a problem that needs to be analyzed and "solved." Often, the referral source's definition of a "solution" involves an intervention which decreases the referred child's maladaptive or target behaviors that are interfering with that child's psychological (or other) development or with the referral source's sense of "normality" or "equilibrium." This solution or intervention plan actually represents only one step of

Howard M. Knoff. Department of Psychological and Social Foundations of Education, School Psychology Program, University of South Florida, Tampa, Florida.

a four-step problem-solving process which most effectively addresses any referral problem. The four problem-solving steps are (*a*) problem identification, (*b*) problem definition and analysis, (*c*) the development of intervention plans, and (*d*) the evaluation of the implemented interventions. This process has been used previously in personality assessment (Knoff, 1983a), consultation (Bergan, 1977; Meyers, Parsons, & Martin, 1979), and individual psychotherapy (Goldfried & Davison, 1976).

Within the personality assessment process, each problem-solving step becomes the foundation and guide for the next step. For example, a practitioner's intervention plans cannot be effectively developed and implemented with any reasonable chance of success unless the problem has been fully analyzed and understood from all relevant perspectives and directions. Similarly, the problem analysis is meaningless unless the *entire* problem has been identified by the practitioner through, for example, interviews with the referral source and significant others. Below, the conceptual components of each problem-solving step are detailed. The ultimate goals of the problem-solving process are (*a*) to comprehensively understand the referral problem, its context and validity, and its dynamics, interactions, and implications; and (*b*) to intervene to change the problem's content, conceptualization, environment, or manifestations.

Problem Identification

Assuming that a referral has been accepted for some kind of action, the primary goals of the problem identification process are (*a*) to initially identify the referral problem and potential areas for further analysis and assessment, and (*b*) to determine the appropriateness of individual personality assessment with the referred child to identify specific problems and to prepare for potential interventions and problem resolution directions. This process actually requires responses to four questions:

1. Does this referral reflect a problem specific to the referred child or is it a problem which includes the child but has a broader context?

2. Does this problem occur in only one (or in a limited number of) environment(s) or does it occur wherever the child is?

3. What are the environmental and/or child-specific components or characteristics of the problems?

4. What are the assessment goals?

The Appropriateness of a Referral

The initial question involves a "reality-testing" procedure for both the referral source and the practitioner whereby the validity of the referral as a problem unique and specific to the referred child is investigated. Often, direct consultation with the referral source uncovers larger or associated problems involving the referral source (e.g., the classroom teacher or parent) and specific environments (e.g., the playground during recess, a low-income neighborhood) in addition to the individual child who is initially referred as the focus of the problem (Caplan, 1970; Conoley, 1981; Meyers *et al.*, 1979). For example, consultation with a teacher who has referred a student for "verbal and physical aggressiveness" might reveal an insecure, novice teacher who is forced to teach in an overcrowded classroom without proper materials. Here, the practitioner might hypothesize that the teacher's inexperience may be contributing to the referred student's inappropriate behavior and/or that the teacher has misperceived entirely the student's "inappropriate" behavior. The environmental characteristics of the classroom (overcrowded, few appropriate materials) might be evaluated separately for their contributions to the referred behavior, or an analysis of their interaction with the teacher's inexperience might be necessary. The practitioner could analyze and discuss these hypotheses during an ongoing consultation interaction with the teacher, attempting to help him or her develop more effective teaching skills and to implement changes in the environment or organization. Contrasted with the initial referral and problem specification, this broader understanding of the "referred child" and the comprehensive understanding of the problem situation suggest that consultation may be a more appropriate and effective direction than an individual personality assessment.

As another example, a court referral may request a personality assessment to evaluate an adolescent's "compulsive stealing behavior." Discussions with relevant social agencies and social workers might reveal the divorce of the adolescent's parents, his or her current destitute situation in a home which is often without food and heat, and his or her residence in a high-crime neighborhood. While this does not legally excuse the behavior, it is more likely that this adolescent is a victim of a larger, more complex problem than that originally stated. Thus, an individual personality assessment for the given referral problem may or may not be warranted. Further, the referral as stated is inappropriate, or at least incomplete.

To briefly summarize, when assessing the appropriateness of a referral, problem identification first identifies its accuracy and completeness as initially stated. Inaccuracies may originate from or indicate "blaming the victim" (Ryan, 1976), self-fulfilling prophecies, theme interference (Caplan, 1970), or referral source problems such as lack of understanding, skill, experience, confidence, and objectivity (Meyers, 1981). Pragmatically, this identification process is accomplished by considering the referred child from two distinct perspectives: (*a*) a normative perspective, and (*b*) a developmental perspective.

The Normative Perspective

In the normative perspective, the referred problem is analyzed in the environment where it occurs to determine if it is unique to the referred child or typical of other children in that setting. Nonnormative behavior constitutes an appropriate referral that probably requires an individual personality assessment.

To accomplish this normative comparison, many authors (Nelson, 1981; Sulzer-Azaroff & Mayer, 1977; Tombari, 1980) recommend a behavioral approach whereby the behavioral characteristics of the targeted problem behaviors (i.e., the frequency, duration, and intensity) are observed and quantified objectively in their relevant environments. By systematically observing the referred child and a few randomly sampled "typical" peers across the target behaviors and characteristics, the presence of nonnormative versus normative behaviors (for that environment) can be identified. If the referred student's target behaviors significantly differ from those of the normative peer group, then the referral likely *does* reflect a child-specific problem which may require personality assessment or at least further study. However, if the target behaviors are typical or consistently observed within the peer or sampled group, the referral of this individual child may be inappropriate; that is, the referred "problem" may be a typical or common behavior in this environment and therefore of minimal concern (except for the referral source's significant misperception). Or, the problem truly may be a major problem in this environment, but should have been referred as a group problem for analysis and intervention.

The use of behavioral observation as a personality assessment technique is discussed further by Keller (Chapter 11 of this volume). The normative perspective is easily evaluated when the referral or target behaviors occur in the classroom setting, because of the availability of a typical peer comparison group. When the target behavior occurs in the family or community, a valid and reliable comparison is more difficult to obtain and to evaluate.

The Developmental Perspective

The developmental perspective uses the child, adolescent, and abnormal psychology literatures to compare referred children or adolescents' target behaviors or psychological issues to their chronological age or developmental expectations. Significant discrepancies between the target behaviors and the developmental expectations indicate some form of a child-specific problem that may require individual personality assessment. The lack of a discrepancy may indicate an inappropriate referral or a comparison that is insensitive to the specific problems inherent to the referral.

A developmental discrepancy involves behavior or characteristics that are typical of a child significantly younger than the referred child. For example, while crying or fearful behavior may be expected from a very young child when confronted by a stranger, such behavior would be developmentally inappropriate from a latency-aged child. In the latter case, a referral for personality assessment or further investigation would be appropriate, if not necessary. Ames, Metraux, Rodell, and Walker (1974) and other authors of major texts in developmental psychology describe specific personality characteristics or behaviors typical of various chronological age groups. These can form a baseline or developmental foundation to determine discrepancies within the problem identification perspective.

To briefly summarize again, the normative and developmental perspectives facilitate the problem identification process by helping to determine the accuracy of a referral and its focus as (*a*) a problem only with the referred child which (*b*) requires further individual analysis. Through these two perspectives and the validation process, the referral problem can be related to specific environmental conditions and/or child-specific characteristics (see Question 2 above).

Environmentally Related Problems

Environmentally related problems involve children whose inappropriate behaviors or psychological issues occur because of external or environmental variables or circumstances which may be out of their control or influence. For example, an elementary school student whose parents are separating and preparing for a divorce may manifest his or her emotional reaction to this stressful situation by hitting peers and swearing at teachers in school. By characterizing this referral as environmentally related, the practitioner has a clearer identification of this problem and a direction which can help organize the problem analysis steps to follow.

Given an environmentally oriented problem, the practitioner can specify the situations, interactions, or variables that need more formal analyses (Question 3 above) by listing, for example, family and ecological systems or characteristics (see Chapters 12 and 13 of this volume, respectively) which appear to significantly influence, support, or maintain the referral problem. Given the example above, the personality assessment could identify the individual dynamics of the elementary student's aggressive behavior and their relationship to the upcoming divorce. It may also focus, however, on the separated parents, their support for the child and the entire family to cope with this stressful situation, and the extended support systems in the child and/or family's circle of friends or community that might need analysis and further understanding. In the end, it is this latter focus on coping with the divorce situation and affected environments that will likely decrease the acting out and other school problems.

Child-Specific Problems

The child-specific problem is also an appropriate referral problem, but it involves behaviors or issues which appear inherent and specific to the child. For example, child-specific problems may include children who aggressively attack peers for no reason and with no remorse or children who persistently self-abuse or self-mutilate. As noted above, this characterization of the referral problem shapes the practitioner's direction and preparation for problem analysis.

Given this focus, the practitioner can use many of the child-specific classification systems described in Chapter 1 of this volume to characterize or specifically define the referred problem. This hypothesized classification can be tested during the problem analysis step and, if supported, may provide specific, relevant, and well-researched intervention programs to address the problem. Given the example of the aggressive, attacking child above, DSM-III's conduct disorder (undersocialized, aggressive) could be hypothesized during problem identification, investigated during problem analysis, and eventually (if confirmed) used to facilitate an appropriate intervention program.

To summarize, a problem's designation as child specific assumes that some referred behaviors occur due to a child's individual, ''intrapsychic'' personality or psychological constitution. Naturally, some practitioners, due to their theoretical beliefs that, for example, all behavior is environmentally determined, may totally reject this characterization. Further, there will be complex problems that are both environmentally related *and* child specific. Certainly, a child-specific problem characterization does not preclude considerations of the child's family or ecological circumstances. Such a focus could still facilitate intervention directions and the identification of environmental implications.

Identifying Personality Assessment Goals

The last problem identification question involves an initial delineation of the personality assessment goals. These goals will be reviewed and revised continually throughout the problem-solving process as the practitioner observes the referred child, interviews and conferences with significant individuals, and obtains a full sense of the pertinent referral issues and characteristics.

At the problem identification stage, the practitioner generally is working with only one or two referral sources (e.g., a parent, or a parent and a teacher), and the referred problem has been confirmed as appropriate only through classroom observations and discussions (the normative perspective) and/or through comparisons with typical developmental behavior (the developmental perspective). At this point in time, the assessment goals are defined as those activities which address those behaviors or issues that the referral source(s) wants to change. For example, the referral source may want the child to decrease acting-out, aggressive, or self-abusive behaviors, to feel better about him- or herself, or to understand and cope with an upcoming divorce and its dramatic change of family composition and status. While these changes structure the personality assessment goal(s) for the referral source, the practitioner will have to operationalize these goals to create more professionally specific assessment and intervention goals. As these goals change during the assessment process, the changes need to be discussed by the practitioner and those whom he or she feels need to be involved (e.g., the original referral sources). These discussions ultimately may become a significant aspect of the intervention and the referred problem's ultimate solution.

Problem Analysis

Problem analysis encompasses an organized set of procedures, strategies, and assessments tailored to define, describe, and comprehensively understand a referral problem in both its individual child and situational or environmental contexts. As noted above, most practitioners approach personality assessment using procedures or models based on their theoretical and conceptual background and their clinical experience. Significantly, practitioners' adherence to a particular theoretical or conceptual position of personality and social–emotional development often structure or dictate their problem analysis questions and procedures. This may help them to organize their problem analyses, but it also may bias their perspectives, restricting the comprehensiveness of their analyses.

The analysis of personality is historically tied to the different systems of psychology (e.g., empiricism, functionalism, structuralism) and to the personality theories and explanations of behavior which explicate these systems. These systems and theories, as well as the analyses of children and adolescents' referred problems and problem environments, can be considered within a general statement of personality and behavior: $B = f(P, E)$. Translated, this means that behavior is a function of complex interactions between person (or individual) and environmental (or situational) variables (Mischel, 1977). In its fullest sense, this statement suggests an interaction of children's behaviors and ecological circumstances.

In reality, different personality theorists explain personality and behavior by emphasizing different parts (or all) of this statement. For example, some view behavior only as a function of the person (Rogers, 1980), some only as a function of the environment (Goldfried & Kent, 1972; Ross, 1980; Travis & Violato, 1982), and some as a complete situational interaction (Bowers, 1973; Ellett & Bersoff, 1976; Endler & Magnusson, 1976; Mischel, 1977).

Recently, Bandura (1978) broadened the implications of the $B = f(P,E)$ statement further by suggesting that behavior, person, and environmental characteristics are actually all interactionally dependent on one another. Bandura's reciprocal determinism model, schematically represented as

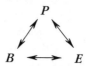

and based on his social learning theory perspective, views personality development as a complex, continuous, and reciprocal process. As Bandura defines the "person" (P) dimension as including an individual's cognitions, beliefs, values, and perspectives, the reciprocal determinism model uses behavioral, ecological, *and* internal or cognitive personality perspectives. According to Bandura (1978),

> [M]ost external influences affect behavior through intermediary cognitive processes. Cognitive factors partly determine which external events will be observed, how they will be perceived . . . and how the information they convey will be organized for future use. . . . By altering their immediate environment, and by arranging conditional incentives for themselves, people can exercise some influence over their own behavior. An act therefore includes among its determinants self-produced influences. It is true that behavior is influenced by the environment, but the environment is partly of a person's own making. By their actions, people play a role in creating the social milieu and other circumstances that arise in their daily transactions. *Thus, from the social learning perspective, psychological functioning involves a continuous reciprocal interaction between behavioral, cognitive, and environmental influences.* (p. 345, emphasis added)

The reciprocal determinism model is the most comprehensive perspective of human behavior and personality development. As such, it will be the theoretical foundation of this entire book. To obtain a comprehensive definition, description, and understanding of a referral problem, the practitioner needs to use the information gathered during the problem identification step and fit it conceptually into the reciprocal determinism model to identify what problem analysis approaches are necessary. To date, seven theoretical analysis approaches which emphasize different parts of the

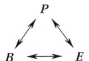

model are available to analyze emotionally and behaviorally disturbed children (Hallahan & Kauffman, 1982; Van Evra, 1983): the neurobiological, psychoanalytic, humanistic, cognitive–developmental, behavioral, psychoeducational, and ecological approaches.

Hopefully, even though committed to a specific theoretical orientation, the practitioner might be eclectic enough to consider any of these analysis approaches when they facilitate a more comprehensive understanding of the referral problem. While the seven approaches were discussed in greater detail in Chapter 1 of this volume, their primary problem analysis procedures will be briefly restated here within the context of the reciprocal determinism model.

The Neurobiological Approach

This approach highlights the importance of genetic, chromosomal, biochemical, neurological, and physiological characteristics, variables, and predispositions to typical and atypical behavior and personality development. While the neurobiological approach primarily emphasizes the interaction of behavior and person characteristics, the notion of predisposition suggests that environmental factors (e.g., stress, highly creative and stimulating settings) can "trigger" neurobiological reactions which may not have otherwise been manifested. The practitioner using the neurobiological approach as one component of a problem analysis might complete a neuropsychological assessment battery, observe and assess the relevant settings where target behaviors are evident, request a medical or pediatric and neurological consultation, and evaluate the child's psychological reactions to any (possible) organic involvement (Alexander, Roodin, & Gorman, 1980; Van Evra, 1983).

The Psychoanalytic Approach

This approach, in the Freudian tradition, explains emotionally disturbed behavior as a dynamic imbalance among the id, ego, and superego components (or constructs) of a referred child's personality. The child is assumed to possess significant underlying psychological conflicts and anxieties which cause the variety of referred inappropriate behaviors and emotional issues. These conflicts can be analyzed through psychoanalysis, symbolic play therapy, projective testing, and the psychoanalytic interpretation of family dynamics. Disturbed behavior is thought to reflect any number of defense mechanisms or symptom substitutions which are protecting the child from a psychotic breakdown. Psychoanalytic practitioners believe that personality development is completely determined by person variables and characteristics (e.g., past events during childhood).

The Humanistic Approach

Those advocating this approach (Maslow, 1962; Rogers, 1980) believe that emotionally disturbed behavior occurs when children lose their sense of reality, develop feelings of negative self-concept, and perceive significant discrepancies between desired and actual relationships and life events. Educationally, these children do not and eventually refuse to "fit into" or adapt to the traditional classroom and curriculum. Humanistic theorists view personality development primarily as a function of person characteristics, although an interactive relationship with behavior does exist. Even though disturbed children evaluate their success or failure through personal and environmental interactions, humanists believe that it is a child's inappropriate or inaccurate perceptions between what is and what should be that causes emotional disturbance. Problem analysis techniques here include "nondirective" counseling, play therapy, and assessments of self-concept through rating scales or Q-sort techniques.

The Cognitive-Developmental Approach

This approach emphasizes the importance of cognitive processes on a child's perceptions and interpretations of self and environmental events. Because cognitive development progresses through qualitatively different stages, typical behavior and behavioral expectations will change across the life span. For children, these changes occur primarily through the assimilation and accommodation processes which help to encode cognitive conceptualizations or representations of elements in their environments. Disturbed behavior occurs when these cognitive structures fail to properly influence age- or setting-specific appropriate behavior. Thus, the cognitive-developmental approach views personality development as a function of person, behavior, and environmental characteristics, although the individual's perception and ability to interpret the environment is the most important aspect of that interaction.

Given its developmental perspective, this analysis approach also draws upon the child and adolescent psychology literatures to suggest "baselines" of age-expected personality and behavioral characteristics. While the child's cognitive development and status is most critical, other areas of development (e.g., physiological, perceptual, socialization) may secondarily influence disturbed behavior. Thus, analyses within this approach may include norm and criterion-referenced assessments of cognition, intelligence, and personality; standardized and non-standardized tests; and formal and informal tools. Use of adaptive behavior scales, behavior rating scales, social skill analyses, parent, teacher, students, and significant other interviews, and other assessment approaches also would be appropriate.

The Behavioral Approach

Advocates of the behavioral approach believe that emotionally disturbed behavior results from inappropriate modeling, social learning, operant and respondent contingencies, and/or reinforcement schedules from (those in) the environment. The recent expansion of behavioral theory and intervention into cognitive and covert processes (Meichenbaum, 1977) also is included in and consistent with this environmental focus as covert behavior is defined and assessed through its observable or tangible manifestations. The behavioral practitioner examines primarily the interaction between behavioral and environmental variables. For example, using the principles and paradigms of operant and respondent conditioning, emotionally disturbed behavior is caused, influenced, and supported by people or characteristics of the environment. Behavior is changed by altering the relevant environmental variables or consequences affecting the child's behavior.

Behavior analysis shares some techniques with other approaches (e.g., interviewing, observation, rating scales), but behavioral practitioners emphasize the quantification and specification of overt behavior. As discussed within the normative problem identification perspective, behavior analysis includes the observation, counting, charting, and comparison of target behaviors exhibited by a referred child with samples of randomly chosen, "typical" peers in the same setting. Other behavior analysis procedures include objective personality inventories, behavioral checklists, samples from psychometric assessments, and observations of referred children in controlled, structured environments (e.g., free-play situations).

The Psychoeducational Approach

This approach (Fagan, 1979; Long, Morse, & Newman, 1980; Morse, 1975) integrates a psychiatric view that emotionally disturbed behavior is caused by conflicts both within children and due to relationships and stresses in their environments, and an educational view that the academic achievement process and its success is important to children and adolescents' well-being because it facilitates positive self-concept, social–emotional growth, and interpersonal change. According to this approach, then, personality development is determined by an interaction of all three reciprocal determinism variables and influences with an emphasis on the classroom as a critical environment and children's academic progress as a critical behavior. Thus, of all the approaches, this one specifically looks at the Psychology (or mental health) × Education (or achievement) interaction.

Problem analysis procedures within the psychoeducational approach include interviews with parents, teachers, the referred student, and significant others; classroom observations; any psychoeducational or social–emotional assessments which analyze significant academic strengths, weaknesses, attitudes, and aspirations; and assessments of family history, expectations, attitudes, and influences. Again, these problem analysis procedures are common to many of the theoretical approaches discussed here, and many of these procedures are independent of any one theoretical perspective. Thus, the psychoeducational (or any other individual) approach's philosophical and theoretical tenets influence the use and interpretation of these analysis procedures.

Other analysis procedures that are particularly useful within the psychoeducational approach come from the group process and social psychological literatures. These procedures investigate the impact of interpersonal dynamics and group development on classroom norms and individual student behavior. Schmuck and Schmuck (1979) describe the importance of analyzing the stages of classroom (group) development across six variables: teacher and student expectations; school, class, and interpersonal norms; communication processes; leadership; attraction; and cohesion-building interactions. Other processes that affect student behavior include the establishment of classroom goals and agenda, how classroom decisions are made, and conflict-management procedures, that is, how serious issues are identified, evaluated, and resolved (Schein, 1969; Schmuck, 1982).

These group process variables ideally facilitate a positive classroom environment where individuals are able to experience academic success and develop and maintain positive self-concepts. Children's emotionally disturbed behavior, in this context, may indicate a significant breakdown of effective group process in the classroom which causes inappropriate behavior or, cyclically, which may have been caused by earlier behavior that caused the group process breakdown. This environmental breakdown may be exacerbated by children's intrapersonal conflicts, misperceptions, or negative self-concept (failure) experiences in classroom or academic domains.

Group process/social psychological analyses may include questionnaires or surveys of students, parents, or teachers, sociograms or social interaction assessments, diagnostic observations of classroom group processes, structured and open-ended group discussions, or practitioner discussions with the referred child (Flanders, 1970; Fox, Luszki, & Schmuck, 1966; Schmuck, 1982). These analyses also require some knowledge of social psychological theory and literature, organizational consultation, and process consultation (Jerrell & Jerrell, 1981; Schein, 1969; Schmuck, Runkel, Arends, & Arends, 1977).

The Ecological Approach

This approach (Hobbs, 1966, 1975; Knoff, 1983a; Rhodes, 1967, 1970; Swap, 1978) fully embraces the person × environment perspective of emotional or behavioral disturbance. According to this approach, emotional disturbance occurs when significant environmental, familial, interpersonal, or intrapersonal stresses create dysfunctional ecological systems. Thus, disturbed or inappropriate behavior by referred children indicates a dysfunctional system, and the system, *not* the individual child, becomes the focus of analysis and change. Depending on the referral source and problem, however, an ecological analysis *can* focus on a referred child in a school, community, or family environment (or microsystem). This procedure, nonetheless, eventually assesses the child in a broader context which does fully consider the entire ecological system of the child. This context includes the macrosystem, exosystem, and mesosystem interactions, as well as the specified microsystem where the referral problem seems to be most prevalent or focused (see Chapter 1 of this volume for a description of these subsystems).

To operationalize the ecological analysis approach further, the four ecological systems will be described within a school-based referral. Because the referral problem is "owned" by or is a function of the entire system, the analysis should

generate descriptions of system strengths and weaknesses, should investigate interactions which explain or support the maladaptive behaviors or psychological issues related to the referral, and should identify previous successful and/or unsuccessful interventions and strategies. For example, an ecological analysis completed
to analyze a referred student would identify the classroom or school building as
the microsystem, components of the family and community as the exosystem, the
community, state, and/or country's societal expectations and values as the macrosystem, and the interactions among all relevant subsystem people, characteristics,
and variables as the mesosystem. Thus, the analysis might investigate significant
interactions among the student, relevant classroom characteristics (the teacher,
peers, curriculum, physical facilities), and school building or school district characteristics (administrators, mental health practitioners, district policies for emotionally disturbed students); pertinent family members (nuclear and extended),
and relevant community organizations (social service agencies, legal or police personnel, religious institutions); and the effects of societal expectations, values, and
mores. A family-oriented referral would have the family as its microsystem, while
the community would comprise the microsystem for community-based referrals
and mental health issues.

As evident above, each of the seven major approaches addressing emotional
and behavioral disturbances favors certain assessment procedures and evaluation
strategies. Some are unique to a specific approach, while others are used by a
number of approaches and may vary primarily by the philosophical and theoretical tenets and perspectives of the individual approach. A composite of these
unique and "generic" procedures and strategies are available in Part II of this book
in far more specific detail and explanation than in this chapter. Briefly, the unique
procedures covered in this volume relate to projective assessment (the Rorschach—
Chapter 5; Thematic Apperception Techniques—Chapter 6; Projective Drawing
approaches—Chapter 7; and Incomplete Sentence Blank approaches—Chapter 8);
objective assessment (the Personality Inventory for Children—Chapter 9); behavioral assessment (Behavior Rating Scales—Chapter 10; Behavioral Observation approaches—Chapter 11); family assessment (Chapter 12); and ecological assessment
(Chapter 13). More generic procedures include diagnostic interview procedures
(Chapter 4) and actuarial and automated assessments (Chapter 14).

Consultation skills and processes are also integral to the problem analysis
process. Utilizing skills (such as empathy, confrontation, clarification, and summarization) and appropriate consultation models (such as the behavioral, mental
health, process, psychoeducational models) as guides, the practitioner can effectively define and analyze referral problems as well as support and direct the referral source(s) toward intervention and change. Because consultation is so important
to the overall change process, it will not be discussed further here. The consultation and change process is addressed in Chapter 16 of this volume as part of the
discussions on intervention.

Given an appropriate personality assessment referral as determined by the
problem identification process, the practitioner must decide how to integrate the
seven analysis approaches (by using one or a combination of approaches) into the
reciprocal determinism model. As noted above, the practitioner may need to use
more than one approach to comprehensively analyze a referred problem, and this
may "force" the practitioner to consider theoretical models or actual analysis procedures that do not conform with his or her training or conceptual orientation
or bias. Lazarus (1981) rationalizes this by discussing the "technical eclectic," the

practitioner who is adept at using techniques from different orientations because they strengthen problem analysis (or intervention), but who does not necessarily adhere to the theoretic foundations underlying these techniques. Despite their conceptual and practical differences, the seven problem analysis approaches can be organized such that they are at least considered with every referral even if they are not used.

Across the seven approaches, the cognitive-developmental approach should be the foundation of any problem analysis because it compares referred children's behavior to "typical" child (or adolescent) behavior and development, identifying a developmental baseline or reference point. This reference point, for example, in socialization or play skills, provides a developmental context and understanding of the problem, a sense of how discrepant, maladaptive, or atypical it is given a child's chronological age, and appropriate and realistic developmental expectations and directions for child-focused intervention. To wit, an intervention technique that necessitates a junior high school level of cognitive understanding would be inappropriate to use on a junior high school adolescent with an elementary school cognitive level.

Along with the cognitive–developmental approach, the neurobiological approach should be considered. While a neurobiological assessment may not have direct educational implications, it may have behavioral or temperamental implications, or it may be useful to discount possible neurobiological conditions or syndromes. This is *not* to say that all personality assessment referrals require a neurobiological analysis and consultation. Rather, the practitioner must decide whether this approach is necessary, why it is necessary, and what specific questions should be answered by its completion.

The ecological approach, after one's use or consideration of the two approaches above, can help to organize the remainder of the analysis. By identifying the relevant focus of the referral (the microsystem), the significant interacting systems and subsystems can be mapped out and specific interactions identified for more in-depth analysis. Subsystems that involve organizations or organizational units (e.g., a classroom, a family's children) might utilize the behavioral or psychoeducational analysis approaches. Subsystems that involve individuals (e.g., the referred child, his or her mother or teacher) might use any combination of the psychoanalytic, humanistic, behavioral, or psychoeducational approaches. At all times, however, these approaches and the analysis as a whole are guided by the interactions and interdependencies that operationalize the reciprocal determinism model.

Intervention

Too often, practitioners, pressured by their administrators and supervisors or by their own needs to seek quick therapeutic change, begin the problem-solving process with the intervention step. Intervention success is determined primarily by good problem identification and sound problem analysis. The problem identification and, especially, the problem analysis steps should generate logical directions for intervention which are based on the strengths, weaknesses, and resources of the referred child, the referral source(s), and any relevant interacting subsystems and environments. Previous successful and unsuccessful interventions should be identified during the problem analysis along with the reasons why they succeeded or failed, respectively. New interventions should utilize available ecosystem strengths and resources and should be consistent with the approaches used during the problem analysis process. Finally, interventions can be implemented individually by a practitioner or can be part of an integrated institutional, hospital, community, or school district plan implemented coordinately by therapy staff, mental health professionals or practitioners, teachers, parents, and the referred child him- or herself.

As noted immediately above, interventions should be consistent within the reciprocal determinism paradigm and should follow directly from those problem analysis approaches that are used for a specific referral; that is, for example, a neurobiological problem analysis should suggest neurobiological interventions, behavioral analyses should suggest behavioral interventions, psychoeducational analyses psychoeducational interventions, and so on. Because intervention is such an important component of the personality assessment process, two entire chapters of this book (Chapters 16 and 17) have been devoted to their discussion. This chapter, however, will suggest a procedure for choosing interventions generated from the problem analysis data and results.

Regardless of the theoretical approach(es) used in the problem analysis step, practitioners still should follow systematic problem-solving approaches when designing the comprehensive intervention plans. As discussed above, an ecological analysis of the referred problem can organize this problem-solving process by identifying system and subsystem interactions that significantly involve the referral problem interactions which are analyzed further by one or more of the other theoretical approaches. These analyses generate data and, ultimately, specific recommendations structured by the ecological interaction investigated *and* the theoretical approach used. For example, a referred problem that requires an analysis of the family subsystem, the classroom subsystem, and the referred child's individual psychological makeup might use a combination of the psychoeducational, behavioral, and cognitive-developmental analysis approaches. The family subsystem analysis will result in family-oriented interventions tailored to that subsystem and consistent with the analysis approaches used; that is, behavioral analyses of the family subsystem will generate behavioral interventions, psychoeducational analysis will generate psychoeducational interventions, and so on. Ultimately, all of the recommendations and interventions suggested by these separate analyses for the family, classroom, and individual child subsystems, respectively, must be integrated and synchronized into an intervention package that addresses the referral problem in its largest, most efficient ecological context. Maher (1981) recommends an excellent decision-making model which facilitates this complex and delicate process.

First, each specific subsystem recommendation or intervention is rated independently for its probability of success in the subsystem it was generated for *and* for its ability to address significant problems or issues occurring in the larger ecological system. A list of possible interventions, rank-ordered by their probabilities of success, results. Then the practitioner rates each intervention for its probability of implementation. This decision is based on the practitioner's (*a*) knowledge and analysis of the referral environment and situation, (*b*) ability to implement or ensure the implementation of the recommendations based on the resources, skills, and commitment of those responsible for or participating in the intervention program, and (*c*) assessment of the intervention's potential effectiveness alongside other specific interventions. When the probability of success (based along a − 1.00 to + 1.00 continuum) and the potential for implementation (based on a 0 to 100 continuum) are multiplied together for each intervention, the resulting final rank-ordering suggests the most potentially effective interventions for the specific referral problem and ecological analysis.

The practitioner then must decide how many of the highest ranked recommendations will most effectively address the referral problem and situation. At this time, no answer is available on the "right" number of interventions for any one specific problem; this is an empirical question which will hopefully be answered in the future. For now, however, this approach by Maher (1981) offers a probability-oriented model which can integrate the often qualitative and subjective process of choosing multifaceted intervention strategies for multifaceted ecosystem needs and analyses. Further, this approach provides an empirical procedure for more empirical study.

Two final comments are necessary to conclude this discussion. First, interventions are conceptualized and implemented within a probability model; that is, interventions are chosen because they have the greatest probability for success given the referral problem, situation, environment, and analysis. If the intervention program is unsuccessful, the practitioner should not be disheartened because the *only* intervention approach has been tried. Instead, the practitioner should reevaluate the analysis approaches and results, or even the original problem identification and conceptualization, and try again. Interventions may be unsuccessful, but the practitioner rarely, if ever, "fails." There should be no blame associated with unsuccessful interventions; there are just too many intervening variables which can negatively influence what may actually be an appropriate intervention.

Second, practitioners should be aware of their intervention expectations for themselves, their therapy and mental health staffs, teachers, parents, and/or referred children. To focus an intervention program on one person's participation or influence is unwise; problems referred for personality assessment are usually so complex that they require multiple intervention participants. This warning is especially sounded for private or community agency practitioners who may feel completely responsible for an intervention program which may be restricted in time to one therapy hour per week. This situation may not only induce practitioner burnout, but also may be very unrealistic and ineffective.

Evaluation

Evaluation is an integral part of the entire personality assessment process. The practitioner should not accept a subjective opinion or impression that an intervention is successful, especially when the intervention is complex, multifaceted, and directed toward numerous interdependent systems and subsystems. Evaluation must include both subjective (e.g., attitude surveys, interviews) and objective data. Further, it must continue beyond the initial intervention period, extending as long as logically necessary (e.g., through the end of a school year, until the child is mainstreamed from a special program or unit). Finally, the evaluation should investigate intended and unintended effects. An example of an unintended effect might involve the negative changes in a peer group resulting from an individual intervention program for a referred child (Payne, 1982).

Process versus Product and Formative versus Summative Evaluations

The evaluation of an intervention program for emotionally or behaviorally disturbed children or adolescents should include both product and process evaluations and formative and summative evaluations. Product evaluations focus on changes in those behaviors or issues targeted during problem identification and addressed during problem analysis and intervention, and/or changes in environmental conditions which significantly affect or influence these target behaviors or issues. Process evaluations assess the interpersonal and social psychological processes between the practitioner, the referral parties, the referred child, and significant others, which affect attitudes and feelings toward the intervention and problem-solving process' success (Knoff, 1982b). Thus, a product evaluation might investigate how a target behavior has changed from its baseline, while a process evaluation might assess the referral source's satisfaction with the practitioner's problem-solving skills and ability to effect change.

Formative evaluation continues through an intervention to determine intermediate levels of success and areas where an intervention needs "fine tuning" to ensure greater success. Summative evaluation occurs when an intervention program is completed or otherwise discontinued (e.g., at the end of the school year) and a final evaluation of its utility and accomplishment is required. This evaluation can be used later to determine the intervention program's potential success with similar problems that reappear in the referred child or that are manifested by other children at risk or referred for individual personality assessments. Additional information on the evaluation of intervention programs and personality assessment processes appears in Conti and Bardon (1974), Knoff (1982b), and Stufflebeam *et al.* (1971).

The success of the entire personality assessment, problem-solving process is most dependent on the use of formative evaluation. If an intervention is not successful (or less successful than expected or desired), this evaluation may identify interpretive or procedural errors across the entire process (at problem identification, problem analysis, or intervention) which need reconsideration or correction. The practitioner must not hesitate to review and reanalyze any of these previous steps. Because personality problems are often complex reflections of the reciprocal determinism model, formative evaluations help to identify missed information or interactions, or changes in systems or subsystems which have occurred since an initial analysis. Practitioners must recognize that for some referrals, the personality assessment process may be never-ending. Further, they must prepare those working with them for the problem-solving process discussed above and for the necessary investment and commitment such a process requires.

Utilization of Personality Assessment Approaches and Techniques in the Field

Upon reviewing the authors' perspectives and interpretations of their data, the most recent studies evaluating personality assessment are undecided on its status and increasing or decreasing popularity in the psychology and mental health fields. For example, clinical psychologists (Fein, 1979; Wade, Baker, Morton, & Baker, 1978) and school psychologists (Prout, 1983; Ramage, 1979) report that personality assessment has remained an important skill and activity in the field, yet that many training programs have decreased their emphasis in courses and supervised experiences. For those who use personality assessment techniques in clinical, agency, or institutional settings, the most used tools were (not in order) the Minnesota Multiphasic Personality Inventory (MMPI), Rorschach, Bender Gestalt Test, Draw-A-Person and Human Figure Drawings, Thematic Apperception Test (TAT), Sentence Completion tests, and the House–Tree–Person (H–T–P) technique (Brown & McGuire, 1976; Lubin, Wallis, & Paine, 1971; Piotrowski & Keller, 1978; Wade & Baker, 1977).

School psychologists often have not been included in surveys investigating the training and use of psychological and personality assessment techniques. Two major studies specific to school psychology, however, have been reported in the literature. Goh, Teslow, and Fuller (1981) described a national survey of school psychologists, their typical assessment requirements, and their typical personality assessment batteries. Given their usual batteries, the respondents' most used assessment areas were (in order) intellectual, achievement, perceptual, personality, and behavior rating scales assessments. These school psychologists used personality assessment techniques in approximately one-half of their cases with their most used techniques being (in order) the Bender Gestalt Test, Sentence Completion techniques, the H–T–P, TAT, Children's Apperception Test (CAT), the Draw-A-Person, the Rorschach, and self-concept scales.

Prout (1983) also completed a national survey of school psychology practitioners to evaluate what personality assessment approaches and techniques they most used. He also surveyed school psychology training programs to assess what approaches and techniques were most emphasized during graduate, precertification training. The practitioners rated the importance of five personality assessment approaches (from most to least important) as follows: behavioral observation, clinical interview, projective techniques, behavior rating scales, and objective techniques (e.g., the MMPI or Personality Inventory for Children). Behavioral observation received a 2.14 rating and objective tests a 3.84 rating along a 1 to 5 (most to least important) scale. The percentages of practitioners who utilized the various approaches were as follows: behavioral observation, 90%; clinical interview, 83%; projective techniques, 74%; behavior rating scales, 44%; and objective tests, 50%. The trainers of school psychologists rated their emphases of the five approaches as follows: behavioral observation, 1.95, 96%; clinical interview, 2.51, 80%; behavior rating scales, 3.34, 66%; projective tests, 3.52, 64%; and objective tests, 3.66, 64%.

The most used personality assessment techniques by Prout's practitioner sample were (in order) clinical interviews, informal classroom observations, Human Figure Drawings, Bender Gestalt Test, Sentence Completion techniques, structured classroom observations, H–T–P, clinical analyses of IQ tests, behavior rating scales, and Kinetic Family Drawings (all rated as either frequently or always used). The trainers reported that they most emphasized (in order) clinical interviews, informal classroom observations, Human Figure Drawings, Bender Gestalt Test, structured classroom observations, Sentence Completion techniques, the TAT, clinical analyses of IQ tests, H–T–P, and behavior rating scales. Interestingly, there was a great deal of conformity between the two ratings despite the fact that the practitioners, on average, completed their training in 1974 and the trainers completed their survey in 1983.

The results of the various surveys, across both school and clinical psychology, do not clarify whether different components of personality assessment are increasing or decreasing in their use or popularity in the field. Nor do we get a firm sense of which analysis models (out of the seven discussed above) are guiding practitioners' personality assessments. It *is* clear that the behavioral model is being used quite regularly as both a theoretical perspective and an assessment technique. Yet, for the other assessment techniques, the guiding theoretical models are not known. Certainly the projective techniques could be analyzed from psychoanalytic, humanistic, cognitive-developmental, behavioral, psycho-educational, and/or ecological perspectives. Other tools (e.g., IQ tests, the Rorschach, Bender Gestalt Test) have been used by the neurobiological perspective, yet also by the other nonmedically oriented theoretical models.

In summary, personality assessment is currently at a crossroad where a practitioner's orientation or perspective does influence interpretations of the various techniques used. The following chapters discuss specific assessment techniques or diagnostic approaches and characterize their versatilities, liabilities, and ultimate utilities to the personality assessment process.

A Pragmatic Approach toward Personality Assessment

Above, the conceptual components of the personality assessment problem-solving process were discussed in detail. One additional conceptual model, Lazarus' BASIC ID, will be added in Chapter 16 of this volume to round out the problem analysis to the intervention process. Nevertheless, the reciprocal determinism model and seven theoretical approaches were outlined and integrated in this chapter across the problem identification, problem analysis, intervention, and evaluation steps.

In this section, a more pragmatic personality assessment process is presented which details the practical steps that a practitioner completes from a problem's referral to its intervention or consultation follow-up. While closely associated, these steps will be presented from both the practitioner-in-the-schools versus the independent practitioner-in-the-community-or-agency perspectives. The complete step-by-step process involves the (a) Referral or Intake, (b) Family and School Background Information Forms and Interviews, (c) Preassessment Conference, (d) Home and School Observations, (e) Child-Involved Assessments, (f) Personality Assessment Report, (g) Feedback Conference, and (h) Follow-up Contacts.

Referral or Intake

In the School

The initial personality assessment referral to a practitioner who is employed by a school district could take one of two directions, depending on its severity and the prospects for placement into special education. If the referral is presented to evaluate a child's signficant emotional or behavioral problems (e.g., school phobia, a transient emotional reaction to a parent divorce) and a special education placement decision is irrelevant or premature, the practitioner (school psychologist) can accept and respond to the referral independently, that is, without any formal special education or regulatory (PL 94-142) considerations. If a special education placement decision might be required, the referral should be presented to the school building or district child study team for formal discussions among the involved multidisciplinary professionals.

Given either referral direction, the intake procedure should specify the referral source and the nature of the problem, document previous intervention attempts, successes, and lack of successes, investigate previous contacts with other community agencies, child study teams, or mental health practitioners, and identify the most recent contacts with the referred child's parents to discuss the presented problems. At this referral step, the practitioner or child study team must, minimally, go through the problem identification procedures outlined in the previous section to determine the validity of the referral for personality assessment.

In the Agency

The referral to a private or community agency should be handled by a professionally trained mental health practitioner. With child or adolescent referrals, an agency should accept the referral only if the referred individual manifests emotional or behavioral styles, needs, or issues which cannot or are not being accommodated by a school's program and/or staff, either through regular or special education. Or, an acceptable referral may involve a child who needs services concurrent with an educational program or to supplement school-based mental health services. In either case, the intake will involve the same questions and information as the school intake above, although the services previously provided in the school system should be investigated and documented. Some referrals may not be accepted, not because they are inappropriate, but because the agency does not have the focus or expertise necessary to address the referred problems most effectively. In these cases, the agency should suggest, if possible, two or more agencies or individuals who could provide the necessary expertise to the child and the referral source.

Some agencies do not accept referrals that involve school and family issues unless both school personnel and family members agree to participate together, regardless of the referral source. These and other issues (e.g., payment, minimum number of sessions, the legal and ethical rights of the referred child and referral source) need to be discussed and agreed upon as part of an assessment contract *before* any services are actually delivered. A sample intake form from a university-based psychoeducational clinic addresses some of these procedures and is reproduced in Appendix I. An appropriate intake form for a school-based practitioner or child study team could easily be adapted from this outline.

School and Family Information Forms

In the School and Agency

These forms, also reproduced in Appendix I, could have exactly the same formats, differing only with the respondent and the information sources. For the school referral, the school information form could be completed by relevant members of the child study team or, with a non-special education referral, the practitioner could consult with the referred child's teacher and/or guidance counselor and review the child's cumulative education folder. For the agency referral, a liaison or contact person in the school system should be identified, and he or she can become responsible for the form's completion.

The completion of these forms encompasses and may initiate some of the problem analysis procedures. Once this occurs, the referred child has become singled out for investigation and evaluation. Therefore, the practitioner may want to obtain formal, written parental permission before commencing this procedure, even if the forms' completions are only for the school's benefit or in-house attention. For an agency to receive school-completed information, a written release (see Appendix I) from the parents which gives the school legal permission to divulge the relevant information is necessary.

The School Information Form obtains general information about the school and asks for descriptions of the child's academic performance levels, strengths and weaknesses, past and current academic standing, prior remedial and special help programs, classroom assets and liabilities, classroom behavior, prior psychoeducational assessments and results, the school's perceptions of the home environment, and significant factors affecting the child's learning progress.

The Family Information Form obtains general information about family attitudes, values, and routines; parent occupations; sibling interactions; family medical and educational histories; and family reactions to the child and his or her difficulty. Also surveyed are the child's educational, medical, social–emotional, and developmental histories; previous psychoeducational assessments and/or diagnoses; perceptions of the school; and the child's strengths and weaknesses.

The practitioner, school or agency based, and/or the child study team can utilize the Information Forms to identify potential assessment directions; previous successful and unsuccessful remedial strategies; areas of possible conflict between the parents, school, child, and significant others; and issues to pursue in subsequent interviews and conferences. The Information Forms also constitute a "public" commitment of sorts by the participating parties to the personality assessment process. This commitment, given the social psychology literature, may facilitate the entire problem-solving process, especially the development and implementation of an interdependent intervention program (Freedman, Carlsmith, & Sears, 1970; Schellenberg, 1970).

School and Family Interviews

In the Schools

From the practitioner or child study team's perspective, there is no single "school interview" with significant staff people, nor does it necessarily occur at exactly this chronological point in the assessment process for every referral. School interviews, both formal and informal, are occurring continuously when a child is considered at risk. These interviews occur before the referral, in preparation for the referral, and after the referral. They involve conferencing, consultation, data collection, and prereferral interventions. Finally, they may involve teachers, principals, specialists, or paraprofessionals.

From the school practitioner's perspective, family interviews may involve all pre- and postreferral conferences with the parents (with the referring teacher also present at times) which discuss the referred student, investigate family history and issues relating to referral problems, and document the referred child's unique history and development within the family context. For the school practitioner, the family interview offers an opportunity to ecologically analyze a problem which may be manifested at school, yet originate from specific family system issues. The family, meanwhile, may not appreciate this intrusion from an educational institution into personal family matters. This may simply reflect the family's belief that there should be a separation between schools and the community at large, that is, that schools are limited to educational, not social and mental health domains. Or, this may be a defensive reaction whereby the family rejects any responsibility for the referred child's difficulties. Regardless of the reason, such family resistance must be identified by the practitioner and resolved as much as possible through direct, indirect, or strategic approaches. Other issues that should be considered by the school practitioner and the family are confidentiality, the discussion and use of family information that occurs but is irrelevant to the referred problem, legal requirements (e.g., to report child abuse or neglect), and/or the process of recommending community-based psychotherapy services or other resources if deemed necessary.

In the Agency

In some ways, the agency's participation in school and family interviews is even more complex than for the school practitioner. For example, some personality assessment requests are actually mandated by the family or judicial court systems or a social service agency. In these cases, the agency or private practitioner often must work doubly hard to facilitate smooth relationship-building and an atmosphere of trust and openness with all concerned so that information is received quickly and accurately. When a parent or school official initiates the referral to the agency and the agency requires both parties to participate jointly, both parties should be forewarned that the interview process may take some time and that cooperation and patience are necessary. At other times, for example, when the referral involves an independent assessment for a due process hearing, school or family cooperation may actually be impossible or ill-advised and the interview process may be quicker.

Despite these considerations, the agency must clearly identify its primary client—the referred child, the referral source, the larger system (family or school) represented by that referral source—during the contract negotiations which occur before the referral's acceptance and discuss the implications of working for/ with that client. This identification of the referred child as the primary client may help the agency practitioner to explain the interview and assessment procedure to the referring and nonreferring parties in the most nonthreatening context. Given this circumstance, the practitioner can be perceived by both school and parents as relatively independent—that is, caring for the child's needs and not the special interests of either the school or family. Within the initial interviews, the agency practitioner must also discuss issues of confidentiality, use and security of information and data gathered, legal implications or regulations, and agency roles and responsibilities.

In General

The school and family interviews are formal and informal interactions between school or agency practitioners (or child study teams) and referral sources and/or significant others, respectively. These interviews can also include the referred child, his or her entire family, or individuals who have worked therapeutically with the child. These interviews can be part of both the problem identification or problem analysis procedures, depending on when they occur in the problem-solving process, and they can suggest and ultimately direct the intervention program.

The School Interviews occur with significant in-school personnel (e.g., teachers, principals, school psychologists, resource teachers, speech or reading specialists). The School Interview attempts to define the school's perspective and attitudes toward the child, his or her family, and the child's learning difficulties; define potential remedial suggestions and analyze previous remedial strategies; identify school, district, and community resources and their potential benefits for the child; and build rapport and a comfortable professional relationship with the school staff.

The Parent Interview investigates the child's developmental history: pregnancy, dimensions of the birth process and delivery, the neonatal course, infant feeding and sleeping characteristics, toilet training, speech and motor development, general health, educational history, play activity and socialization experiences, expression of feelings and personality development, home discipline, typical family relationships and interactions, and family feelings and concerns about home and school issues.

Nuttall and Ivey (Chapter 4 of this volume) expand this discussion of the diagnostic interview both theoretically and pragmatically.

Preassessment Conferences

In the Schools

Knoff (1982a), in an empirical study investigating the efficacy of an independent psychoeducational clinic's services, found that the surveyed parent and school clients agreed on only 57% of the referral problems on any shared case even after the case had been completed. Recommendations that practitioners convene a joint preassessment conference with parents and appropriate school staff resulted from the study with clear applicability to both school and agency organizations and practitioners.

In the school, the school staff relevant to a referral problem is easily accessed, and often this conference is organized simply by inviting the parents to a meeting. If the referral is not special education related, the practitioner can invite the appropriate school staff along with the parents and chair the meeting. Thus, the meeting could be held as a generic, non-special education child study team. If special education related, the parents are automatically considered members of the child study or special education team (as by PL 94-142), and their inclusion comprises a formal part of the problem analysis procedure. At times, this special education preassessment conference actually initiates the problem analysis procedure, and the parents must give permission as to whether an assessment in this context should occur.

In the Agency

For the agency practitioner, the preassessment conference may constitute the first joint meeting of the most relevant parties (e.g., school and parents) to a referral. Because of their third-party status, these practitioners may observe the interactions and dynamics between these parties and collect important qualitative information which may influence both problem analysis and intervention directions. These observations are more difficult for the school practitioner who may be heavily invested in the school's perspectives and agenda or who is unable to assume an unprejudiced, impartial role. Along a separate dimension, the preassessment conference is not a legally mandated activity required of agency practitioners, yet it may be more important for them than for the school practitioners.

Often, only one party initiates a referral to an agency (e.g., either parents or school personnel). After the first contacts and a personal perspective of the referral problem from the referral source, the agency practitioner may have formed or heard biases which can generalize into inappropriate problem definitions and analysis directions. The preassessment conference offers the practitioner an opportunity to test these impressions from both school *and* parent perspectives, and to decrease any biases which are incorrect and/or which may interfere with the conceptualizations and directions of the personality assessment and problem-solving process. This activity, therefore, can facilitate a broader understanding of the child's referral problem and increased insight into parent and school interactions and dynamics. These perspectives may be necessary to the development of multifaceted interventions which involve both family and school subsystems and individuals.

The preassessment conference should address the goals and procedures of the personality assessment process; summarize the initial referral questions and concerns, the Family and School Background Information Forms and Interviews, and the problem identification and analysis impressions to date; and initiate a discussion among family members and school staff personnel on their respective reactions to everything thus far. Ultimately, the preassessment conference will clearly define the referral problems and the personality assessment directions that both parties feel are important. This consensus or agreement will (*a*) permit the separate parties to explore conflicting observations and perspectives of the referred child's developmental and educational history, (*b*) address the child's current psychoeducational and social–emotional behaviors and styles, and (*c*) discuss previous disagreements, conflicts, and incorrect perceptions or interpretations. Finally, this consensus can maximize the conclusions and interventions suggested by the problem analysis and assessment process, because an agreed upon set of referral problems has been targeted to address both parents' and school staffs' specific concerns. A final, secondary outcome involves the preassessment conference's ability to engender trust among the family and school participants, to nurture constructive, cooperative communication, and to solidify the participants' commitment to the problem-solving personality assessment process such that the referred child's best interests may be served.

Home and School Observations

Observations of the referred child in home and school environments as well as observations of important people and characteristics (e.g., parents, siblings, teachers, peers, attention to the child, interactive styles) in those environments supplement the parent and school interviews. In a sense, the practitioner is always observing and evaluating these and other environments relevant to the referral; thus, this activity's formal acknowledgment and placement in the problem-solving chronology is artificial. Nonetheless, when formal planned observations (see Keller, Chapter 11 of this volume) are used to differentially analyze a referred child's behaviors and others' behaviors that affect the child psychologically and developmentally, this activity is placed correctly and logically here in the assessment process.

These observation procedures have some of the same school versus agency differences discussed in the interview section above. Further discrepancies will be elaborated by Keller in Chapter 11 of this volume.

Child-Oriented Assessments

In the School and Agency

Most child-involved assessments will be completed at either the school or agency; it is very rare to assess a child with various tests or techniques in his or her own home. Generally, the assessment room should be comfortable, well lit, temperature-controlled, free of visual or auditory distractions, adequately equipped with furniture and other necessities, and conducive to its assessment (or other) purposes. Often, agency facilities have the additional benefits of an adjacent observation room equipped with one-way mirrors, and videotaping and audiotaping capabilities. This permits parents and school staff to observe the assessment process, as well as allowing the preparation of a documented, videotaped record of the process for later more careful observation and analysis.

The test-by-test assessment procedure will not be discussed here. Certainly practitioners have or should develop their own assessment style, format, and options. To present a personal, preferred assessment order would be self-serving and noninstructive. The reader is referred to the above theoretical and conceptual discussions of the seven assessment approaches (neurological, psychoanalytic, humanistic, cognitive–developmental, behavioral, psychoeducational, and ecological) and to the chapters in Part II of this book which discuss the various assessment tools and techniques. Two assessment topics, however, will be discussed: the use of projective techniques and intellectual assessment within the personality assessment battery and process.

The use and utility of projective techniques has been much debated in the professional literature (Batsche & Peterson, 1983; Knoff, 1983b). My use of projective techniques is founded upon three primary assumptions. First, projective assessment is just one approach to personality assessment. It can be strategically coordinated with objective personality assessment approaches, behavioral approaches, psychoeducational and neurobiological approaches, as well as the other approaches previously discussed. Practitioners need to choose the assessment procedure to accomplish their goals; projective techniques are simply another available assessment resource. Second, projective techniques do not reliably facilitate differential diagnosis and generally should not be used for the psychoeducational placement of a referred child. Projective assessments are best used to identify issues or interactions that are significant to a referral or a referred student. Thus, they may be useful for developing intervention strategies. Third, personality assessment is a skill developing over time with training, supervision, and experience. Projective techniques *do not* make a practitioner effective; only experience and the integration of their results with other approaches and successful interventions constitute effectiveness.

Projective techniques usually round out a comprehensive personality assessment, but a comprehensive battery of projective assessments does not have to always be administered. The projective battery is, in fact, time-consuming—to administer, to score, and to interpret. Further, it is usually used inappropriately—to confirm a psychologist's impressions rather than to clarify confusing ones. Thus, a projective battery is recommended when (*a*) the referral problem is so confusing that projectives will facilitate a better understanding of the issues and dynamics and/or suggest appropriate interventions, (*b*) the referred student (or individuals related to the referral problem) is resistant to discussing/disclosing important psychological issues relevant to his or her current social–emotional status, and (*c*) a practitioner needs confirmation of his or her diagnostic/clinical impressions for legal or ethical reasons. A projective battery should *not* be completed when (*a*) the psychological issues specific to the referral are clear, (*b*) it is requested by an administrator who wants evidence to support a (placement) decision that is (probably) already made, and (*c*) it is requested to convince, for example, parents or teachers of the seriousness of a child's problems. Generally, the significant psychological issues specific to a referral problem can be identified through interviewing the referred student and significant others, short-term, diagnostic counseling with a related mental health practitioner (i.e., psychologist, counselor, social worker), behavioral observation and behavior rating scale approaches, and teacher (and other) consultation. In most cases, a practitioner should not accept a referral or complete a projective assessment until these procedures have been completed.

Often, an intellectual and/or cognitive assessment is critical to the comprehensive evaluation of a referred child. An intellectual assessment provides not only a developmental and classification status (e.g., mentally retarded, average, gifted) for the child, but it also suggests the child's learning style, problem-solving capacity, and contact with reality. Given the former, a child's intellectual status will significantly affect the developmental and social–emotional expectations of him or her. For example, a retarded child may not understand the concept of nonaggression and self-control, let alone be able to practice them. Given the latter, there are some (see Ogdon, 1982) who believe that scatter and profiles within an intellectual assessment can predict, or even constitute, certain emotionally disturbed styles, behaviors, or classifications. Some of this literature is highly speculative.

Although the intellectual assessment domain will not be specifically addressed further in this chapter or book, the practitioner should, nonetheless, be aware of its very important presence in the (personality) assessment battery. Additional information is available from Allison (1978), Kaufman (1979), and Sattler (1982).

The Personality Assessment Report and Feedback Conference

The Personality Assessment Report and the Feedback Conference both symbolize that point in the process where problem analysis is finishing, an intervention program is being formulated, and intervention directions must be agreed upon. The report should be sent to the relevant family members, school personnel, and significant others prior to the Feedback Conference. The report is ultimately the final, official document describing the results and recommendations derived from the assessment results and data.

The Feedback Conference uses the content and ideas in the Assessment Report to focus the discussion and planning process as participants are encouraged to accept, adapt, or reject any information or ideas. The Conference should be a working session which blends brainstorming, group processing, reality testing, intervention planning, and negotiation, all leading toward interventions that are agreeable to those involved. The practitioner in the Conference, therefore, becomes an information provider, process observer and consultant, and advocate as interventions in the referred child's best interests are developed. These two steps in the personality assessment process are explored in greater detail in Chapter 15 of this volume.

Follow-Up Contacts

Follow-up by the practitioner, whether in a school or agency setting, may involve on-going contacts with members of the intervention team to facilitate, reassess, or adapt various strategies, or it may involve periodic telephone calls to determine if a more formal contact is needed. Follow-up procedures, therefore, can be part of the intervention program or of either a formative or summative evaluation. Follow-up generally increases the probability that an intervention program is implemented (White & Fine, 1976), and it is an important procedure which assesses the utility and effectiveness of the entire personality assessment process. Further discussion of this activity is delineated above in the evaluation section of this chapter.

School versus Agency Referrals

While some practical differences between school and agency referrals were presented throughout the personality assessment discussion above, one major conceptual difference remains for elaboration. Personality assessment in the schools often uses a conceptual model that differs subtly yet significantly from the more "clinical" child- or family-centered approaches used by mental health agencies or private practitioners in the community. Conceptually, school-based personality assessment often reflects a Psychology × Education interaction. Unlike the community agency, which often focuses solely on psychological processes and interpersonal concerns, the school practitioner must balance school-related psychological concerns (e.g., Why is this student so depressed at school?) with educational concerns (e.g., Why is this child also not progressing academically?). Procedurally, the school practitioner completes a personality assessment as one part of a comprehensive evaluation involving a multidisciplinary child study team of educators asking primarily educational questions. With parental permission, the private practitioner has access to a school's child study team, but generally is working independently on psychological or social–emotional, not educational concerns.

In some ways, the Psychology × Education interaction "forces" the school practitioner to comprehensively assess the student referred for emotional or behavioral difficulties. Psychologically, the school practitioner must consider the referral problem in the context of the child's present and future mental health in and out of the school environment. Again, this suggests an ecological systems approach (Bronfenbrenner, 1979): a systematic analysis of the referral problem as it relates to the child, significant environmental subsystems (e.g., the school, home, community), and Child × Environmental subsystems interactions. Educationally, the school practitioner evaluates a subset of the ecological analysis: the Child × School interaction. Here, the practitioner analyzes the referral problem as it relates to the child's academic, social, and prevocational progress, and as it interfaces with the school environment (i.e., the students, the professional staff, and the educational process).

Agency or private practitioners, when dealing with school-aged children and adolescents, should also consider their assessments and interpretations within the Psychology × Education interaction. This is a necessary and important step toward analyzing and addressing referral problems comprehensively, ecologically, and in the most informed and least biased way.

Summary

The present chapter has discussed both a conceptual and pragmatic approach toward personality assessment referrals. The conceptual approach described a problem-solving model that focuses on seven theoretical approaches which help an understanding, analyzing, and intervening process with emotionally or behav-

iorally disturbed children and adolescents. The pragmatic approach went through
: step-by-step or activity-by-activity process of personality assessment. Also highlighted in this chapter were surveys of practitioners' and trainers' use of various
personality assessment techniques and approaches, a discussion of projective techniques and intellectual assessment and their uses and utility, and a conceptual contrast of school versus agency assessment perspectives. Ideally, both school and
agency practitioners will use this chapter to make their personality assessment
processes more comparable, comprehensive, and effective.

Appendix. Intake, Information, Interview, and Release Forms and Examples[a]

Telephone Intake Form

Date: _____

Child's Name: _____

Address: _____

Telephone: _____

Parent's Name: _____

Referred By: _____

        Address: _____

        Telephone: _____

Nature of Problem: _____

_____

_____

_____

_____

Present or Previous Contacts with other Agencies: _____

_____

_____

Diagnostic Procedure and Remedial Facilities Explained? _____
Family Information Form Sent to Parents? _____
School Information Form Sent to Parents (if relevant)? _____
Other Information Requested? _____ _____
Referral Acknowledgment letter sent to referral source? _____
Has it been explained that action on the referral will begin only when the family has returned its form and the school has returned the School Info form? _____

Filled out by: _____

[a]All forms are courtesy of Corrine R. Smith, Ph.D., Director, Psychoeducational Teaching Laboratory, Syracuse University, 805 South Crouse Avenue, Syracuse, New York 13210.

<u>Family Information Form</u>

Date sent: _____

Date returned: _____

Name: _____ Birthdate: _____ Age: _____ Sex:_____

Information supplied by: _____ Relationship: _____ Date:____

***** ****

Any prior contact with this clinic? (who and when): _____

Who suggested you consult this clinic? _____

Why? _____

Any special help from a tutor or other agencies and clinic (who and when): ___

_____

Did your child ever repeat a grade? _____ Highest grade completed ____

Regular or special class? _____

Family Doctor: _____ Address: _____

Child under medical care of: _____

I. <u>HISTORY</u>:

   Any complications during pregnancy? _____

   Walked at: ___months. Talked at: ___months. Any speech problems? _____

   Natural or adopted? _____ Single or multiple births? _____

   Ever been unconscious? (cause and duration): _____

   Any malformations or operations? (specify): _____

   Serious illnesses? (specify): _____

   Frequent colds? _____ Frequent headaches? _____

   Frequently fatigued ? _____ How is appetite? _____

Date of last physical exam: _____ Circumstances and results: _____

Date of last vision check: _____ Any corrections or training? _____

Date of last hearing exam: _____ Current weight _____ Hours of sleep

per night: _____

Any medicine being taken now? (what and why): _____

_____

Any language other than English spoken in the home? _____

Parents: (both natural or specify relationships) _____

II. FAMILY:

	Mother	Father
Name:	_____	_____
Age:	_____	_____
Occupation:	_____	_____
Highest School Level Completed:	_____	_____
General Health:	_____	_____
Serious Illnesses:	_____	_____
Learning Problems?	_____	_____

Parent(s) Marital Status and appropriate dates:

Married _____   Separated _____   Divorced _____

Single _____   Mother or Father Remarried? _____

Does mother and/or father live outside the home? If so, give address:

_____

Persons living in home where child lives:

	Name	Relationship	Birth Date	Occupation or School & Grade	Employer
1.					
2.					
3.					
4.					
5.					
6.					
7.					
8.					

Other siblings living outside of home:

	Name	Relationship	Birth Date	Occupation or School & Grade	Employer
1.					
2.					
3.					
4.					
5.					

Is there or has there been any psychiatric/psychological counseling for anybody in the family? If so, who, when, where, why?

_____

_____

_____

Have any other members of the family (parents or siblings) has serious illnesses or specific learning problems?

_____

_____

_____

III. PRESENTING PROBLEM(S)

1. What is currently concerning you about your child or family?

2. When did the problem(s) start?

3. What happened that led you to come here?

4. What changes in your family have you noticed since this problem began?

5. What would you like to change?

6. Do both parents see the problem the same way?

7. Does the child agree that there is a problem?

8. What major changes have occurred in your family over the past few years (moves, changes in income or employment, changes in family composition?

IV. <u>RELATIONSHIPS WITH PARENTS</u>:

    A. Child's relationship with father:
       1. Describe nature of contacts with father in home:

       2. Have there been separations?
          a. How old was child at time of separation?

          b. How often does father see child?

          c. Under what circumstances?

    B. Child's relationship with mother:

       1. Describe nature of contacts with mother in home:

       2. Have there been separations?
          a. How old was child at time of separation?

          b. How often does mother see child?

          c. Under what circumstances?

    C. Discipline:
       1. What kinds of things does child do that mother disciplines him for?

       2. What does she do about it?

       3. What kinds of things does child do that father disciplines him for?

       4. What does he do about it?

Feelings between parents and the child:

1. Do you like being with the child? (Elaborate)

2. Do you find it difficult to be with child? (Elaborate)

3. What things do you most enjoy about the child?

4. What does the child do well?

LEGAL PROBLEMS

1. Has child ever been in trouble with the law?

2. If so, how many times?

3. Give approximate date(s):

4. What was the court's disposition?

5. Is the child currently on probation?

6. If yes, who is the probation officer? Telephone:

7. Is there any legal action currently pending?

Please comment on any other behaviors or attitudes that you feel might be important for me to know.

SCHOOL INFORMATION FORM   Date Sent: _____
                                                 Date Returned: _____

    The person listed below has been referred to us. We will need the following information. Please be as thorough as possible in filling out the form, and add any further information you feel would help.

****

Name:_____ Birthdate:_____ Age:_____ Grade:_____

Parents:_____ Phone:_____

Address:_____ City:_____ Zip:_____

School:_____ Phone:_____

School Address:_____ City:_____ Zip:_____

Name of Principal:_____

_____
_____

What is the general academic performance level? _____

_____

What are the strongest and weakest academic performance areas? _____

_____

_____

Has child ever repeated a grade?_____ When?_____ What grade?_____

How effective was the non-promotion? _____

Is non-promotion or exclusion now an issue or under consideration?_____

_____

_____

Has the child previously had special help through the schools? (By whom, date,
purpose and results, if known)? _____

_____

_____

_____

Has the child been seen by any other service or referral agency or by a private
tutor? (By whom, address, date, for what (reading, speech, emotional, etc.):

_____

_____

_____

_____

Other information relevant to problems (i.e. behavior, medical history, siblings,
relations, home situation, excessive absences, etc.): _____

_____

_____

_____

_____

_____

_____

Describe any extra or special methods or materials used in the classroom to
aid this child: _____

_____

_____

_____

What is the greatest problem presented in the classroom? _____

_____

_____

_____

Describe classroom behavior: _____

_____

_____

Is the child now receiving special services? _____   Where? _____

Purpose: _____

_____

     Please list all test results in space provided below and on following page. Wherever possible, please include photo copies of the test data. Please add any additional comments which will help us to better understand this child's problems.

Standardized Test Results

   Intelligence

Name of test	Date	C.A.	M.A.	I.Q.	Examiner

  Achievement

Name of test	Date	Age Norm	Grade Placement	Examiner

Other

Name of Test (Please include any relevant data):

_____

_____

_____

Do other children in the family attending your schools present problems?

Explain: _____

_____

_____

_____

Signature: _____

Title: _____

Date: _____

INITIAL PARENT INTERVIEW

Identification

Name _____ Age _____   D.O.B. _____

Address _____   Sex _____

_____   Phone _____

Family

Father _____   Mother _____

Occupation _____   Occupation _____

Education _____   Education _____

Age _____   Age _____

Siblings _____   Ages _____   Sex _____

_____   _____   _____

_____   _____   _____

_____   _____   _____

Entrance Complaint: Parental Description of Problem

What are the child's problems/problem?
When did they/it begin? Why?
How does the family react to problem?
What has been done to alleviate the problem? (i.e. other referrals,
  clinics, professional help? etc.)
Describe a typical day of the child's.

Pregnancy

Past pregnancies and results.
Medications taken during these pregnancies.
Were the pregnancies planned?
What was the mother's health condition during pregnancies?
Any sickness? (excessive vomiting, measles, etc.)
Were any drugs taken during the pregnancy? What? When?
Who administered pre-natal care?
What was the length of the pregnancy?
Where was the child delivered? (hospital, home, etc.)

Birth

Was the birth spontaneous, induced, or Ceasarian?
Was there anethesia? What kind?
Were forceps used during delivery?
Forceps marks on child? Where?
How long was labor?
Any complications?
Weight of child at birth, injuries?
Condition of child at birth. (Jaundiced, blue, yellow, etc.)
At birth did the child cry immediately, or need oxygen?

Neonatal Course

How long was mother in hospital?
How long was baby in the hospital?
Any special procedures used? (incubator, intravenous feeding, given oxygen?)
Was the sucking reflex strong?
Breast or bottle fed?

Feeding

Any colic?
Did child have trouble eating or good appetite?
Were any special diets required?
Age of weaning.

Sleeping

What age when child slept all night?
Are there any sleep problems, past or present? (nightmares, restlessness,
     sleep walking, etc.)
Is there rocking behavior, head banging?
Where does the child sleep? With parents, with siblings?

Toilet Training

When did training begin? Bowel-Bladder.
When was toilet training completed?
What were the methods used?
Attitudes of parents to training.
Child's responses. (resistance, smearing)
Does child wet or soil now? When?

Speech

Vocalization as infant?
At what age did child speak?
What language is used in the home?
Problems, if any, with speech. (stuttering, no speech, reversals)

Motor development

What age did child roll over, sit with support, no support, crawl, walk?
What type of coordination does the child have? (slow, sluggish, quick,
    level of activity)
What is the child's preferred activity? What does he like to play with
    the best?

Health

How is the child's general health?
Accidents? When? What?
Child's response to accident.
Illnesses? When? What?
At what age did these illnesses occur?
Hospitalization? When? Where? Why?
Operations.
Effect of hospitalization on parents, on child.
Is child taking any medications? Past medications?

School History

Pre-school or nursery?   Age?   Where?
Kindergarten?
Reaction of child to beginning school?
Feeling of child towards school?
Separation anxiety?
Strongest and weakest academic areas.
Relationship with teachers.
How well does child get along with classmates?

Play Activity

Does child play well with others, or prefer to play alone?
Will he share things easily?
Are the child's friends, older, younger, or the same age?
Does the child frequently play by himself?
Favorite play activity.

Expression of Feeling

Does the child show affection easily?
Is the child's personality: shy, sociable, even-tempered, tantrums,
    moody, reserved, aggressive?
Does the child strike out at parents or siblings?
What does parent do when child shows aggressive behavior?

Discipline

Who administers discipline?
What approach is used?
Parents attitudes.
Child's responses.

Relationships

Who is the child closest with?
How does the child relate to: Parents, siblings, relatives, teachers?
Does the child have any special relationships? (Teacher, neighbors, etc.)

Special Comments

Are there any events that would be significant in affecting the child's
    development?
If so, what were the child's responses to these events?

Re: _____

Birthdate: _____

    Kindly release to this office photocopies of any confidential
educational, psychological or medical information on the above named
client. The parent's release is signed below.

                          Howard M. Knoff, Ph.D.
                          Licensed Psychologist

    I hereby give permission to furnish Howard M. Knoff, Ph.D. with
information in your files about the above referenced person.

                          Signature _____

                          Relationship _____

                          Address _____

                          Date _____

I hereby give permission for a report of all confidential

information about _____ in the files of
                        (name)
Howard M. Knoff, Ph.D. to be released to the following:

                           _____

                           _____

                           _____

                           _____

SIGNATURE   _____

RELATIONSHIP   _____

NAME   _____

ADDRESS   _____

DATE   _____

References

Alexander, T., Roodin, P., & Gorman, B. (1980). *Developmental psychology*. New York: Van Nostrand.

Allison, J. (1978). Clinical contributions of the Wechsler Adult Intelligence Scale. In B. B. Wolman (Ed.), *Clinical diagnosis of mental disorders* (pp. 355–392). New York: Plenum Press.

Ames, L., Metraux, R., Rodell, J., & Walker, R. (1974). *Child Rorschach responses: Developmental trends from two to ten years*. New York: Brunner/Mazel.

Bandura, A. (1978). The self-system in reciprocal determinism. *American Psychologist, 33*, 344–358.

Batsche, G. M., & Peterson, D. W. (1983). School psychology and projective assessment: A growing incompatibility. *School Psychology Review, 12*, 440–445.

Bergan, J. R. (1977). *Behavioral consultation*. Columbus, OH: Charles E. Merrill.

Bowers, K. S. (1973). Situationism in psychology: An analysis and a critique. *Psychology Review, 80*, 307–336.

Bronfenbrenner, U. (1979). *The ecology of human development*. Cambridge, MA: Harvard University Press.

Brown, W. R., & McGuire, J. M. (1976). Current psychological assessment practices. *Professional Psychology, 7*, 475–484.

Caplan, G. (1970). *The theory and practice of mental health consultation*. New York: Basic Books.

Conoley, J. C. (Ed.). (1981). *Consultation in schools: Theory, research, procedures*. New York: Academic Press.

Conti, A., & Bardon, J. I. (1974). A proposal for evaluating the effectiveness of psychologists in the schools. *Psychology in the Schools, 11*, 32–39.

Ellett, C. D., & Bersoff, D. N. (1976). An integrated approach to the psychosituational assessment of behavior. *Professional Psychology, 7*, 485–494.

Endler, N. S., & Magnusson, D. (1976). Toward an interactional psychology of personality. *Psychological Bulletin, 83*, 956–974.

Fagan, S. A. (1979). Psychoeducational management and self-control. In D. Cullinan & M. Epstein (Eds.), *Special education for adolescents: Issues and perspectives* (pp. 235–272). Columbus, OH: Charles E. Merrill.

Fein, L. G. (1979). Current status of psychological diagnostic testing in university training programs and in delivery of service systems. *Psychological Reports, 44*, 863–879.

Flanders, N. A. (1970). *Analyzing teacher behavior*. Reading, MA: Addison-Wesley.

Fox, R., Luszki, M. B., & Schmuck, R. (1966). *Diagnosing classroom learning environments*. Chicago, IL: Science Research Associates.

Freedman, J. L., Carlsmith, J. M., & Sears, D. O. (1970). *Social psychology*. Englewood Cliffs, NJ: Prentice-Hall.

Goh, D. S., Teslow, C. J., & Fuller, G. B. (1981). The practice of psychological assessment among school psychologists. *Professional Psychology, 12*, 696–706.

Goldfried, M. R., & Davison, G. C. (1976). *Clinical behavior therapy*. New York: Holt, Rinehart, & Winston.

Goldfried, M. R., & Kent, R. N. (1972). Traditional versus behavioral personality assessment: A comparison of methodological and theoretical assumptions. *Psychological Bulletin, 77*, 409–420.

Hallahan, D. P., & Kauffman, J. M. (1982). *Exceptional children* (2nd ed.). Englewood Cliffs, NJ: Prentice-Hall.

Hobbs, N. (1966). Helping disturbed children: Psychological and ecological strategies. *American Psychologist, 21*, 1105–1115.

Hobbs, N. (1975). *The futures of children*. San Francisco, CA: Jossey-Bass.

Jerrell, J. M., & Jerrell, S. L. (1981). Organizational consultation in school systems. In J. C. Conoley (Ed.), *Consultation in schools: Theory, research, procedures* (pp. 133–156). New York: Academic Press.

Kaufman, A. S. (1979). *Intelligent testing with the WISC-R*. New York: Wiley-Interscience.

Knoff, H. M. (1982a). Evaluating consultation service-delivery at an independent psychodiagnostic clinic. *Professional Psychology, 13*, 699–705.

Knoff, H. M. (1982b). The independent psychodiagnostic clinic: Maintaining accountability through program evaluation. *Psychology in the Schools, 19*, 346–353.

Knoff, H. M. (1983a). Personality assessment in the schools: Issues and procedures for school psychologists. *School Psychology Review, 12*, 391–398.

Knoff, H. M. (1983b). Justifying projective/personality assessment in school psychology: A response to Batsche and Peterson. (1983). *School Psychology Review, 12*, 446–451.

Lazarus, A. A. (1981). *The practice of multi-modal therapy*. New York: McGraw-Hill.

Long, N. J., Morse, W. C., & Newman, R. G. (Eds.). (1980). *Conflict in the classroom* (2nd ed.). Belmont, CA: Wadsworth Press.

Lubin, B., Wallis, R. R., & Paine, C. (1971). Patterns of psychological test usage in the United States: 1935–1969. *Professional Psychology, 2*, 70–74.

Maher, C. A. (1981). Decision analysis: An approach for multidisciplinary teams in planning special service programs. *Journal of School Psychology, 19*, 340–349.

Maslow, A. (1962). *Toward a psychology of being*. New York: Van Nostrand.

Meichenbaum, D. H. (1977). *Cognitive-behavior modification: An integrative approach*. New York: Plenum Press.

Meyers, J. (1981). Mental health consultation. In J. C. Conoley (Ed.), *Consultation in schools: Theory, research, procedures* (pp. 35–58). New York: Academic Press.

Meyers, J., Parsons, R. D., & Martin, R. (1979). *Mental health consultation in schools*. San Francisco: Jossey-Bass.

Mischel, W. (1977). On the future of personality measurement. *American Psychologist, 32*, 246–254.

Morse, W. C. (1975). The education of socially maladjusted and emotionally disturbed children. In W. M. Cruickshank & G. O. Johnson (Eds.), *Education of exceptional children and youth* (3rd ed., pp. 553–612). Englewood Cliffs, NJ: Prentice-Hall.

Nelson, C. M. (1981). Classroom management. In J. M. Kauffman & D. P. Hallahan (Eds.), *Handbook of special education* (pp. 663–687). Englewood Cliffs, NJ: Prentice-Hall.

Ogdon, D. P. (1982). *Psychodiagnostics of personality assessment: A handbook*. Los Angeles, CA: Western Psychological Services.

Payne, D. A. (1982). Portrait of the school psychologist as program evaluator. In C. R. Reynolds & T. B. Gutkin (Eds.), *The handbook of school psychology* (pp. 891–915). New York: Wiley.

Piotrowski, C., & Keller, J. W. (1978). Psychological test usage in Southeastern outpatient mental health facilities in 1975. *Professional Psychology, 9*, 63–67.

Prout, H. T. (1983). School psychologists and social-emotional assessment techniques: Patterns in training and use. *School Psychology Review, 12*, 377–383.

Ramage, J. (1979). National survey of school psychologists: Update. *School Psychology Digest, 8*, 153–161.

Rhodes, W. C. (1967). The disturbing child: A problem of ecological management. *Exceptional Children, 33*, 637–642.

Rhodes, W. C. (1970). A community participation analysis of emotional disturbance. *Exceptional Children, 36*, 309–314.

Rogers, C. (1980). *Freedom to learn*. Columbus, OH: Charles E. Merrill.

Ross, A. O. (1980). *Psychological disorders of children* (2nd ed.). New York: McGraw-Hill.

Ryan, W. (1976). *Blaming the victim*. New York: Vintage Books.

Sattler, J. M. (1982). *Assessment of children's intelligence and special abilities*. Boston, MA: Allyn & Bacon.

Schein, E. H. (1969). *Process consultation: Its role in organization development*. Reading, MA: Addison-Wesley.

Schellenberg, J. A. (1970). *Social psychology*. New York: Random House.

Schmuck, R. A. (1982). Organization development in the schools. In C. R. Reynolds & T. B. Gutkin (Eds.), *The handbook of school psychology* (pp. 829–857). New York: Wiley.

Schmuck, R. A., Runkel, P. J., Arends, J. H., & Arends, R. I. (1977). *The second handbook of organization development in schools*. Palo Alto, CA: Mayfield.

Schmuck, R. A., & Schmuck, P. A. (1979). *Group processes in the classroom* (3rd ed.). Dubuque, IA: Wiliam C. Brown.

Stufflebeam, D., Foley, W., Gephart, W., Guba, E., Hammond, R., Merriman, H., & Provus, M. (1971). *Educational evaluation and decision making*. Itasca, IL: F. E. Peacock.

Sulzer-Azaroff, B., & Mayer, G. R. (1977). *Applying behavior-analysis procedures with children and youth*. New York: Holt, Rinehart, & Winston.

Swap, S. (1978). The ecological model of emotional disturbance in children: A status report and proposed synthesis. *Behavioral Disorders, 3*, 186–196.

Tombari, M. L. (1980). Assessing the emotionally disturbed. In T. Oakland (Ed.), *Nonbiased assessment modules*. Austin: University of Texas Press.

Travis, L. D., & Violato, C. (1982). A possible path past some personality study problems. *Alberta Journal of Educational Research, 28*, 19–30.

Van Evra, J. P. (1983). *Psychological disorders of children and adolescents*. Boston, MA: Little, Brown.

Wade, T. C., & Baker, T. B. (1977). Opinions and use of psychological tests: A survey of clinical psychologists. *American Psychologist, 32*, 874–882.

Wade, T. C., Baker, T. B., Morton, T. L., & Baker, L. J. (1978). The status of psychological testing in clinical psychology: Relationships between test use and professional activities and orientation. *Journal of Personality Assessment, 42*, 3–10.

White, P. L., & Fine, M. J. (1976). The effects of three school psychological consultation models on selected teacher and pupil outcomes. *Psychology in the Schools, 13*, 414–420.

II

Personality Assessment Approaches and Techniques with Children and Adolescents

Within the problem-solving personality assessment process, the problem identification and problem analysis steps facilitate a comprehensive understanding of referred problems while leading toward logical intervention recommendations. There are many diverse approaches, tests, and techniques which can provide this comprehensive understanding. In this section, many of the most common are presented through reviews of their research and descriptions of their administration (or assessment) procedures, scorings, and interpretations. Included are interview procedures; projective techniques (the Rorschach, thematic approaches, drawings, and sentence completion techniques); objective assessment tests (the Personality Inventory for Children), behavioral approaches (rating scale and observation approaches); and family, ecological, and actuarial or automated personality assessment approaches.

4

The Diagnostic Interview Process

Ena Vazquez Nuttall
Allen E. Ivey

The Role of the Interview

The purpose of assessment is the construction of models. Through the personality assessment process, the model is built describing a referred elementary school student, adolescent, or family. A model is by definition a representation of reality. Thus, the assessment picture is never fully complete. Nonetheless, our task is to develop as complete and comprehensive a portrayal as possible. This occurs through an examination of files and records, observation, formal testing, and, most directly, through the diagnostic, clinical interview. While the other procedures provide critical and essential data, only the clinical interview provides an overall frame of reference which guides the entire assessment process. The interview, then, is the core of the assessment process—the *model* that we are modeling.

Critical to a constructionist view of assessment is the assumption that school psychologists, therapists, and other mental health practitioners are describing reality through their assessments. This is actually somewhat presumptuous, for the best these practitioners can do is to present their picture of the child or adolescent with the full recognition that this picture is incomplete. Because test scores are concrete and specific and at best approximate reality, it is tempting to rely on them. Indeed, our awareness of the complexity and ambiguity of the clinical interview encourages this overreliance on tests. Our training and experience have cautioned us of the unreliability of the interview: Can we trust what we see, hear, and feel?

This chapter discusses the clinical interview as a critical part of the assessment process. Despite all its limitations, the clinical interview is still the centerpiece of assessment. Without it, one cannot determine strategies for testing, one cannot determine context, one cannot describe reality.

Recent work in interviewing training provides specific information on how

Ena Vazquez Nuttall and Allen E. Ivey. Counseling and School Psychology Program, University of Massachusetts, Amherst, Massachusetts.

to obtain more useful and reliable results. Some of this information will be discussed later in the context of microcounseling training using data generated by the second author. Generally, the results indicate that the interview process can be made more predictable. But inherent in this predictability issue are several problems. The most important of these is the presence and effect of sexual, racial, and ethnic biases within the process. For this reason, cross-cultural therapy and counseling are on the upswing (Marsella & Pedersen, 1981; Sue, 1981). Derald Sue and a group of seven colleagues (Sue *et al.*, 1982) from the Division of Counseling Psychology of the American Psychological Association (APA) have noted that cross-cultural issues somehow affect virtually all counseling, interviewing, or testing sessions. Table 4-1 presents their summary of recommendations, an essential set of guidelines for effective assessment and helping.

Based on this introduction, this chapter has three purposes: (*a*) to point out that assessment results are models rather than reality itself, (*b*) to provide guidelines toward more effective and predictable interviewing in personality assessment, and (*c*) to discuss and emphasize that the entire assessment process, including the diagnostic interview process, operates in a cross-cultural context.

Table 4-1
Characteristics of the Culturally Skilled Counseling Psychologist[a]

Beliefs/attitudes	Knowledge	Skills
1. The culturally skilled counseling psychologist is one who has moved from being culturally unaware to being aware and sensitive to his/her own cultural heritage and to valuing and respecting differences.	1. The culturally skilled counseling psychologist will have a good understanding of the sociopolitical system's operation in the United States with respect to its treatment of minorities.	1. At the skills level, the culturally skilled counseling psychologist must be able to generate a wide variety of verbal and nonverbal responses.
2. A culturally skilled counseling psychologist is aware of his/her own values and biases and how they may affect minority clients.	2. The culturally skilled counseling psychologist must possess specific knowledge and information about the particular group he/she is working with.	2. The culturally skilled counseling psychologist must be able to send and receive both verbal and nonverbal messages accurately and "appropriately."
3. A culturally skilled counseling psychologist is one who is comfortable with differences that exist between the counselor and client in terms of race and beliefs.	3. The culturally skilled counseling psychologist must have a clear and explicit knowledge and understanding of the generic characteristics of counseling and therapy.	3. The culturally skilled counseling psychologist is able to exercise institutional intervention skills on behalf of his/her client when appropriate.
4. The culturally skilled counseling psychologist is sensitive to circumstances (personal biases, stage of ethnic identity, sociopolitical influences, etc.) which may dictate referral of the minority client to a member of his/her own race/culture.	4. The culturally skilled counseling psychologist is aware of institutional barriers which prevent minorities from using mental health services.	

[a]From Sue, D., Bernier, J., Duran, A., Feinberg, L., Pedersen, P., Smith, E., & Vazquez-Nuttall, E. (1982). Cross-cultural counseling competencies. *Counseling Psychologist, 10,* 45–52. Reprinted by permission.

Background of the Interview

Definition

Many have tried to define what an interview is. Matarazzo (1978) defines it as a "deliberately initiated conversation wherein two persons, and more recently more than two, engage in verbal and nonverbal communication toward the end of gathering information which will help one or both parties better reach a goal" (p. 47). The most important elements of this definition are the fact that the interview is a conversation between two or more people and that it is conducted for the purpose of obtaining information.

While in the past most interviews were face to face, this process now includes telephone interviewing (Dillman, 1978) and computer interviewing (Myers & Cairo, 1983; Veldman, 1967). The purpose and type of information pursued during the interview vary among professions and work settings. Medical doctors, nurses, personnel workers, newspaper reporters, survey researchers, political poll takers, psychiatrists, social workers, and psychologists all use interviewing to achieve different goals and obtain different kinds of information.

In this chapter, clinical interviewing around referred children's problems is the focus of attention. This type of interviewing is used in schools to obtain information from students, teachers, other support staff, and parents about the academic, social, and psychological problems experienced by such referred students. Parents are usually interviewed about the developmental and school history of these children and about their perceptions of the child's referred problems. School staff are queried about their perceptions of the problem, past attempts to solve the problem, and strategies indicated for the future. And referred children are asked about their points of view regarding the presenting problem and possible solutions. Within this process, telephone interviews may also be conducted with outside professionals such as pediatricians, psychiatrists, community agencies personnel, and other mental health practitioners.

In hospitals and community mental health centers, interviewing is used to obtain intake and case history information. Generally, the client(s) and their families, singly or conjointly, are interviewed in these settings. Telephone interviews with school personnel, other hospital personnel (especially medical specialists), community agencies personnel, and court staff often supplement these initial interviews.

Strengths of the Diagnostic Interview

In school and community settings, diagnostic interviewing has decided advantages over other assessment procedures such as testing, observing, and using questionnaires. Among the strengths of interviewing are the following:

It is flexible. A competent interviewer can probe more deeply or widely when conducting an interview. He or she can proceed quickly or slowly, omit questions, or reword them. Observation and formal (standardized) testing do not offer this range of flexibility.

Covert processes can be ascertained. Through interviews, one can find out how clients define their subjective experience and what they perceive as significant people and events in their environment. Observation and testing do not yield this type of information.

It offers personal contact. Face-to-face or telephone contact increases the opportunity to develop a good relationship between interviewer and interviewee. This can prove extremely important later on when recommendations are made and treatment plans implemented. Often, the client will also be more receptive to follow-up contacts which examine the status of these recommendations and treatment programs. Observation, questionnaires, and group tests do not necessarily facilitate this process.

It is the best method for obtaining historical data. Important information about a client's personal developmental, school, and occupational history is best obtained through a case history interview because it allows unique information to be assessed and permits deep probing into expected (and uncovered) areas.

It provides opportunity for observation. Like individual testing and observation, face-to-face interviewing also provides the opportunity to observe nonverbal behavior, body language, tone of voice, pauses, the other relevant dimensions.

Weaknesses of the Diagnostic Interview

Interviewing has some drawbacks, however. These include the following issues:

Expense. Compared to group testing and to written questionnaires, interviewing can be expensive, since it requires the personal attention of the professional.

Time. Scheduling, traveling to the interview site, and interviewing can be time-consuming. Asking people to come to your office can lessen the amount of time spent; however, the opportunity to observe the person in his or her own environment is lost. Leaving scheduling to another lower-paid person may result in a substantial loss of opportunity for building rapport.

Bias. While every assessment procedure incurs some bias, interviewing can be perhaps the most dangerous, because bias in interviewing is harder to identify, prove, and control. Biases inherent in diagnostic tests can be identified, often empirically, by inspecting the normative sample, the context of the test, procedures for administration, or differential performances of targeted groups. However, very few interviews conducted in the real world are ever routinely documented (e.g., via audiotape or videotape) and empirically analyzed for such biases. Thus, the impact of nonverbal behavior, tone, and pauses, and the effects of ageism, racism, classism, sexism, and other important factors present between interviewer and interviewee are unavailable for evaluation.

Conflict generation. While interviewing provides an opportunity for face-to-face encounter and the development of interpersonal rapport, it can also initiate unproductive and negative relationships. For example, issues of power and social conformity within the interview context can destroy the productivity of the encounter, such as when a young child discusses "acceptable" topics rather than "what's bothering me" because he or she perceives the adult interviewer as someone who should be obeyed and who "may think I'm bad for having these problems and feelings." Transference can also interfere with the effectiveness of the interview. For example, a teenager who is experiencing difficulties with his or her teachers and principal in school will have to be convinced by an adult interviewer that their relationship is founded on objectivity and confidentiality.

While the strengths and weaknesses of the interview vis-à-vis other methodologies have been discussed, the values of these other methodologies should not be devalued or dismissed. We subscribe to a constructionist philosophy of assessment that is multimethod, multisource, and multidimensional. A good personality assessment battery should contain observation, examination of documents, objective and projective tests, and interviewing.

Within this context, interviewing should involve as many individuals as necessary to obtain the clearest understanding of the referred problem's interactions and scenarios. For instance, if a referred problem involves a child who is not doing well in school, interviews with the child, parents, homeroom teacher, special education teachers, the counselor, and whoever else is deemed important should occur. Further, the assessment and interview process should investigate as many personality dimensions as necessary to clarify the focus of any broader personality problems. Thus, if a mental health practitioner wants to study those personality dimensions affecting school performance, he or she should include questions addressing students' academic status and attitudes, their self-concepts and sense of control, their perceptions of teachers' and parents' attitudes toward their problems, the influence of peers, and/or their previous experiences with success or failure in the area. Only after several methods are used to obtain data, several sources of information are included, and several dimensions of personality are evaluated through the assessment process will a good construction of the reality of a referred child's problem occur which minimizes or balances any existing biases or prejudices.

The History of the Diagnostic Interview

The history of the clinical interview as a diagnostic tool is closely tied to the history of interviewing techniques in psychotherapy (Matarazzo, 1965, 1978). Freud, Sullivan, and Rogers have contributed greatly to the development of the individual psychotherapeutic interview. This section provides an overview of the contribution of these three thinkers to the crystallization of this personality assessment method. Many other approaches have been left out, notably those of behavioral and systems-oriented interviewers. Other chapters in this book address these two approaches more fully.

The Dynamic Interview

After initially relying on hypnosis with their clients for significant personality-related information, Breuer and Freud in the 1890s began to ask their patients to talk (1957). Freud found that with some help his patients could talk freely and that he could derive insights into their "unconscious" memories and impulses of personality. Freud called this technique the "talking out cure" or "free association." Therapeutically, this interviewing technique was designed to help patients explore their conscious and unconscious personalities in order to reconstruct them (Matarazzo, 1965).

The free-association method demands that the patient talk about everything and anything that occurs to him or her, without restraint and without any attempt to produce a logical, organized, meaningful discourse (Hall & Lindzey, 1957). The patient usually reclines on a couch in a quiet room while the therapist listens and prods occasionally when the flow of conversation dries up.

To Freud, the interviewer was not a neutral participant in the interview, but an integral and dynamic catalyst in the interaction. Through such concepts as "transference," "countertransference," "resistance," and others, Freud pioneered the concept of the interviewer as an important diagnostic and therapeutic human instrument (Matarazzo, 1965). This methodology led to his conceptualization of the psychosexual developmental stages; the dynamics of personality; the role of transference, resistance, and anxiety in personality development; and the mechanisms of defense.

Sullivan's Interviewing Technique

According to Matarazzo (1965), Sullivan's interpersonal theory of personality development and its application to psychotherapeutic interviewing is used by today's "dynamic" clinical psychologists, nonpsychoanalytic psychiatrists, and social workers more than the theory and techniques of Freud. Sullivan's view of personality is sociopsychological. To him, personality is conceptualized as "the relatively enduring pattern of recurrent interpersonal situations which characterize human life" (Sullivan, 1953, p. 11).

The psychiatric interview as conceptualized by Sullivan consists of a "system or series of systems of interpersonal processes, arising from participant observation in which the interviewer derives certain conclusions about the interviewee" (Sullivan, 1954, p. 128). In the *Psychiatric Interview* (1954), Sullivan divides the interview into four stages: (*a*) formal inception, (*b*) reconnaissance, (*c*) detailed inquiry, and (*d*) termination. The interview is primarily a vocal communication between two people in which the interviewer listens not only to what the client says, but to how he or she says it. Chief sources of information for the interviewer are intonation, rate of speech, changes in volume, and other expressive behaviors. Sullivan's interviewer is an expert in interpersonal relations whose goal is to uncover what is troubling the client.

In the inception stage, the interviewer acts primarily as an observer, asking few questions yet trying to formulate the reasons why the client needs consultation and what the specific nature of the problem is. During the period of reconnaissance, the interviewer finds out who the client is through an intensive interrogation into his or her past, present, and future. The period of detailed inquiry is dedicated to testing and validating the hypotheses formulated during the previous stages. And, during the termination phase, the interviewer makes a final statement of what has been learned, prescribes a course of action for the client to follow, and assesses the probable effects of the prescription on the client's life.

Whenever there are difficulties in communication during these stages, they are attributed to the impact of the interviewer's attitudes upon the client's capacity to communicate. Sullivan assumes that a great deal of reciprocity occurs between the interviewer and interviewee during an interview, with each individual continually reflecting the feelings of the other. He defines this process as "reciprocal emotion," a process that can both facilitate and interfere with effective interviewing. Thus, to Sullivan, who was influenced greatly by the anthropologists Sapir and Benedict, the interview is an immense challenge to the participant observer who must maintain accurate observation perceptions despite this reciprocity (Hall & Lindzey, 1957).

The Rogerian Interview

Rogers's therapeutic approach is generally known as the "client-centered" approach. Its primary theoretical construct is the self. Rogers postulates that the self develops out of an organism's interaction with the environment. The self strives for consistency, perceives inconsistency as threatening, and develops as a result of maturation and learning. The person, according to Rogers, is the best source of information about him- or herself; the individual's internal frame of reference, then, is the best point from which to understand his or her behavior. Self-reports, therefore, are the best sources of psychological data. Testing and observation are considered inadequate personality assessment procedures because they provide a limited view of a person's phenomenological field. The interview is thought to provide the most complete view of this field; it is the method par excellence for obtaining information about people.

Some consider Rogers and Dymond's (1954) *Psychotherapy and Personality Change* the single most important research publication impacting on interviewing in the 1960s. Rogers is also credited with the first verbatim transcript of a psychotherapy session (Matarazzo, 1965). He and his followers (Covner, 1944; Snyder, 1961) have contributed significantly to the study of the structure and dynamics of the interview.

Rogers's interviewing approach is characterized by the recognition and clarification of feelings expressed by the client, the nonjudgmental acceptance of his or her statements, and the delivery of "structuring" statements where the interviewer explains the client's and his or her role. Generally during the interview, the client-centered counselor tries to avoid giving information, giving advice, using reassurance and persuasion, asking direct questions, offering his own interpretations, and giving criticism.

Psychometric Issues and Types of Interviews

Interviewer and Interviewee Bias

Bias in the interview can emerge from three different sources: the interviewer, the interviewee, and the content of the interview itself. When children are the interviewees, the potential for bias is greater because of the greater difference in power, age, cognitive development, education, and other factors between interviewer and interviewee.

Among the many variables that contribute to bias on the part of the interviewer and the interviewee, social class and political attitudes, cultural background, uses of interpreters, stages of cognitive development, age, gender, and the degree of training will be discussed.

The social class of the interviewer greatly determines the type of information obtained and the interpretation given to it. For example, Rice (1929) found that interviewers who were prohibitionists tended to attribute poverty to the excessive use of alcohol, while Socialist interviewers generally blamed indigence on bad economic conditions. In a 1942 study, Katz found that interviewers from working-class backgrounds consistently obtained more radical opinions from respondents than did middle-class interviewers. Thus, in judging information obtained through interviews, practitioners should be aware that the social-class background of the interviewer may affect the nature of the information obtained. Interviewers should be aware of their own social-class biases and work hard to minimize them.

Cultural and ethnic background exert great potential influence on the interviewing process; however, research studies documenting this influence are sparse. In a study of interviewer effects, Robinson and Rohde (1946) investigated attitudes toward Jewish interviewers by using two experimental groups—one Jewish in appearance and the other not. The interviewers who appeared Jewish obtained significantly fewer anti-Semitic attitudes and remarks than did the interviewers who appeared to be non-Jewish. In a study involving Mexican American migrant parents and their children, interviewees' degree of self-disclosure during the interview varied with age and cultural background. Zusman, Olson, and Garcia (1975) found that children interviewees, when asked about the best and worst aspects of their educational systems, gave more extensive negative information. The parents, on the other hand, gave more detailed explanations when reporting on positive, rather than negative, characteristics.

These studies underscore the need to be aware of cultural differences during an interview. Lack of awareness may lead to incorrect conclusions that a specific behavior is caused by an individual's personality dynamics rather than by the individual's cultural background or upbringing.

Increasingly in America, however, mental health practitioners are serving clients who not only come from different cultures, but who also speak a language other than English. When confronted with this situation, most English-speaking practitioners resort to colleagues who speak the native language or to interpreters. While no studies that focus on the use of interpreters in interviewing are available, studies on the use of interpreters in testing (Vazquez-Nuttall, Goldman, & Medeiros, 1983) point out the difficulties encountered in such situations. First, it is hard to find interpreters who are totally bilingual, and accurate translations between two separate languages are hard to achieve. Next, different languages do not use all words with the same frequency, making some words more difficult to understand in one language than in another. Finally, the meaning of some words also differs from culture to culture. For example, when people talk about ''family'' in Spanish, they mean the extended family. They refer to the nuclear family as ''mi casa,'' meaning ''those people who live in my house'' (Vazquez-Nuttall, Avila-Vivas, & Morales-Barreto, 1984).

The stage of cognitive development of the interviewer is crucial, especially when interviewing children. As explained later in this chapter, the interviewer functioning at a formal operations level will have to change his or her language in order to meet the needs of children operating at a concrete operations level. Such an interviewer will need cognitive flexibility and linguistic versatility in order to communicate validly and usefully with his or her clients.

How a child responds to an adult interviewer also depends on the social norms governing relationships between people of different ages. As Yarrow (1960) points out, an adult interviewer has to exercise special care to avoid influencing and reinforcing a child to give a response motivated only by social conformity and the expectation of adult approval. Adults who treat adolescents on an equal basis will establish easier rapport and obtain better information than those who enact parental, teacher, police, or other authority roles.

In the past, the use of structured interviews with children was generally frowned upon because of this age variable (Yarrow, 1960). However, recent research by Herjanic, Herjanic, Brown, and Wheatt (1975) has found children to be reliable reporters. In their study, 50 children, ranging in age from 6 to 16, and their mothers were interviewed using the same structured interview, which was similar in content to a psychiatric evaluation. When comparing the answers of the two groups, the researchers found 80% agreement between children and adults on all questions. Girls were more reliable than boys, and there was greater agreement on factual information and less agreement on questions dealing with mental status. Judging from this research, therefore, it seems that interviewing children can be used more comfortably in personality assessment. Children seem to be as good in responding to an interview as to a formal test.

The effect of the interviewer's gender may vary with the age and sex of the child. While women analysts have worked with apparent success with latency-age boys (Yarrow, 1960), Fleming and Snyder (1947) found, during nondirective therapy, that 10-year-old boys did not respond as well to a female versus a male therapist. This study indicates that these variables should be considered when choosing an interviewer for a child, and that some interviews may be affected by a less-than-favorable child–interviewer match.

Finally, the level of the interviewer's training and competence is another important factor potentially affecting the interview process. With the advent of more systematic training packages (Ivey & Authier, 1978), interviewer performance can be improved considerably and more reliable and valid information can be obtained. Practitioners who want to become competent interviewers should take advantage of these new training programs.

The Open and Standardized Interview

Clinical interviews are usually organized into two types: open and structured (or standardized). In the open interview, the interviewee is encouraged to talk freely and at length on topics that may be flexibly worded and organized by the interviewer to suit the occasion and the responses to previous questions (Dyer, 1976). The open interview is usually used in case studies of individuals, families, programs, or institutions, and its goal is to explore the interviewee's thinking and experience in great depth. Significantly, the open interview requires a great deal of clinical expertise and training.

The standardized interview is typically conducted by interviewers who are specially trained to follow a standard set of procedures and questions. This process ensures as much as possible that the answers given by all respondents can be readily compared (Dyer, 1976). The best example of the standardized diagnostic interview is the individual intelligence test. In this type of interview, clinicians are provided with a set of questions sometimes accompanied by tasks to present to the interviewee. Then they observe, evaluate, and record each response according to a prescribed coding scheme which is available because of the controlled nature of the questions. As interviewers can be trained extensively in the administration and scoring of the instrument, this pattern of interviewing can yield more reliable and valid data and comes close to the degree of objectivity attained by personality scales, checklists, and self-report (paper and pencil) measures.

Reliability

In the context of the clinical interview, reliability usually refers to the consistency of scores or diagnoses obtained when an interview is examined by different practitioners. Technically, the two (or more) practitioners' scores or diagnoses can be statistically correlated with the resulting correlation coefficient identified as a measure of interrater reliability (Anastasi, 1982). Most of the reliability studies using the interview as a personality assessment tool have focused on the consistency of psychiatric diagnosis, that is, whether two or more clinicians interviewing the same persons at the same time or in close proximity assign them to the same diagnostic categories.

Early studies investigating this type of reliability gave interviewing a reputation of *un*reliability. However, later studies (Matarazzo, 1978) using clearer diagnostic systems such as DSM-III or the Research Diagnostic Criteria (RDC) report test–retest correlations in the .70s, .80s, and .90s—levels consistent with the best psychometric tests available, such as the Wechsler intelligence scales. This improvement in the reliability of the diagnostic interview stems from the clearer and more specific operationalizations of psychiatric diagnostic categories as exemplified by DSM-III and research completed by Helzer, Clayton, Pambakian, Reich, and Wish (1977). Psychiatric conditions have been more clearly defined by including characteristics, symptoms, time variables, and absences of other conditions. With this increased clarity and precision, clinicians are more likely to define categories in the same way. Similarly, training of personnel in the use of these categorizations has become more systematic and well planned (Webb, DiClemente, Johnstone, Sanders, & Perley, 1981).

Another improvement in this research has been the use of the kappa statistic (K) (Spitzer, Cohen, Fleiss, & Endicott, 1967). The kappa statistic takes into account the base rates for different diagnoses. The base rate of a specific diagnosis affects the degree of predictability of a diagnostic category. Use of this new statistic helps researchers improve the quality of their work and the reliability and validity of the psychiatric interview.

Validity

The question of validity in the structured interview concerns what the interview measures and its measurement effectiveness (Anastasi, 1982). All procedures used to determine an interview's validity compare the information gathered from the structured interview with other independently observed facts related to the referral problem under consideration. The validity and reliability concerns of the open interview will not be discussed, since this type of interview is too individualized and unstandardized to meet the requirements of the psychometric paradigm.

There are three major categories for determining the validity of the standardized interviews: content validity, criterion-related validity, and construct validity. Of these, criterion-related is the one most pertinent to the clinical interview. This type of validity evaluates the effectiveness of a structured interview to predict an individual's behavior in specified situations. Behavior and performance assessed in the interview are compared to a criterion—a direct and independent measure consistent with the behavioral and performance concerns the interview is designed to predict. Thus, if an interview's goal is to determine a person's psychological fitness for college, a long-range criterion would be his or her successful graduation from college 4 years later and a short-range criterion would be academic performance (grade-point average) during the first semester.

Most of the research assessing the validity of clinical interviewing has been based on two types of criterion-related validity, concurrent and predictive validity (Matarazzo, 1978). Concurrent validity refers to an external criterion that is obtained at approximately the same time as the interview with characteristics that hopefully correlate well with the descriptive or diagnostic intent of the interview; predictive validity refers to an outside measure obtained after a set period of time which hopefully correlates with the behavior or performance that the interview has predicted. While studies on the reliability of the clinical interview have shown a decided improvement because of the objectively standardized, operationally defined, differential psychiatric diagnostic classifications, the evidence of the interview's validity remains mixed. Briefly, the clinical interview is most valid when used to make general predictions instead of fine discriminations, and when the samples used contain heterogenous populations, including severely impaired people.

Several studies conducted by Hunt and his co-workers (Hunt, 1951, 1955; Wittson & Hunt, 1951) have demonstrated the validity of the psychiatric interview. A study typical of their research style (Hunt, Herrman, & Noble, 1957) used a large group of new recruits who had begun training at the Great Lakes Naval Training Center. Each recruit was given a brief psychiatric screening interview as part of his intake physical examination. The interviewer then assigned each recruit to one of four categories: (a) free of psychiatric defect and fully qualified for duty; (b) mild, transient, or mildly severe dysfunction; (c) more moderate chronic dysfunction; and (d) unsuitable for service. Three years later, 2,406 recruits were followed up. Of the 617 recruits found to have no psychiatric condition, only 1% were discharged for psychiatric reasons, 2.43% for medical reasons, and 1.64% for bad conduct. Recruits receiving a rating for a mild psychiatric defect had an attrition rate of 8.33%, and those given a rating as moderately disturbed had an attrition rate of 11.24%. The success of the brief interview was greater in differentiating category (a) from categories (b) and (c) and not as successful for differentiating between categories (b) and (c), which involve finer discriminations and judgments.

Research where clinical interviewing has proved invalid has involved judgments for specific personality traits and fine discriminations within groups of essentially very healthy subjects, such as the prediction of success in the Peace Corps (Fisher, Epstein, & Harris, 1967), in clinical psychology training, and in later professional work (E. L. Kelly & Goldberg, 1959). The failure of differential diagnosis in the legal arena is also well documented. For example, Ennis and Litwack (1974) did a study consisting of several follow-ups of 967 patients who were diagnosed in clinical interviews as criminally insane and dangerous patients. They found that 147 had been discharged to the community and 702 presented no special problems to hospital staff. Only 7 of the original 967 were found to be so difficult to manage or so dangerous that they had to be recommitted.

In summary, the reliability of the clinical interview has increased while much work on its validity remains to be done. Improvements in reliability studies stem partially from more clearly defined taxonomic systems and better training methods. The next section discusses the microcounseling training package which has greatly helped to improve the interviewing performance among counselors and school psychologists.

The Structure of the Assessment Interview

This section summarizes a skills-based training program, microcounseling, and its particular relevance to the assessment interview. The basic argument presented here is that specific skills of helping and interviewing can be identified, organized into specific sequences, and taught such that relatively predictable interview outcomes will occur. It is important to note that the basic framework presented here tends to be oriented to the middle-class and Western culture. Work with varying cultural groups reveals that this set of skills and structures must be modified to meet the specific needs of these groups.

Microcounseling and Microcounseling Skills

Microcounseling (Ivey, 1971; Ivey & Authier, 1978) is a skills-based framework for teaching the interview process. Beginning students are taught specific interviewing skills in a social learning format consisting of (*a*) the introduction or overview of the specific skill, (*b*) the presentation of video, audiotape, or live models demonstrating the skill, (*c*) a reading/didactic presentation outlining the skill and its implications, (*d*) practice of the skill to a demonstration or mastery level, and (*e*) planned generalization of the skill to daily life and work. The specific skills of microtraining are presented in the "microskills hierarchy" in Figure 4-1.

Attending behavior and client observation are the foundation skills of interviewing and helping. Included here are sensory-motor data that the interviewer can see, hear, and feel. A conscious awareness of cultural differences in behavior is important here. Many training programs, unfortunately, still teach direct, forthright eye contact as the most appropriate mode of helping. Different individuals and different cultures, however, have widely varying modes of visual communication. For example, particularly with children, not looking at the teacher or counselor may be a sign of respect rather than the typical white middle-class sign of defiance.

Microcounseling next stresses the basic listening sequence of open and closed questions, encouraging, paraphrasing, reflection of feeling, and summarization. Here, students learn that specific results may be anticipated as a result of accurate listening. Two levels of listening competence (Ivey, 1983) are particularly important to note: (*a*) demonstration mastery, in which the trainee simply demonstrates the skill (i.e., does the trainee actually ask an open question after training?), and (*b*) active mastery, which is far more important. Here, the trainee's competence is measured by the specific impact produced by using the skills with the client. For example, with an open question, does the client actually provide more data of a specific type? The basic listening sequence's goal is to elicit client facts, feelings, and thoughts about a situation and then to summarize them accurately to the client's satisfaction.

This results-oriented teaching approach leads to a precision in the interview that is not usually anticipated. But with this precision comes increased responsibility for awareness of individual and cultural differences. Merely asking a question to a person of a different culture may be more intrusive than we realize. For example, some black clients may see an interviewer's questioning as white space intrusion, and the resulting data may be inappropriate or inaccurate for assessment and diagnostic purposes. Research and clinical experience in microcounseling clearly reveal that the data obtained in an interview are as much a construction of the interviewer as of the interviewee. It is for this reason, the risk of cultural imperialism, that microtraining gives special attention to both listening skills and the awareness of cultural differences in response to those listening skills. Assessment, based on listening, is best when it most closely represents the constructions and values of the client rather than of the assessment interviewer.

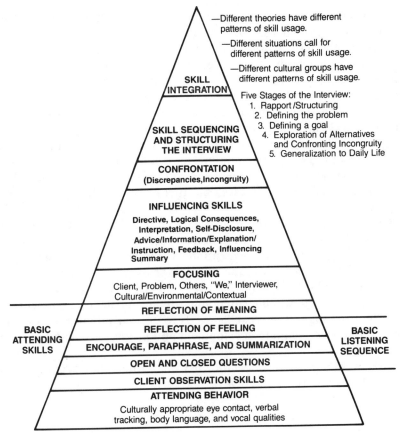

—Different theories have different patterns of skill usage.

—Different situations call for different patterns of skill usage.

—Different cultural groups have different patterns of skill usage.

Five Stages of the Interview:
1. Rapport /Structuring
2. Defining the problem
3. Defining a goal
4. Exploration of Alternatives and Confronting Incongruity
5. Generalization to Daily Life

SKILL INTEGRATION

SKILL SEQUENCING AND STRUCTURING THE INTERVIEW

CONFRONTATION
(Discrepancies,Incongruity)

INFLUENCING SKILLS

Directive, Logical Consequences, Interpretation, Self-Disclosure, Advice/Information/Explanation/ Instruction, Feedback, Influencing Summary

FOCUSING
Client, Problem, Others, "We," Interviewer, Cultural/Environmental/Contextual

REFLECTION OF MEANING

REFLECTION OF FEELING

ENCOURAGE, PARAPHRASE, AND SUMMARIZATION

OPEN AND CLOSED QUESTIONS

CLIENT OBSERVATION SKILLS

ATTENDING BEHAVIOR
Culturally appropriate eye contact, verbal tracking, body language, and vocal qualities

BASIC ATTENDING SKILLS

BASIC LISTENING SEQUENCE

1. Attending behavior and client observation skills form the foundation of effective communication, but are not always the appropriate place to begin training.

2. The basic listening sequence of attending skills (open and closed questions, encouraging, paraphrasing, reflection of feeling, and summarization) is often found in effective interviewing, management, social work, physician diagnostic sessions, and many other settings.

Figure 4-1. The microskills hierarchy. [From Ivey, A. E. (1983). *Intentional interviewing and counseling* (p. 5). Monterey, CA: Brooks-Cole. Copyright 1982, Allen E. Ivey, Box 641, N. Amherst, MA 01059. Reproduced by permission.]

While listening and attending skills form the foundation of microtraining, reflection of meaning (adapted from Frankl's logotherapy) and influencing skills such as interpretation are important. Microtraining gives special attention to the interrelation between reflection of meaning and interpretation, attention that is critical to effective assessment. Given a set of data presented by a client (e.g., a child having difficulty in school), the assessment interviewer may have an idea as to what is "really" happening and what it "really means." Whenever the interviewer thinks he or she has an interpretation of the client's construction of reality, it may be time for a reflection of meaning to validate the interpretation (rather than assume it is correct).

One can reflect meaning fairly simply. For example, the interviewer can initially ask the client questions relating to value and meaning ("What values are important in your family?" "What does your daughter's behavior *mean* to you?" "What sense do you make of it?"). Out of such questions, the client's construction of the situation may be generated. At this point, the interviewer may reflect meaning by using variations of the paraphrase or reflection of feeling ("I sense the meaning of this to you was. . . . "). Interpretations come from the interviewer's construction of the world, not from the client's. To assess, one must first understand the constructions of the other. The tendency in assessment (further emphasized in testing) is to depend too much on theory and psychological constructions rather than on the more direct experience of the client.

Microcounseling, then, facilitates an understanding of the client's experience by identifying the client's unique frame of reference either during assessment or counseling/therapy. During the assessment interview, the interviewer tries to enter the client's frame of reference with minimal impact through a reality-testing procedure. Later, the assessment officer may interpret and draw conclusions (always with cross-cultural sensitivity and care), but first he or she must understand the client's frame of reference.

Within this understanding (of the frame of reference) and the assessment process, influencing skills such as interpretation and self-disclosure are not as important as the attending skills. Again, exceptions due to cultural expectations must be noted. Self-disclosure, honesty, and interpersonal openness may be more important than the best listening skills with some lower-income people who have learned not to trust the questioning/attending/listening mental health practitioner. As such, the entire range of microskills needs to be available to the assessment practitioner if one is to facilitate development and promote growth for all individuals.

Microskills do not provide specific answers; rather, they provide specific tools that may lead to more comprehensive and accurate constructions and models of the client.

Constructing a Well-Formed Interview

At the top of the microskills hierarchy (see Figure 4-1) is the integration of skills. The word "top," however, is quite misleading. In a sense, the foundation skills of attending and client observation are the top skills, for without them nothing else is possible. Too many individuals involved in assessment jump to the mythical top, conduct interviews, and make conclusions when their foundation skills of listening and cultural understanding are inadequate.

Given this caution, the issue of structuring a well-formed interview is addressed. The five stages of the interview as taught in microtraining are outlined in Table 4-2. The interview presented here is a problem-solving interview and is considered a metamodel (Ivey & Matthews, in press) for other helping interviews. The metamodel implies that this particular set of interview stages occurs in many types of interviewing. Whether one is conducting a Rogerian therapy session, a psychodynamic dream analysis, or assertiveness training, this metamodel may be used to frame the session. Ivey (1983) discusses these points in greater detail. He uses the microtraining framework described in the previous section to teach entire methodologies of interviewing. For example, in teaching dream analysis to advanced students, the five steps of microtraining are followed: (*a*) an overview of theory of dreams is presented; (*b*) a videotape demonstrating a dream analysis section is shown broken down into the five stages of the interview presented here; (*c*) the tape is analyzed and discussed with theory; (*d*) students practice dream analysis; and (*e*) generalization plans for use of the larger set of skills are negotiated.

A review of the five stages of the interview in Table 4-2, however, indicates that the assessment model requires more important variations for success. It would seem appropriate at this point to consider each stage and the implications of skills and stages for assessment procedures. As we begin this review, it is important to recall that the stages are a road map, not a specific route that one must follow. According to various needs of the client, different roads must be taken to meet individual and cultural differences.

Stage 1. Rapport/Structuring

The first task of any interviewer is to establish rapport and to structure the session. Rapport may be instantaneous, or it may take several interviews to nurture. Rapport is manifested in the sensory-motor data of eye contact, vocal tone, and mirroring postures. It exists when an easy conversational flow occurs. The routes toward developing rapport are as many as the number of clients and assessment interviewers. The case study below provides an instance where rapport occurs quickly and spontaneously.

The interviewer in that session also moved quickly to structure the session meaningfully for the client by giving accurate information about why they were meeting. This, of course, is a distinction between therapy interviews and assessment interviews where the client may often be more directly involved in the nature of structuring. It is critical that the purpose and general structure of the assessment interview be presented explicitly for the client.

Stage 2. Problem Definition/Asset Definition

Assessment interviews almost always occur because the clients have problems and difficulties. However, one can talk about problems freely only if one feels sure of oneself. Bringing out the positive characteristics and resources of the individual being interviewed, the child who is being discussed, or the total referral situation fairly early in the session, therefore, facilitates this feeling. Otherwise, the session often remains in a downward spiral of concern and trouble.

In the interview at the end of this chapter, note that Mrs. Rivera at section 6 (page 134) spontaneously talks about some positive aspects of her daughter. Why did that happen? Did it really occur spontaneously? At section 4, Mrs. Rivera talks about difficulty in ballet and only one positive statement occurs: "She likes ballet and I was successful in sending her to ballet." Rather than following up the more troubling aspects of Mrs. Rivera's situation, the assessment interviewer commented, "She is beginning to adjust." This is an example of a "positive reflection of meaning" skill in that the interviewer reflected the positive meaning inherent in Mrs. Rivera's statement. Another positive reflection of feeling occurs at section 7 when the interviewer notes, "You are really enjoying her." This provides a solid base for the exploration of current problems that then follows. Clients can talk very freely in an atmosphere of listening and respect. Critical to the entire process of this interview were these quick, seemingly unimportant comments by the interviewer. From this point on, the client talks freely from *her* frame of reference about her situation.

Most assessment interviews are, of course, concerned with problem definition, yet are balanced by definitions of the client's assets and resources. The goal of an assessment interview is to obtain the client's frame of reference concerning the referral problem through a variety of open and closed questions. In the following section is a simple outline for thinking through important referral issues which suggests assessment questions.

Table 4-2
A Simple Five-Stage Structure for the Interview[a]

Definition of stage	Function and purpose of stage	Commonly used skills
1. Rapport and structuring. "Hello."	To build a working alliance with the client and to enable the client to feel comfortable with the interviewer. Structuring may be needed to explain the purpose of the interview. Structuring functions to help keep the session on task and to inform the client what the counselor can and cannot do.	Attending behavior to establish contact with the client, and client observation skills to determine appropriate method to build rapport. Structuring most often involves the influencing skill of information giving and instructions.
2. Gathering information, defining the problem, and identifying assets. "What's the problem?"	To find out why the client has come to the interview and how he or she views the problem. Skillful problem definition will help avoid aimless topic jumping and give the interview purpose and direction. Also to identify clearly positive strengths of the client.	Most common are the attending skills, especially the basic listening sequence. Other skills may be used as necessary. If problems aren't clear, you may need more influencing skills. The positive asset search often reveals capabilities in the client that are useful in finding problem resolution.
3. Determining outcomes. Where does the client want to go? "What do you want to have happen?"	To find out the ideal world of the client. How would the client like to be? How would things be if the problem were solved? This stage is important in that it en-	Most common are the attending skills, especially the basic listening sequence. Other skills used as necessary. If outcome is still unclear, more influencing skills may

(*continued*)

Stage 3. Determining Outcomes

Most assessment interviews stop with problem assessment; a few add the assessment of client assets. Even fewer assessment interviews ask the critical question, "Given all these data, where do you want things to go?" An all-too-common tendency in assessment is to assess the client-related difficulties and look to the past. Returning to the road map analogy, it is as if a person comes to us asking how to get to the next town, but instead of answering, we spend our time asking where they have been.

Client assessment, of course, must ask clients where they have been and how they got there. But assessment is incomplete unless we find out where clients want to go. Where you think a client or a client's child should go may not be where they want to or are willing to go.

Thus, the assessment interviewer's question at section 37 of the case study is particularly important: "Do you have any further questions or concerns, particularly as to what you want for the future?" Mrs. Rivera's response provides some very specific information. It shows that the client understands that some

**Table 4-2
(Continued)**

Definition of stage	Function and purpose of stage	Commonly used skills
	ables the interviewer to know what the client wants. The desired direction of the client and counselor should be reasonably harmonious. With some clients, skip phase 2 and define goals first.	be helpful. With clients from other cultures and those who are less verbal, this phase should often precede phase 2.
4. Exploring alternatives and confronting client incongruities. "What are we going to do about it?"	To work toward resolution of the client's issue. This may involve the creative problem-solving model of generating alternatives (to remove stuckness) and deciding among those alternatives. It also may involve lengthy exploration of personal dynamics. This phase of the interview may be the longest.	May begin with a summary of the major discrepancies. Depending on the issue and theory of the interviewer, a heavy use of influencing skills may be expected. Attending skills still used for balance.
5. Generalization and transfer of learning. "Will you do it?"	To enable changes in thoughts, feelings, and behaviors in the client's daily life. Many clients go through an interview and then do nothing to change their behavior, remaining in the same world they came from.	Influencing skills, such as directives and information/ explanation, are particularly important. Attending skills used to check out client understanding of importance of the stage.

*a*From Ivey, A. E. *Intentional interviewing and counseling.* Monterey, CA: Brooks-Cole. Copyright 1982, Allen E. Ivey, Box 641 N. Amherst, MA 01059. Reproduced by permission.

psychological support is needed by her child, and indicates that she supports the school system toward achieving common objectives.

Mrs. Rivera's statement is followed by a positive reflection of feeling/meaning and feedback on what already has been done for the children. Mrs. Rivera then provides even more specific data about what she wants for her child. Goal setting is an important part of assessment; unless we ask our clients for their goals, we are in danger of constructing goals for them that are totally inappropriate.

Stage 4. Generating Alternatives/Confronting Incongruity

This stage in the interviewing process is, of course, *not* a part of the typical assessment interview, at least in the early stages. Practitioners conduct assessments, hold evaluative sessions, and plan groups so that they may present the results of assessments and *then* generate alternatives. Thus, this phase of the interview is actually part of the larger assessment process. The stage at which tests, interview data, observations, and other information obtained from files are brought together (often in a case conference) is the direct analogue to the working stage of the therapeutic interview. When the client joins the assessment practitioner or team for a presentation of assessment results, he or she actually becomes part of the treatment approach where, considering this an additional interviewing session, alternatives for action are generated and the basic incongruity of a referral situation is confronted.

Stage 5. Generalization/Transfer of Learning

In the case study, the assessment interviewer very briefly at section 43 brings the interview to a close and summarizes specific plans for follow-up after the session. For this stage of the helping process, the brief transfer of learning statement is probably sufficient. Needless to say, for assessment efforts to be meaningful, final assessment meetings should be followed with careful follow-up to ensure implementation and generalization of the assessment plan. We are suggesting here, of course, that follow-up and generalization are again direct analogues of what occurs in the effective interview. Thus, once again, it is important to understand the basic structure of the interview to ensure that, in both assessment interviews and in the structure of the larger treatment plan which results from the assessment process, reasonably sensitive and efficient action will follow.

The structural analysis above fails to consider the basic content of the assessment interview. This is considered in the next section.

The Content of the Assessment Interview

"If you don't know what's wrong with a client, ask. He (or she) may tell you" (G. Kelly, 1955, p. 201). The most fundamental element or process in the assessment interview is the act of questioning. Two questions are most basic: "What's wrong?" (stage 2 of the interview), and "What do you want done about it?" (stage 3 of the interview). Sometimes within these two questions are important cultural differences. Middle-class assessment procedures most often focus on "What's wrong?". However, careful examination of other cultures reveals that the goal-setting agenda implicit in "What do you want done about it?" may be more important and helpful. So, even in the most basic structure of the interview (i.e., questions) lie critical cultural differences to which one must be sensitive.

George Kelly (1955) presents a simple, but important, model of assessment that may be useful to beginning (or many advanced) assessment practitioners. The model is an amplification of the newspaper rule of thumb of "who, what, where, when, how, and why." The newspaper rule of thumb is itself a useful checklist to ensure that the assessment practitioner has considered the most critical issues. Kelly's model (G. Kelly, 1955, pp. 777–779), paraphrased below, is critical for ensuring that you have considered the most basic issues. Careful coverage of his points generally takes a full assessment hour.

1. What is the client's presenting problem? What does the client think is wrong? What are the results of the problem?

2. How does the client view the world? What are the client's constructs and key words? How does this construction of the world bear on the problem?

3. What is the client's environmental and situational context? What effect do issues such as socioeconomic class, housing, and environment have on constructions and life?

4. To maintain personal clarity, what are your (the practitioner's) basic theories and constructs in regard to this particular client? What does this client mean to you? How can you avoid imposing your constructions?

5. What do you and the client do next? Is it clear to each of you or is it a mystery? Will you and the client follow up on agreed goals? (This point is critical; unless clients know what is going on, very little will happen.)

As you consider the case study of the assessment interview, look to see if these five questions are answered. Note that assessment often works only with the first of these five questions; the concept of the client's unique constructions of the world is often missing. In the assessment interview presented here, the interviewer consistently supports/reinforces the client's constructions of the world from her own cultural base. The sensitivity to culturally different constructions is particularly important to effective assessment.

Also important in the client-oriented model is the interviewer's awareness of possible bias and distortion. Only through examining our own constructions of the world and our own biases and beliefs can we better hear someone else's. Without this honest self-examination, any assessment fails.

When working with young people such as children and adolescents, it is not as easy to follow this format, and the practitioner may need to vary his or her style so that the important diagnostic issues are covered. The five points above, however, will serve as a useful checklist to help ensure that as much data as possible have been obtained. Below are some specific suggestions for using the Kelly model with a younger population.

1. Focus on the young person's construction of the world: Everyone construes reality and the world differently and this is even more true of children. It is far too easy to impose your diagnosis on the willing (or rebellious) youngster. Remember your first task in assessment is to ground yourself in the frame of reference of the child or adolescent. To "get into their shoes," you must see the world as they do. This will be critical for your work in assessment.

2. Through the use of listening skills, discover what the child thinks is wrong. Develop rapport; spend a good deal of time obtaining a picture of the problem from the youngster's frame of reference. With some children or adolescents, questions are fine. In other cases, questions will create barriers, and you will have to use your own self-disclosure or simple patience to obtain the youngster's point of view and feelings.

3. Note key words the youth uses. These may be repeated words that are sometimes so common that their importance is missed. You may, for example, find a child discussing everything in terms of "big" or "little." This is a classical Kelly-type polar set of constructs which is common with children. Spend some time elaborating on those words and listening to their deeper meaning. You may find that these key words are attached differently to different people and objects. Words relating to the mother and the child's experience with the mother, for example, may be heavily laden with the word "big." Find out through listening and minimally encouraging direct repetition ("Big?") the deeper meanings of key words to the youngster.

The issue here is to listen to the WORDS. The importance of key words that indicate how the child or adolescent construes an event cannot be overstated. The most direct route toward understanding key words is repeating the word (the encourage or minimal encourage) and then noting the response which represents the deeper meaning or structure underlying that key word.

4. Draw out socioeconomic and housing issues as they relate to the child. Again, you may find that your original diagnosis changes as you listen carefully to the child's construction of his or her environment.

5. Maintain an awareness of your own theoretical system. You have patterns of key words and constructs which repeat, just as the youngster does. Note the reports you write. You will find personal patterns which repeat across almost all of the youngsters with whom you work. Some argue that theory sometimes blinds us to our own perceptions of the world. Are you allowing theory and your own construction of the client to become reality? The answer to this problem is awareness and self-study.

Each person is unique. The goal of effective assessment is to avoid stereotyping. Repeating patterns in your diagnoses and reports take the uniqueness out of the child and situation. They may also signal serious "burn-out" on your part. Unfortunately, all too often assessment staff fall into the very trap that they are trying to avoid.

6. Determine the child's goals. This is perhaps the most important activity of all. Assessment is much too often concerned with the past as long lists of problems are obtained to be solved. Much time can often be saved by determining the child's goal(s), a task that can be obtained via an infinite array of procedures. For example, you may directly ask the youngster how he or she would like things to be. Often, this results in child-specific goals that are very similar to those which you would set. At other times, the child may give socially appropriate goals which he or she expects are "correct." An important task for you is to decide whether the stated goal is indeed the child's personal goal or one designed to please you and the parents.

Other possible procedures for obtaining children's goals include fantasy ("Imagine the perfect day." "Close your eyes and think how you might feel if things were the way you wanted them to be."), asking the child for negative goals ("How could things be worse?" "What would be the worst possible thing?"), play-therapy, role-playing, and a variety of other counseling and clinical interventions. Interestingly, negative goals can add humor and may later be translated into positive directions.

These six suggestions provide only an introduction to the process of discovering a young person's construction of a referred problem. As noted above, this process is a central part of any efficient and complete child assessment, and a child's construction of a referred problem is best obtained through the clinical interview. Unless a complete and, hopefully, accurate picture of the child's construction of the problem is identified, the assessment is empty.

When the child's construction of the problem is determined, it may be combined with several other components to form a more complete assessment picture. These components include the construction of the problem by the child's parents, the teacher (or other professionals), and by the mental health practitioner. Ultimately, the correct construction of the referral problem will be that one which is based on the reality of these different parties; a construct need not be supported by tests and theory. Finally, the practitioner must guard against accepting just a personal view of a child's problems; the assessment process must be geared toward the integration of everyone's constructs into an accurate, unified, and accepted perspective of the referral problem.

Summary

The section has presented the systematic training framework of microcounseling skills and interviewing structure and has explained how these concepts may be relevant to the assessment process. It has emphasized the important cultural differences that are present in some form in virtually all interviews and has noted that without cultural awareness, the assessment interview may easily reflect interviewer biases or inappropriate psychological practice. It suggests that the structure of the interview is one in which many types of interviewing procedures may be clarified. Specifically, the assessment interview is concerned with Stages 1, 2, and 3, but the long-term assessment process follows the basic structure of the entire five-stage process with careful plans for follow-up and generalization. The content of the assessment interview can vary, but the newspaper model (who, what, when, where, why, and how) and George Kelly's systematic model provide basic guidelines.

Developmental Issues and the Assessment Process

Does the model of interview-oriented assessment presented here "work" with people of different developmental levels and conceptual abilities? The answer is yes, with specific qualifications. For example, open questions may be useful with highly verbal clients. With a resistant client or child, however, they may be totally ineffective; closed questions or patient waiting may be the preferred alternative with these individuals. The structure of the interview likewise is appropriate for many different types of people, but again must be modified to meet specific needs. A child is not likely to sit still for a lengthy problem assessment, while the parents may provide more data than one can assimilate or use. Different people of different developmental levels present themselves for the assessment process, and the process must be adapted to them.

Ivey (in press) has recently generated a model based on Piagetian theory relating counseling/therapy and interview assessment to varying developmental stages. In the process, he has incorporated person/environment models of relating to microskills and the interview structure. A brief summary of the model follows, with indications of some practical implications for immediate practice.

Four Epistemological Foundations of Development

Piagetian theory is ultimately concerned with how we know and how we know what we know (ad infinitum). Assessment, similarly, is concerned with discovering and analyzing how clients know or construct their worlds. Thus, questions of epistemology and the nature of knowing are critical for accurate assessment.

Sensory-Motor

In Piagetian theory, children first learn their world through their senses. They see, hear, and feel their world. Through primary circular reactions, they gradually coordinate the means of movements (e.g., eye–hand coordination). Their epistemology or way of knowing is sensory-motor. For counseling purposes, Ivey points out that we never fully transcend sensory-motor experience. Underlying "higher" cognitive functions are concrete data gained through sensory experience. Thus, all assessment procedures must ultimately be grounded in concrete reality.

The assessment interviewer grounds the interview in rapport (which itself is basically sensory-motor) and matches the physical movements of the interviewee (eye contact, posture, breathing).

Preoperational

A second mode of knowing is preoperational, in which children learn to name objects and form elementary relationships between them. Linear causality and conservation of knowledge do not exist in children at this age; often they make "magical" connections between events. A child may say, for example, "The way you looked at me caused me to trip."

The preoperational mode of knowing is not restricted to children. Most of our counseling and therapy clients come to counseling or therapy in some preoperational way. They have made magical, incorrect connections such as, "It is the child's fault." An alcoholic, for example, may deny his or her alcoholism. And so on. The task of assessment and change in counseling and therapy is to raise the developmental level or mode of thinking/epistemology.

For the practitioner conducting an assessment at this level, it is useful to recognize preoperational thinking. Then preoperational thinking and magical connections can often be raised to a more concrete level through asking the question, "What did you see, hear, or feel that led you to that conclusion?" Note that this question first returns to concrete, sensory-motor experience, then encourages the experiential developmental level of the client to rise to early concrete operations—a more systematic and accurate way of knowing.

No one, according to Piagetian theory, can truly function beyond his or her current and predominant stage. Thus, for assessment procedures, it is critical to note where development has momentarily or more permanently stopped and why.

Concrete Operational

Concrete operations, of course, is the next level of Piagetian development. With conservation of knowledge, the child (or parent) is beginning to understand cause and effect: "If I do this, then that will happen." At this point, the individual separates self from other objects. Ordinarily occurring around ages 5 to 7, the developmental timing of concrete operations interestingly parallels that of the Freudian Oedipal complex, which also requires a separation of self from object (mother). Thus, the separation of self from object as required in concrete operations is a particularly important aspect of development, and the assessment interview uses it to provide an opportunity to note developmental stages of children and parents.

According to Ivey (in press), counselors move peoples' preoperational thinking to concrete operations through the question, "What, specifically, happened?" To answer that question, the client must use, at a minimum, early concrete operations. For assessment purposes, it is also important to remember that the observer affects the observed, and the act of questioning changes what is being assessed.

Formal Operational

Late concrete operations adds the dimensions of causality and more accurate linear thinking: "I did this *because.* . . . " Repeating patterns of linear causality provide the transition to formal operational thinking that allows the individual to think about self-thinking. For example, if a family discovers that it is repeating a pattern it once thought unique, it has moved to the act of thinking about thinking itself or formal operational thinking.

Formal operational thinking is manifested when our clients join us in thinking about their situation. However, it is readily apparent that most children are not really able to engage in this type of thinking. Many families are incapable as well, particularly as they encounter difficult interpersonal issues.

Ivey suggests that different counseling/interviewing styles are required for the varying developmental levels if one is to have successful therapy or successful assessment. He suggests first utilizing sensory modality matching, regardless of developmental level or stage. This can be followed by naming the problem/asset in a preoperational sense using simple, forthright, and direct closed questions to assess the situation as it is. To facilitate the move to concrete operations, the all-important "Could you give me a specific example?" or, "What did you see, hear, or feel that led you to that conclusion?" questions provide impetus. Early evidence suggests that individuals at the concrete operational stage will do better with behavioral approaches to counseling and possibly cognitive behavioral approaches like Ellis's. As clients and their families move to formal operations and thinking about thinking, Rogerian therapy and the reframing therapies such as logotherapy or psychodynamic therapy may be more useful.

The evaluation of an entire family requires assessing and understanding a mixture of constructions and epistemologies. There may be a preoperational child, a concrete operational father, and a formal operational mother. Each has distinctly different epistemologies and ways of knowing the world. Further, even while the mother may be individually capable of formal operations, she may be preoperational in how she copes with her family. The assessment practitioner and the treatment team follow the interviewing and testing process by analyzing a family's different constructions and epistemologies. Perhaps the treatment team's greatest value is its ability to generate the mixture of treatment plans and strategies that address these family differences and most likely will be required for meaningful and effective intervention.

A more detailed review of these ideas may be found in Ivey (1983) and the most recent discussion in Ivey (in press). The next section discusses the case history interview, which deals with the process of development and its unique content for each person evaluated.

The Case History Interview

The case history interview is the most frequently used of all personality assessment techniques (Prout, 1983). However, due to the "test-centered" emphasis of current assessment practices (Maloney & Ward, 1976), it is the least discussed in the literature. Anastasi (1982), in her now classic introduction to psychological testing, dedicates half a page to a discussion of the case history interview.

Interviews centered on obtaining case history information are performed in both schools and community settings and for both children and adolescents. This interview provides much needed information about the past and present context in which the client is operating. The client's family structure and dynamics, support systems, early developmental history, and school and social history are extremely important pieces of the diagnostic puzzle. In many cases, the data obtained are important not only for diagnostic purposes, but also for the design of treatment options. A good illustration of this point involves cases of suspected mental retardation where eliciting the client's achievement of developmental milestones is diagnostically important, and where the presence of a strong support system would significantly influence recommendations for living arrangements.

Formal Systems

Although most case histories are obtained through semistructured interviews, a few formal systems have been developed. Generally, these formal systems have been adaptive behavior scales or medical histories. Best known among these scales are Mercer's (1979) Adaptive Behavior Inventory for Children (ABIC) and her Medical History and Sociocultural Scales of the SOMPA (System of Multipluralistic Assessment), the AAMD Adaptive Behavior Scale (Lambert, Windmiller, Cole, & Figueroa, 1975), and the Vineland Adaptive Behavior Scales (Sparrow, Balla, & Cicchetti, 1984). These standardized interviews are most often used in the diagnosis of mental retardation or other significant educational deficits.

Semistructured Systems

Case histories are usually conducted in a semistructured way, addressing specific areas of concern while leaving room for issues that may emerge during the conversation. (A list of general areas for interviewing parents and adolescents is presented in Appendix I.) Case history interviewing is a skill of great importance to the mental health practitioner. Some professions, such as social work and psychiatry, rely almost solely on the case history to formulate diagnoses and treatment plans. Psychologists use the case history to provide information about the context in which the client functions, to generate hypotheses to be tested by more formal testing, and to help determine appropriate treatment options.

Taking a Case History

The way a case history is taken depends on the setting and age of the client. In the case of referred children, most case history material is obtained from the parents, especially the mother. In some ethnic groups, grandparents may provide this information. Once at the adolescent stage, the referred individuals are themselves capable of providing a great deal of the information, except for early developmental history data. The mother is the best source of prenatal history and medical information; this will be especially important information if the child or adolescent has a specific or hypothesized handicap.

The Effect of the Setting

School Setting

Schools, hospitals, and community mental health centers are different because of their unique functions, internal environments, and organizational structures. Schools must be responsive to parents and the community, and need to keep personal information confidential. Further, their main or sole function is not to assess and maintain the mental health of their young charges. For these reasons, the mental health practitioner in the school has a more difficult time obtaining information for a case history. Parents sometimes are reluctant to air private information to school personnel, fearing that it may become part of the child's cumulative record or it could be passed on to inappropriate school personnel. The current practice of interviewing parents in their homes has helped alleviate some of this distrust. However, sometimes this creates separate difficulties with parents who are even more resentful of school personnel entering their homes.

Writing up the findings of a case history interview for a school file is a challenge to the tactfulness and sensitivity of the professional. What to include and in what depth are questions one has to wrestle with when working in a school setting. Practitioners should bear in mind that their write-ups are open to the public, stay in the child's records for many years, and can be summoned by a court. One recommendation for newcomers to a setting is to examine case reports of competent workers who are experienced in the system to determine the boundaries of confidentiality. The practitioner working in a school should include only information that is essential to the understanding of the child's difficulties in school, and should write this information in ways that will not be construed as offensive by the family or the teachers.

Mental Health Center or Hospital Settings

Settings whose major function is to provide mental health care to their clients have an easier time obtaining and reporting information. Generally, clients who contact these settings have been directed there by other, sometimes school mental health professionals. Clients usually come with the sole purpose of obtaining help, and they actually anticipate being interviewed, since medical care has a longstanding tradition of being preceded by the taking of a medical history. Thus, it is easier in this setting to delve directly into intimate matters. One drawback, however, when working in mental health and hospital settings is that the interviewer is often working with more difficult cases. The client's reluctance to disclose important aspects of his or her background will emerge not for fear of confidentiality, but because of pain, fear of legal reprisals, or distrust of the interviewer.

How to Conduct the Case History Interview

Initial Telephone Call

The case history interview should begin with a telephone call from the practitioner to the couple or parent to be interviewed. At this time, the interviewer introduces him- or herself to the client, explains the purpose and nature of the interview, and inquires about where and when they would prefer to be interviewed. Because the initial contact is so important and sets the tone for future encounters, it should be conducted by the practitioner and not left to a secretary. Thus, the building of rapport starts here. Through this call, the professional learns whether the parents are relaxed and eager to be interviewed, anxious and worried about the meeting, or hostile and resistant to the query. Taking into consideration this initial reading of parental attitudes, the interviewer plans strategies for a successful case history interview.

When a child or teenager is going to be interviewed, this initial phase often does not occur because the arrangements have been made through the child's parents, teacher, or counselor.

Beginning the Interview

At the beginning of the case history interview, the interviewer introduces herself or himself and explains the purpose of the interview. Once this has been accomplished, the interviewer asks a general question to find out the concerns that prompted the parents to refer the child. If the school initiated the referral, the first question to ask would be how the parents perceive the concerns of the school. Questions such as "What concerns you about your son?" or "What prompted you to refer your child?" are good starting points. In this initial part of the interview, the most important thing to keep in mind is to develop rapport with the interviewees by communicating that you are trying to be helpful and are either neutral or on their side. Sections 1–11 of the case study below (with a middle-class Hispanic single mother whose daughter was experiencing difficulties in school) exemplify some of these principles. This interview was conducted in the presence of the school counselor. Prior to the meeting, the author had contacted the mother, introduced herself, and explained the purpose of the meeting. The interview started with greetings and introductions at the door and with Mrs. Rivera expressing discomfort at having to speak in English about intimate emotional matters. The counselor assured her that she could switch to Spanish whenever she felt necessary and that she was there only as a participant observer.

As can be seen from the interview, this client started the interview by describing the worries that she had about her daughter during the past 6 years (this information is given while the structure, dynamics, and history of the family are being described). This client displayed openness and a high level of self-disclosure because her own personal therapy had augmented her level of self-assertiveness and because of the cultural and linguistic similarities between the interviewer and the mother. These factors helped make the interview very easy to conduct. The interviewer was careful not to interrupt the flow of the interview, since the mother was furnishing her with the information needed to understand the family context in which the child had developed. The interviewer summarized the points previously covered to keep the interview in focus.

In school interviews, it is often hard to ask questions about divorce and its consequences because parents are afraid of revealing confidential material. It is easier to explore the divorce issue if the mother brings up the subject spontaneously. In the case of children and at the early stages of intervention, it is not necessary to obtain in-depth information about divorce. It is sufficient to know that the child has gone through the process. When the mother does not mention the issue of divorce spontaneously, a general question asking about how many people live in the house will usually reveal the absence or presence of the father. A follow-up question inquiring where the father lives usually leads to an explanation of why he does not live with the family.

Family History, Structure, and Dynamics

In this section, the interviewer wants to obtain information about the number and spacing of children, the family history, extended family, and education and places where the parents work. It is also useful to obtain information about the internal climate of the home, especially affect and power dimensions (Kantor & Lehr, 1975): How do the parents and children show affection? Who disciplines the children? What activities are prohibited and which are encouraged? In cases where the parents are not divorced or the family has not undergone drastic changes, such as unemployment, death, sickness, or accidents, this part of the interview can be completed fairly easily. In school cases, some of this information is already in the cumulative folder or is known to the teachers in the school.

In the case study interview with Mrs. Rivera, the client provided a lot of information on her own. The interviewer needed only to ask her specific questions about financial assistance and visitation rights (see sections 11 to 12) to establish the parameters of the divorce situation.

In cases of adoption, specific follow-up questions about the adoption process, such as the time and circumstances, might be necessary if the client does not offer this information. Similar questions or prompts establish other circumstances such as family death, illness, accident, migration, or job loss.

Developmental History

Information about the early developmental history of the child is vital for a complete diagnostic workup. In the diagnosis of mental retardation, learning disabilities, and emotional disorders, it is crucial to establish the age at which the child achieved his or her developmental milestones. Thus, it is imperative to include in this section questions determining the ages when the child talked, walked, and was toilet trained, and about his or her prenatal history. When children suffer from medical problems, a more formal medical history should be taken, such as the one developed by Mercer (1979) as part of the SOMPA. Questions about the personality of the baby should also be included. Attendance at nursery school and friendship patterns during those preschool years should be ascertained. Sections 15–17 of the interview with Mrs. Rivera illustrate these points clearly.

School History

Obtaining information about performance in school is very important for both children and adolescents. A child who consistently has been doing well academically and suddenly begins to do poorly is very different from a child whose schoolwork has been characterized by poor performance from the very beginning and throughout.

Elementary School Years

School life begins formally with kindergarten. It is important to find out whether and where the child attended kindergarten, and how well she or he did. Did the teacher observe anything remarkable? How did the child relate to other children?

First grade is crucial to the process of learning to read. If the interviewer is assessing children suspected of emotional difficulties, learning disabilities, or mental retardation, questions about the ease or difficulty with the learning-to-read process are important. Inquiring whether the child has repeated any grades or received special help is also imperative. Again, the child's socialization development is important: Did the child make friends easily? How did he or she get along with children in the neighborhood?

If the child is bilingual, it is vital to obtain information about the amount of English the parents know, the child's dominance and proficiency in both English and his or her native language, the language he or she learned to read in first, and whether he or she has ever attended a bilingual program. A grade-by-grade account of the educational history of this child is needed, especially if the child has shifted from a school with a bilingual program to a school that does not offer such options. Sections 32–40 of the Rivera case demonstrate the type of information usually obtained in the case of a bilingual child.

If an English-speaking child is referred for learning problems, a grade-by-grade rundown should be obtained. Difficulties experienced in math, reading, or with peers should be ascertained.

Junior and Senior High School

With an adolescent in junior or senior high school, it is important to determine academic status and progress as well as to inquire about participation in sports, work, arts, dating patterns, career interests, college or vocational plans, drug and alcohol habits, and hobbies. The youngster's reactions to his or her physiological changes and appearance and his or her feelings about sexual identity are critical areas to investigate. Areas of conflict with parents, such as independence versus dependence, money, relationships with the opposite sex, grades, and college attendance, should also be investigated.

This information can be obtained directly from the adolescent or his parents. When interviewing the adolescent, the practitioner should start with nonthreatening questions such as career interests, sports, work, or arts participation, and college or vocational plans before delving into more private matters such as relationships with parents or dating patterns.

Case Study: Mrs. Rivera

Family Background and Developmental History

The Rivera family is composed of Mrs. Rivera and her three children, Maria, Juan, and Carmen. Ten years ago, Ana Rivera came to this country from Puerto Rico to do graduate work in the sciences. She had just divorced Mr. Rivera, who was then a medical student and who is now practicing medicine on the island. While in Puerto Rico, the children were appointed by the court to visit with him every other weekend. Now, they spend a month with him during the summer. At present, Mrs. Rivera is being visited by her parents who came to help her take care of the children while she prepares for her comprehensives and dissertation. In the past they have served as her major support system, taking care of the children while she worked and looking after the two youngest children in Puerto Rico when she first came to settle in the United States.

Mrs. Rivera described Maria's first 4 years of life as normal and happy. She walked at 8 months and talked early, too. She was an independent child who liked to wander in the neighborhood and visit different homes. She loved to dance. At age 4½, she attended a day-care center while her mother finished her bachelor's degree at the university. She had a good year while she attended kindergarten. First grade, however, was difficult. Her parents were in the midst of divorce proceedings and her teacher was an uncaring, insensitive, irritable woman. Maria did not want to go to school. Although she learned to read easily, she hated math intensely. She refused help from her mother and was unwilling to do her homework.

Socially, she felt unliked by everyone and preferred the company of only one friend. She was very possessive and refused to share her friend with anyone else.

When Maria came to this country, she was in shock: She regressed and became very dependent on her mother, refusing to leave her presence and insisting on sleeping with her. She attended a bilingual summer program and later was placed in a bilingual classroom. Mrs. Rivera became uncomfortable with the isolation of the children in the program and insisted that the children be changed to the regular classroom while receiving assistance from the ESL teacher. Her ESL teachers were very good, but her regular teacher was not. This teacher let Maria vegetate the whole year in her classroom. Maria did nothing for the whole term. Maria missed the protection and companionship offered by the children in the bilingual class.

In the meantime, the two children were subjected to considerable name-calling and racial abuse from their classmates. They came home one day crying because the children were calling them "pigs." They did not understand that the children were actually calling them "spics." Mrs. Rivera explained to the children what was really happening and reminded them that their classmates were just jealous of the fact that they could speak two languages. She is very proud of her heritage and has instilled in her children ethnic pride.

Maria learned to speak English slowly. She seemed to block and was not able to learn anything. However, learning to read in English was easy because she could use the skills she had developed learning to read in Spanish. Mrs. Rivera has insisted that the children speak only Spanish at home.

The mother's major worry about Maria is her low self-esteem and her unwillingness to share her friends. Mrs. Rivera has had a serious relationship with a classmate that terminated last September. The children had become used to her friend and she fears that her breakup has affected them. She worries about how the loss of their father and of her boyfriend may influence the mental health of her children, particularly her daughter. She reports that Maria has difficulty expressing and identifying her feelings. Her lack of sharing of these feelings concerns Mrs. Rivera.

Academically, Maria's understanding of mathematical and time concepts is an issue for her mother. She feels that her teacher has helped her a great deal and instilled in her a sense of self-confidence. She would like to keep her in the present school, but is contemplating transferring her other children to a more structured school. She reports that her son's makeup is more consonant with that teaching style. She would like him to be evaluated as well.

Background to the Interview

This interview took place at 8 o'clock in the morning in the office of an elementary school counselor serving a suburban school system. Present during the interview were the counselor, the mother, and the first author. The counselor had requested to be present because she was going to be in charge of helping the mother and her children during their stay at the school. The mother was a graduate student in her mid-30s who was the single parent of three children. Her 10-year-old daughter Maria had been referred to the author because of difficulties in language and in asserting herself in class. The family spoke both Spanish and English and arrived in this country 3 years ago.

Transcript of the Interview

Counselor: While Dr. Nuttall sets up the tape recorder, I will take the opportunity of explaining to you what happens during a core evaluation. At this meeting the psychologist, the counselor, the reading specialist, the teacher, and the principal get together with the parent to discuss the results of the assessment each person has done. The parent is asked for any information which he or she deems relevant. You can bring a friend or relative to the evaluation if you want to. Parents tend to feel sometimes uncomfortable about the sheer number of professionals who are present. Each professional gives his or her input and plans are developed for the education of the child. Do you have any questions about the process, Mrs. Rivera?

Mrs. Rivera: No, I do not. I am glad that we are doing this for my daughter.

1. *Dr. Nuttall:* Mrs. Rivera, these meetings are sometimes hard for parents because they feel outnumbered and overwhelmed by the number of school staff. However, the staff of this school are very nice and well meaning and they try their hardest at making parents feel comfortable. I will help you as much as I can. I would like now to begin with my interview. What concerns you about Maria?

2. *Mrs. Rivera:* At the beginning, I was worried. I was worried in Puerto Rico, too. In the first grade she did not have a good experience, too. Here was a new experience. She was real scared, insecure. She became unusually dependent, will not let me out of her presence.

3. *Dr. Nuttall:* She regressed.

4. *Mrs. Rivera:* Yes. She would walk around the house. Hard to deal with three kids. But thank God her teacher Mrs. X noticed it, too. I am very insecure, too. She was blocked. She would say, "I can't do it, I do not want to study." I tried to help her. She likes ballet, and I was successful in sending her to ballet. There, she showed the same insecurity, clinging to me and not wanting me out of sight. It has changed a lot.

5. *Dr. Nuttall:* She is beginning to adjust.

6. *Mrs. Rivera:* Yes. She come to school without her homework. Now, she does it. Her self-esteem is much better. Now she says, "I know I can do it." Our relationship is much better. I am enjoying her so much. She likes to dress up. Makeup.

7. *Dr. Nuttall:* You are really enjoying her!

8. *Mrs. Rivera:* Yes. Before she was very dependent. Now she wants me to recognize her as a teenager. Before she would say she was older, acting like a mother with her brother and sister. I tried to deal with that. I wanted her to just be a child. She protected her brother and sister a lot. She does not want me to scold her. She works a lot at home. She is acting like an older girl. I have accepted her like that.

9. *Dr. Nuttall:* She seems to want to help you.

10. *Mrs. Rivera:* She is very aware of everything, especially in crisis with father. When she was in first grade, father would come to the house and shout. She was aware. She did not say anything. She seems OK with me. It is better. She says it is more pleasant not having ma and pa together. She saw one versus the other. After she spend a month in Puerto Rico, it was awful. Ramon is a very cold man and the children are like me. They are always touching. I hug, kiss, and touch my children all the time. Ramon called me on the phone and told me the children were driving him crazy because they are too physical. He and I are very different. He is very lonely. He needs to get along with the children. Maria knows he is boring, he is not tender, but he is papa.

11. *Dr. Nuttall:* She seems to have learned to accept her father as he is. Does he help you with the children financially?

12. *Mrs. Rivera:* I was pushed to explain my financial situation to the children last year. He had only given me $175 in 3 years. I was desperate. I didn't have money. It was very hard. It was my fault. I always solved everything. I was like a superwoman. He is a physician and took advantage. Last summer I took him to court. Now am getting $325 a month. That is still not enough.

13. *Dr. Nuttall:* That can barely pay the rent. What are his visitation rights?

14. *Mrs. Rivera:* Every other weekend. He was not doing it. He never saw them. He started establishing a relationship with Maria here. She is very sharp. It was hard. They did not want to see him. The children did not know Ramon. When he was going to medical school he spent all the time studying. Afterwards he spend his time studying for the licensing board exam and setting up his practice. They would cry. They thought he was going to keep them. It was very uncomfortable for 6 months. I decided to come to the States. I brought Maria. Carmen, her younger sister, was left with my parents. She is very happy with them. Right now, my parents are with me. Carmen sits on their laps. She is their nurse, brings their medicines. They play a lot with her. She is marvelous. She is the apple of their eyes. She stayed with them for 6 months. It was real hard for Maria and I. I am very appreciative of the teacher. She helped her a lot. I could not help her. I can do it now. I have never been by myself. Last year I was going out with Manuel, a classmate. I started therapy. I used to cry a lot. I am "mine" now. I stopped therapy a month ago. My parents came up to help me finish my dissertation.

15. *Dr. Nuttall:* You are interviewing yourself. You have told me a great deal about the family environment that has surrounded Maria during her life. I would like to know now what are some of her developmental milestones. When did she walk?

16. *Mrs. Rivera:* Maria? She was 8 months. I have a film of her walking. She talked early, too. She was very independent. She would put a towel to help her climb places. I was breast-feeding. I would carry her around. I would talk to her. She was too independent. I had to watch her. She would go to a little store and buy things. Well liked by everybody in the neighborhod. They would ask her to come in. Real nice life for her first 4 years. She liked to dance a lot. She has had four and a half years of formal ballet.

17. *Dr. Nuttall:* Did she attend nursery school?

18. *Mrs. Rivera:* When she was four and a half in—I was working and studying in Ponce. She went to a day-care center from 9 to 12. Then she would go to my parents and I picked her up there.

19. *Dr. Nuttall:* Where did she go to kindergarten?

20. *Mrs. Rivera:* In Ponce. She attended the—School in—. This is a very good place. Parents buy books for the kids, paper towels. A lot of parent involvement. Something between a private and public school, but they do not pay the teachers.

21. *Dr. Nuttall:* How was kindergarten for Maria? How did she do?

22. *Mrs. Rivera:* Wonderful. She was with a beautiful teacher. The experience was good.

23. *Dr. Nuttall:* What about first grade? How did she like it?

24. *Mrs. Rivera:* First grade was hard. Last semester was hard. The crisis in the marriage. Verbal battles. Ramon would get physical. He would hit me and push me. The teacher was going through a similar situation. I found out too late. She was always shouting at the children. Maria did not want to go to school. I called a psychologist friend of mine. She suggested that I play teacher with her. I did. The teacher would shout at the kids "I am going to tear your hair off!" ("Te voy a halar por las grenas.") I tried hard to help her. I have a big sense of hierarchy. I was afraid of asking for her to be changed.

   I am in the same position in school right now. I have talked to Mr. Smith, the principal, about Juan not saluting the flag. I am making them stand for their own culture. All those are acts of responsibility. They have had a chance to be proud about their own culture. I am trying to make them feel proud, and saluting the flag does not help it. Juan is afraid because of what the other children may say.

25. *Dr. Nuttall:* It is good that you make your children proud of their own culture. You should bring that point up with the principal. Now, let's see where we are. You have told me about Maria's early childhood, child care, kindergarten, and first grade. Did she have any difficulty learning in first grade?

26. *Mrs. Rivera:* Hard to consider school evaluation. I do not care much about grades. I am more interested in whether the children are developing skills.

27. *Dr. Nuttall:* I do not mean grades. I mean was she learning to read and do math?

28. *Mrs. Rivera:* She learned to read easily. Math—she hated it. She didn't like it at all. Didn't want to do the homework. When I tried to help her she would say, "You are not my teacher, you are my mother." I talked to the teacher, but it did not help. In second grade was different. She had an older teacher. She was good. She helped her a lot. Maria was tired of school.

29. *Dr. Nuttall:* How did she get along with her peers?

30. *Mrs. Rivera:* She would say, "Nobody likes me. Nobody likes to play with me." She preferred to have one friend. Did not want to share her with anyone else. She was very possessive until last year. She has started to share.

31. *Dr. Nuttall:* What happened in third grade?

32. *Mrs. Rivera:* I thought it would be good to be in a bilingual classroom. We came in August. Hard for us. Summer camp was real good and supportive. She went half-day to give myself half-day. She would not get to bed by herself. Her teacher knew Spanish and practice her Spanish with her. She took her to many places in —. I took her to first-grade bilingual program in —. Instead of integrating the children, they formed a little separate group. I was not feeling good about her program. I told them. They placed her in ESL. It was a good decision. Maria felt protected by teacher. Teacher would let her wear her shoes. They went to school and they would call them names. They came crying home. "They are calling us pigs." I told them it was not pigs, but "spics." I told them that they were just jealous because they could speak two languages and that made people uncomfortable. Even the man in the bus didn't care. He told me that was not part of his job to scold the children.

    After I changed them to regular class, they spent a whole year doing nothing. Juan did OK. His teacher liked and helped him. Maria vegetate, doing nothing. She missed the bilingual class because they felt protected by the teacher and the other children.

33. *Dr. Nuttall:* How did she pick up English?

34. *Mrs. Rivera:* It took her time to learn. It wasn't that easy. Mr. X helped her a lot. When she got here she used to understand almost anything. But she blocked, she could not learn anything. TV helped a lot. She is very visual.

35. *Dr. Nuttall:* How did she learn to read English?

36. *Mrs. Rivera:* It was easy because she knew how to read in Spanish. It wasn't very tense. At home, they can't speak English. Language at home is Spanish.

37. *Dr. Nuttall:* I feel that you have given me enough information about Maria's background and educational history. Do you have any further questions or concerns, particularly as to what you want for the future?

38. *Mrs. Rivera:* My main concerns are Maria's self-esteem. Most important. Painful to deal with her. I feel so good with her now. I worry about her tendency to feel possessive and jealous about her friends. Definitions of feelings are hard for her. Expressing her feelings. She tells me, "Mama, I don't know how I feel." Carmen is voluntarily outspoken. Juan is hard to ask, too. Manuel and I split last semester. We broke off last October. He used to visit them, take them back to his apartment. Now we are not giving them double messages. She likes him. She tells me that she prefers to live with me alone, but that she knows I love him. So it is OK if I live with him. I know it affects them. They lost their father and now they have to get used to another loss.

39. *Dr. Nuttall:* It is hard on the children, but you also have to take care of yourself. You have done a great deal for your children.

40. *Mrs. Rivera:* I am concerned with concepts related to math. Time measurement. She has been doing much better. When she came in, she did not understand concepts such as 10 years, a century. Next year I would like to move my two youngest children to a more structured school. Juan would like more structure. The other day I told him (Juan), "Why do I always have to remind you many times to take out the trash, to do things for me?" He said, "Ma, I like you to remind me, I need it." That is why I think he needs a more structured school. For Maria, it would be good to stay. At home we

have flexible structure. Last night the grandparents were telling the children stories about their childhood. It was 9:30 and the children were not in bed.

41. *Dr. Nuttall:* I know how you worry about your children being tired for school, but their grandparents are not going to be around forever and it is good for the children to have good relationships with them. This situation does not happen all the time.

42. *Mrs. Rivera:* That is true and my parents are here to help me finish. With them here I will be able to make more progress. I will like Juan to have a workup just like Maria's. I want to know how he's doing. I must go now. I have to teach a class in 15 minutes. Thank you.

43. *Dr. Nuttall:* Thank you. I will try to do all I can to help you. The information that you gave me is going to be very useful for our testing. I will see you Tuesday.

Counselor: Thank you, Mrs. Rivera, for allowing me to sit for this meeting. I learned a lot about Maria. See you Tuesday.

Epilogue

In the context of the total evaluation workup performed on this child, this interview provided much needed information to formulate the case study and to create a model of this child, her family, and her school. Because the interview was conducted by an educated person from the same ethnic and linguistic group and sex as the interviewee, rapport was easily established and a general atmosphere of trust was created which pervaded the whole session. The high level of education of the mother and her past experience in therapy also contributed to the positive nature of the interaction. These conditions yielded data that we feel were reliable, valid, and useful in formulating a program for this child. If Freud had been present during this interview, he would have described it as "cathartic."

From the mother's report, we concluded that emotional factors were a very important component of the problems that this child was experiencing in school. Because her early development as described by the mother was normal, we were able to rule out the possibility of an organic basis for her problems. Facts obtained about her educational history helped us to better understand her present adjustment to school.

The mother's description of the present and past family situation made us aware of the many stresses that this child had faced and was facing. Her way of describing the problems also informed us that the mother was caring, emotionally stable, and ready to do anything to help her daughter. This knowledge was extremely important in designing educational and psychological treatment plans for this child.

The positive nature of the interview set the tone for the team meeting that followed and later encounters with the mother which centered around finding an appropriate therapist for her daughter. This case history interview demonstrates that when conducted properly, they contribute greatly to a useful and informative personality assessment.

Appendix

Suggested Case History Interview Areas and Questions

Clarifying Referral Questions
  What brings you here?
  What is happening?

What concerns you?

Family Background

Family size: If divorce, death, adoption, or separation have occurred (ask when, reaction of child, frequency child sees other parent)

Sibling order

Occupation of parents

Education of parents

How long in present home?

Where did you live before?

What language do parents speak at home?

How well do parents speak English? Other languages spoken at home?

Family support systems

Development: Infancy

When did child walk?

When did child talk?

When was child toilet trained?

What was child like as a baby? Colicky? Easy?

Were there any complications during pregnancy and delivery?

Has child had any serious illnesses or operations?

What was the child's personality like? Happy/optimistic? Sad/pessimistic? Outgoing/introverted? Calm/jumpy? Flexible/stubborn? Leader/follower?

Did child attend nursery school? What kind? Were there any problems?

Does child have any friends in neighborhood? Nearby relatives? School friends?

What does child do in free time?

Parental Values during Infancy

How do you discipline your child when he or she does something you feel is wrong?

When child pleases you, how do you let him or her know?

Do you help your child with schoolwork? How?

Childhood

Nursery school attendance: When? Where? What type?

Peer relationships: Played with outside children? Stayed in backyard and played with siblings?

Kindergarten: Any problems? Any strengths?

School: Graded obtained, repeated, any problems

Subjects liked or disliked

Friendships: Loner? Many friends?

Membership in formal recreational or academic groups: Dance? Sports? Scouts?

Informal groups: Neighborhood? Family?

Hobbies

Parental Values during Childhood

Parents' feelings about children's school performance?

Do they demand responsibility?

Restrictions? Autonomy?

Discipline?

Adolescence

Academic grades

Subjects enjoyed, subjects disliked

Subjects failed

Study habits

Nonacademic school activities: sports, drama, art

Peer relationships

Leadership qualities

Relationship to parents

Difficulties with alcohol? Drugs?

Reaction to physical changes and physical appearance

Gender identity

Independence vs. dependence

Work experience

Money and allowances

Hobbies or special interests

Career interests or goals
College or vocational plans
Parental Values during Adolescence
  Sexuality
  Independence
  College attendance

References

Anastasi, A. (1982). *Psychological testing*. New York: Macmillan.

Breuer, J., & Freud, S. (1957). *Studies on hysteria*. New York: Basic Books.

Covner, B. J. (1944). Studies in phonographic recordings of verbal materials, IV. Written reports of interviews. *Journal of Applied Psychology, 28*, 89–98.

Dillman, D. A. (1978). *Mail and telephone surveys: The total design method*. New York: Wiley.

Dyer, H. S. (1976). *The interview as a measuring device in education*. Princeton, NJ: ERIC Clearinghouse on Tests, Measurement and Evaluation, Educational Testing Service.

Ennis, B. J., & Litwack, T. R. (1974). Psychiatry and the presumption of expertise: Flipping coins in the courtroom. *California Law Review, 62*, 693–752.

Fisher, J., Epstein, L. J., & Harris, M. R. (1967). Validity of the psychiatric interview. *Archives of General Psychiatry, 17*, 744–750.

Fleming, L., & Snyder, W. W. (1947). Social and personal changes following non-directive group play therapy. *American Journal of Orthopsychiatry, 17*, 101–116.

Hall, C. S., & Lindzey, G. (1957). *Theories of personality*. New York: Wiley.

Helzer, J. E., Clayton, P. I., Pambakian, R., Reich, T., & Wish, E. D. (1977). Reliability of psychiatric diagnosis. II. The test-retest reliability of diagnostic classification. *Archives of General Psychiatry, 34*, 136–141.

Herjanic, B., Herjanic, M., Brown, F., & Wheatt, T. (1975). Are children reliable reporters? *Journal of Abnormal Child Psychology, 3*, 41–48.

Hunt, W. A. (1951). An investigation of naval neuropsychiatric screening procedures. In H. Guetzkow (Ed.), *Groups, leadership, and men* (pp. 245–256). Pittsburgh, PA: Carnegie Press.

Hunt, W. A. (1955). A rationale for psychiatric selection. *American Psychologist, 10*, 199–204.

Hunt, W. A., Herrmann, R. S., & Noble, H. (1957). The specificity of the psychiatric interview. *Journal of Clinical Psychology, 13*, 49–53.

Ivey, A. (1971). *Microcounseling*. Springfield, IL: Charles C Thomas.

Ivey, A. (1983). *Intentional interviewing and counseling*. Monterey, CA: Brooks/Cole.

Ivey, A. (in press). *Genetic epistemology and developmental counseling and therapy*. San Francisco, CA: Jossey-Bass.

Ivey, A., & Authier, J. (1978). *Microcounseling* (2nd ed.). Springfield, IL: Charles C Thomas.

Ivey, A. E., & Matthews, W. (in press). A five stage meta-model of the interview. *Journal of Counseling and Development*.

Kantor, D., & Lehr, W. (1975). *Inside the family*. San Francisco, CA: Jossey-Bass.

Katz, D. (1942). Do interviewers bias poll results? *Public Opinion Quarterly, 6*, 248–268.

Kelly, E. L., & Goldberg, L. R. (1959). Correlates of later performance and specialization in psychology: A follow-up study of the trainees assessed in the VA Selection Research Project. *Psychological Monographs, 73* (12, Whole no. 482).

Kelly, G. (1955). *The psychology of personal constructs*. New York: Norton.

Lambert, N. M., Windmiller, M., Cole, L., & Figueroa, R. A. (1975). Standardization of a public school version of the AAMD. *Mental Retardation, 13*, 3–7.

Maloney, M. P., & Ward, M. P. (1976). *Psychological assessment: A conceptual approach*. London & New York: Oxford University Press.

Marsella, T., & Pedersen, P. (1981). *Cross-cultural counseling and psychotherapy*. Oxford: Pergamon.

Matarazzo, J. D. (1965). The interview. In B. J. Wolman (Ed.), *Handbook of clinical psychology* (pp. 403–451). New York: McGraw-Hill.

Matarazzo, J. D. (1978). The interview: Its reliability and validity in psychiatric diagnosis. In B. J. Wolman (Ed.), *Clinical diagnosis of mental disorders: A handbook* (pp. 47–96). New York: Plenum Press.

Mercer, J. (1979). *SOMPA (System of Multicultural Pluralistic Assessment): Technical manual*. New York: Psychological Corporation.

Myers, R. A., & Cairo, P. C. (Eds.). (1983). Computer assisted counseling. *Counseling Psychologist, 11.*

Prout, H. T. (1983). School psychologists and social-emotional assessment techniques: Patterns in training and use. *School Psychology Review, 12,* 377–383.

Rice, S. A. (1929). Contagious bias in the interview. *American Journal of Sociology, 35,* 420–423.

Robinson, D., & Rohde, S. (1946). Two experiments with an anti-semitism poll. *Journal of Abnormal Social Psychology Quarterly, 41,* 136–144.

Rogers, C. R., & Dymond, R. F. (1954). *Psychotherapy and personality change.* Chicago, IL: University of Chicago Press.

Snyder, W. U. (1961). *The psychotherapy relationship.* New York: Macmillan.

Sparrow, S. S., Balla, D. A., & Cicchetti, D. V. (1984). *Vineland Adaptive Behavior Scales.* Circle Pines, MN: American Guidance Service.

Spitzer, R. L., Cohen, J., Fleiss, J. L., & Endicott, J. (1967). Quantification of agreement in psychiatric diagnosis. *Archives of General Psychiatry, 17,* 83–87.

Sue, D. (1981). *Counseling the culturally different.* New York: Wiley.

Sue, D., Bernier, J., Duran, A., Feinberg, L., Pedersen, P., Smith, E., & Vazquez-Nuttall, E. (1982). Cross-cultural counseling competencies. *Counseling Psychologist, 10,* 45–52.

Sullivan, H. S. (1953). *The interpersonal theory of psychiatry.* New York: Norton.

Sullivan, H. S. (1954). *The psychiatric interview.* New York: Norton.

Vazquez-Nuttall, E., Avila-Vivas, Z., & Morales-Barreto, G. (1984). Working with Latin American families. In B. Okun (Ed.), *Family therapy with families with school related problems* (pp. 74–88). Rockville, MD: Aspen Systems Corporation.

Vazquez-Nuttall, E., Goldman, P., & Medeiros, P. (1983). *A study of mainstreamed limited English proficient handicapped students in bilingual education.* Newton, MA: Vazquez-Nuttall Associates.

Veldman, D. J. (1967). Computer-based sentence completion interview. *Journal of Counseling Psychology, 14,* 153–157.

Webb, L. J., DiClemente, C. C., Johnstone, E. E., Sanders, J. L., & Perley, R. A. (1981). *DSM III training guide.* New York: Brunner/Mazel.

Wittson, C. L., & Hunt, W. A. (1951). The predictive value of the brief psychiatric interview. *American Journal of Psychiatry, 107,* 582–585.

Yarrow, L. J. (1960). Interviewing children. In P. H. Mussen (Ed.), *Handbook of research methods in child development* (pp. 561–603). New York: Wiley.

Zusman, M. E., Olson, A. O., & Garcia, G. (1975, March). *Gathering complete responses from Mexican-Americans by personal interview.* Paper presented at the annual meeting of the Southwestern Sociological Association, San Antonio, TX.

Assessing Children and Adolescents with the Rorschach

Irving B. Weiner

The first Rorschach study published in the United States described the personality characteristics of mentally retarded children examined in the New York City Children's School on Randall's Island (Beck, 1930). Over the years, a great many articles and numerous books have specifically addressed the Rorschach assessment of children and adolescents (e.g., Ames, Learned, Metraux, & Walker, 1973; Ames, Metraux, & Walker, 1971; Exner & Weiner, 1982; Halpern, 1953; Levitt & Truumaa, 1972). Despite this long history and extensive literature, however, reliable information on young persons' Rorschachs has only recently begun to accumulate.

The slow progress in this area has been due largely to the fact that since the 1930s there has not been any one Rorschach test. Instead, several different methods of using the 10 inkblots published with Rorschach's (1921/1942) monograph have evolved. These several methods or "systems" prescribe different ways of administering the test and coding or "scoring" subjects' responses. Work by Exner (1974, chap. 2) has demonstrated that these differences produce significant variations in the data that are obtained.

For example, the number of percepts that subjects report depends on how the test is administered. If Rorschach's original instructions are used (presenting the inkblot and asking, "What might this be?") and some encouragement is given on the first card if the child provides only one response ("You may see some other things if you look at it a little longer"), subjects give an average of 23.9 responses. This is the administration procedure suggested by Klopfer and Davidson (1962). If, instead, the examiner says, "Tell me everything that you can see" and offers encouragement on each of the first five cards if only one response is given, subjects give an average of 31.2 responses. These are Beck's (1950) instructions, and the resulting number of responses is significantly ($p < .05$) greater than with Klopfer's instructions.

Many Rorschach summary scores also vary with the method that is used. A

Irving B. Weiner. Office of Academic Affairs, Fairleigh Dickinson University, Rutherford, New Jersey.

"flying bat" is scored *FM* (Animal Movement) in Klopfer's system and *F* (Form) in Beck's system; some location choices that involve most but not all of a blot are scored as a "cutoff" *W* (Whole) by Klopfer but as a *D* (Common Detail Response) or *Dd* (Unusual Detail Response) following Beck. These and other differences between these two (and other) Rorschach systems can generate wide disparities in how Rorschach responses are coded by examiners of different persuasions. To complicate this problem further, many psychologists have combined elements from different systems in their teaching and use of the test and have even added idiosyncratic "wrinkles" of their own (Exner & Exner, 1972; Jackson & Wohl, 1966).

When scientists use the same terms in different ways and practitioners apply generic labels to their own uniquely evolved methods, they create serious obstacles to building a systematic knowledge base for either clinical or research purposes. This is not to deny or disparage a practitioner's ability to derive accurate impressions of personality functioning from a self-styled Rorschach approach. However, chaos is a big price to pay for this, and effective communication to enhance the skills of others and foster cumulative knowledge requires something more: It requires strict adherence to a method of administration and scoring prescribed by some standard published system and to uniform interpretation of results in light of normative data developed within that system.

The presentation in this chapter will follow the Rorschach Comprehensive System (Exner, 1974; Exner, Weiner, & Schuyler, 1978). Aside from the widespread familiarity of psychodiagnosticians with this system, two important substantive considerations recommend its use in the personality assessment of younger people. First, all of the scoring codes in the Comprehensive System have achieved substantial interscorer agreement (correlations of .85 or more) among trained examiners. This means that readers acquainted with the system will know exactly what is meant by scores, percentages, and ratios mentioned in the presentation, since they will be virtually identical to the scores, ratios, and percentages they would have obtained working with the same responses.

Second, an extensive data bank compiled in the development and continuing refinement of the Comprehensive System includes detailed normative information on the Rorschach performance of children and adolescents. These developmental norms are based on the protocols of 1,870 nonpatient young people, 5 to 16 years old, tested by 147 examiners in different parts of the country. In proportions roughly comparable to United States census data, this sample includes males and females, white and minority youngsters, members of different socioeconomic groups, and residents of urban, suburban, and rural homes. The number of records at each of the 12 age levels from 5 to 16 ranges from 105 to 150 (Exner & Weiner, 1982, chap. 3). These normative data, together with considerable additional Comprehensive System data on the Rorschach performance of young people with various kinds of adjustment difficulties, provide valuable points of comparison in interpreting the records of children and adolescents.

Although a brief review will follow, this chapter will assume knowledge of the basic principles of administering, scoring, and interpreting the Rorschach within the framework of the Comprehensive System. The primary goal of this chapter is to demonstrate the effectiveness of the Rorschach in assessing child and adolescent personality functioning. To that end, the discussion will address (*a*) the nature of the Rorschach method and why it provides valid information about people, (*b*) special considerations in interpreting the Rorschach responses of younger subjects, (c) the use of Rorschach indices in identifying some major patterns of developmental psychopathology, and (d) the analysis of a Rorschach protocol in an illustrative case.

The Nature of the Rorschach

In conducting personality assessments with the Rorschach method, clinicians need to recognize that it was originally developed and still operates primarily as a perceptual–cognitive task. Subjects are presented with 10 inkblots and asked, "What might this be?" As subjects respond during this Free Association phase of the test, the examiner records all of their responses verbatim. After completing all 10 blots, the examiner goes back through the cards again, reading aloud each response and asking the subject which part of the blot was used for it ("Where did you see it?") and what suggested this particular response ("What made it look like that?"). This is called the Inquiry Phase, and it provides the information to help score the subject's responses. For records of average length, it takes approximately 45 minutes to complete the Rorschach administration in this fashion.

The Response Process

In a literal sense, there is only one correct response to the administration directions: "An inkblot!" But this is not an acceptable response. Instead, subjects are required to misperceive the blot—to see it as something that it is not. How they respond in this problem-solving situation is a function of certain interactions between what they see (perception) and what they decide to articulate (cognition). Both the perceptual and the cognitive elements of this interaction are influenced by several factors that constitute what has come to be known as the response process (Exner, 1978, chap. 2; 1983). The four chief factors in the response process are the following:

1. The nature of the stimulus itself, particularly with respect to compelling features of the blots or "stimulus pulls" that lead most people to classify the blots in certain ways.
2. Subject concerns about making a particular kind of impression or behaving in a socially desirable manner such that they censor their responses, expressing some of their percepts and keeping others to themselves.
3. Various personality traits that dispose people to structure their experience in individually characteristic ways.
4. Situational psychological states that affect how people structure their experience at the time they are being examined.

These features of the response process provide a critical context for Rorschach interpretation. As an introduction to interpretive principles, a review of the basic scoring categories in the Comprehensive System is in order.

Scoring

Each individual response to a Rorschach card is scored or, technically, coded. The Comprehensive System currently includes some 90 possible scores organized into seven major categories: Location, Determinant(s), Form Quality, Organizational Activity, Popularity, Content(s), and Special Scores. A Structural Summary, which shows all of the possible system scores, plus various ratios, percentages, and derivations that summarize these scores or codes, can be seen in the Case Study at the end of this chapter.

The Location score uses one symbol to describe the part of the blot used by the respondent (*W* for the whole blot, *D* for a common detail, *Dd* for an uncommon detail, and *S* for white space) and a second symbol for the developmental or cognitive quality of the responses ($\pm$ for synthesized, *o* for ordinary, *v* for vague, and $-$ for arbitrary). The Determinant scores code the features of the blot or the subject's impressions of it that contributed to the formulation of the response. The symbols and criteria used for these determinants and for several other summary scores are listed in Table 5-1. A *Z* score is assigned if the response has been organized in some way; *P* (popular) is assigned if the response is one that is very commonly given; and the Content(s) are simply abbreviations for various categories of objects (e.g., *H* for human, *A* for animal, *Na* for nature, etc.). Several Special Scorings denote unusual verbal material (e.g., *PSV* for perseveration, *MOR* for morbid content, *DV* for deviant verbalizations).

All seven (potentially) of the scoring categories are organized in a specific order such that any response can be coded. For example, a response to Card II of "It's a couple of clowns in a circus dancing around together, and they've got these black costumes on and they've hurt themselves, because it's red and bloody down here" would be scored as follows:

$$W+ \qquad Ma.FC'.CFo \qquad (H),Cg,B1 \qquad 4.5 \qquad MOR$$

Here the *W +* denotes that the whole blot was used in a synthesized fashion. The *Ma* indicates active human movement blended with an *FC'* or form-dominant achromatic color (the black costumes) and a *CF* or color–form (the blood). The *o* denotes perceptually accurate use of the blot with respect to the form quality of the response. The content scores refer respectively to the less-than-real human figure, the clothing, and the blood included in the response. Finally, there are a 4.5 *Z* (organizational) score for use of the entire blot and a MOR for the morbid quality of being hurt and bloody.

Interpretation

Given the factors discussed above that influence a subject's response process, Rorschach interpretation is guided by two assumptions. First, we assume that the manner in which subjects articulate their impressions of the inkblots provides a representative sample of how they structure other kinds of perceptual–cognitive experience. In other words, to the extent that the Rorschach is a problem-solving situation, people will attempt to solve it in the same manner as they attempt to solve problems in their lives, and they will utilize the same kinds of coping mechanisms or styles that they employ whenever they are faced with making decisions or taking action. Consistent with the trait–state distinction, moreover, some features of Rorschach behavior will reflect characteristic ways in which subjects cope with experience, whereas other features will reflect more transient, situationally determined tendencies to deal with the Rorschach in a particular manner.

The second interpretative assumption is that, if we can identify the psychological corollaries of structuring the Rorschach task in certain ways, we can

Table 5-1
Scoring Symbols Used in the Rorschach Comprehensive System[a]

Symbol	Explanation
F	*Form answers.* To be used separately for responses based exclusively on the form features of the blot, or in combination with other determinant scoring symbols (except *M* and *m*) when the form features have contributed to the formulation of a percept.
M	*Human movement response.* To be used for responses clearly involving a kinesic perception, the content of which involves behavior restricted to human or, in animals, is human-like.
FM	*Animal movement response.* To be used for responses involving a kinesthetically marked movement involving animals. The movement perceived must be congruent to the species identified in the content.
m	*Inanimate movement response.* To be used for responses involving the movement of an inanimate, inorganic, or insensate object.
C	*Pure color response.* To be used for responses based exclusively on the chromatic color features of the blot. No form is involved.
CF	*Color–form response.* To be used for responses that are formulated because of the color features of the blot or blot area and the form involved is of secondary importance.
FC	*Form–color response.* To be used for responses that are formulated because of the form of the blot area and in which color is used secondarily for purposes of clarification and/or elaboration.
Cn	*Color naming response.* To be used when the colors of the blot or blot area are identified by name with no form involved and with the intention of presenting a response.
C'	*Pure achromatic color response.* To be used when the response is based exclusively on the gray-black-white features of the blot or blot area, as they are identified as color. No form is involved.
C'F	*Achromatic color–form response.* To be used when the response is based primarily on the gray-black-white features of the blot or blot area, as they are identified as color, and where the form has been involved secondarily.
FC'	*Form–achromatic color response.* To be used when the response is based primarily on form and the achromatic coloring of the blot or blot area is used for purposes of elaboration and/or clarification.
T	*Pure texture response.* To be used for responses where the shading components of the blot are interpreted as representing a textural phenomenon with no involvement of the form of the blot.
TF	*Texture–form response.* To be used for responses where the shading features of the blot or blot area are interpreted as texture, and form is used secondarily for purposes of elaboration and/or clarification.
FT	*Form–texture response.* To be used for responses in which form is a primary determinant and the shading is interpreted as textural for purposes of clarification and/or elaboration.
V	*Pure vista response.* To be used when the shading features of the blot or blot area are interpreted as depth or dimensionality with no form involvement.
VF	*Vista–form response.* To be used for responses in which the shading components of the blot or blot area are interpreted as depth or dimensionality and the form features are used for purposes of clarification and/or elaboration.
FV	*Form–vista response.* To be used for responses in which form is the primary determinant and the shading features are included secondarily to represent depth or dimensionality.
Y	*Pure shading response.* To be used for responses based exclusively on the light–dark features of the blot that are completely formless and do not involve either reference to texture or vista.
YF	*Shading–form response.* To be used for responses based primarily on the light–dark features of the blot or blot area in which the form features are used for

(continued)

Table 5-1
(Continued)

Symbol	Explanation
	purposes of elaboration and/or clarification.
FY	*Form–shading response.* To be used for responses that are based primarily on the form of the blot or blot area in which the shading features are used for purposes of clarification and/or elaboration.
FD	*Form-based dimensional responses.* To be used for responses that are identified as having depth or dimensions based exclusively on the form features of the blot or blot area. No shading is involved.
(2)	*Pair response.* To be used for responses in which the content includes two objects identified and that are based on the symmetrical features of the blot or blot area. The objects identified must be similar in all respects, but must not be identified as "reflected" or "mirror images."
rF	*Reflection–form response.* To be used for responses in which the blot or blot area is perceived as a reflection (because of the symmetry), and the content or object reflected has no specific form requirements.
Fr	*Form–reflection response.* To be used for responses in which the blot or blot area is identified because of its form and is also perceived as reflected or "mirrored" because of the symmetry features.
a : p	*Active–passive ratio.* This is a ratio that shows the number of active and passive movement responses in the record. All types of movement are included (*M, FM,* and *m*).
Afr	*Affective ratio.* This represents the proportion of response occurring to the last three cards. It is obtained by dividing the number of responses to Cards VIII–X by the number of responses to Cards I–VII.
3r + 2/R	*Egocentricity index.* This represents the proportion of reflection and pair answers in the record. It is obtained by dividing the sum of three times the number of reflections plus the number of pairs by the total number of responses.
L	*Lambda.* This represents the ratio of pure *F* responses in the record to all non-pure *F* responses; it is obtained by dividing the former by the latter.
X + %	*Form quality.* This percentage represents the proportion of good form quality responses appearing in the record. It is calculated by dividing the sum of all plus and ordinary form quality responses by the total number of responses.
Sum C	*Weighted color use.* This score is obtained by adding 0.5 points for each *FC* scored in a record, 1 point for each *CF*, and 1.5 points for each *C*.
Zd	*Incorporation index.* This is a difference score obtained by subtracting the estimated *Z* score for a record, as based on the frequency of organized responses, from the sum of the *Z* scores obtained. The ratio of the sum of the human movement determines (*M*), including those in blends, to the weighted sum of the chromatic color determinants (*Sum C*).
EB	
EA	The sum of the two elements in the *EB: M + Sum C*. The ratio of the sum of *FM*
eb	plus *m* determinants to the sum of all shading and achromatic color determinants.
ep	The sum of the two elements in the *eb: FM + m +* all *T +* all *Y +* all *V +* all *C'*.
Four Square	Reference to the four summary scores of *EB, EA, eb*, and *ep*.

[a]Based on Exner, Weiner, and Schuyler (1978).

draw valid inferences from subjects' responses concerning their characteristic dispositions and current emotional and attitudinal states. A few examples should help to clarify these concepts and illustrate the interaction between what people see in the inkblots and what they decide to articulate during the response process.

To begin with location choice, the subject must initially scan or encode the stimulus inkblot. We know from eye-tracking studies that subjects typically scan every part of an inkblot within less than a second of its presentation (Exner, 1983). Yet very few subjects deliver responses that account for every detail of every blot. Instead, people vary in how much organizing activity they undertake in formulating their Rorschach responses. Some use the entire blot or combine several parts of it into their responses, in which case they have a high Z (organizing) frequency; others, even though they also have scanned the blots entirely, decide to use only isolated details in their responses, which results in a low Z frequency.

This difference suggests that the first kind of person tends to deal with experience by focusing on broad issues and by formulating relationships between events, perhaps at the expense of losing sight of individual trees in the forest. The second kind of person, by contrast, prefers to focus on narrow issues and discrete events, perhaps sometimes losing sight of the forest for the trees. Since Z frequency is a stable index of response preference, with a retest reliability of .83 among nonpatient adults, the differences between these two kinds of people, as represented in their Rorschach behavior, probably identifies abiding dispositions that have in the past and will in the future characterize their individual coping styles.

Looking at determinants, there is a good reason to believe that almost every subject who says "Bat" on Card I is being influenced by the gray–black features of this blot. If Card I is presented to subjects in some chromatic color, the frequency of the popular "Bat" response decreases dramatically; in fact, when this stimulus was shown as blue to one large sample of adults, not one of them classified it as a bat. Yet only 1 in 100 subjects who report a bat on Card I articulate the gray–black features as helping them see it—*unless* they happen to be depressed, in which case 22 per 100 subjects articulate C' or Y in giving a bat response (Exner, 1959, 1983).

The psychological corollaries of C' and Y include feelings of gloom and helplessness. Hence, the difference between being influenced by the gray–black features of Card I and articulating these features as the determinant of their response appears to be at least partly a function of whether the subject is experiencing depressive affect. Additionally, since C' is only a moderately stable determinant (retest reliability of .67 among nonpatient adults) and Y is fairly unstable (retest reliability of .41), a subject's inclination to articulate in this way suggests a state of depressed affect rather than a trait of being prone to persistent or recurrent depression.

As an example related to content, research indicates that most adults have little difficulty seeing a penis at the top of Card VI and will say as much if they are led to believe that this is an acceptable percept commonly reported by well-adjusted people (Exner, 1978, chap. 2). Under conditions of standard Rorschach administration, however, this response is rarely given. In the absence of special instructions to the contrary, most subjects apparently feel that saying "penis," even if they clearly see it, would be inappropriate and give a bad impression. Hence they censor this and other sex responses, unless (*a*) they are being examined by someone they know well, such as their own therapist, in which case the frequency of sex responses goes up (Exner, Armbruster, & Mittman, 1978); (*b*) they are struggling with sexual anxieties or preoccupations that override their concerns about propriety; or (*c*) they are suffering from some loss of control over their ideation or some impairment of their capacity for social judgment. Accordingly, sex responses appearing in a standard administration with an examiner who is a stranger to the subject, especially when they are numerous or dramatic, suggest one of these latter two circumstances.

In this way, through all of the location, determinant, and content categories (and all of the ratios and percentages in the Rorschach Structural Summary), interpretation proceeds by identifying idiographic, nonnormative features of a subject's responses and then drawing on known psychological corollaries of these features to formulate hypotheses about the subject's personality characteristics. In addition to using the structural data to generalize from the subject's way of coping with the Rorschach to how he or she is likely to cope with other life situations, clinicians may also find clues to a person's underlying attitudes and concerns in their thematic imagery. Administered properly, the Rorschach calls only for subjects to indicate "What might this be?" and to help the examiner " . . . see it the way you saw it." At times, however, subjects embellish their responses on their own initiative as if questions appropriate to the TAT had been asked, such as who the figures are, what they are doing, what led up to the situation, and what will happen next. Thus, a response to Card III might be, "Two stupid people who don't like each other very much, and they've just had an argument, and they're thinking about why they can't find a way to get along better."

Such thematic embellishments in Rorschach responses often reveal how people feel toward important figures in their lives, what they hope or fear might happen in the future, the kind of self-image they have, and how they regard previous experiences that have shaped their lives. Added to the inferences about personality traits and states that can be derived from the structural data, hypotheses about such personality dynamics based on thematic imagery enrich Rorschach interpretations and help provide a three-dimensional picture of the subject.

Two considerations should govern the interpretation of content elaborations, however. First, hypothesizing about personality dynamics on the basis of thematic imagery is a more highly inferential and subjective process than drawing general conclusions about coping styles from the subject's style of coping with the Rorschach as a specific problem-solving task. Hence, practitioners need to exercise more caution and express less certainty when they are working from content elaborations than when they are generalizing from the structural data (see Exner & Weiner, 1982, chap. 1; Goldfried, Stricker, & Weiner, 1971, chap. 13; Weiner, 1977).

Second, although content elaborations enrich a Rorschach protocol, they are not crucial to forming valid and useful impressions of personality functioning. Clinicians who regard the Rorschach primarily as a measure of fantasy may consider a record with meager thematic imagery as too "sterile" or "guarded" to indicate very much about the subject's personality. To the contrary, however, a record will not be too sketchy to interpret meaningfully so long as the subject has given close to an average number of responses and has articulated some range of location choices, determinants, and content categories.

The Rorschach is primarily a measure of perceptual–cognitive style, in which the subject's problem-solving approach reflects key dimensions of his or her psychological traits and states. Hence, detailed personality descriptions, diagnostic formulations, and treatment prescriptions can often be formulated in the absence of content elaborations and independently of them even when they are abundant. For this reason, the recommended approach to interpretation with the Comprehensive System involves first identifying the salient features of a subject's personality structure as indicated by the data in the Structural Summary, and then generating whatever additional hypotheses about the subject's personality dynamics that may be suggested by the available thematic imagery.

Interpreting the Rorschach Responses of Younger Subjects

Clinicians trained and experienced in using the Rorschach with adults are sometimes hesitant to interpret the records of younger people. Such hesitancy is largely unwarranted because the psychological corollaries of Rorschach response styles are identical among persons of all ages; that is, a particular aspect of Rorschach behavior has the same general meaning whether the subject is a child, an adolescent, or an adult. There is only one set of interpretive principles for examiners to learn, and, once mastered, these principles can be applied in clinical work regardless of the age of the client.

On the other hand, the general meaning of Rorschach behaviors can have different specific implications for people in different circumstances or at different ages. For example, indications that a subject feels a high level of distress usually have positive implications if he or she is about to enter insight-oriented psychotherapy, since initial anxiety promotes involvement and continuation in this form of treatment. The same indications usually have negative implications for a person who is in psychotherapy and is being evaluated for termination, since continuing high anxiety suggests that the treatment is not yet finished (Horowitz, 1974; Weiner, 1975, chaps. 2 & 12). Similarly for people of different ages, the same psychological corollaries of Rorschach behavior may signify different degrees of normative development and adaptive coping.

Accordingly, to understand the implications of personality traits and states manifested by a young person at a specific chronological or developmental age, clinicians evaluating children and adolescents need to be familiar with (*a*) normative expectations for Rorschach behavior at various ages, (*b*) normal and abnormal patterns of development that commonly characterize childhood and adolescence, and (*c*) trends toward stability and change in dimensions of personality that affect predictability of behavior from one age to another.

Normative Expectations

As noted earlier, extensive normative data using the Comprehensive System are available for the Rorschach responses of subjects from age 5 to 16. These norms provide the basis for determining the specific implications for a young person's personality functioning in light of the psychological corollaries of his or her responses.

As an example, consider the relationship between the number of *FC* and *CF* responses a subject gives. *FC* responses reflect a fairly controlled and restrained approach to expressing affect, and *FC* emotions tend to be relatively deep and enduring; *CF* responses reflect a fairly spontaneous and labile affective display, and *CF* emotions tend to be relatively shallow and fleeting. With respect to general meaning, the ratio between these two determinants indicates whether any person at any age is more likely to be emotionally reserved or emotionally demonstrative.

In terms of specific implications, however, what do we know about developmental differences from a normative perspective? We expect adults to control their emotional expression most of the time and to form deep and enduring affective attachments as a feature of their maturity. Correspondingly, nonpatient adults average two to three times as many *FC* as *CF* responses (Exner, Weiner, & Schuyler, 1978, Table 7). By contrast, we expect young children to be emotionally spontaneous and demonstrative, not controlled and reserved. Consistent with this expectation, nonpatient 7-year-olds give twice as many *CF* as *FC* responses, and 6-year-olds give three times as many. Only 8% of 6-year-olds give more *FC* than *CF* responses. This proportion increases with age, but even by age 16 only a little more than half (56%) of young people are giving more *FC* than *CF* (Exner & Weiner, 1982, chap. 3).

The implication of these normative data is clear. A predominance of *CF* over *FC* responses in a record is an index of emotional lability. Since emotional lability is expected in children, this Rorschach finding has no special significance in describing a child's personality functioning. On the other hand, a predominance of *FC* over *CF* responses, which would be normative and adaptive for an adult, is not typical of a child's record. Rather, in young people it often identifies maladaptive emotional inhibition or reserve and is associated with problematic peer-group relationships—although overcontrolled, uptight *FC*-dominant children who have difficulty mixing it up with their peers are sometimes praised by adults for their "maturity" and "self-control."

In comparable ways, the normative implications of many Rorschach interpretations change gradually from one age to the next. Practitioners need to take account of these changes while also keeping in mind implications that remain the same regardless of age. Most important among these is the significance of a low form level as an indication of impaired reality testing. Normative data indicate that the average $X + \%$ among nonpatient adults is 81 and that $X + \%$ also averages in the low 80s at every age from 5 to 16. Hence the pathological implications of impaired reality testing are identical and equally serious among children, adolescents, and adults.

Normal and Abnormal Development

Rorschach assessment contributes to clinical practice by providing information about a client's personality functioning. However, identifying personality characteristics is rarely the purpose of a clinical evaluation. Psychodiagnostic consultants are usually being asked to shed some light on a client's problems and suggest helpful interventions. Differential diagnosis and treatment planning thus become the goals of consultation, with Rorschach assessment of personality functioning being one means to these ends.

To translate personality characteristics identified by the Rorschach into diagnostic formulations and treatment suggestions, clinicians must be conversant with current concepts and research relating to psychopathology and psychological intervention. The example above of using Rorschach indices of subjectively felt distress (such as *ep* substantially larger than *EA*) to predict involvement in insight-oriented psychotherapy in one situation and recommend continued treatment in another is a case in point. Clinicians who work with children and adolescents need to be especially knowledgeable about developmental psychology and developmental psychopathology. What kinds of psychological disturbances are likely to appear in children and adolescents, for example, and how are these disturbances likely to be colored by a young person's level of maturation? What are the primary developmental tasks that young people face, and what kinds of concerns are likely to capture the attention of boys and girls at different ages? What physical and social contexts influence the lives of young people at home, in school, and among their peers, and how do these contexts change over time?

Such information about normal and abnormal development (see Elkind &

Weiner, 1978; Weiner, 1982) helps examiners determine and effectively communicate the implications of a young persons' unique psychological traits and states and the interventions that seem indicated. Without such knowledge, even experienced Rorschachers will be handicapped in providing useful diagnostic consultation in child and adolescent cases.

Stability, Change, and Predictability

A long-standing question of whether the Rorschach is a reliable measuring instrument has been put to rest by extensive studies with the Comprehensive System of the temporal stability of structural variables. In the first of these studies, 100 nonpatient adults were retested after a 3-year interval with no allowances made for whatever events may have occurred in their lives. Of 19 structural variables examined, 13 showed retest correlations of .75 or higher, and 7 of these correlated .85 or higher. Only two of the variables examined, m and the sum of gray–black and shading responses, had stability coefficients below .70. These variables appear to reflect transient or situational states that are expected to fluctuate over time (Exner, Armbruster, & Viglione, 1978).

Among 6- and 9-year-old children, the retest correlations for these 19 variables over a 24- to 30-month interval are much lower than for adults (Exner & Weiner, 1982, p. 24). However, this result does not mean that the Rorschach cannot provide a reliable assessment of younger subjects. Children are, after all, in the process of developing their adult personalities, and the developmental psychology literature provides abundant reason to expect that personality characteristics—and test indices of these characteristics—will be less stable among younger people than among adults. Nonetheless, to consider the Rorschach reliable with children and adolescents, (a) the temporal stability of Rorschach structural variables should increase with age during childhood and adolescence, consistent with what is known about personality development; and (b) when briefer retest intervals are used in examining younger subjects, stability coefficients should reach a satisfactory level.

Findings of both kinds have in fact been obtained. When retesting is done at a 9-month interval, 7-year-olds show stability coefficients above .75 for only 4 of the 19 variables examined. By age 15, however, 9-month retesting approaches adult levels of stability; 10 of the 19 variables reach correlations of .75 or higher and only 4 fall below .70 (m, sum of gray–black and shading, passive movement, of a longer list of 23 variables were examined over an 18- to 21-day period among of a longer list of 23 variables are examined over an 18- to 21-day period among adults and 9-year-olds. As shown in Table 5-2, 18 of the stability coefficients were at .75 or higher and 10 at .85 or higher for the adult subjects, with only 4 below .70 (m, C', Y, and ep). Among the 9-year-olds, 19 variables retested at .75 or higher, with 14 of these at .85 or higher; just two (m and Y) fell below .70 (Exner, 1983, p. 84).

These and other retest studies by Exner and the present author establish the Rorschach's ability to provide a reliable assessment of current child and adolescent personality functioning. At the same, the retest findings have some very important implications for the time perspective that can be attached to interpretations. The most obvious of these involves distinguishing those variables that are most stable (and hence most likely to reflect abiding dispositions of the individual) from those that are relatively unstable (and likely to measure transient states rather than

Table 5-2
Stability Coefficients for 23 Rorschach Variables among
Adults and Children Retested after an 18- to 21-Day Interval[a]

		35 Adults (r)	35 9-year-olds (r)
Variable	Description		
R	Response	.84	.87
P	Popular	.81	.89
Zf	Z frequency	.89	.92
F	Pure form	.76	.80
M	Human movement	.83	.87
FM	Animal movement	.72	.78
m	Inanimate movement	.34	.20
a	Active movement	.87	.91
p	Passive movement	.85	.88
FC	Form color	.92	.84
CF + C + Cn	Color dominant	.83	.92
Sum C	Sum weighted color	.83	.87
T	Texture	.96	.92
C'	Achromatic color	.67	.74
Y	Diffuse shading	.41	.17
V	Vista	.89	.93
FD	Form dimension	.86	.81
Percentage	Ratio		
L	Lambda	.76	.84
X + %	Extended good form	.87	.92
Afr	Affective ratio	.85	.91
3r + (2)/R	Egocentricity index	.90	.86
EA	Experience actual	.84	.87
ep	Experience potential	.59	.70

[a]From Exner (1983). Reprinted with permission of John Wiley & Sons.

persistent traits). In addition, the extent to which a young person's Rorschach protocol predicts his or her future personality depends on the person's age and how far the prediction extends into the future. Generally speaking, inferences about personality functioning will increase in stability as a child or adolescent gets older and as the time period used for a prediction of the future gets shorter. Conversely, the younger the subject, the more caution must be exercised when drawing inferences from the Rorschach and when describing anything but short-term personality functioning.

This relationship is documented in Table 5-3, which also provides some specific details concerning ages at which certain Rorschach variables become reasonably predictive of subsequent personality characteristics. The data are based on the responses of 57 subjects who were tested five times at 2-year intervals (at ages 8, 10, 12, 14, and 16); the four columns of correlations indicate each variable's predictability from the first four testings, respectively, to the final assessment at age 16. In almost every instance, the similarity of the subjects' structural data to their protocol at age 16 increases steadily over the course of the prior four testings; the most striking exceptions to this progressive trend involve the two variables already identified as largely situational and state-related, *m* and *Y*. At age 8, *X* + % is the only variable correlated above .75 with the results at age 16. At age 10, there are 4 variables correlated above .75 with performance at age 16;

at age 12, there are 7; and by age 14, there are 13 variables showing this level of long-term (2-year) stability. These data suggest which features of a young person's personality functioning, as reflected in his or her Rorschach responses, are likely to become persistent character traits or dispositions and which features are still relatively fluid. This distinction is especially important in formulating diagnostic impressions that have long-term implications.

Identifying Patterns of Developmental Psychopathology

Rorschach assessment of psychological disorder in young people is an extensive subject that cannot be covered within the limits of this chapter (see Exner & Weiner, 1982). However, some brief illustrations of the diagnosis of developmental psychopathology from Rorschach indices of personality characteristics are provided below. The discussion will focus on four forms of disorder that must often be considered in evaluating children and adolescents with behavioral problems. Two of these are the traditional diagnostic categories of schizophrenia and depression; the other two are clusters of behaviors identified in empirical approaches to classification and referred to as anxiety-withdrawal and conduct disorder.

Table 5-3
Retest Correlations (r) for 57 Subjects Tested Five Times at 2-Year Intervals, Comparing Each of the First Four Tests with the Last Test[a,b]

Variable	Test 1 vs. 5 (ages 8 & 16)	Test 2 vs. 5 (ages 10 & 16)	Test 3 vs. 5 (ages 12 & 16)	Test 4 vs. 5 (ages 14 & 16)
X + %	**.78**	**.83**	**.81**	**.85**
Popular	.64	.72	**.84**	**.82**
a (active movement)	.72	**.80**	**.86**	**.83**
V (vista)	.47	**.87**	**.84**	**.92**
FD (form dimension)	.62	.71	.74	**.86**
T (texture)	.54	**.77**	**.81**	**.91**
p (passive movement)	.41	.48	.70	**.78**
R (responses)	.41	.61	.74	**.80**
L (lambda)	.26	.37	.59	**.78**
Zf (frequency)	.29	.38	.65	**.79**
M (human movement)	.43	.70	**.76**	**.77**
FM (animal movement)	.53	.67	**.77**	**.81**
Afr (affective ratio)	.10	.23	.42	**.76**
Sum C (weighted)	.16	.29	.63	.69
CF + C (color dominant)	.11	.37	.67	.72
FC (form dominant)	.09	.41	.69	.73
S (space)	.17	.14	.27	.18
C' (achromatic)	.06	.16	.40	.69
Y (diffuse shading)	.12	.27	.16	.13
m (inanimate movement)	.21	.18	.10	.06
3r + 2/R (egocentricity)	.28	.34	.56	.73
Zd (Z difference)	.54	.38	.19	.70
Sum 5 special scores	.24	.29	.51	.66

[a]From Exner, Thomas, and Mason (1985). Reprinted with permission of the Society for Personality Assessment.
[b]Boldface correlations = .75 or greater; p at .01 = .331.

Schizophrenia

Schizophrenia consists of a serious breakdown in a person's cognitive, interpersonal, and integrative capacities. This breakdown leads to several kinds of functioning impairment that define the nature of this condition, including disordered thinking, inaccurate perception of reality, interpersonal ineptness, and inadequate control over ideation, affect, and behavior (Weiner, 1966, 1982, chap. 5). Numerous features of a Rorschach protocol identify such impairments and thus help to assess the possible existence of a schizophrenic disorder in children and adolescents (Exner & Weiner, 1982, chap. 7).

Among these Rorschach features are (a) an accumulation of five Special Scores (Deviant Verbalization, Incongruous Combination, Fabulized Combination, Autistic Logic, and Contamination) that reflect illogical reasoning, especially when the more serious of these indices (FABCOM, ALOG, and CONTAM) outnumber the milder ones (DV and INCOM); (b) poor form level as an index of impaired capacity to perceive the world as most people do, especially when $X + \%$ falls below 70 and minus forms are more numerous than weak forms; (c) the presence of $M-$ responses, which reflect distorted impressions and poor judgment in interpersonal situations; and (d) bizarre or gruesome content as an indication of loss of control over ideation.

Thorough differential diagnosis of schizophrenia requires attention to many features of the Rorschach other than these four. Nevertheless, as elaborated elsewhere, these four bits of data capture the essence of schizophrenic impairment and provide a highly valid initial screening device in both adult and younger clients (Exner, 1983; Exner & Weiner, 1982, chap. 7; Weiner, 1966). Table 5-4 shows the results achieved in the Rorschach assessment of 43 subjects, ages 9 to 16, who were admitted to an inpatient psychiatric facility. Twenty of these subjects were subsequently identified as schizophrenic by the hospital staff and by the Research Diagnostic Criteria of Spitzer, Endicott, and Robins (1978). The Rorschachs were administered within 10 to 15 days after each subject's admission and were considered independently of the other evaluative procedures, which did not pro-

Table 5-4
Agreement between Rorschach and RDC Diagnosis of Schizophrenia among Inpatient 9- to 16-Year-Olds[a]

	RDC diagnosis	
Rorschach diagnosis	Schizophrenic (N = 20)	Nonschizophrenic (N = 23)
Actuarial sort with four variables positive[b,c]		
Called schizophrenic	16	0
Called nonschizophrenic	4	23
Unanimous agreement among three blind judges working with complete Rorschach and brief history[d]		
Called schizophrenic	18	0
Called nonschizophrenic	2	23

[a]Based on data reported by Exner and Weiner (1982, chap. 7).

[b]Four variables: Sum of five critical Special Scores greater than 5; FABCOM + ALOG + CONTAM greater than DV + INCOM; $X + \%$ less than 70; sum minus greater than Sum weak.

[c]Difference significant at $p < .001$ (χ^2 of 36.1875 with 1 df).

[d]Difference significant at $p < .001$ (χ^2 of 45.4615 with 1 df).

duce the final staff diagnosis until long after the Rorschach impressions had been recorded.

The data indicate that an actuarial sort based just on four Rorschach indices of the key dimensions of disordered thinking and inaccurate perception can agree closely with a very carefully determined final diagnosis. Indeed, 16 of the 20 schizophrenic youngsters were correctly identified (80%), and there were no false positives, so that the process yielded a total correct classification rate of 90.7%. In a situation more comparable to actual clinical practice, three adequately trained psychologists working with the complete Rorschach and a brief history, but "blind" to the final diagnosis, were even more accurate than this: Their unanimous agreements correctly identified 18 of the 20 schizophrenic subjects, with no false positives, for a total correct classification rate of 95.3%.

Depression

Depression is primarily a disorder of mood characterized by persistent feelings of sadness, loss of interest in people and previously enjoyed pursuits, and a diminished ability to experience pleasure. Other common dimensions of depression include (a) negative attitudes that result in low self-esteem, pervasive pessimism, and a sense of helplessness and hopelessness; (b) a depleted energy level that results in lethargy, a slowed pace of thinking and acting, reduced effort, and difficulty concentrating; and (c) an exaggerated concern with bodily functions that results in feeling physically weak, vulnerable, and in poor health (Weiner, 1982, chap. 7).

In assessing possible depression as well as other psychological disorders, practitioners need to keep in mind that the Rorschach is a measure of personality processes, not diagnostic categories. Rorschach data help to identify forms of psychopathology only to the extent that they identify personality characteristics associated with various types of disorder. This conceptual perspective on Rorschach diagnosis cautions against merely developing checklists of signs for use in making differential diagnoses. No matter what level of empirical validity such checklists achieve, they fail to provide any basis for understanding how certain psychological traits and states account for relationships between Rorschach behavior and some diagnosable disorder.

This conceptual approach was followed in the preceding discussion of schizophrenia, in which a compilation of personality impairments associated with this disorder was used to identify Rorschach indices that assist in evaluating its presence. The resulting list of indices is empirically valid and can be applied effectively in differential diagnosis, but it is hoped and strongly recommended that clinicians using this list will not lose sight of its conceptual foundation. Similarly, the following discussion provides not merely a checklist of Rorschach features linked to depressive disorders (although it can be used that way), but a set of Rorschach behaviors that suggest depression because they reflect personality characteristics associated with depressive disorders.

Among Rorschach variables that identify dimensions of depression in subjects of all ages are (a) the presence of any color-shading blends and an elevated C' which are indices of dysphoric affect and difficulty experiencing pleasure; (b) the presence of any V, an elevation of Y, and a low Egocentricity Ratio, corollaries of which are low self-esteem and feelings of being helpless to improve one's situation; (c) less productivity and complexity than would be expected from the subject's intellectual capacity, including low R (total number of responses), very long reaction times, slow delivery of responses, few blends, limited organizational activity, and a narrow range of content categories, all of which reflect a depleted energy level; and (*d*) morbid content, especially in anatomy responses, which suggests bodily concerns and feelings of vulnerability.

The precise definition of what constitutes an "elevated" or "low" score in these categories may vary with a subject's age. Hence, for several variables in the preceding list, diagnostic significance is defined by having a score substantially above or below average for one's age. For example, the mean Egocentricity Ratio in nonpatient subjects at age 6 is .60, with a standard deviation of .13, and .43 (standard deviation .09) at age 14. For 6-year-olds, then, an Egocentricity Ratio less than .47 is likely to suggest seriously deficient self-esteem, whereas among 14-year-olds, problematically low self-esteem is not indicated until the Egocentricity Ratio falls below .34. In the normative data base for the Comprehensive System, the actual figures show 8.6% of 6-year-olds and 15.7% of 14-year-olds, with Egocentricity Ratios falling more than one standard deviation below the mean for their age (Exner & Weiner, 1982, chap. 3).

Working with the above Rorschach indices for different dimensions of depression and judging their significance in light of age norms, practitioners can draw valid inferences concerning the extent to which subjects are depressed. Some evidence to this effect is reported for 74 11- to 15-year-old patients examined within 2 weeks of being admitted for hospitalization or to outpatient care (see Table 5-5). One-half of these subjects were subsequently diagnosed as having significant depressive features, based on DSM-III criteria and without reference to the Rorschach data. The other half were diagnosed as having forms of adjustment, substance abuse, or personality disorder, but without depressive features. The table shows statistically significant differentiation between these groups for each of four key Rorschach indices associated with dimensions of depressive disorder.

Table 5-5
Some Rorschach Variables Associated with Depressive Disorder in 11- to 15-Year-Olds[a]

	DSM-III diagnosis		
Rorschach variable	Depressed (N = 37)	Nondepressed (N = 37)	X^2
Vista + dimensionality			
One or more present	32	15	
None present	5	22	17.8448*
Color–shading blends			
One or more present	28	7	
None present	9	30	25.4214*
Egocentricity ratio			
Less than .35	29	9	
.35 or higher	8	28	22.8445*
Experience base			
$T + Y + V + C'$ more than $FM + m$	33	11	
$FM + m$ more than $T + Y + V + C'$	4	26	29.5379*

[a]Based on data reported by Exner and Weiner (1982, chap. 6).
*$p < .001$ with 1 df.

Anxiety-Withdrawal

Schizophrenia, depression, and most of the other diagnostic categories in DSM-III and other standard nomenclatures represent an approach to classification based on identifying and describing dimensions of disorder. Disordered thinking as an indication of schizophrenia and disturbed mood as an indication of depression are two examples of how types of psychopathology are formulated in terms of the inferred impairments that help to identify them.

An alternative to this approach involves classification schemes that are based on identifying and describing dimensions of behavior. In this approach, extensive data from observations of how people behave are analyzed with multivariate techniques to determine what kinds of behavioral descriptions cluster together. When certain characteristics are regularly found to occur in tandem, they are given a label that seems to fit them. The classification scheme that emerges from this approach is thus empirically based, in contrast to the conceptually based classification scheme represented by most traditional nosology.

The advantages and disadvantages of these two approaches to classification and the various issues they raise are an important topic in child and adolescent clinical psychology (see Achenbach & Edelbrock, 1978; Quay, 1979; Weiner, 1982, chap. 2). Within the context of the present chapter, psychodiagnosticians should recognize that the Rorschach can be utilized effectively in assessing young people regardless of one's preferred classification scheme. So long as referral questions can be answered in terms of personality or behavioral characteristics that are corollaries of certain kinds of Rorschach behavior, the test findings can be expressed in whatever terminology is favored by those involved with the case.

This broad applicability of the Rorschach can be illustrated by applying it to two empirically derived dimensions of developmental psychopathology identified by Quay (1979): anxiety-withdrawal and conduct disorder. Although these categories may overlap with some DSM-III categories and closely resemble others, all that matters for the present discussion is that (a) these are commonly observed dimensions of youthful behavior disorder that child and adolescent clinicians should be able to identify, (b) each involves a specified set of defining characteristics, and (c) many of these characteristics are reflected in Rorschach data that, in turn, can be used to help identify the presence of the disorder.

As described by Quay (1979), children with a pattern of anxiety-withdrawal show the following four characteristics, among others: They are likely to be anxious, fearful, and tense; they tend to be shy and timid, to be withdrawn and seclusive, and to have few friends; they appear or report feeling sad and depressed; and they suffer from feelings of inferiority, worthlessness, and low self-confidence. Although certain other characteristics of this disorder would usually have to be observed outside of a single testing session (such as a tendency to cry frequently), these four are often reflected in features of the Rorschach data.

First, a state of tension and anxiety is indicated when ep exceeds EA by a substantially greater degree than is age appropriate. Subjects in whom elevated ep scores result from other than just an accumulation of m and Y responses are especially likely to be persistently susceptible to inordinate stress. As noted earlier, m and Y are temporally unstable determinants that point to situational rather than chronic stress. Fearfulness is suggested when subjects give morbid content and convey in their thematic imagery that they anticipate being victimized by hostile people or forces in the environment.

Second, reluctance to engage in emotional interchange with others, hesitancy to initiate social interactions, and a loss of interest in being with or thinking about people are suggested by a low Affective Ratio and the absence of *H* (Human) responses.

Third, depressed mood constitutes part of depressive disorder. As already noted in discussing depression, color-shading blends and an elevation of *C'* point to feelings of sadness and difficulty in experiencing pleasure.

Fourth, negative self-attitudes also cut across anxiety-withdrawal and depressive disorder. Whichever terminology is used, the Rorschach data will provide the same answer. In asking whether a young person has an anxiety-withdrawal disorder, as in asking whether he or she has a depressive disorder, a low Egocentricity Ratio and the presence of *V*, as indices of low self-esteem, will support an answer in the affirmative.

One caution should be repeated before proceeding. The above brief summary does not paint the full picture of anxiety-withdrawal disorder, nor does it tell the whole story of how the Rorschach might be used to help identify its presence. Within the space available, the text can only illustrate clinical application of the Rorschach and provide some preliminary guidelines for differential diagnosis. Hence, the discussion in this section identifies relationships between just some of the central features of the disorder and some of the Rorschach characteristics that reflect them.

Conduct Disorder

As in the case of anxiety-withdrawal, the pattern of conduct disorder that emerged from Quay's cluster analysis includes some behaviors that can be documented only from the case history (e.g., recurrently getting into fights, destroying property, lying, and stealing). Some other characteristics of this disorder are not directly measured by the Rorschach, but may appear in how a subject relates with the examiner or complies with the requirements of being examined. These include being disobedient, defiant, impertinent, uncooperative, argumentative, and profane. The remaining characteristics, which also constitute central features of undersocialized conduct disorder and antisocial personality, as defined in DSM-III, can often be identified as corollaries of Rorschach response styles.

These remaining characteristics describe conduct disorder individuals as angry, irritable, inconsiderate, negativistic young people who show frequent temper tantrums, tease and bully others, and call attention to themselves by dominating whatever situations they happen to be in. In the language of personality functioning, these characteristics involve having an expressive style of coping with experience (i.e., a preference for doing things rather than thinking about them), being emotionally labile, feeling hostile toward the environment, being self-centered, and lacking concern for the welfare of others. The likely presence of conduct disorder is therefore indicated in part by the following several Rorschach features.

An expressive as opposed to an ideational or reflective coping style is apparent when *Sum C* exceeds *M* by 2 points or more. Emotional lability is indicated by an excess of *CF + C* over *FC* responses, especially when *C* responses are present and the extent of lability goes beyond what would be age appropriate. Occurring in combination, these Rorschach patterns identify a person who prefers to deal with experience by taking action or venting affect and who does so without much effort at restraint or self-control.

Concerns about hostility are reflected in the articulation of dangerous or threatening contents and in thematic elaborations of aggressive interactions among human and animal figures. When a subject appears to view such events from the perspective of a perpetrator rather than a victim of aggression, the combination of such imagery with an expressive, labile coping style suggests a propensity for angry, assaultive behavior. An elevation of S (white space responses), as an index of oppositional behavior, often lends weight to this propensity.

Self-centeredness appears on the Rorschach in the form of a high Egocentricity Ratio that includes one or more Reflection responses. This pattern identifies a degree of narcissism that leaves little room for paying attention to the needs of others or surrendering center stage to anyone else. Such selfishness tends to become especially problematic when the subject's record contains no Texture responses, since T is an index of interest in sharing warm, close, nurturant relationships with other people. Hence, an individual with a high Egocentricity Ratio and no T responses is likely to have little regard for the rights or needs of others, little interest in having interpersonal relationships except for the purpose of dominating or exploiting people, and little hesitation about running roughshod over whomever seems to stand in his or her way.

Case Study

The subject is an 11-year-old boy being evaluated in consultation to a family court. Two weeks prior to this examination he was caught setting fire to a neighbor's garage, which burned to the ground. Although this was the first known instance of fire-setting, he has had a history of aggressive behavior. He is regarded as a bully at school and has often been reprimanded for pushing and shoving classmates during recess and on the school bus. On two occasions during the past year he threatened another boy with a jackknife; the second time this happened, the school principal called the police. The boy's mother promised the police that she would discipline her son, and they let the matter drop. Following this recent fire-setting incident, however, the boy was arrested and charged. He has been removed from school and placed in his mother's custody by the family court, pending further judgment.

The family at home consists of the mother, age 33, who works regularly as a nurse's aid, and a sister, age 9. The boy's father is a construction worker who changes jobs frequently. Over the years he has alternated between moving the family from one place to another on short notice and leaving them behind while he goes off to work in some other city. When away from home he sends back money only occasionally, and the family has often had to go on public assistance. His last departure was 2 years ago. He was supposed to send for the family after he got settled in his new job, but he has not been heard from since.

The mother, who is supporting the family with her salary and some public assistance, has no particular interest in finding the father ("He probably got killed in some accident") or in becoming involved with other men. She works at her job, has several close women friends in the neighborhood, and, by her report, spends most of her evenings home watching television. She says that she has not been able to "handle" her son since her husband left, and she complains that "he is always picking on his sister and doesn't do well in school." She adds that she and her daughter have always gotten along well, but that she has been thinking about having her son placed in a foster home. In separate interviews with the children, both report that their mother has a ''bad temper'' (which she denies) and has been threatening to leave them. A visiting social worker who talked with neighbors got the impression that the mother is away from home much more than she or the children admit.

The boy is currently in the fifth grade and speaks openly about ''hating'' school and some of the children there. When confronted with the seriousness of the knife and fire-setting incidents, he acknowledges that they were ''dumb,'' but does not otherwise seem particularly concerned. He expects the court will put him ''on probation'' and not send him anywhere. He says he would like to be a police-man when he grows up. He talks about his father and says he expects him to appear at any time. He says that his mother is ''nice'' and that he likes to play with his sister. The questions being asked by the family court are what kinds of problems does he have; is he dangerous; should he remain with his mother, be placed in a foster home, or be sent to a detention facility or a psychiatric treatment center; and what kind of treatment might be helpful?

Rorschach Protocol

Rorscbach Protocol

Card	Free association	Inquiry	Scoring
I:5″	1. Mayb a bat, yeah a bat w the wgs out, zippin along	E: (Rpts Ss resp) S: I d.kno, it just does E: I kno it does but help me to c it too S: Here's the wgs & the body & the littl feet	Wo Fm^{a}o A P 1.0
	2. Thts lik a dancer in the midl	E: (Rpts Ss resp) S: Well s.times dancers hav skirts lik u can c thru & here, c here's her legs & her skirt & her hands r up lik she was doing a boggie or s.thg E: U can c thru the skirt? S: Yeah, c here she is, her legs (D3), u kno lik on TV specials & her skirt comes out here, the liter part	D+ M^a.FVo H,Cg P 4.0 PER
II:5″	3. A mask I guess	E: (Rpts Ss resp) S: The white parts r for the eyes & here, ths white is for u'r nose & its got like red for a beard, like for halloween & red ears like a devil mask E: Devil mask? S: Yeah, the pointed ears, they hav em lik tht	WS − FC − (Hd) 4.5
	4. Its lik a spaceship too, lik lifting off, like Columbia	E: (Rpts Ss resp) S: Well the white is the main part & ths black tip is lik the nose cone, thts where the crew stays & the fire is coming out down here, ths red is the fire, lik its just lifting off	Dds+ m^a.FC' .CFo Rocket 4.5
III:8″	5. Mayb a coupl of puppets, its lik sometimes they let the lines loose, they sorta sag down, lik in a dance or when thy hav em jumping around	E: (Rpts Ss resp) S: Thy do, c the legs & the head & their arms r sorta droopy, I don't kno wht ths is down here, forget tht, just a coupl puppets	D+ M^{p}o (2) (H) P 4.0
	6. Tht ll some bld up there	E: (Rpts Ss resp) S: Its just red lik a couple of blood spots	Dv C (2) Bl

(continued)

Rorschach Protocol
(Continued)

Card	Free association	Inquiry	Scoring
IV:4″	7. Thts lik some guy from space invadrs	E: (Rpts Ss resp) S: All big bulky lik, bug feet & a scrunchd down head	Wo Fo (H) 2.0
	v8. Ths way its lik Dracula, kinda w his wgs out lik he's ready to take off w his big black cape, tht turns into his wgs	E; (Rpts Ss resp) S: Yeah, he's neat, I watch him & Frankenstein on TV, he turns into a bat lik ths w tht big cape, its his wgs & away he goes, anywhere he wants	W + M^a.FC'o (H),Cg 4.0 PER
V:3″	9. Hey thts lik Dracula too, just lik he just landed w his wgs all out	E: (Rpts Ss resp) S: Yeah, in the other one he was taking off & now he's just landg, c the big cape & he still hasn't changed back all the way E: Changed back all the way S: Well he's still got big ears & funny feet	W + M^{a}o (H), Cg 2.5 PSV
VI:15″	10. Thts lik a space gun, lik a big space ray gun or s.thg	E: (Rpts Ss resp) S: This (D3) is the barrel & ths big part is lik the main part w the handles out here	Wo Fw Gun 2.5
	11. Right up at the top is a fist	E: (Rpts Ss resp) S: Rite here (points) just lik u mak a fist like ths (demonstrates) if u'r gonna fite	Do M^{a}o Hd PER
VII:3″	12. Tht just ll a lotta smoke	E: (Rpts Ss resp) S: I d.kno, it just does E: But help me c it lik tht S: Its all grey lik smoke	Wv C' Fi
	v13. Ths part up here ll a face, lik in the Planet of the Apes, thts a movie	E: (Rpts Ss resp) S; Yeah, it really does ll an ape face lik in tht movie, I saw it twice, c the ears & the nose & the eyes	D – F – (Ad) PER
III:5″	14. The top ll the pyramid	E: (Rpts Ss resp) S: It just does, its formed lik the pyramid	Ddo Fo Ay
	<15. Ths ways its lik a lizzard climbg ovr some rocks & he's all down here too, lik in a water reflection	E: (Rpts Ss resp) S; C his legs & head & tail, he's going ovr thes rocks & thgs & the blue I guess is lik water & he's all being reflected & the rocks too E: I'm not sur why it ll water S: Its blue, thts lik water	W + FM^a.Fr.CFw A,Na,Ls 4.5
IX:17″	16. Just a blob of paints, thts all I can c here, its a mess	E; (Rpts Ss resp) S: Just lik s.b thru some paint & it all splotched this way, all the colors, lik paint	Wv C Paint MOR
X:5″	17. Hey, thts lik Darth Vader	E: (Rpts Ss resp) S: Up here, just lik him in Star Wars, its the way he looks, just lik it, I've got a poster of him E: Help me to c it S: Sur, c the peak & the white part is eyes	DdSo Fw (Hd) 6.0 PER
	18. Mayb a frog, 2 of em	E: (Rpts Ss resp) S: C out here, the brown, frogs r brown lik ths & the legs r out, just frogs	D – FC – (2) A
	19. Tht pink is lik somethg, lik s.k. of candy mayb. some on each side	E: (Rpts Ss resp) S: Well, I can't thk of it, but lik s.k. of candy we get sometimes, its just pink chewy stuff, lik u pull it apart, its not gum, just pink candy, I don't rem the name, but its lik tht	Dv C (2) Fd PER

(continued)

Rorschach Protocol
(Continued)

Card	Free association	Inquiry	Scoring
20.	Thos littl thgs in the cntr ll 2 bells, lik hang down ovr the door of a store, theres some lik thos in the grocery store on our corner, c ths is the door & the handles Thts all I can c, thts enuff	E: (Rpts Ss resp) S: Yeah, thy ll tht, the old guy who runs it put em there so he knows if anyone comes in, c rite here, they kinda hang ovr the door E: I'm not sur about the door S: Well u draw it in the white lik ths & ths blue part is the handles on the door (S outlines)	DdS – / + F – (2) Bells 6.0 PER

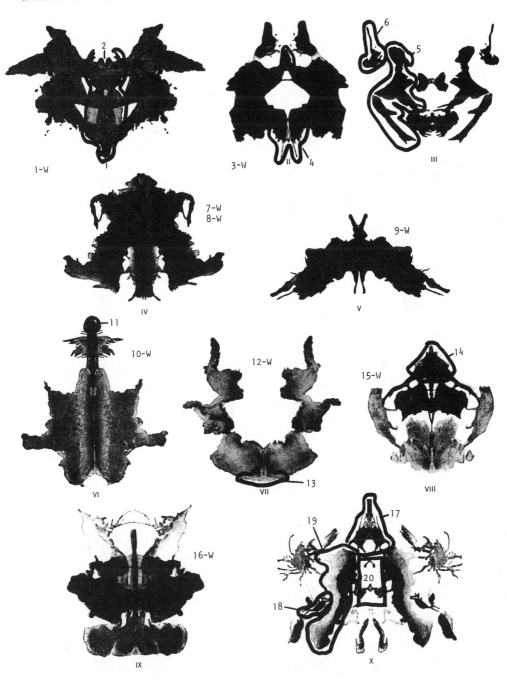

Case Study Response Locations. Use of Rorschach Ink Blots Is with Permission of Hans Huber, Berne, Switzerland.

Sequence of Scores

Card	RT	No.	Location		Determinants (S)		Content (S)		Pop	Z Score	Special
I	5"	1	Wo	1	FM^{a}o		A		P	1.0	
		2	D +	4	M^a.FVo		H,Cg		P	4.0	PER
II	5"	3	WS –	1	FC –		(Hd)			4.5	
		4	DdS +	99	M^a.FC'.CFo		Rocket			4.5	
III	8"	5	D +	9	M^{p}o	(2)	(H)		P	4.0	
		6	Dv	2	C	(2)	Bl				
IV	4"	7	Wo	1	Fo		(H)			2.0	
		8	W +	1	M^a.FC'o		(H),Cg			4.0	PER
V	3"	9	W +	1	M^{a}o		(H),Cg			2.5	PSV
VI	15"	10	Wo	1	Fw		Gun			2.5	
		11	Do	7	M^{a}o		Hd				PER
VII	3"	12	Wv	1	C'		Fi				
		13	D –	11	F –		(Ad)				PER
VIII	5"	14	Ddo	99	Fo		Ay				
		15	W +	1	FM^a.Fr.CFw		A,Na,Ls			4.5	
IX	17"	16	Wv		C		Paint				MOR
X	5"	17	DdSo	99	Fw		(Hd)			6.0	PER
		18	D –	7	FC –	(2)	A				
		19	Dv	9	C	(2)	Fd				PER
		20	DdS – / +	99	F –	(2)	Bells			6.0	PER

Case Study: Structural Summary

R = 20   Zf = 12   ZSum = 45.5   P = 3   (2) = 5

Location Features		Determinants (Blends First)		Contents				Contents (Idiographic)	
W = 9	**DQ**			H = 1		Bl = 1		Bells	.... =
D = 7	+ = 6 (7)	M.FV = 1		(H) = 4		Bt =		Gun	
Dd = 4	o = 6	M.FC' = 1		Hd = 1		Cg = 0,3			
S = 4	v = 4	FM.Fr.CF = 1		(Hd) = 2		Cl =		Paint	.... =
DW =	— = 4	m.FC'.CF = 1		A = 3		Ex =		Rocket	
				(A) =		Fi = 1			
		M = 3		Ad = 1		Fd = 1		.... =
Form Quality		FM = 1		(Ad) =		Ge =		
FQx		m =		Ab =		Hh =		
+ = 0	FQf	C = 3		Al =		Ls = 0,1		.... =
		CF =		An =		Na = 0,1		
o = 9	+ = 0	FC = 2		Art =		Sx =		.... =
w = 3	o = 2	C' = 1		Ay = 1		Xy =		
— = 4	w = 2	C' F =						**Special Scorings**	
NO FORM = 4	— = 2	FC' =		**S-CONSTELLATION**				DV =
		T =		.... FV+VF+V+FD > 2				INCOM =
M Quality		TF =		.... Col-Shd Bl > 0				FABCOM =
+ = 0		FT =		.... 3r+(2)/R < .30				ALOG =
		V =		.... Zd > ± 3.5				CONTAM =
o = 5		VF =		.... ep > EA				
w = 0		FV =		.... CF+C > FC				CP =
		Y =		.... X+ % < .70				MOR = 1
— = 0		YF =		.... S > 3				PER = 7
NO FORM =		FY =		.... P < 3 or > 8				PSV = 1
		rF =		... H < 2				=
		Fr =		.... R < 17				
		FD =		.... TOTAL				
		F = 6						

RATIOS, PERCENTAGES, AND DERIVATIONS

ZSum-Zest = 45.5-38.0	FC:CF+C = 2:5	Afr = .54
Zd = + 7.5	W:M = 9:5	3r+(2)/R = .40
EB = 5:7.5 EA = 12.5	W:D = 9:7	Cont:R = 10:20
eb = 3:4 ep = 7	L = .46	H+Hd:A+Ad = 8:4
(FM = 2 m = 1 T = 0 c = 3 V = 1 Y = 0)	F+% = .33	H+A:Hd+Ad = 6:0
Blends:R = 4:20		(H)+(Hd):(A)+(Ad) = 8:4
	X+% = .45	XRT Achrom = 6.0 "
a:p = 7:1	A% = .20	XRT Chrom = 8.0 "
Ma:Mp = 4:1		

Structural Interpretation

The record contains 20 responses, which is average among 11-year-olds and indicates that the norms for this age can be applied without any adjustments for record length. Beginning with the Four Square (*EB, EA, eb*, and *ep*), which summarizes many of the key data relating to personality style, we see from the *EB* (5 : 7.5) that he has well-developed capacities for both ideational and expressive ways of dealing with experience, but has formed a preference for the latter. His inclinations to discharge affect or take action in coping situations is underscored by the distribution of his color responses: two *FC*, two *CF*, and three pure *C*. Compared to expectation at age 11 (when the mean for pure *C* is just .4 and only 23% of subjects give any at all), this excess of poorly modulated color use signifies considerable propensity for emotional outbursts and impulsive behavior. Although the two *FC* reflect some capacity for adaptive self-control, the evidence for a prevailing tendency to let his feelings flow freely and his actions run unchecked is among the striking features of this record.

The *eb* shows expected frequencies on the left side (*FM* and *m*), but an elevation among the achromatic and shading determinants on the right side. The three *C'* and one *V* suggest that he is feeling a bit sad or gloomy and is harboring some negative attitudes toward himself. Since these are two common characteristics of depression, a scan of the Structural Summary for indices of other aspects of depression is in order. This scan reveals that he has a color–shading blend (*FC.CF*), which identifies some difficulty in experiencing pleasure. Otherwise, however, his Egocentricity Ratio is a bit low, but within normal limits for his age, which argues against chronically low self-esteem; he has only one morbid content and no *An* (anatomy), which argues against bodily concerns or feelings of vulnerability; and his average response total, average number of blends (4), higher than average *Z* frequency (12), wide range of content categories (10), and lower than average lambda (.46) argue against a low energy level.

Hence, we would infer that he is experiencing some depressive affect, but probably does not have a major or even minor depressive disorder. For an additional perspective on whatever depressive feelings he is experiencing, note that his *EA* is substantially higher than his *ep* (12.5 : 7). This tells us that he is comfortable with being the kind of person he is and usually satisfied with his capacity to think or act as he sees fit. He is not experiencing more concerns than he feels he can handle adequately, nor is he contemplating changes in how he behaves. When such a pattern of prevailing self-satisfaction and freedom from subjectively felt distress appears in a person who is having adjustment difficulties, it suggests some relatively stable and persistent form of personality or character disorder rather than any relatively acute or transient form of anxiety or neurotic disorder.

Another dramatic feature of the record revealed in analyzing the Four Square is the absence of *T* responses, which normatively are given by 92% of 11-year-olds. Failure to give a single *T* points to a serious deficit in the capacity to reach out to other people for warm, close, nurturant relationships. As would be true of a person at any age with a *T*-less record, this boy seldom expects mutually caring and supportive relationships to enter his life; to the contrary, he anticipates little love from others and offers little love to them.

As further evidence of a disinterested, distrustful attitude toward intimate interpersonal involvement, his Affective Ratio of .54 falls far below expectancy, and his one *H* (human) response is far outnumbered by seven (*H*) (whole fictional or mythological human), *Hd* (human part or detail), and (*Hd*) (fictional or mythological human detail) responses. The former points to withdrawal from emotional interchange with the environment, and the latter suggests some fearfulness or at least caution in dealing with people in their full human capacity (as opposed to their being segmented, diminished, or dehumanized in some way). Indeed, his high frequency of Personal responses (7 compared to normative expectation of 1–3) suggests he has some strong needs to protect and reassure himself in interpersonal interactions by self-aggrandizing references to how much he knows and how much he has done. With respect to this and other aspects of his coping style, the heavily one-sided nature of his Active–Passive ratio (7 : 1) suggests rigidity; he is an 11-year-old who is already fairly set in his ways and not very open to considering new or different ways of living his life.

A further striking feature of the Structural Summary is his poor perceptual accuracy ($X + \% = .45$), which identifies impaired reality testing. Together with his low number of Populars (3), this tells us that he does not see the world the way most people do and is prone to serious errors of judgment in assessing the impact and consequences of his behavior. This helps to account for his believing that the court will let him off, that his father will be returning shortly, and that he will become a policeman, when most people would view the facts of the situation as making any of these events unlikely.

Although the poor reality testing he shows is among the characteristics of schizophrenia, there is little evidence of other personality impairments associated with this condition. Most significant in this regard are (a) the absence of any of the five Special Scores that reflect disordered thinking, and (b) the good form quality of all five of his M responses, which means that he is not suffering any basic deficit in his capacity to size up and understand other people correctly.

Two other summary scores are noteworthy. First, the Zd of 7.5 identifies this boy as an overincorporater. More so than most people who are inclined as he is to behave impulsively, he tends to scan his surroundings extensively and attend to more features of the environment than he can organize efficiently. Like his five good Ms and two FCs, this feature of his record reveals some underutilized personality resources that should not be overlooked in formulating the treatment plan. Second, his frequent S (white space) responses (4) suggest some tendency to stubborn or oppositional behavior that also needs to be taken into further account.

Sequence of Scores

The most significant aspect of the sequence of scores is the deteriorating performance as the record proceeds. With respect to the structure of his responses, his best card is the first one, on which his percepts are organized (Wo and $D+$), controlled (form-dominant), accurate (good form), and attuned to conventional reality (2 Populars). The only other cards with consistently good form are IV and V, but he misses the Populars on both of these and perseverates his single response to Card V from Card IV.

His worsening performance over time also appears in the number of signs of difficulty in coping that accumulate in Cards VII–X. Because the 10 inkblots vary in their card-pull, no two groups of them constitute parallel forms for purposes of comparison. Nevertheless, we have to be struck by the fact that the last four cards include three of his four minus responses, two of his three pure C, three of his four vagues, and four of his seven Personals, but none of his three Populars, none of his five M, and only three of his twelve Z responses.

Ordinarily subjects become more comfortable and less defensive during the course of the Rorschach, as they become familiar with the task, gain confidence in being able to formulate responses, and draw reassurance from the supportive, nonthreatening stance of the examiner. If anything, then, changing records usually show fewer signs of distress or incapacity near the end than in the beginning. When the opposite occurs, as in this case, the subject is likely to be operating with a veneer of adequacy that wears away during prolonged exposure to problem-solving or self-disclosing situations. In addition to identifying a greater extent of coping difficulty than is initially apparent, deteriorating performance suggests that the subject is threatened rather than comforted by becoming closely involved with an interested and supportive person.

Hence, this boy's sequence of scores poses an obstacle in getting him involved in a treatment program. Psychological treatment typically proceeds with the expectation that the client's relationship with a warm, genuine, and understanding therapist who is trying to be of help will facilitate efforts to implement behavior change (Weiner, 1970, chap. 9; Weiner, 1975, chap. 3). In this case, relying on the treatment relationship as a vehicle for promoting therapeutic involvement and behavior change is likely to alienate rather than appeal to him, at least initially, and a developing relationship may make him feel increasingly uneasy rather than more secure.

Content Elaborations

The content elaborations reveal something more about the nature of this boy's concerns and about how his defensive style gets him into behavioral difficulties. He begins Card I in fine fettle. In addition to the structural adequacy of his handling of this card, he has the popular bat "zippin' along." There is a flavor in this phrase of sailing through life and getting where you want to be, without a care in the world.

He opens Card II with the only minus that appears in the first half of the record, and this response of a "devil mask" suggests some heightened concerns he has about the world being a hostile, dangerous place. The "spaceship" that follows is a fairly typical response for an 11-year-old boy, but Card III begins an interesting sequence starting with "puppets, it's like sometimes they let the lines loose . . . or when they have 'em jumping around." To the extent that he is identifying himself with these puppets, he may well feel that he is being manipulated by other people or is in danger of having this happen to him. The clear reference to the "they" who are pulling the strings points to his being the puppet rather than the puppeteer in this image; in contrast to the carefree, self-determined "zippin' along" in Card I, there is now a concern about being jerked around at the whim of others.

The succeeding percepts suggest that he responds to the prospect of being jerked around by others first by getting angry (on response 6 he literally "sees red" in giving a pure C blood response) and then by asserting power and self-determination. On Card IV, he seems to identify first with a "guy from space invaders" who is "big" and "bulky"—presumably someone powerful you wouldn't want to mess with. Next, he projects an image of "Dracula," whom anyone in his right mind would fear, and idealizes him as "neat." And what does Dracula do? With his "big cape" and "wings," "away he goes, anywhere he wants." So much for doing away with being a puppet on a string.

For good measure—and as evidence of how important it is for him to assert power, even at the expense of maladaptive coping—he perseverates the Dracula response on Card V while ignoring the easy popular. He continues this theme on Card VI, arming himself with a "big space ray gun," and then seeing the top detail as "a fist." In the inquiry for this response, he leaves little doubt concerning whether he sees himself as a perpetrator or victim in these aggressive images: "Just like you make a fist like this (demonstrates) if you're gonna fight." To avoid being pushed around in this world, he appears to be saying, you have to show people how tough you are, and you have to get them before they get you.

It is after this fist response that the record changes character. Along with showing less structural adequacy than the first 11 responses, the last 9 responses reflect a relaxation of the power assertion theme. To be sure, there is a response of "Darth Vader" on Card X, which might involve his continuing to identify with powerful, menacing figures. However, it is "just the way he looks," without any further elaboration of strength or domination. There is a "pyramid" on Card VIII, which could have some symbolic association with the might of the Pharaohs; however, there is nothing in what he says that lends weight to this particular association as opposed to many other possibilities. And there is an "ape face" from the Planet of the Apes on Card VII, but this movie features benign as well as aggressive apes, and there is no indication concerning which he has in mind.

As for the rest of the last nine responses, two are formless ("smoke" on Card VII and "blob of paints" on Card IX), which tell us only that he is backing off from formulating any revealing thematic imagery; two are insignificant animals (a lizard on Card VIII and two frogs on Card X); and the final two are so far removed from aggressive assertion that they merit special comment. Response 19 is candy, "pink chewy stuff," and response 20 describes the grocery store on his corner. The most common corollary of this kind of attention to food and its sources is a clearly felt need to depend on other people.

What seems to be happening, then, is that he handles the Rorschach task reasonably well while he is being defensively assertive and reactively aggressive. When these defenses desert him or he flirts with lowering his guard in the latter part of the record, underlying concerns about not being so powerful and needing to depend on others start to emerge. Then he becomes upset and less able to cope with the Rorschach task in an organized and realistic manner. He makes a final feeble effort to reassert himself ("That's all I can see, that's enough"), but calling it quits after having given four responses on the last card and a total record of average length conveys an effort to please as much as an effort to resist complying.

Summary

The Rorschach findings strongly suggest that this boy has an undersocialized conduct disorder with aggressive features and is on his way to developing an antisocial personality. He has some difficulty perceiving reality the way most people do, and he is currently experiencing some depressive affect. However, aside from showing poor judgment in anticipating the consequences of his and others' actions, he does not present evidence of a schizophrenic disorder that could account for his problem behavior, nor does he display other features of a primary depressive disorder that might be motivating him to engage in dramatic or attention-seeking misconduct.

Instead, his aggressive acts toward other people and their property appear to result from a combination of asocial attitudes and a disinclination to exercise self-control. He is a loveless boy who neither offers nurturance nor expects to receive it from others; to the contrary, he sees the world as a hostile environment in which the best way to protect yourself against the aggression and exploitation of others is to strike first, without caring too much about how they may be hurt in the process. He is an impulsive boy who tends to say and do what occurs to him without giving much thought to alternatives, and he can be expected to do as he pleases most of the time, without being much concerned about how others regard his behavior.

These personality characteristics and the usually persistent nature of an undersocialized conduct disorder suggest that this boy is likely to continue behaving aggressively, especially in situations that threaten him with being victimized or manipulated. Furthermore, his mistrust of people, his comfort with himself, and his oppositional attitudes and rigidity indicate that it will not be easy to get him involved in a treatment program. On the other hand, he does have some adaptive capacities for perceptive interpersonal relatedness (2 *Mo*), for well-modulated affective expression (2 *FC*), for wide-ranging attention to the environment (*Zd* of + 7.5), and for logical reasoning (absence of critical Special Scores) that he is not fully utilizing. Although these personality resources are presently playing second fiddle to his maladaptive tendencies, they are nevertheless available to be tapped and strengthened in the course of therapy.

Regarding disposition, the circumstances of the case would caution against merely returning this boy home or to a foster family, even if outpatient therapy with him and/or his family were implemented. His type of conduct disorder is ordinarily difficult to modify through occasional clinical visits, and his home environment, with an absent father and detached mother, could not be expected to lend much support to a treatment program. With rare exceptions, detention facilities are unlikely to provide a setting that would help this kind of boy move psychologically in any direction except toward an adult antisocial personality disorder. The best prospects for him to change his developmental course and learn more self-control and less interpersonal distrust would probably emerge in a residential treatment setting. Although residential placements for young people are often hard to find, the Rorschach findings suggest that this would be the best advice to give the family court.

References

Achenbach, T. M., & Edelbrook, C. S. (1978). The classification of child psychopathology: A review and analysis of empirical efforts. *Psychological Bulletin, 85*, 1275–1301.

Ames, L. B., Learned, J., Metraux, R. W., & Walker, R. N. (1973). *Child Rorschach responses* (rev. ed.). New York: Brunner/Mazel.

Ames, L. B., Metraux, R. W., & Walker, R. N. (1971). *Adolescent Rorschach responses* (rev. ed.). New York: Brunner/Mazel.

Beck, S. J. (1930). The Rorschach test and personality diagnosis. *American Journal of Psychiatry, 10*, 19–52.

Beck, S. J. (1950). *Rorschach's test. I. Basic processes* (2nd ed.). New York: Grune & Stratton.

Elkind, D., & Weiner, I. B. (1978). *Development of the child.* New York: Wiley.

Exner, J. E. (1959). The influence of chromatic and achromatic color in the Rorschach. *Journal of Projective Techniques, 23*, 418–425.

Exner, J. E. (1974). *The Rorschach: A comprehensive system.* New York: Wiley.

Exner, J. E. (1978). *The Rorschach: A comprehensive system: Vol. 2. Current research and advanced interpretation.* New York: Wiley.

Exner, J. E. (1983). Rorschach assessment. In I. B. Weiner (Ed.), *Clinical methods in psychology* (2nd ed., pp. 58–99). New York: Wiley.

Exner, J. E., Armbruster, G. L., & Mittman, B. L. (1978). The Rorschach response process. *Journal of Personality Assessment, 42*, 27–38.

Exner, J. E., Armbruster, G. L., & Viglione, D. (1978). The temporal stability of some Rorschach features. *Journal of Personality Assessment, 42*, 474–482.

Exner, J. E., & Exner, D. E. (1972). How clinicians use the Rorschach. *Journal of Personality Assessment, 36*, 403–408.

Exner, J. E., Thomas, E. A., & Mason, B. (1985). Children's Rorschachs: Description and prediction. *Journal of Personality Assessment, 49,* 13–20.

Exner, J. E., & Weiner, I. B. (1982). *The Rorschach: A comprehensive system. Vol. 3. Assessment of children and adolescents.* New York: Wiley.

Exner, J. E., Weiner, I. B., & Schuyler, W. (1978). *A Rorschach workbook for the comprehensive system* (rev. ed.). Bayville, NY: Rorschach Workshops.

Goldfried, M. R., Stricker, G., & Weiner, I. B. (1971). *Rorschach handbook of clinical and research applications.* Englewood Cliffs, NJ: Prentice-Hall.

Halpern, F. A. (1953). *A clinical approach to children's Rorschachs.* New York: Grune & Stratton.

Horowitz, L. (1974). *Clinical prediction in psychotherapy.* New York: Jason Aronson.

Jackson, C. W., & Wohl, J. (1966). A survey of Rorschach teaching in the university. *Journal of Projective Techniques and Personality Assessment, 30,* 115–134.

Klopfer, B., & Davidson, H. H. (1962). *The Rorschach technique: An introductory manual.* New York: Harcourt, Brace, & World.

Levitt, E. E., & Truumaa, A. (1972). *The Rorschach technique with children and adolescents: Application and norms.* New York: Grune & Stratton.

Quay, H. C. (1979). Classification. In H. C. Quay & J. S. Werry (Eds.), *Psychopathological disorders of childhood* (2nd ed., pp. 1–42). New York: Wiley.

Rorschach, H. (1942). *Psychodiagnostics* (5th ed.). Bern: Hans Huber. (Original work published 1921)

Spitzer, R. L., Endicott, J., & Robins, E. (1978). Research diagnostic criteria: Rationale and reliability. *Archives of General Psychiatry, 35,* 773–782.

Weiner, I. B. (1966). *Psychodiagnosis in schizophrenia.* New York: Wiley.

Weiner, I. B. (1970). *Psychological disturbance in adolescence.* New York: Wiley.

Weiner, I. B. (1975). *Principles of psychotherapy.* New York: Wiley.

Weiner, I. B. (1977). Approaches to Rorschach validation. In M. A. Rickers-Ovsiankina (Ed.), *Rorschach psychology* (2nd ed., pp. 575–608). Huntington, NY: Krieger.

Weiner, I. B. (1982). *Child and adolescent psychopathology.* New York: Wiley.

6

Thematic Approaches to Personality Assessment with Children and Adolescents

John E. Obrzut
Carol A. Boliek

Thematic personality assessment techniques have achieved widespread clinical and empirical use, along with a growing theoretical acceptance. These techniques attempt to identify the conscious and unconscious factors which affect the psychological functioning of the individual (Korchin & Schuldberg, 1981) and the underlying dynamic factors (constructs, drives, needs, or traits) which form the structure of the personality (Goldfried & Kent, 1972) and which are considered to be major determinants of behavior. Further, as Howes (1981) suggests, thematic techniques raise psychological testing above the mere collection of information and routine computation of IQ scores by providing insight into the dynamics of individual human personality. These tests view personality in a global, holistic manner rather than portraying it segmentally, as more structured personality inventories sometimes do. Blatt (1975) suggests that children and adolescents' responses to thematic procedures may offer us the opportunity to study their styles and contents of thinking and perceptions, information which may not be readily accessible through observational procedures.

Historically, the period from the 1930s through the early 1960s saw a tremendous upsurge in the development and application of thematic techniques, as the major professional activity of mental health practitioners focused on the skills of assessment. In recent years, however, these techniques have been subjected to criticism regarding their use for personality assessment. Obrzut and Zucker (1983) state, "not only have they (thematic techniques) weathered the storms of criticism, but now, in the sixth decade, the field is thriving, with techniques in various stages of development and with varying degrees of established validity and reliability" (p. 85). Indeed, recent surveys of personality assessment indicate that thematic techniques have become increasingly valuable as primary assessment techniques (Goh, Teslow, & Fuller, 1981; Lubin, Wallis, & Paine, 1971; Prout, 1983; Wade, Baker, Morton, & Baker, 1978), despite the criticisms about these

John E. Obrzut. Department of Educational Psychology, University of Arizona, Tucson, Arizona.
Carol A. Boliek. School Psychology Program, University of Northern Colorado, Greeley, Colorado.

techniques' apparent lack of reliability and validity (Anastasi, 1982) and the competitive growth of behavioral psychology (Cummings, 1982).

Reviewing these personality assessment surveys in greater detail, Goh *et al*. (1981) found that psychologists working in school settings tend to prefer "quick, easy-to-use procedures (Bender–Gestalt, Sentence Completion, H-T-P) over more comprehensive, time-consuming techniques such as the TAT and Rorschach" (p. 14). They also noted that objective techniques (e.g., MMPI, CPQ) were not ranked among the most frequently used personality measures. In contrast, Wade *et al*. (1978) found, in their survey of clinical psychologists, that both objective and projective tests were used with high frequency with the Rorschach and Thematic Apperception Test (TAT) recommended approximately 30% more often than objective tests by those actually practicing (rather than in training or research) in the field. Levy and Fox (1975), in their survey of clinical employers, determined that 84% expected job applicants to have skills in the area of projective techniques, including thematic techniques. Wade and Baker (1977) similarly found that clinical psychologists recommended that students familiarize themselves with these techniques. Thus, thematic techniques seem to be recommended by practitioners for both the current and the future practice of personality assessment.

In summary, thematic methods continue to thrive in clinical settings as does the controversy surrounding their use. Some of the controversy is related to the appropriate use and interpretation of these techniques. Their use requires a sound theoretical background in the psychodynamic approach to personality development. It is imperative for the practitioner to understand the assumptions underlying these techniques and to acknowledge the problems of standardization, reliability, and validity. Thus, the purpose of this chapter is to examine several issues regarding the clinical use of the TAT and other thematic techniques. In the concluding section, comments will be offered on the use of thematic techniques with children and the role of these approaches in the assessment process.

Historical Perspective

According to Piotrowski (1957), the ancient Greeks were the first to discuss the effect of stimulus ambiguity on the perception of reality, while Leonardo da Vinci alluded to the usefulness of ambiguous stimuli in the creative process. The first formal projective technique, however, was suggested in 1879 by Sir Francis Galton, who used words to stimulate verbal associations. Jung followed Galton's ideas and developed the word-association technique in an effort to better understand the unconscious motivation of his clients (Exner, 1976).

Near the turn of the century, Alfred Binet and Victor Henri suggested using inkblots to study visual imagination. In particular, William Dearborn in 1897 examined imaginative productions as a means of understanding an individual's early life experiences; this is much of what one does today with projective techniques. Sharp, in 1899, was the first to develop typologies on the basis of imaginative responses, while Edwin Kirkpatrick in 1900 attempted the development of age norms. In 1910, G. M. Whipple used inkblots to test "active imagination" as part of his battery of physical and mental tests; Sir John Herbert Parsons in 1917 reported detailed age and sex differences in associations to a standard series of inkblots (Rabin, 1968). Finally, in 1910, Hermann Rorschach began his study of inkblot interpretations as a way to differentiate between various types of psychopathology. The monograph *Psychodiagnostik*, published in 1921, reported the results of his "experiment" on various modes of perception and their relation to personality and psychopathology.

In addition to the inkblot technique, some authors attempted to elicit individuals' meaningful responses to pictures. In 1905, Binet and Theodore Simon used responses to pictures to assess intellectual development, while Brittain in 1907 reported his investigations of systematic sex differences in stories told by his subjects, relating them to the individual's broader social environment. In 1908, Libby used similar procedures with children and adolescents, and Schwartz in 1932 developed the Social Situation Test as an aid in interviewing delinquent boys (Bellak, 1975; Rabin, 1968).

The most significant development in this area occurred when Henry Alexander Murray introduced the TAT. This indicated a shift in emphasis from the perception of single visual stimuli that needed interpretation (i.e., Rorschach) to more structured visual stimuli that required different interpretation formats. While the TAT was first described by Morgan and Murray (1935), it was not until 1938 when Murray published *Exploration in Personality* that it began to gain in popularity. The TAT has led to the development of a variety of other thematic techniques which permit the assessment of individuals with the different ages, cultural backgrounds, and socioeconomic levels found in both educational and clinical settings.

Assumptions of Thematic Approaches as Projective Techniques

The most central assumption of thematic techniques is that an individual will "project" (or reflect) his or her needs, desires, and/or conflicts when asked to impose meaning or order on an ambiguous or unstructured stimulus. Inherent in this hypothesis is the notion that all behavior manifestations are expressions of an individual's personality. For example, the story that is solicited from a TAT card may directly or indirectly reflect the client's emotional–social needs, environmental presses, and/or coping styles. This basic assumption appears to be well supported in the literature (Lindzey, 1952).

From this central assumption, several corollary assumptions have been derived. Murstein (1961, 1965) suggests that projection is directly related to the amount of stimulus ambiguity. Moderate ambiguity, where two or more psychological interpretations of a stimulus are possible, is thought to elicit the greatest amount of projective response. Murstein suggests that moderately ambiguous situations often provide enough cues to elicit verbalizations in a desired direction or area, but not so many as to preclude individual response variations.

A second central assumption of thematic techniques suggests that the strengths of individuals' psychological needs are positively related to their direct or symbolic manifestation in thematic technique responses. Murstein (1961) contends that an individual's thematic responses are a function of projective stimulus properties; the perceived purpose of the testing; the individual's experiences, needs, and expectations; and the examiner's instruction and his or her interpersonal influence or bias. This assumption, and Murstein's perspective of it, related directly to the thematic technique's validity; this will be discussed in greater detail below. For now, however, it is quite clear that such factors as willingness to self-disclose, ego involvement in the task, specific stimulus properties of the projective materials, test situation/examiner effects, and the examiner's framework are all factors that must be considered when interpreting a projective protocol.

The third central assumption posits a parallel between thematic technique behavior and responses and individuals' behavior in the environment. Four studies (Kagan, 1956; Lesser, 1957; Murstein & Wolf, 1970; Mussen & Naylor, 1954) have supported this assumption. Mussen and Naylor (1954) hypothesized that lower class children who show a high amount of fantasy aggression and a low fear of punishment relative to those fantasies would display more overt aggression than children with few fantasy aggressions and a high fear of related punishment. Their hypothesis was strongly supported ($p < .003$), indicating the need to consider variables other than the need strength alone (Assumption 2 above).

Lesser (1957) examined environmental factors that would increase the accuracy of predicting aggressive behavior from thematic fantasy. He found a larger correlation between thematic fantasy and overt aggression in children whose mothers encouraged aggression than in children with maternal disapprovals. Kagan (1956), meanwhile, found a significant positive relationship between thematic fantasy and overt aggression in children when (*a*) the stimulus material was suggestive of aggressive content, and (*b*) when overt and fantasy behavior were similar in their mode of expression (i.e., predicting fighting behavior from fighting themes rather than from swearing themes). Kagan further suggested that anxiety over the overt expression of aggression may inhibit its verbalization, even if the stimulus is strongly cued in that direction.

Finally, Murstein and Wolf (1970) reported a significant correlation between amount of projection and the degree of psychopathology as rated by trained clinicians. They noted that normal subjects were able to censor their responses, projecting more "unconscious" material to highly ambiguous tests such as the TAT. Psychiatric patients, on the other hand, expressed an equal degree of projection regardless of the degree of stimulus structure.

Leary (1957) has suggested a multilevel framework for viewing personality which can incorporate these central assumptions. Level I considers how the individual is perceived by others (observable behavior); Level II involves the individual's self-perception (the conscious self-concept); Level III considers unconscious processes, and according to Leary, is measured by projective techniques. Any projective technique, however, will likely tap several levels of personality simultaneously.

Using Leary's approach, one may be working with a child who is not viewed as aggressive by classmates or the teacher (Level I), who does not perceive him or herself as aggressive (Level II), yet whose projective responses reveal a great deal of anger (Level III). A thorough understanding of the child would include consideration of all three levels. The child may be seething with anger, yet may repress it. Thus, he or she might be unaware of and "protected" by these urges due to the anxiety or guilt aroused by their expression.

Major Thematic Approaches

Thematic picture techniques are the most widespread projective techniques used with children and adolescents. These techniques are but one component of a thorough assessment of personality, which is already one aspect of the total psychoeducational or clinical assessment process. In general, the goal of this entire process is to make "informed decisions" (Korchin, 1976; Korchin & Schuldberg, 1981). In that context, any test (or technique) should provide significant data to facilitate valid educational (including personality) diagnosis. The test should yield information pertinent to the development of appropriate interventions and be able to document change as a function of treatment. If a given test does not accomplish these functions, its presence in the test battery should be seriously questioned. Therefore, the role(s) that thematic picture techniques play in an assessment battery needs definition and discussion (Obrzut & Cummings, 1983).

The Thematic Apperception Test

One of the most prevalent thematic techniques for children and adolescents is Murray's TAT (Murray, 1938). Murray (1938) introduced the term "projective test" to describe methods that attempt to "discover the covert (inhibited) and unconscious (partially repressed) tendencies of normal persons by stimulating the imaginative processes and facilitating their expression in words or in action" (Rabin, 1968, p. 8).

In developing the TAT, Murray (1938) selected 31 cards which primarily show people in implied actions or human interactions. These cards can be organized to create sets particularly for male and female children, adolescents, and adults. In general, approximately 10 cards that are expected to elicit potentially meaningful projective material are administered in a single session to a specific subject. Each individual's spontaneously verbalized stories to the cards are recorded verbatim as they are given, with scoring and interpretation based on the content of these stories. Murstein (1963) summarized a variety of content and quantitative scoring and interpretive analyses for thematic techniques. Quantitative analyses also have been developed through various research endeavors (McClelland, Atkinson, Clark, & Lowell, 1953; Zubin, Eron, & Schumer, 1965). These analyses, however, have been useful for research purposes, but appear to have little clinical application (Lanyon & Goodstein, 1982). Most clinicians, therefore, tend to use qualitative approaches to interpretation.

The TAT manual provides instructions for its administration (Murray, 1943). Basically, the instructions for children and adolescents are as follows:

> This is a story telling test. I have some pictures here that I am going to show you, and for each picture I want you to make up a story. Tell what has happened before and what is happening now. Say what the people are feeling and thinking and how the story will end. You can make up any kind of story you want. Do you understand? Well, then, here's the first picture. (pp. 3–4)

The exact wording of these instructions may be altered to suit the age, intelligence, personality, and circumstances of the subject.

Since the practitioner presents a subset of 10–12 of the 31 TAT cards, decisions must be made regarding which cards to administer (Murstein, 1968). Symonds (1939) suggests that pictures that are ambiguous and minimally detailed are the most useful. This suggestion is especially appropriate if the practitioner wishes to decrease the predominantly sad characteristics and the dark, gloomy tones that many (e.g., Murstein, 1963; Ritzler, Sharkey, & Chudy, 1980) have noted in the

TAT cards. Indeed, Goldfried and Zax (1965) have reported that more ambiguous cards have been typically rated as less sad and somber.

Another important consideration in the selection of TAT cards is the child's ability to relate favorably to those chosen. Specific TAT cards are recommended below for certain age levels and issues based on the age and sex of the central figure in the TAT card and the card's general "stimulus pull." Implicit in these recommendations is the assumption that individuals will relate best to cards depicting characters of the same sex, comparable age, and like inter- or intrapersonal issues. Note also that some TAT cards show scenes involving these similar inter- and intrapersonal issues, yet they are individualized for boys (B), older or adult males (M), girls (G), and older or adult females (F). Other TAT cards are appropriate for any age or sex because of their depicted scene or stimulus pull and not due to their central characters.

The cards best suited for children between 7 and 11 years of age include cards 1, 3BM, 7GF, 8BM, 12M, 13B, 14, and 17BM. The content categories of the stories told by children at these ages usually concern achievement and status goals (1, 8BM, 14, 17BM), aggression to and from the subject (3BM, 8BM, 12M, 14, 17BM), concern with parental nurturance and rejection (3BM, 7GF, 13B, 14), and parental punishment and attitudes toward parents (1, 3BM, 7GF, 14) (Rabin & Haworth, 1960). With adolescents, productive TAT cards include cards 1, 2, 5, 7GF, 12F, 12M, 15, 17BM, 18BM, and 18GF. To these basic sets of TAT cards, practitioners should add one or two additional cards which elicit themes that may be necessary for a better understanding of the particular child or adolescent. For example, if the adolescent appears depressed, those TAT pictures related to depression and suicide should be included. Other psychological conflicts or issues may be similarly investigated by using flexibility and economy in choosing TAT cards.

An inquiry or a series of clarifying questions is completed after each TAT story to generate additional data which may facilitate a more complete analysis or understanding of the child. These questions may be specific or neutral in content. Bellak (1975), who opposes this procedure, suggests that the inquiry process be conducted only after all the stories have been told. He argues that this procedure may then become a free association process and, thus, part of an initial psychotherapeutic intervention. Regardless of the procedure used, the practitioner must keep in mind that the more questions that are asked, the less projective is the material obtained; that is, the use of direct questions tends to structure the nature of responses, not allowing the projective process to freely occur.

Two possible inquiry process directions involve questions about the generated story or questions about *how* the story was generated. In the former, questions could further clarify identified characters' feelings, thoughts, desires, or beliefs. In the latter, the practitioner may ask children for the sources of their ideas, or whether the story themes were derived from their own private experiences, from the experiences of others, or from environmental events (e.g., movies or books). For either inquiry process direction, children can be reminded of the plot of each significant story and encouraged to speak freely and openly.

Regardless of the scoring approach, TAT stories are presumed to reveal some of the individual's dominant drives, emotions, traits, and conflicts by identifying significant interpersonal needs, presses, and themas (Murray, 1971). According to Murray, a "need" represents the significant determinants of behavior (motives or forces) within the person, while a "press" represents the significant determinants of behavior in the environment. The press can either facilitate or impede the efforts of the individual to reach a given goal. Examples of needs are abasement, achievement deference, dominance, order, sex, and succorance; examples of press include family insupport, danger or misfortune, rejection from others, deception, or betrayal (see Hall & Lindzey, 1978, for a more thorough review).

A thema is a molar and interactive behavioral unit. It deals with the interaction between need and press and permits a more global and less segmented view of behavior. Combinations of simple themas which interlock or form a sequence are called complex themas. As Murray (1943) indicates, when used loosely, thema means the plot, theme, or principal dramatic feature of the TAT story. Themas also may be viewed as assessing defense tendencies and indices of conflict. Thus, the TAT technique explores personality dynamics rather than differential diagnosis.

Several scoring systems have been developed for use with TAT data. Morgan and Murray's (1935) system was composed of frequency tallies and weighted scores for needs and presses. Needs were said to be expressed in stories as impulses, wishes, intentions, or descriptions of overt behavior. According to this scoring system, each need is rated on a scale from 1 to 5 when it occurs in a story, with the actual rating being determined by the intensity, duration, frequency, and importance that the particular need manifests in the story. Presses are also scored on a 5-point scale according to the criteria of intensity and frequency. In addition to these weighted scores for needs and presses, this approach also identifies and analyzes the sex of the heros (the characters whom the subject identified with the most), the prevailing kinds of outcomes, the consistency of simple or complex themes, and the repetitive expression of interests and sentiments (Exner, 1976). This scoring approach, therefore, assumes that the elements of greatest importance to the subject will occur most frequently across the composite of the TAT stories. Thus, Murray did not intend the TAT to be a diagnostic tool, but an instrument to explore an individual's personality in some detail.

Bellak (1947) devised a TAT scoring system that focuses exclusively on content analysis. Bellak argues that the strength of the TAT lies in its ability to elicit the content and dynamics of interpersonal relationships and, thus, psychodynamic patterns. His method of interpretation and scoring categories, therefore, are primarily concerned with these dimensions. Bellak's system contains 10 scoring categories: main theme, main hero, main needs and drives of the hero, conception of the environment, what the figures are seen as, significant conflicts, nature of anxieties, main defenses against conflicts and fears, nature of punishment for offenses, and ego integration. Bellak suggests that the 10 scoring variables should be used primarily as a frame of reference and that not all aspects will be relevant to every story.

In contrast to the approaches above, Eron (1950) uses a very formal quantitative/normative approach in which rating scales evaluate each TAT story for emotional tone and outcome. Expanding upon this, Murstein (1963) suggested that TAT pictures be scaled for each of the specific personality dimensions they are designed to tap. Along this line, McClelland et al. (1953) used the TAT to examine achievement motivation exclusively. Pragmatically, however, the task of scaling each card is very time-consuming, and its clinical utility has not been demonstrated as yet. Indeed, this approach may be more suitable for research as opposed to practitioner purposes.

The present authors recommend the inspection technique as the simplest and, perhaps, most useful for TAT interpretation. Here, the practitioner treats the stories as meaningful psychological communications simply noting data that seem significant, specific, or unique. In dealing with the content of stories, the practitioner should analyze each story by identifying the hero; the motives, trends, and feelings of the hero; the forces within the hero's environment; the outcome of the stories; simple and complex themes; and interests and sentiments attributed to the hero. The manner in which a child or adolescent tells a story is also highly significant. It may reflect his or her cognitive style, expressive language, organization of thoughts, and ability to identify and elaborate on aspects of a TAT picture's plot (Kagan, 1960).

The Children's Apperception Test

The popularity and utility of the TAT prompted the development of other, similar thematic picture tests designed for the personality assessment of different age groups. The Children's Apperception Test (CAT; Bellak & Bellak, 1949) was designed for young children who are 3 to approximately 10 years of age. The 10 cards, depicting animal rather than human characters, are thought to elicit meaningful projective material from individual children. The CAT was designed especially to assist in the understanding of a child's relationship to important figures and drives (Bellak, 1975). Bellak also intended the stimulus cards to elicit such problems as sibling rivalry, aggression, and a child's personality structure, defenses, and social–emotional reactions to and coping with problems of growth.

The CAT administration parallels that of the TAT; that is, the child is asked to tell what happens prior to the CAT picture, what is currently taking place, and what will occur beyond the present activity. Bellak's (1975) approach to CAT interpretation is essentially the same as his system for the TAT. He recommends that practitioners analyze CAT content for the status of the hero and for the primary conflict and outcome themes manifested in the stories, especially those which relate to the status of the hero. McArthur and Roberts (1982) suggest using the CAT only with very young children who generally respond "seriously" to pictures with animals; older children may give stereotyped or less useful CAT responses because they have difficulty relating to the animal-based scenes.

The Blacky Pictures Test

The Blacky Pictures Test (Blum, 1950) was designed to explore "personality dynamics" and to validate the psychoanalytic theory of psychosexual development. This is accomplished through a chronologically presented series of cards which represent the traditional psychosexual stages of development. This projective technique can be utilized with children as young as 5 years of age, and its age range extends through adulthood. The pictures, in the form of cartoons depicting events in the life of a family of dogs, present Blacky (the central dog figure) as the hero or character with whom the child or adolescent should identify. Blacky is shown in possible (psychosexual) conflict situations with Papa, Mama, or Sibling Dogs. For example, Card 8 portrays sibling rivalry as Blacky is at the side of the picture watching the mother and father dog be affectionate to the younger puppy, Tippy.

Each Blacky Test card is introduced to the child by providing a brief description of who or what role each character is playing in the particular scene. Eleven total cards are administered with essentially three components to each card: (*a*) the child tells a spontaneous story about the card similar to that of the TAT, (*b*) the child answers a series of multiple-choice questions, and (*c*) the child chooses the most- and least-liked cards. The manual recommends that scoring be done on four elements (spontaneous story, answers to inquiry, cartoon preferences, and related comments), and 13 separate dimensions such as oral eroticism, Oedipal intensity, and positive identification are analyzed. In addition, Blum (1962) proposed a 30-variable scoring system based on factor analysis.

Studies have demonstrated that the proposed Blacky Test scoring system has sufficient reliability for research, but remains inadequate for individual clinical assessment (see Sappenfield, 1965). Further, Sappenfield (1965) suggests that the breadth of projective information may be limited for the Blacky Test because (a) only a single central character is used throughout the 11-card series, (b) Blacky's general identification as a "male" character by children of both sexes may limit those psychosexual processes related to female roles and individuals (especially for female examinees), and (c) the presentation of the Blacky cards may not be chronologically ordered to follow Freud's psychosexual developmental stages. Specific to the last point, Blum (1950) assumed that children's responses would "mature" as the picture sequence moved to developmentally older situations. Sappenfield (1965), however, suggests that a "regressive or infantile" response set could persist throughout the entire test administration, inhibiting the instrument's effectiveness with older children and adolescents.

In general, the Blacky Pictures draw information regarding children's self-perceptions, their attitudes toward family members, and their coping strategies. The test is interpreted qualitatively, based on one's knowledge of psychoanalytic theory and projective techniques. Research does indicate good interrater, test–retest, and split-half reliability (Granick & Scheflin, 1958). Perhaps the major strength of the Blacky Pictures Test is the careful development of its manual, including the well-defined scoring instructions (Sappenfield, 1965).

The Make-A-Picture Story Test

The Make-A-Picture Story Test (MAPS; Shneidman, 1952) is essentially a variation of the TAT for individuals 6 years old to adulthood. Initially, children or adolescents make their own pictures by selecting one or more human-like or animal cutouts from a variety of figures, placing them on pictorial backgrounds selected by the practitioner. The child is then required to tell stories about the pictures that he or she created. While there are a total of 22 background scenes (including a bedroom, bathroom, and schoolroom), usually not more than 10 are utilized for any one assessment. For example, the practitioner might present the schoolroom background and have the child choose any number and combination of male/female adults and children of various ethnic origins, of animals, or of legendary or fictitious characters. With respect to scoring the MAPS protocol, a variety of quantitative schemes are available; however, they generally require a good deal of the practitioner's time (Jensen, 1965). Thus, like other thematic approaches used in assessment settings, qualitative analysis is practiced most often.

One of the MAPS' basic assumptions is that the variety of cutouts and backgrounds offers more extensive stimulus variability than the TAT. However, because of this variability, attempts to standardize the test or assess its validity are very difficult. The MAPS has had the greatest clinical use with young children who are hyperactive or resistant to the TAT's administrative format. The MAPS technique allows for many variations, such as the use of plastic and wooden figures; this procedure resembles some of the techniques used in play therapy (Obrzut & Zucker, 1983).

Contemporary Thematic Techniques

The utilization of the TAT and CAT as personality assessment tools with children and adolescents has spawned the development of similar verbal and picture tests designed to improve or adapt this assessment process. These thematic tests include the School Apperception Method, the Michigan Picture Test–Revised, and the Roberts Apperception Test for Children.

The School Apperception Method

The School Apperception Method (SAM; Solomon & Starr, 1968) was developed for children in kindergarten through ninth grades. The SAM consists of 22 cards of detailed drawings depicting school-related and classroom scenes. For example, Card 1 shows a group of children forming a line on a school playground. A monitor is standing next to the group. On Card 2, a boy is standing and reading a book in the classroom. In the background, another girl and boy are conversing as they appear to be looking at the boy who is reading. Transparencies for group administration of the SAM are available.

The SAM is designed to elicit information pertaining to children's significant emotional and academic adjustment difficulties in school. These difficulties include or involve how the child perceives teachers and peers, attitudes toward academic activity, conceptualizations of punishment, frustration and aggression indicators, and coping skills in the school environment. The authors suggest presenting 12 SAM stimulus cards to a child, requiring a story with a beginning and an end for each picture. One of the main assumptions of the SAM is its situational relevance; that is, the behavior of children in school settings is more directly and efficiently measured using projective stimuli which are relevant to school situations (where these behaviors occur) than with stimuli of more general environments and situations.

Solomon and Starr (1968) state that SAM responses can be formally scored using Bellak's (1947) guidelines for the TAT or CAT. In addition, they present a framework for the qualitative analysis of the SAM, including the liberal use of questions during the child's story narration (see pp. 14–16, Manual). While reliability, validity, and normative data are unsubstantiated, useful clinical data regarding the child's perception of his or her school environment can be obtained from the SAM. This information, in combination with other personality data, can assist the practitioner in making school- or clinically related decisions.

The Michigan Picture Test–Revised

The Michigan Picture Test–Revised (MPT–R; Hutt, 1980) is a thematic instrument designed for children from 8 to 14 years of age or in grades 3–9. The major objective of the MPT–R is to differentiate children with emotional maladjustment from those who have "satisfactory" emotional adjustment (Hutt, 1980, p. 3). This is accomplished with the MPT–R's 15 cards and the recommended administration of a basic "core" set of 5 cards as a minimal battery, with up to 7 additional cards as supplements. Procedurally, the child is asked to tell a story about what has happened in the picture and how the story will end. Directions for both quantitative and qualitative analysis (including scoring and norms) are provided in the Manual (see pp. 37–57).

Using the recommended scoring criteria, a Tension Index (similar to Murray's needs, 1971, as expressed on the TAT), a Tense Score (tenses used in the stories), a Direction of Forces Index (outward, inward, or neutral actions of the central character), and a Combined Maladjustment Index (probability of maladjustment) can be derived. In addition, information can be numerically scored regarding psychosexual levels, interpersonal relations, personal pronouns, and popular objects. While the author suggests that these latter four variables are not statistically significant in discriminating between adjusted and maladjusted groups, they can provide useful inter- and intraindividual dynamic information to the practitioner.

The MPT–R was standardized and normed on a representative sample of children from public school populations and children with behavioral and personality problems from child guidance clinics. Hutt (1980) reported interrater reliability on the Tension Index at .98. Initial discriminant analyses completed by the author on the Tension Index, Tense Scale, Direction of Forces Index, and the Combined Maladjustment Index demonstrated that each of the four scales significantly discriminates adjusted from maladjusted children. These preliminary findings are hopeful, yet further research is needed to establish the MPT–R's construct, concurrent, and predictive validity.

The Roberts Apperception Test for Children

The Roberts Apperception Test for Children (RATC; McArthur & Roberts, 1982) is the most recently developed thematic approach designed for children 6–15 years of age. The purpose of the RATC is to assess children's perceptions of interpersonal situations, including their thoughts, concerns, conflicts, and coping styles (McArthur & Roberts, 1982). Pictorially, the RATC goes beyond other thematic approaches by including cards depicting parental disagreement, the observation of nudity, parental affection, aggression situations, and school and peer relationships. The RATC is made up of 27 stimulus cards, of which 16 are administered at any one time. Eleven cards have both male ("B"-boy) and female ("G"-girl) versions, respectively. The administration is similar to the TAT; that is, the child is required to create a story about the picture, including what led up to the depicted scene and how the story ends.

The RATC manual includes an explicit scoring system which yields adaptive scales, as well as five clinical scales (anxiety, aggression, depression, rejection, and unresolved). The Adaptive Scales consist of eight individual scales, including reliance on others, support to others, support of the child (self-sufficiency and maturity), limit setting (by parents and other authority figures), problem identification (the child's ability to formulate concepts beyond the scope of the stimulus card), and three resolution scales indicating how the child resolves particular problems included in a story.

The clinical scales are comprised of five individual scales that, when taken together, represent a child's feelings about the self or about the environment. The Anxiety scale measures guilt, remorse, apprehension, self-doubt, and the themes of illness and death. Aggression is the second of the clinical scales, measuring either physical or verbal expressions of anger. Depression is designed to measure stories with themes of sadness, despair, and/or physical symptoms related to depression. The Rejection scale measures themes involving separation and feelings of being left out, jealousy, and discrimination.

In addition to the adaptive and clinical scales, critical indicators such as atypical responses, maladaptive outcomes, and card rejections or refusals are also included in the scoring system. An Interpersonal Matrix (interactions with significant others), Ego Functioning Index, Aggression Index (child's ability to deal with situations needing some kind of aggressive response), and Levels of Projection scale (cognitive and ego development) can also be obtained.

The RATC has been standardized on a sample of 200 "well-adjusted" children of both sexes, with efforts to include a representative cross section of lower, middle, and upper socioeconomic families. Analyses of individual children's scores can be obtained by converting the obtained raw scores to T scores and placing these on profile norms that have been divided into four age groupings (ages 6–7, 8–9, 10–12, and 13–15). Psychometrically, interrater and split-half reliabilities have been reported to be in the acceptable range (Hersh, 1978; Kaleita, 1980; McArthur & Roberts, 1982; Muha, 1977). According to the test authors, interrater agreement between doctoral level raters was generally high across all 16 profile scales and indicators (86% for the high-difficulty protocol to 93% for the low-difficulty profile; see manual, p. 76). Also, children's scores on the various scales and indicators are reported to be reasonably consistent across stratified, split-half versions of the test. The scales with the highest reliability estimates are Limit Setting, Unresolved, Resolution 2, Resolution 3, Problem Identification, and Support.

Both convergent and discriminate validity have been obtained for the RATC. The authors' data demonstrate a high degree of interrelatedness among the RATC scales using subgroups of 200 well-adjusted and 200 clinic children. Yet, the results also reveal the relative independence of certain scales such as Aggression, Depression, and Rejection. A principal component factor analysis with varimax rotation suggested that three factors combined account for approximately 45% of the common variance. Factor I was defined as Unresolved (global psychological functioning, including telling unresolved stories); Factor II as a specific clinical factor (significant negative loadings on the clinical scales, excluding unresolved); and Factor III was defined by two scales, Limit Setting and Resolution I (elementary problem-solving strategies, reflecting age trends). In addition, a multiple regression discriminant analysis conducted on the clinic and nonclinic groups of children resulted in a multiple R of .79, which was highly significant, indicating that approximately 62% of the variance in group membership was accounted for by the 13 profile scales. Finally, some attempt was made to obtain concurrent and predictive validity (see manual, pp. 85–91), but more studies need to be conducted in these areas. In summary, preliminary research findings indicate that the RATC profile scales are useful for differentiating the adaptive and maladaptive functioning of children of different ages.

McArthur and Roberts (1982) suggest that the reliability and validity studies noted above represent a "first step" in establishing the RATC's clinical utility and psychometric soundness. They describe a variety of areas that require future investigation. These include the examination of appropriateness of the RATC for younger children, as well as for children from various ethnic and socioeconomic backgrounds; and additional comparisons, beyond the "well-adjusted" children used in the standardization groups, to include more representative samples of "average" or "typical" children.

"Home-Made" Thematic Techniques

Hypothetically, any picture could be used as a thematic technique. As long as the child or adolescent can relate to the picture as a psychological or social–emotional stimulus, the potential for eliciting responses that provide insight and understanding of that individual exists. Ritzler *et al.* (1980) created an alternative to the TAT when they selected both positively and negatively toned pictures from the *Family of Man* photo essay collection. Their intent was to elicit a more balanced view of the subject's personality. In comparing responses from the standard TAT and their variation, they found that subjects generated stories of comparable length, thematic variety, and type of characters. However, the standard TAT stories more frequently were classified as reflecting Eron's (1950) "disequilibrium." In contrast, the Ritzler *et al.* (1980) version produced stories with comparable proportions of "equilibrium" and "disequilibrium." This was a preliminary investigation, however, with a small sample of undergraduate students. As noted by the test authors, more research is needed with emotionally disturbed children before the real merit of this variation on the TAT can be determined.

Thematic Adaptations for Specialized Populations

In the past, psychologists have designed special sets of pictorial stimuli to explore particular themes important in understanding children and adolescents' personality development. Some of the more recent research investigations, however, assuming that stimulus properties sometimes influence responses, have developed alternative thematic stimuli appropriate for different populations. In particular, these researchers argue that there are significant influences due to similarities between examinees and certain characteristics of the TAT figures. Indeed, Thompson (1949), using the Black TAT that he devised, found that blacks provided more responses when using the TAT with black stimuli than when using the traditional TAT stimuli. However, it should be noted that Thompson's findings were not replicated by subsequent researchers (Korchin, Mitchell, & Meltzoff, 1950; Riess, Schwartz, & Cottingham, 1950).

More recently, Constantine, Malgady, and Vazquez (1981) provided a modification of the TAT stimuli, the Tell-Me-A-Story (TEMAS), for urban Hispanic children. The inclusion of culturally relevant characters resulted in increased verbal responsiveness to the stimuli. Caution, however, should be observed until more research can confirm and generalize these findings.

In general, research findings with apperceptive methods have shown that specialized adaptations do not necessarily elicit longer or more productive stories than the traditional figures that differ from children in age, sex, and race (Bailey & Green, 1977; Weisskopf-Joelson, Zimmerman, & McDaniel, 1970). However, there does appear to be a need for projective techniques that include more balanced selections of stimulus pictures, that is, ones that reflect our multicultural society. Further, studies are needed to explore the thematic productions of special diagnostic groups such as the physically handicapped. Without specific thematic stimuli and investigations with these diagnostic groups, practitioners should be cautious when making interpretive statements from data obtained with the traditional TAT (or any other thematic) technique.

General Strengths and Limitations of Thematic Techniques

Thematic picture techniques are content tests that tap personality structure and the dynamics of interpersonal relationships by verbal means. These techniques elicit basic data on individuals' relationships to male and female authority figures, and they frequently provide insight into family relationships. In addition, projective thematic techniques may reveal underlying personality structures, motives, conflicts, needs, values, and attitudes toward others and selves. Indeed, the intensity of a child or adolescent's attitudes or needs is often directly or symbolically evident in the themes of generated stories. Finally, picture techniques analyze individuals' perceptions of their environments and differences in these perceptions across people in the same environment. This helps the practitioner's understanding of a child's unique interaction with the external and internal determinants of personality across the past, present, and future times of his or her life.

Although thematic picture techniques facilitate explorations into personality dynamics, the problem of relating latent thematic data to overt behavior requires considerable attention. Lanyon and Goodstein (1982) suggest caution when interpreting responses to thematic picture stimuli because of the difficulty in predicting that individuals will manifest thematic-related needs or personality characteristics in their overt behavior. Bellak (1975) also recognizes this dilemma, calling it the problem of overt and latent needs. Certainly, the practitioner must be aware that a need expressed in a story might be, minimally, at a fantasy level or at an emergent behavioral level. Bellak suggests that background information, observations, and interviews help to substantiate and guide interpretation along these levels and dimensions.

Some of the problems inherent to all tests also apply to the TAT and other thematic approaches to personality assessment. Since tests are by design relatively limited samples of behavior, the problem associated with the representativeness of the sample is always present. Especially with thematic techniques, one must be cognizant of the role that recent experiences play in the construction of stories. For example, a given theme may be the result of a recent exposure to a television show or to an event-specific transitory state (e.g., fear and grief, respectively). This suggests that the multimethod approach emphasized in this book may best protect the practitioner from undue diagnostic hypotheses or conclusions.

Psychometric Properties with Thematic Techniques

In addition to the weaknesses discussed above, many critics who adhere to strict psychometric standards claim that projective techniques lack adequate reliability and validity (Exner, 1976). Advocates of projectives, however, feel that this psychometric issue is semantical, not statistical, in nature. As Schwartz and Lazar (1979) point out, projective interpretation deals with the possible meaning of a response, not its probabilistic (in a statistical sense) status. Thus, as thematic analysis involves "the overlap of connotative meaning across responses," the practitioner is interested in common themes or consistencies that emerge across an entire protocol and an entire assessment process. Semantics aside, many studies have shown various projective techniques to have considerable reliability and validity, particularly when used in clinic settings.

Reliability Studies

Clinical diagnosis skills with projective techniques are often experientially obtained by working with various kinds of psychopathology, sorting clients into global categories. The reliability of this categorization process occurs when those working with professionals, who employ these categories consistently, internalize their procedures and conceptualizations. However, as Blatt (1975) suggests, (*a*) current diagnostic concepts are only gross categories, and (*b*) clients usually transcend any single psychological category because they function on several levels of psychological organization. Thus, when evaluating the reliability of projective techniques, one must consider the nature of the variable being measured.

Test–retest reliability, or consistency over time, can only be considered relevant if the variable being measured is also consistent over time. Most of the traits and characteristics that are measured with projective devices are motivational and emotional in nature; there is no reason to assume that these characteristics are temporally stable. With internal consistency (split-half reliability), meanwhile, questions regarding motivation, ego defense, and control must be considered. An emotional, cathartic release on Card 1 of the TAT may prompt a more controlled and benign story on Card 2. Thus, when clients pull back and regroup in the face of exceptionally provocative stimuli, they also create potentially unreliable results—especially when a technique's split-half consistency is being evaluated. While critics may cite poor split-half reliabilities as shortcomings of projective techniques, none of these methods is designed with equivalence of stimuli as a goal. Rather, specific parts of the projective technique or battery are expected to contribute to the entire evaluation, but not necessarily with the same weight or with the same impact for each subject (Exner, 1976).

Numerous studies with adult populations demonstrate substantial reliability for specific variables on the TAT, even when lengthy periods exist between testings (Exner, 1976). However, there are relatively few studies that primarily and specifically address these issues with child and adolescent populations. A number of studies with the TAT and various other thematic approaches, however, are worth noting.

Sutton and Swenson (1983) conducted a study using the TAT, an unstructured interview (INT), and the Sentence Completion Test of Ego Development (SCT; Loevinger, 1976) to examine both the reliability and concurrent validity of assessing ego development. Seventy subjects were placed into six groups, including juveniles from a detention center (12–17 years of age), junior high school students (14–16 years of age), high school students (16–19 years of age), undergraduate students (20–35 years of age), college graduates and graduate students (22–47 years of age), and retired university professors (67–82 years of age). Each subject received all three tests, and each test was rated similarly to the SCT using ego development theory and Loevinger and Wesler's (1970) scoring techniques.

The results indicated that interrater reliability, using this scoring system for the TAT, was .95. Utilizing sum scores for each instrument, correlations between the different instruments were .79 between SCT and TAT, .89 between SCT and INT, and .81 between TAT and INT, all significant at $p < .01$. Newman-Keuls Sequential Range Tests, used to test for differences between the ego level scores of each group and each instrument, revealed no significant differences for groups 1, 2, and 3 (ages 12–19). However, the mean TAT score was significantly higher than the SCT score for groups 5 and 6 (ages 22–82), with $p < .01$ and $p < .05$, respectively. As hypothesized by the authors, groups with older subjects scored higher on the INT and TAT. The authors concluded that these three instruments demonstrated acceptable reliability as well as adequate concurrent validity. They stated that the TAT appears to be a reliable alternative to assess ego development, more so with older populations. Finally, they suggested that Loevinger's (1976) self-training exercises be used with the TAT to assist the practitioner in assessing ego development.

In another study with the TAT, Slemon, Holzworth, Lewis, and Sitko (1976) constructed an Associative Elaboration Scale and an Integration Scale to evaluate the TAT protocols of randomly selected individuals aged 7–15. While the interrater reliabilities for the Associative Elaboration Scale were satisfactory (.91), those for the Integration Scale were found to be too low for clinical use in individual assessment. Overall, the reliability was not affected by stories stimulated by different TAT cards, even when given by different age groups.

With other thematic techniques, Schroth (1977) reports high interscorer reliabilities for specific CAT scoring categories and suggests that interscorer reliability may increase as the age of the child increases. Kelly and Berg (1978) report test–retest reliability and internal consistency coefficients in the 70s for a group of 488 fourth- and eighth-grade children using the Family Story Test. Rosenzweig (1978) examined the retest and split-half reliabilities of the Rosenzweig Picture Frustration (P-F) Study (Children's Form) for two groups of subjects aged 10–11 and 12–13 years; each group was tested twice at an interval of 3 months. Test–retest reliability for all scoring categories (except O-D) was significant, while reliability by retest was consistently higher than by the less appropriate split-half methods. Finally, Kinard (1982) also used the Children's Form of the Rosenzweig P-F Study with 30 physically abused children and 30 control nonabused children. When interrater reliability scores were calculated as percentage agreements across subjects for each of the 24 pictures, agreements ranged from 84% to 98%, with the majority above 90%.

In an attempt to obtain higher TAT interrater reliability coefficients, Squyres and Craddick (1982) recently showed that judges were able to discuss scoring differences during training and at various times during a research project until agreement was reached. These authors suggested that this training, used as an adjunct with periodic assessment of raters' reliability, could improve reliability coefficients to within a range acceptable for research purposes.

Validity Studies

Projective methods also have been criticized for their apparent lack of validation. While many studies have shown various picture techniques to have considerable validity (Singer, 1968), others have demonstrated their invalidity. Part of the problem arises from the divergent dimensions used to operationalize the concept of validity, for example, construct and predictive validity. Different authors or researchers consider validity in the context of (*a*) a test's correlation with some criterion measure (psychiatric diagnosis or another "validated" instrument), (*b*) the correlation coefficients between raw and "true" (error-free) scores, (*c*) diagnostic and predictive accuracy in relation to the test user's purpose, and/or (*d*) the utility or interpretability of test scores (Ebel, 1961).

Criterion-related or concurrent validity is most commonly used in evaluating projective techniques. Here, one evaluates a test's validity by its ability to agree or correlate with some other measure (criterion). While projective tests often fare poorly in predicting psychiatric diagnosis, studies have shown that the failure is related to the criterion measure, not to the inadequacy of the projective instrument. Not only does psychiatric diagnosis differ from setting to setting, but it varies considerably between practitioners within the *same* setting. For example,

Schmidt and Fonda (1956) report nearly 80% agreement between pairs of psychiatrists on three major clinical categories (organic, psychotic, and characterological), yet "agreement with respect to diagnosis of the specific subtype of a disorder occurred in only about half of the cases and was almost absent in cases involving personality patterns, trait disorders, and the psychoneuroses" (p. 266). In addition, diagnostic and classification schemes change over time. As Schwartz and Lazar (1979) indicate, patients characterized as paranoid in the past may now be viewed as examples of a manic-depressive syndrome. Similarly, the current "borderline" group now includes patients described previously in other symptomatic terms.

Construct validity is an internal measure of a test's validity; sometimes it is used when a practitioner has no single alternative criterion known to measure a specific trait. The American Psychological Association's (APA) *Standards for Educational and Psychological Tests* (APA, 1974) describes a psychological construct as "a dimension understood or inferred from its network of interrelationships. . . . Evidence of construct validity is not found in a single study; rather, judgments of construct validity are based upon an accumulation of research results" (pp. 29–30).

Idiographically, a construct may be more appropriately applied to an entire assessment battery than to a specific assessment technique; this allows the practitioner to make inferences about an individual's collective personality and behavioral style. Similarly, the process of validating a projective technique seems more comparable to validating an experimental hypothesis (about the "whole person") than to validating a more traditional psychological/educational test (Ainsworth, 1951); that is, no single statistical coefficient or correlation can fully represent the validity of a particular projective technique. Validity coefficients are situation-specific and may support specific hypotheses about a particular technique and/or the underlying traits or processes it is presumed to measure. As noted above, a projective technique's accumulated research and interrelated network of data best support its construct validity; this then supports the validity within the entire projective battery and personality assessment.

Although a projective approach might logically emphasize construct validation, it appears that most studies have focused on single traits or characteristics of personality. Empirical data analyzing multiple dimensions of the individual are lacking. For example, in order to establish this validity with the TAT, it would be necessary to show that the needs or presses (traits) described by Murray (1938) are related to the characters in children's fantasy productions, and that these many traits motivate behavior in various environments across time.

Assessing the predictive validity of projective techniques is also questionable, in part because of the erroneous assumption that projective methods should have special predictive capabilities. The value of using projectives is to understand the person "as he or she is" in contrast to how "he or she will be." Thus, the overall goal of projective testing is to gain an understanding of the total personality, that is, the assessment of an individual's strengths, weaknesses, and defenses in an understanding of the individual's primary needs, desires, and degrees of satisfaction or frustration in meeting those needs (Exner, 1976).

Despite the perspective above, there are predictive studies where clinically appropriate differentiations were successfully related to carefully specified projective technique criteria. Werner, Stabenau, and Pollin (1970) investigated the parent–child interactions of 10 schizophrenic, 10 delinquent, and 10 normal children by using 240 TAT stories told by their parents. These authors found that distinct patterns of parent–child interactions characterized the three sets of parents: "Normal parents are more personally involved, child-centered, and flexible; delinquent parents are more impersonal, autocratic, task- rather than child-oriented, and inflexible; whereas, schizophrenic parents are overinvolved, oriented to parent vs. child needs and rigidly demanding" (p. 143). Similarly, Sharp, Glasner, Lederman, and Wolfe (1964) noted differences in the family interactions of sociopaths versus schizophrenics. The responses of the sociopaths' parents regarding their sons were classified as "unconcerned and rejecting," while responses from the parents of schizophrenic patients were classified as "egocentrically or pathologically concerned."

Beck (1960) also found that children in "well" families were growing up within psychological environments that had more "nutritive," growth-promoting effects than those for families with schizophrenic children. Finally, Matranga (1976) investigated how fantasy mitigated the overt expression of male adolescent juvenile offenders' aggression by examining the relationship between their aggressive behavior and their aggressive TAT story contents. Results supported the hypothesis that an inverse relationship exists between hostile content on the TAT and behavioral measures of aggression in adolescent males.

Other studies investigating other types of validity are presented below. For example, Lehmann (1959) administered the CAT to 160 kindergarten children from four different socioeconomic areas to learn (a) the manner and extent to which certain personality dynamics (aggression, fear, toileting, cleanliness, and orality) were elicited by the CAT pictures; (b) whether the pictures elicited the themes for which they were designed; and (c) whether there were any significant differences among the four groups in the themes investigated. First, it was found that 33% of the initial responses were descriptive in nature, while 67% of these responses were interpretive; the theme of orality was the most pronounced. Second, the CAT pictures did not consistently elicit the dynamics they were designed to tap. Third, only the theme of fear significantly differed among the four groups. Children from the high SES group exhibited more frequent fear responses than those from the low SES-broken group.

Mazumdar and Solanski (1979) studied the TAT/CATs' utilities as screening devices to differentiate emotionally disturbed (ED) and normally adjusted children. Children aged 10–18 years old, selected from child guidance clinics and children's hospitals, were administered 10 selected cards from the TAT/CAT. The results indicated that ED children reported more "unfavorable presses," had more conflicts of security versus insecurity, were not likely to look at the future with optimism, and used more defense mechanisms of rationalization than did the normal subjects. The study concluded that there is some support for the use of the TAT/CAT to screen for and diagnose emotional disturbance in children.

Bachtold (1975) studied the adaptive functioning of 20 boys, aged 13–16 years old, who were placed in self-contained classrooms for emotionally disturbed learners with the TAT. The protocols were scored for $_p$Aggression (environmental press toward aggression), $_p$Dominance, $_n$Aggression (need for aggression), $_n$Achievement, and $_n$Autonomy. The findings indicated that interactions between these disturbed adolescents and their environment were most likely to involve aggression and dominance. These adolescents' themes were least likely to involve achievement, despite their average intelligence.

May (1975) conducted four studies to explore the construct validity of a sex-linked difference in Deprivation/Enhancement TAT fantasy patterns. The results, both with various clinical groups (hysterical, obsessive–compulsive, field dependent–field independent) and with normal children, supported the notion that Deprivation/Enhancement fantasy patterns are meaningfully related to sexual identity and sex role development. In addition, these sex-linked patterns were found to appear by age 6 and were well established by age 10.

Another projective picture technique used with referred students to assess their personality functioning is the Bene–Anthony Family Relations Test (FRT; Bene & Anthony, 1957). This projective method is designed to explore the perception of one's feelings toward other family members. Although few studies have been carried out with ED students (Frost, 1969; Kauffman, 1971; Swanson, 1969), one recent study is worth mentioning. Phillip and Orr (1978) studied the clinical ability of the FRT to discriminate between ED inpatients, ED outpatients, and normal control children aged 9–13 years. The authors found that both ED groups more frequently identified family members as sources of negative feelings than normal controls. However, the FRT did not appear to effectively discriminate between the inpatient and the outpatient groups.

Another specialized picture technique is the Rosenzweig Picture-Frustration (P-F) Study, "a limited projective procedure for disclosing certain patterns of response to everyday stress" (Rosenzweig, 1978, p. 483). This technique was used to measure the direction of aggression in a sample of 30 physically abused children and 30 nonabused, control children (Kinard, 1982). Results indicated that the abused children were more likely to express extrapunitive aggression and less likely to express impunitive aggression than their nonabused counterparts. This, however, occurred only in situations where another child was the frustrating agent.

In summary, several points need to be stressed regarding the validity and use of projective methods. First, because of the unique characteristics specific to projective techniques (e.g., their differing number of responses, rarity of many categories, interrelatedness of responses, and sensitivity to interpersonal variables), they provide poor psychometric data, but rich ideographic data (Aronow, Reznikoff, & Rauchway, 1979). Second, projective data should only be used in combination with other data. Third, the lack of validity may be due to the inconsistent use of psychodiagnostic labels. Fourth, more studies need to be carried out with children as subjects. And fifth, as Falk (1981) suggests, the questions proposed in research need to be congruent with the realities of clinical practice.

Future research should give serious consideration to improving the psychometric properties of projectives (e.g., limiting the subject to one response, standardizing administration and scoring, using alternate forms) and their idiographic properties (e.g., requiring more association and discussion of percepts; inquiring further about examinees' expectations, perceptions, and general response sets, and their interpretations of their own test responses) (Aronow *et al.*, 1979). Some of this work on the psychometric aspects has already begun. For example, Stang, Campus, and Wallach (1975) examined the impact of exposure length on TAT performance and found a linear decrease in "pleasantness" as a function of exposure length. Further, the reduced pleasantness was thought to affect scoring on such dimensions as affectivity and, perhaps, need achievement or affiliation. In addition, studies need to be conducted that (*a*) provide useful information for understanding individuals' behavior, (*b*) adhere to projective test theory and present a different approach to diagnostic labeling, (*c*) evaluate children and their responses from a developmental perspective, and (*d*) examine the effects of external factors within children's ecosystems as expressed through their projective performances.

Projection in Children

While the purposes of personality assessment and the techniques used may be similar when evaluating both children and adults, there are special considerations when assessing young children. For example, children's perceptions of test situations and the ease of interaction with the examiner may affect, in varying degrees, the nature and content of a child's responses as well as overall productivity of the protocol. Therefore, while a child's age, developmental status, and verbal ability are factors influencing quantity and quality (or richness) of responses, the practitioner should recognize that the child's desire or willingness to reveal his or her personality may be to a large extent dependent on his or her overall mood and ease with the examiner and the (test) situation (Rabin & Haworth, 1960).

Both the child and the projective responses obtained during an assessment must be evaluated from both a developmental and normative perspective. Problems of distinguishing between immature and aberrant responses are correctly regarded as more acute when working with children than with adults (Altman, 1960). What would be considered a distorted response with an indication of pathology in adults may be merely a sign of developmental immaturity in children. Due to their limited knowledge of the social and physical reality around them and their limited verbal/abstract reasoning skills, children's "distorted responses" cannot necessarily be interpreted to indicate defensiveness, regression, or ego disintegration. Finally, young children's projective performances may be more indicative of their developmental statuses than of their personality organizations per se. For example, impulsive responses reflecting poor judgment and tenuous controls may be expected from the 4-or-5-year-old child who is just beginning to exercise control over his or her impulses. It is not until the age of 6 or 7 that one begins to see patterns which reflect the children's general coping styles (construction, withdrawal, aggression).

In summary, the social setting of the test situation, the examiner's effects upon the child (and vice versa), children's shortened attention spans, their limited verbal skills, and their spontaneous and often revealing conversations are all factors that deserve special consideration when testing and interpreting the projective and personality assessment results of children and adolescents.

The following case illustrates the significance of a child's spontaneous verbalizations.

Bobby was 7 years and 3 months old at the time of the psychological evaluation. His mother deserted the family when he was 4 years old and his father had placed him in residential care due to Bobby's uncontrollable outbursts of aggression. Bobby was keenly aware of and distressed by his deficits, particularly his visual–motor integrative difficulties, as evidenced in his poor BenderGestalt reproductions.

In the middle of the WISC-R administration, with the increasing pressure of more difficult items, Bobby began shifting in his chair until he was lying down on it and said he didn't want to do any more. He finally withdrew to sitting on the floor peering out from behind his chair. Even in this silent and frightened state, he could be gently coaxed to continue. From this frozen position he commented, while pointing to a toy (a small toy man inside a plastic container), "This guy's all locked up he can't get out." It was clear that Bobby was vividly describing his own feelings at that moment. His final TAT story revealed his wishes and needs and his ability to experience great satisfaction from very basic pleasures. His face lit up as he told a story (to TAT Card 10) of "a man and a woman going out on a date, happy, eating ice cream, cake, and soda and going home to sleep." (Obrzut & Zucker, 1983, p. 204, reprinted with permission)

Integration and Application of Test Results: A Case Study

The purpose of the personality assessment, the child's background, his or her current test behaviors, and the test results themselves should all be considered when providing personality descriptions, psychodynamic interpretations, diagnostic formulations, or prognoses and recommendations for any given child. The psychological evaluation should be an integration of the available information about the child and should be geared toward a better understanding of the child's present adjustment, behavior, conflicts, strengths, and limitations. The referral problem should guide the selection of instruments, the specific questions to be answered, and the nature of the recommendations.

The following case material exemplifies the integration and application of all these relevant data.

David is a nine year old child who has a history of physical abuse and emotional and medical neglect and who has been in foster care for the past 5 years. He is currently being evaluated for admission into a therapeutic foster care program. His need for additional services beyond those offered by the regular foster care program has been increasingly apparent since the termination of parental rights and the death of his grandmother. Faced with the loss of all of his family, David's behavior became extremely angry, impulsive, and difficult to control. He also exhibited problems with sleeping, eating, and bowel and bladder control.

Records indicate that David has been tested many times because of the complexity of his diagnosis. According to the most recent reports, he is deaf in one ear and has a partial hearing loss in the other with resulting problems in the areas of auditory receptive and expressive skills. This report also indicates that, contrary to the opinion of previous examiners, David is not aphasic and that the preservative, tangential, and inappropriate aspects of David's expressive language are due primarily to emotional disturbance. Examiners have also disagreed about the level of David's intellectual abilities. Given his other disabilities, IQ tests have probably underestimated his ability and he probably could score within the average range or slightly below without such interference. Finally, there has also been disagreement regarding the degree and nature of David's emotional disturbance. An evaluation in 1979 indicated that he was definitely not psychotic and that David had good capacity for attachment. His current therapist at Children's Hospital, however, states that he frequently exhibits signs of borderline psychosis.

David was cooperative throughout the testing process and, in contrast to two years ago, was able to complete both the CAT and Rorschach. He was an appealing child who seemed eager to please, fairly affectionate, and capable of making good eye contact. With effort, it was possible to communicate despite David's hearing loss. He seemed to make good use of lip reading skills and would turn his best ear toward the examiner when he had difficulty hearing. A brief interview was conducted in an attempt to get some feeling for David's perception of his current situation and future placement.

David seemed to have little ability to verbalize the reasons for his out of home placement, but was able to say that "my parents can't help me." He was clearly preoccupied with the many recent losses he has experienced, and spontaneously discussed missing his father, the death of his grandmother, and the upcoming termination meetings with his mother. It is interesting to note that he avoided mention of his previous foster family from whose home he was recently moved. David seemed to understand that his current placement with a foster family was temporary but also engaged in considerable denial with regard to the fact that he may soon be moved from this home. It seemed clear that he preferred to stay in this home primarily because of his need for stability and consistency and his difficulty adjusting to change.

David exhibited some confusion in labeling feelings during the interview. He clearly confused sad and angry feelings and at times simultaneously stated he felt sad and flexed his muscles as if angry. At other times, when the examiner reflected back a statement about sad feelings, he flexed his muscles as if to let the examiner know that it made him angry to get in touch with sad feelings. At other times, David responded to the examiner's questions by reciting a string of feeling-related words (happy, sad, mad, scared) without affect. The examiner got the impression that he had learned what therapists like to hear and that this was an attempt to please the examiner when he didn't understand the question or else wanted to avoid discussing an issue.

TAT stories clearly suggested, through clinical/qualitative analyses, preoccupation with recent losses. David appears to have gone beyond the denial stage and is currently in an angry phase in dealing with his losses. Anger was clearly mixed with sadness and, as noted above, it was often apparent that David was using anger to avoid dealing with pain. A clear example of this was one story which was told in response to a card depicting a family of monkeys. He identified each monkey as a biological family member and stated that a large monkey pointing at a smaller monkey was his Dad pointing at him and stating that "he wouldn't see him any more." Two other monkeys were telling secrets (his mother and sister) and saying that "David stinks," indicating underlying feelings that David perceives his losses as his fault. After telling this story, David became extremely angry and began punching the card and simultaneously saying "David feels mad." It is interesting to note that David was unable to make up a story about the next card which pictures a baby rabbit alone in bed at night and instead returned to the previous family card and continued punching it. Clearly, David is having great difficulty tolerating the pain and loneliness evoked by recent major losses.

David's Rorschach protocol presented a strong contrast to the one he produced two years ago which was during a good period for him when he had settled into his first foster care home. At that time, his responses were characteristic of a child who was delayed in his emotional development but not seriously disturbed. His current Rorschach suggests strong emotional disturbance with a combination of neurotic and psychotic features. He would probably be best characterized at this point as borderline and undergoing a severe regression due to the major losses suffered in the past few months. David perceived no Popular responses on the Rorschach this time (again in contrast to his past performance) indicating that he does not currently see reality the way others do. Some underlying capacity for attachment was evident, but it was clear that he also currently associates perception of the human figure with body damage and injury, thus indicating that he feels damaged on a very primitive level by recent losses. Thus, for example, responses showed a preoccupation with blood inside his body and gushing forth due to injury, and bodies with holes in them or fingers missing. Perceptions were often of poor form quality, although recovery on subsequent responses often followed. Thus, David's ability to stay in touch with reality is probably variable at this point. Responses to color cards indicate that David tends to become overwhelmed by his emotions and becomes very impulsive due to his inability to integrate and make appropriate use of his emotions at the present time. He showed some tendency to withdraw from emotional stimuli when overwhelmed as a way of pulling himself together. Behaviorally, this might indicate a tendency to withdraw from emotionally stimulating human contact, whether positive or negative, in order to avoid the feelings which this arouses. Despite the above, however, David is still fairly well in touch with his dependency needs and will probably continue to seek to get these met at some level.

Currently, David is expressing intense anger with regard to these losses at a primitive bodily level in terms of fantasies of injury to himself. Some primary process like thinking seems to be interfering with his ability to understand cause and effect relationships. In addition, like many foster children, David is viewing these losses as his fault and is likely to engage in behavior which will provoke further rejection. Thus, although David's behavior has improved, since placement in a new home, he continues to test limits and act out in this new environment.

Summary

In order to interpret individuals' responses to the TAT and similar thematic techniques, the practitioner should operate from a theoretical framework. Holtzberg (1968) notes, "where there is emphasis on techniques with theory minimized, there is danger of developing diagnostic technicians rather than scientist clinicians" (p. 18). Thematic picture techniques may be interpreted from numerous theoretical perspectives. Whether the practitioner's orientation is psychoanalytic, behavioral, or eclectic, the theoretical framework is critical in order to provide purpose and cohesiveness to the diagnostic/intervention process.

Projective tests in general may be most valid when used as a type of structured clinical interview. In this context, projective tests facilitate an understanding of the unique needs, interests, pressures, conflicts, affective and cognitive styles, and coping strategies that characterize each individual adolescent or child. Given their ability to broaden our understanding of a referred child, and in the hands of an experienced user, it is likely that projective tests will continue to flourish and be improved technically over time.

References

Ainsworth, M. G. (1951). Some problems of validation of projective techniques. *British Journal of Medical Psychology, 24*, 151–161.

Altman, C. H. (1960). Projective techniques in the clinical setting. In A. I. Rabin & M. R. Haworth (Eds.), *Projective techniques with children* (pp. 332–349). New York: Grune & Stratton.

American Psychological Association (APA). (1974). *Standards for education and psychological tests*. Washington DC: Author.

Anastasi, A. (1982). *Psychological testing* (5th ed.). New York: Macmillan.

Aronow, E., Reznikoff, M., & Rauchway, A. (1979). Some old and new directions in Rorschach testing. *Journal of Personality Assessment, 63*, 227–234.

Bachtold, L. M. (1975). Perceptions of emotionally disturbed male adolescents on the Thematic Apperception Test. *Perceptual and Motor Skills, 40*, 867–871.

Bailey, B. E., & Green, J., III. (1979). Black Thematic Apperception Test stimulus material. *Journal of Personality Assessment, 41*, 25–30.

Beck, S. J. (1960). Families of schizophrenic and of well children: Method, concepts, and some results. *American Journal of Orthopsychiatry, 30*, 247–275.

Bellak, L. (1947). *A guide to the interpretation of the Thematic Apperception Test*. New York: Psychological Corporation.

Bellak, L. (1975). *The TAT, CAT, and SAT in clinical use*. New York: Grune & Stratton.

Bellak, L., & Bellak, S. S. (1949). *The Children's Apperception Test*. New York: C.P.S. Company.

Bene, E., & Anthony, J. (1957). *Manual for the Family Relations Test*. London: National Foundation for Educational Research in England and Wales.

Blatt, S. J. (1975). The validity of projective techniques and their research and clinical contribution. *Journal of Personality Assessment, 39*, 327–343.

Blum, G. S. (1950). *The Blacky Pictures: Manual of instructions*. New York: Psychological Corporation.

Blum, G. S. (1962). A guide for research of the Blacky Pictures. *Journal of Projective Techniques,* *26,* 3–29.

Constantine, G., Malgady, R. G., & Vazquez, C. (1981). A comparision of the Murray-TAT and a new thematic apperception test for urban Hispanic children. *Hispanic Journal of Behavioral Sciences, 3,* 291–300.

Cummings, J. A. (1982, August). *Research on projective drawings: Implications for practice.* Paper presented at the annual meeting of the American Psychological Association, Washington, DC.

Ebel, E. L. (1961). Must all tests be valid? *American Psychologist, 16,* 640–647.

Eron, L. A. (1950). A normative study of the TAT. *Psychological Monographs, 64* (Whole No. 315).

Exner, J. E. (1976). Projective techniques. In I. B. Weiner (Ed.), *Clinical methods in psychology* (pp. 61–121). New York: Wiley.

Falk, J. D. (1981). Understanding children's art: An analysis of the literature. *Journal of Personality Assessment, 45,* 465–472.

Frost, B. P. (1969). Family Relations Test: A normative study. *Journal of Projective Techniques and Personality Assessment, 33,* 409–413.

Goh, D. S., Teslow, C. J., & Fuller, G. B. (1981). The practice of psychological assessment among school psychologists. *Professional Psychology, 12,* 696–706.

Goldfried, M. R., & Kent, R. N. (1972). Traditional versus behavioral personality assessment: A comparison of methodological and theoretical assumptions. *Psychological Bulletin, 77,* 409–420.

Goldfried, M. R., & Zax, M. (1965). The stimulus value of the TAT. *Journal of Projective Techniques and Personality Assessment, 29,* 46–57.

Granick, S., & Scheflin, N. A. (1958). Approaches to reliability of projective tests with special reference to the Blacky Pictures Test. *Journal of Consulting Psychology, 22,* 137–141.

Hall, C. S., & Lindzey, G. (1978). *Theories of personality* (3rd ed.). New York: Wiley.

Hersh, J. A. (1978). *A concurrent validation of the Roberts Apperception Test as a measure of the therapeutic progress of children.* Unpublished doctoral dissertation, California School of Professional Psychology, Los Angeles.

Holtzberg, J. D. (1968). Psychological theory and projective techniques. In A. I. Rabin (Ed.), *Projective techniques in personality assessment* (pp. 18–63). New York: Springer.

Howes, R. J. (1981). The Rorschach: Does it have a future? *Journal of Personality Assessment, 45,* 339–351.

Hutt, M. L. (1980). *The Michigan Picture Test–Revised: Manual.* New York: Grune & Stratton.

Jensen, A. R. (1965). Review of the Make-A-Picture Story Test. In O. K. Buros (Ed.), *The sixth mental measurement yearbook.* Highland Park, NJ: Gryphon Press.

Kagan, J. (1956). The measurement of overt aggression from fantasy. *Journal of Abnormal and Social Psychology, 52,* 390–393.

Kagan, J. (1960). Thematic apperception techniques with children. In A. I. Rabin & M. R. Haworth (Eds.), *Projective techniques with children* (pp. 105–129). New York: Grune & Stratton.

Kaleita, T. A. (1980). *The expression of attachment and separation anxiety in abused and neglected adolescents.* Unpublished doctoral dissertation, California School of Professional Psychology, Los Angeles.

Kauffman, J. M. (1971). Family Relations Test responses of disturbed and normal boys: Additional comparative data. *Journal of Personality Assessment, 35,* 128–138.

Kelly, R., & Berg, B. (1978). Measuring children's reaction to divorce. *Journal of Clinical Psychology, 34,* 215–221.

Kinard, E. M. (1982). Aggression in abused children: Differential responses to the Rosenzweig Picture-Frustration Study. *Journal of Personality Assessment, 46,* 139–141.

Korchin, S. J. (1976). *Modern clinical psychology.* New York: Basic Books.

Korchin, S. J., Mitchell, H., & Meltzoff, J. (1950). A critical evaluation of the Thompson Thematic Apperception Test. *Journal of Projective Techniques, 14,* 445–452.

Korchin, S. J., & Schuldberg, D. (1981). The future of clinical assessment. *American Psychologist, 36,* 1147–1158.

Lanyon, R. I., & Goodstein, L. D. (1982). *Personality Assessment* (2nd ed.). New York: Wiley.

Leary, T. F. (1957). *The interpersonal diagnosis of personality.* New York: Ronald Press.

Lehmann, I. J. (1959). Responses of kindergarten children to the Children's Apperception Test. *Journal of Clinical Psychology, 15,* 60–63.

Lesser, G. S. (1957). The relationship between overt and fantasy aggression as a function of maternal response to aggression. *Journal of Abnormal and Social Psychology, 55,* 218–221.

Levy, M. R., & Fox, H. M. (1975). Psychological testing is alive and well. *Professional Psychology, 6,* 420–424.

Lindzey, G. (1952). Thematic Apperception Test: Interpretive assumptions and related empirical evidence. *Psychological Bulletin, 49,* 1–25.

Loevinger, J. (1976). *Ego development.* San Francisco, CA: Jossey-Bass.

Loevinger, J., & Wesler, R. (1970). *Measuring ego development: I. Construction and use of a sentence completion test.* San Francisco, CA: Jossey-Bass.

Lubin, B., Wallis, R. R., & Paine, C. (1971). Patterns of psychological test usage in the United States: 1935–1969. *Professional Psychology, 2,* 70–74.

Matranga, J. T. (1976). The relationship between behavioral indices of aggression and hostile content on the TAT. *Journal of Personality Assessment, 40,* 130–133.

May, R. (1975). Further studies on deprivation/enhancement patterns. *Journal of Personality Assessment, 39,* 116–112.

Mazumdar, D. P., & Solanski, P. S. (1979). A comparative study of emotionally disturbed and normal children on selected criteria of projective apperception tests (TAT/CAT). *Indian Journal of Clinical Psychology, 6,* 115–117.

McArthur, D. S., & Roberts, G. E. (1982). *Roberts Apperception Test for Children: Manual.* Los Angeles, CA: Western Psychological Services.

McClelland, D. C., Atkinson, J. W., Clark, R. A., & Lowell, E. L. (1953). *The achievement motive.* New York: Appleton-Century-Crofts.

Morgan, C. D., & Murray, H. A. (1935). A method for investigating phantasies: The Thematic Apperception Test. *Archives of Neurology and Psychiatry, 34,* 289–306.

Muha, T. W. (1977). *A validation study of the Robers' Apperception Test as a measure of psychological dysfunction in families.* Unpublished doctoral dissertation, California School of Professional Psychology, Los Angeles.

Murray, H. A. (1938). *Explorations in personality.* London & New York: Oxford University Press.

Murray, H. A. (1943). *Manual of Thematic Apperception Test.* Cambridge, MA: Harvard University Press.

Murray, H. A. (1971). *Thematic Apperception Test: Manual.* Cambridge, MA: Harvard University Press.

Murstein, B. I. (1961). Assumptions, adaption level and projective techniques. *Perceptual and Motor Skills, 12,* 107–125.

Murstein, B. I. (1963). *Theory and research in projective techniques.* New York: Wiley.

Murstein, B. I. (1965). New thoughts about ambiguity and the TAT. *Journal of Projective Techniques and Personality Assessment, 29,* 219–225.

Murstein, B. I. (1968). Effects of stimulus, background, personality and scoring system on the manifestation of hostility on the TAT. *Journal of Consulting and Clinical Psychology, 32,* 335–365.

Murstein, B. I., & Wolf, S. R. (1970). Empirical test of the "levels" hypothesis with five projective techniques. *Journal of Abnormal Psychology, 75,* 38–44.

Mussen, P. H., & Naylor, K. (1954). The relationships between overt and fantasy aggression. *Journal of Abnormal and Social Psychology, 49,* 235–240.

Obrzut, J. E., & Cummings, J. A. (1983). The projective approach to personality assessment: An analysis of thematic picture techniques. *School Psychology Review, 12,* 414–420.

Obrzut, J. E., & Zucker, S. (1983). Projective personality assessment techniques. In G. W. Hynd (Ed.), *The school psychologist* (pp. 195–229). Syracuse, NY: Syracuse University Press.

Philipp, R. L., & Orr, R. R. (1978). Family relations as perceived by emotionally disturbed and normal boys. *Journal of Personality Assessment, 42,* 121–127.

Piotrowski, Z. A. (1957). *Perceptanalysis.* New York: Macmillan.

Prout, H. T. (1983). School psychologists and social-emotional assessment techniques: Patterns in training and use. *School Psychology Review, 12,* 377–383.

Rabin, A. I. (1968). Projective methods: An historical introduction. In A. I. Rabin (Ed.), *Projective techniques in personality assessment* (pp. 3–17). New York: Springer.

Rabin, A. I., & Haworth, M. R. (Eds.). (1960). *Projective techniques with children.* New York: Grune & Stratton.

Riess, B. F., Schwartz, E. K., & Cottingham, A. (1950). An experimental critique of assumptions underlying the Negro version of the TAT. *Journal of Abnormal and Social Psychology, 45,* 700–709.

Ritzler, B. A., Sharkey, K. J., & Chudy, J. F. (1980). A comprehensive projective alternative to the TAT. *Journal of Personality Assessment, 44,* 358–362.

Rosenzweig, S. (1978). An investigation of the reliability of the Rosenzweig Picture-Frustration (P-F) Study, Children's Form. *Journal of Personality Assessment, 42,* 483–488.

Sappenfield, B. R. (1965). Review of the Blacky Pictures. In O. K. Buros (Ed.), *The sixth mental measurement yearbook.* Highland Park, NJ: Gryphon Press.

Schmidt, H. O., & Fonda, C. P. (1956). The reliability of psychiatric diagnosis: A new look. *Journal of Abnormal and Social Psychology, 52*, 262–267.

Shneidman, E. S. (1952). *The Make-A-Picture Story Test.* New York: Psychological Corporation.

Schroth, M. L. (1977). The use of the associative elaboration and integration scales for evaluating CAT protocols. *The Journal of Psychology, 97*, 29–35.

Schwartz, R., & Lazar, Z. (1979). The scientific status of the Rorschach. *Journal of Personality Assessment, 43*, 3–11.

Sharp, V. H., Glasner, A., Lederman, I. I., & Wolfe, S. (1964). Sociopaths and schizophrenics—A comparison of family interaction. *Psychiatry, 27*, 127–134.

Singer, J. L. (1968). Research applications of projective methods. In A. I. Rabin (Ed.), *Projective techniques in personality assessment* (pp. 581–610). New York: Springer.

Slemon, A. G., Holzworth, E. J., Lewis, J., & Sitko, M. (1976). Associative elaboration and integration scales for evaluating TAT protocols. *Journal of Personality Assessment, 40*, 365–369.

Solomon, I. L., & Starr, B. D. (1968). *School Apperception Method (SAM).* New York: Springer.

Squyres, E. M., & Craddick, R. A. (1982). A measure of time perspective with the TAT and some issues of reliability. *Journal of Personality Assessment, 46*, 257–259.

Stang, D. J., Campus, N., & Wallach, C. (1975). Exposure duration as a confounding methodological factor in projective testing. *Journal of Personality Assessment, 39*, 583–586.

Sutton, P. M., & Swenson, C. H. (1983). The reliability and concurrent validity of alternative methods for assessing ego development. *Journal of Personality Assessment, 47*, 468–475.

Swanson, B. M. (1969). Parent and child relations: A child's acceptance by others of others and of self. *Dissertation Abstracts International, 30*(4B), 1890.

Symonds, P. M. (1939). Criteria for the selection of pictures for the investigation of adolescent phantasies. *Journal of Abnormal and Social Psychology, 34*, 271–274.

Thompson, C. E. (1949). *Thematic Apperception Test: Thompson modification.* Cambridge, MA: Harvard University Press.

Wade, T. C., & Baker, T. B. (1977). Opinions and use of psychological tests: A survey of clinical psychologists. *American Psychologist, 32*, 874–882.

Wade, T. C., Baker, T. B., Morton, T. L., & Baker, L. J. (1978). The status of psychological testing in clinical psychology: Relationships between test use and professional activities and orientations. *Journal of Personality Assessment, 42*, 3–10.

Weisskopf-Joelson, E., Zimmerman, J., & McDaniel, M. (1970). Similarity between subject and stimulus as an influence on projection. *Journal of Projective Techniques and Personality Assessment, 34*, 328–331.

Werner, M., Stabenau, J. R., & Pollin, W. (1970). Thematic Apperception Test Method for the differentiation of families of schizophrenics, delinquents, and "normals." *Journal of Abnormal Psychology, 75*, 139–145.

Zubin, J., Eron, L. D., & Schumer, L. (1965). *An experimental approach to projective techniques.* New York: Wiley.

Projective Drawings

Jack A. Cummings

> The drawings of young children fulfill a very different purpose from that of the art products of older children or adults. They must be looked upon as a universal language of childhood whereby children of all races and cultures express their ideas of the world about them. They belong not to the realm of aesthetics, but to the realm of thought and expression. (Goodenough 1931, p. 505)

The present chapter addresses issues and practices associated with the use and interpretation of projective drawings by reviewing (*a*) the historical development of drawing techniques, (*b*) the assumptions underlying their interpretations, (*c*) the frequencies of their clinical uses, and (*d*) the specific types of projective drawings. The drawing techniques covered will include the Draw-A-Person, House-Tree-Person, and Kinetic Drawing System (Kinetic Family and Kinetic School drawing combined) techniques. The discussion of each technique will address each technique's administration, interpretation, and its psychometric qualities. For the purposes of this chapter, psychometric quality will include the concepts of construct validity, and reliability and stability.

Minimally, there are two camps of psychologists or mental health practitioners: those who view drawings as valuable tools investigating children's attitudes, needs, and conflicts; and those who question the assumptions underlying projective drawings. Koppitz's (1983) recent statement reflects the position of many advocates of projective drawings: "Drawing is a natural mode of expression for children age 5 to 11. Long before youngsters can put their feelings and thoughts into words they can express conscious attitudes, wishes, and concerns in drawings. Drawing is a non-verbal language, a means of communication" (pp. 283–284). Another advocate of projective drawings suggests that drawings are a form of symbolic speech that " . . . tap the stream of personality needs as they flood the area of graphic creativity" (E. F. Hammer, 1981, p. 154).

In contrast, Roback (1968) states,

> Many clinicians apparently entertain grandiose delusions that they can "intuitively" gain a great deal of information from figure drawings about the personality structure and dynamics of the drawer. . . . Perhaps in individual cases, they may provide insight into the drawer's perception of himself and others, but in these instances the cases are usually so extreme or the patient so disorganized that one could easily have gotten the same information from a multitude of other sources which would not have necessitated a testing situation. (pp. 16–17)

Jack A. Cummings. Department of Counseling and Educational Psychology, Indiana University, Bloomington, Indiana.

Palmer (1983) suggested that hypotheses developed from drawings are the most tenuous and specious of all clinical predictions. The most extreme comment on projective drawings was made by Martin (1983). He labeled the use of projective drawings unethical and called for a moratorium on their applications in clinical practice.

Rather than focus exclusively on the position of either the advocates or the critics, a more balanced view will be presented by reporting the relevant empirically oriented studies for each drawing technique. In this way, each technique's validity can be assessed in the most objective manner. After reviewing the various drawing techniques, a case study and a conclusion with recommendations for the appropriate uses of projective drawings will follow.

Historical Perspective

Using a quantitative approach and analysis process, Goodenough generally is considered the first psychologist to translate children's drawings into meaningful psychological data. Her classic work, *Measurement of Intelligence by Drawings* (Goodenough, 1926), describes the Draw-A-Man Test and a corresponding scoring system for estimating individuals' levels of intellectual functioning. It is interesting that Goodenough (1931) credits Barnes (1892) as the first to classify children based on the details of their drawings. Barnes asked children to illustrate the poem "Johnny Look-in-the-Air," and analyzed their products developmentally.

The psychological use of drawings has flourished since Goodenough introduced the Draw-A-Man Test. Although Goodenough was primarily interested in quantitatively assessing children's intellectual functioning, E. F. Hammer (1968) reports that practitioners quickly noted a clinical discrepancy in that qualitatively different drawings could still receive the same quantitative credit. Indeed, qualitative characteristics such as facial expression, size, position on page, and boldness of line seemed to reveal important clinical information about the child. According to Hammer, expressions of affect "flooded" the drawings.

Machover's (1949) *Personality Projection in the Drawings of the Human Figure* represented a comprehensive treatment of the qualitative use of human figure drawings. Machover was concerned with the "projective" aspects of drawings, that is, the pictorial representations of individuals' impulses, anxieties, conflicts, and compensations as symbolized in human figures. Based on Machover's experiences with emotionally disturbed male adolescents and adult institutionalized psychotics, a wide variety of interpretive hypotheses were reported for human figure drawings. For example, the mouth of an individual's human figure drawing shown as a single heavy slash was said to communicate aggression. Alternatively, an overly emphasized mouth suggested manifestations of gastric symptoms, profane language, or temper tantrums.

During the same period, Buck (1948) published the House-Tree-Person (HTP) drawing technique as a more thorough measure of intelligence, although it has since become more popular as a projective technique. In 1951 and 1952, Hulse described a family drawing technique, advocating a subjective/intuitive approach to its interpretation. Hulse's portrait-like, noninteracting (or nonkinetic) Family Drawing Test became the precursor to R. C. Burns and Kaufman's (1970, 1972) Kinetic Family Drawing (KFD) technique. The kinetic component of the drawings was added by asking the child to draw a picture of everyone in his or her family *doing* something. Burns and Kaufman hypothesized that activity introduced into the drawings would permit self and family attitudes to become more apparent. Later, the Kinetic Family Drawings spawned an analogous technique applied to the school setting, the Kinetic School Drawing technique (Prout & Phillips, 1974; Sarbaugh, 1983); and finally, the Kinetic Drawing System (Knoff & Prout, 1985a, 1985b) was introduced—an integration of both Family and School Drawing techniques. Regardless of the variant form of the drawing technique, it is important to understand the assumptions underlying the interpretation of drawings.

Assumptions Underlying Projective Drawings

The most basic assumption underlying projective drawings is that a child's psychomotor response (i.e., drawing) contains nonverbal, symbolic messages. Machover (1949) proposed the "body image" hypothesis, which assumes that when a person draws a human figure, it is actually a representation of how he or she views him or herself. Machover stated, "In some sense the figure drawn is the person and the paper corresponds to the environment" (1949, p. 35).

E. F. Hammer refined and extended the body image hypothesis. In 1958, he stated that the interpretation of drawings depends on three theoretical postulates: (*a*) humans view the world in an anthropomorphic manner, that is, in their own images; (*b*) projection is the core of the anthropomorphic view, with projection being the attribution of one's feelings, attitudes, and strivings to people or objects in the environment; and (*c*) distortions result during projection when they serve a defensive function. In other words, projection would be "ascribing to the outer world that which the subject denies in himself" (E. F. Hammer, 1968, p. 369). In the case of an emotionally disturbed child whose perception of the world is inaccurate, the drawing would reveal these distortions.

In contrast to Machover and Hammer, Dennis (1966) takes a sociological perspective on the interpretation of drawing and assumes that drawings capture social values or preferences. By comparing the drawings of children from culturally different groups, he observed differences among drawings by American, Mexican, East Asian, and Middle Eastern children. The differences were on dimensions such as modern versus traditional dress, emphasis on masculinity, the inclusion of work themes, and the diversity of social roles.

Use of Projective Drawings: Frequency and Function

The use of projective drawings has been widespread in psychology and mental health practice. For several decades, drawings have been reported to be among the most frequently used tests by psychologists in clinical practice (Loutitt & Browne, 1947; Lubin, Larsen, & Matarazzo, 1984; Lubin, Wallis, & Paine, 1971; Sundberg, 1961; Wade & Baker, 1977). Further, projective drawings have been among the most frequently used psychological measures within the school setting. Several recent surveys of school psychologists reveal a high frequency of use, especially when children with suspected social–emotional problems must be assessed (Eklund, Huebner, Groman, & Michael, 1980; Fuller & Goh, 1983; Goh, Teslow, & Fuller, 1981; Prout, 1983; Vukovich, 1983). For instance, Prout (1983) found that school psychologists ranked human figure drawings as their third most frequently used technique. Only the clinical interview and informal classroom observation were ranked above the human figure drawings. When these practitioners were asked about the frequency of their human figure drawings use, 41.9% reported that they always use them in social–emotional assessments, 41.3% reported frequent use, 11.6% reported rare use, and only 5.2% reported that they never use these drawings.

In the second part of Prout's survey, university trainers of school psychologists were asked to report the emphasis they placed on 19 techniques for individual social–emotional assessment. Again the clinical interview and informal classroom observations were ranked first and second, with human figure drawings placing third. A total of 76.8% reported that students received clinical training in projective drawings. Only 1.6% reported little or no formal training with drawings.

Piotrowski and Keller (1984) surveyed 80 of the 113 American Psychological Association (APA)-approved clinical psychology programs to investigate patterns of training in psychodiagnostic assessment. They reported a shift in emphasis from "projective" tests (e.g., Thematic Apperception Test, Rorschach, Sentence Completion, and Human Figure Drawings) to more objectively based measures of personality (e.g., the Minnesota Multiphasic Personality Inventory, California Psychological Inventory, 16 Personality Factor Questionnaire). Nevertheless, 79% of the programs devote at least half a required course to the instruction of projective personality assessment.

These recent studies suggest that, despite the zeitgeist of skepticism regarding the utility of personality research and instruments (Berger, 1968; Bersoff, 1973; Cleveland, 1976; Hogan, Desota, & Solano, 1977), projective drawings continue to occupy a place in the mental health practitioner's assessment repertoire and, more specifically, in the training of clinical and school psychologists.

A review of the projective drawing literature suggests that projective drawings have been used for several functions:

1. To allow nonverbal children to express themselves, that is, graphic communication between the child and psychologist through the use of symbols.
2. To gain an understanding of a child's inner conflicts, fears, interactions with family members, and perceptions of others.
3. To understand the child from a psychodynamic perspective, for example, sexual identification, ego strength.
4. To generate hypotheses and serve as a springboard for further evaluation.

The Draw-A-Person Technique

Administration

A blank sheet of 8½″ × 11″ paper and a #2 lead pencil with an eraser are given to the child when administering the Draw-A-Person. The paper should be positioned vertically and the table should be clear. The child is then asked to "Draw a picture of a whole person." To discourage older children from drawing stick figures as a means of avoiding the task, Koppitz suggests adding "It can be any kind of person you want to draw. Just make sure that it is a whole person and not a stick figure or a cartoon figure" (1968, p. 6). The instruction to "draw-a-person'' is superior to ''draw-a-man,'' because it allows for a greater degree of ambiguity and choice; that is, the child may choose to draw a child or adult as well as a male or female. When the child asks questions, noncommital answers are given. For instance, if the child asks whether or not erasures are permitted, the examiner responds by saying, ''It is up to you.'' The examiner thereby attempts to maintain the ambiguity of the situation.

Most children complete a Draw-A-Person in 5 to 10 minutes. After finishing the first drawing, the child is asked to draw another person, but of the opposite sex. With young children it is frequently necessary to ask them whether their first drawing is a boy or girl. Subsequently, they can be requested to draw a picture of a boy or girl. This level of specificity may be necessary with young children, because they may not understand the concept of drawing a figure of the opposite sex.

General Perspectives of Interpretation

Machover's (1949) classic book, *Personality Projection in the Drawing of the Human Figure*, has been the single greatest influence on the interpretation of drawings. The hypotheses developed by Machover have not only guided the clinical use of drawings, but also have served as stimuli for several decades of empirical investigations. Her approach to drawings was based on her intensive study of thousands of drawings.

Overall, Machover suggested that interpretation should be based on a confluence of indicators, not an atomistic analysis of single signs or characteristics. The clinician must detect and analyze the pattern of diagnostic indicators. This is comparable to assembling a jigsaw puzzle; the pieces must be juxtaposed to form a comprehensive picture of the child or adolescent. Machover's most significant contribution was to define the pieces of the puzzle and to offer interpretive hypotheses organized by several features or components of a drawing. While a comprehensive description of these features is clearly beyond the scope of this chapter, Machover's social and contact features of the drawing will be highlighted. The reader is encouraged to consult Machover (1949) for other hypotheses and elaborations.

Machover's social features of the drawing are represented in the parts of a drawing's head. This area of the body is considered the most expressive as well as the center for social communication. Each part of the figure's face may reveal something about the child or adolescent. For instance, closed eyes may suggest an attempt to shut out the world, while eyes with excessive detail may reveal paranoia, or large, dark accentuated eyes may be associated with hostility.

The contact features of the drawing reveal a child's interactions with the environment. Contact features include fingers, hands, arms, toes, feet, and legs. A relative lack of attention to feet and legs or their omission may reveal a child's insecurity or his or her problems dealing with sexual impulses. Clothing (e.g., buttons, pockets, ties, hats, shoes) is another contact feature for which Machover developed symbolic, interpretive hypotheses. For example, Machover states that ''irrelevant emphasis upon pockets is seen in drawings of infantile and dependent individuals'' (1949, p. 79).

In addition to the social and contact features, other structural variables provide insight into the child. Figure size, its placement on the paper, and the theme of the drawing, in part, constitute the category of structural drawing characteristics. Research on these variables will be reviewed in a subsequent section of the chapter.

Elizabeth Koppitz is another psychologist whose writings have been influential in drawing interpretation. Koppitz's (1968) method of interpreting children's human figure drawings is among the most frequently used by clinical and school psychologists. Koppitz distinguishes between signs or drawing characteristics which reflect a child's age or level of maturation, and those which suggest anxiety, social–emotional concerns, and interpersonal or intrapersonal attitudes. The former characteristics comprise "developmental items"; the latter items are "emotional indicators."

Koppitz defines emotional indicators according to three criteria: (*a*) They must have clinical utility and differentiate between drawings of healthy and emotionally disturbed children; (*b*) they should occur at a low frequency in the drawings of healthy children, that is, in less than 6% of the drawings of normal children; and (*c*) their frequency of occurrence should be independent of age and maturation level. Based on a review of Machover (1949) and E. F. Hammer's (1954, 1958) works, Koppitz developed a list of 38 signs which she believed met the above criteria. These emotional indicators were divided into three categories: Quality signs, Special features, and Omissions. Based on a series of studies comparing the drawings of normal children with those of emotionally disturbed children, she reduced the list to 30 indicators (see Table 7-1).

Koppitz believes that the diagnostic significance of emotional indicators is increased by considering their presence in a drawing collectively, rather than individually. For example, when comparing the human figure drawings of 76 pairs of child guidance patients and public school children, approximately three-fourths or 55 clinic children had two or more emotional indicators present in their drawings (Koppitz, 1966). In contrast, only 4 of the 76 public school children included two or more indicators. Further, Koppitz strongly cautions practitioners not to make diagnoses or predictions of children's behavior based on a single emotional sign. Again, the total drawing and combination of signs should be "analyzed on the basis of the child's age, maturation, emotional status, social and cultural background, and should be then evaluated with other available test data" (Koppitz, 1968, p. 55).

Koppitz (1968) points out that a drawing can represent a variety of attitudes and emotions. Joy, anger, fears, fantasies, or past experiences may be expressed in a drawing. When attempting to clinically analyze a drawing, Koppitz suggests that three questions should be posed.

1. How did the child draw the figure(s)? The child's approach to the figure, even if the child reports the drawing to be representative of another person, reflects the child's self-concept. Hence, the signs and symbols associated with the figure provide information about the child's self-concept.

2. Who does the child draw? According to Koppitz, the child draws the most important person to him or her at the time of the drawing. She suggests that children typically draw themselves due to their egocentricity. When another individual is drawn, the person may be associated with (appropriate or inappropriate) concern and/or possible conflict.

Koppitz's notion that children draw the person with whom they are most concerned admittedly contrasts with Machover's sexual identification hypothesis. Machover postulated that children draw the sex with which they identify. Based

Table 7-1
Koppitz's Emotional Indicators for Human Figure Drawings[a]

Quality Signs

Poor integration of parts: One or more parts not joined to rest of figure, part only connected by a single line, or barely touching

Shading of face: Deliberate shading of whole face or part of it, including "freckles," "measles," etc.; an even, light shading of face and hands to represent skin color is not scored

Shading of hands and/or neck

Gross asymmetry of limbs: One arm or leg differs markedly in shape from the other arm or leg. This item is not scored if arms or legs are similar in shape, but just a bit uneven in size

Slanting figures: Vertical axis of figure tilted by 15° or more from the perpendicular

Tiny figure: Figure 2 inches or less in height

Big figure: Figure 9 inches or more in height

Transparencies: Transparencies involving major portions of body or limbs; single line or lines of arms crossing body not scored

Special Features

Tiny Head: Height of head less than one-tenth of total figure

Crossed eyes: Both eyes turned in or turned out; sideway glance of eyes not scored

Teeth: Any representation of one or more teeth

Short arms: Short stubs for arms, arms not long enough to reach waistline

Long arms: Arms excessively long, arms long enough to reach below knee or where knee should be

Arms clinging to body: No space between body and arms

Big hands: Hands as big or bigger than face of figure.

Hands cut off: Arms with neither hands nor fingers; hands hidden behind back of figure or in pocket not scored

Legs pressed together: Both legs touch with no space in between; in profile drawings only one leg is shown

Genitals: Realistic or unmistakably symbolic representation of genitals

Monster or grotesque figure: Figure representing nonhuman, degraded or ridiculous person; the grotesqueness of figure must be deliberate on part of the child and not the result of immaturity or lack of drawing skill

Three or more figures spontaneously drawn: Several figures shown who are not interrelated or engaged in meaningful activity; repeated drawing of figures when only "a" figure was requested; drawing of a boy and girl or the child's family is not scored

Clouds: Any presentation of clouds, rain, snow, or flying birds

Omissions

No eyes: Complete absence of eyes; closed eyes or vacant circles for eyes are not scored

No nose

No mouth

No body

No arms

No legs

No feet

No neck

[a]From Koppitz, E. M. (1968). *Psychological evaluation of children's human figure drawings*. New York: Grune & Stratton.

on her extensive clinical experience and a review of the literature, Koppitz rejected the hypothesis that children's latent or conscious sexual identification confusion is manifested when they draw the opposite sex first.

Finally, when children choose to draw a portrait of the examining practitioner, this was hypothesized to reflect lonely and socially isolated children who are looking for attention, even the attention of a stranger with whom they have interacted for a short period of time.

3. What is the child trying to express via the drawing? Or, what is the message that he or she is trying to convey to the examiner? Koppitz notes that

the message may be a representation of a wish, an expression of attitudes and conflicts, or both. A child's spontaneous story about the drawing could reflect a wishdream. Yet a child's self-figure drawing and corresponding description more likely reflects the child's self-perceptions. A child's drawing of someone else, however, probably reveals attitudes or conflicts toward that given person. While this may appear to contradict the statements in Question 1, Koppitz clarifies this by stating that descriptions of the non-self-figure apply to the depicted individual, while the manner in which the figure was drawn reflects the child's self-attitudes.

Specific Interpretation Issues and Indices

Body Image

In Swenson's (1957) original review of projective drawings, few of the research studies cited supported the body image hypothesis. As noted in the above section on assumptions, the body image hypothesis is central to the interpretation of projective drawings. It states that when an individual is asked to draw a person, the product is that person's image of his or her own body.

Unfortunately, the concept of body image is not a simple one; actually, it is quite complex and difficult to measure. Swenson (1968) poses the question, "Is it (the body image) a photograph, or a verbal self-description, or is the body image a function of the interaction between a person's physical appearance and his self-concept? . . . or a combination of something else?" (p. 23). In Swenson's (1968) follow-up review of projective drawing research, he cites several studies which provide support for the body image hypothesis. For instance, Apfeldorf and Smith (1966) had judges sort 25 drawings and 25 full-length photographs of those who created the drawings. The judges, 30 male graduate students and 30 female art students, were able to match the examinees' drawings and photographs significantly better than chance.

In another study, Nathan (1973) analyzed the drawings of 36 obese and 36 matched (sex, SES, IQ) control children. The sample was composed of equal numbers of males and females, all classified by age. Hence, there were 12 children at ages 7, 10, and 13 in each sample. Obese children were defined as those whose body weight exceeded 30% of their weight by height on the Boston Anthropometic Chart. Children in both the obese and control groups drew figures of various sizes; however, qualitative analysis revealed that those in the latter group drew more "fat" figures. Initially, this may appear to disconfirm the body image hypothesis, but further analyses provide insight into the obese children's drawings. In all three of the age groups, some of the obese children drew stick figures. In contrast, all of the normal controls drew two-dimensional figures. There was also a lack of differentiation between the male and female figures among the obese children and a greater number of bizarre and distorted drawings by this sample. Using the Goodenough–Harris (Harris, 1963) scoring system, significant developmental/maturational differences were observed between the obese and control groups, in favor of the latter. This difference was noteworthy because the groups had been matched based on their verbal IQs from the Wechsler Intelligence Scale for Children.

From the Nathan study, it is clear that obese children represent their figures differently from matched controls. However, a simple linear correlation between these children's weights and the size of their drawn figures did not exist. Nathan suggested that the obese children may have undifferentiated and immature body images, as a function of negative feedback from normal peers and adults. Therefore, it is the undifferentiated body image that is manifested in their drawings of human figures.

The body image hypothesis has also been investigated using mentally retarded children's projective drawings. Wysocki and Wysocki (1973) administered the Draw-A-Person to educably mentally retarded children and a control group of normal children. As expected, the mentally retarded children drew less detailed and more simplistic figures. They were more likely to omit fingers and clothing, yet less inclined to make erasures. While most of the normal group's drawings contained two to five erasures, the mentally retarded children tended to draw over a line instead of erasing it. Finally, while Machover would have predicted that the normal children would create larger figures, an opposite trend resulted as mentally retarded children drew more expansive figures.

Wysocki and Whitney (1965) compared the human figure drawings of crippled and noncrippled children. A significant 36% of the 50 crippled children drew figures with a physical handicap corresponding to their own crippling condition. Significant differences also were evident on the following variables: large head, drawing opposite sex first, oversized figure, shading pressure, and paper rotation. Interpretations of these differences suggested that the crippled children were feeling more inferiority, anxiety, and aggression. This study provides support for Machover's body image hypothesis. Although only slightly more than one-third of crippled children drew figures incorporating their handicapped area, their drawings, as a group, were more likely to include emotional maladjustment. Both anxiety and aggression are normal reactions associated with crippled children's body images.

A more recent study by F. A. Johnson and Greenberg (1978; see also F. A. Johnson, 1972) revealed that 32 convalescing poliomyelitis patients did not isomorphically represent their disability in their figure drawings. However, this study's sample was composed of adults (mean age, 30.4), a significantly different sample from Wysocki and Whitney's (1965) children. Johnson and Greenberg also departed from standard administration procedures in that (a) they had their subjects use a black felt-tip pen instead of a pencil, and, more importantly, (b) they asked their subjects to "draw a person in a bathing suit." Thus, it is inappropriate to conclude that Johnson and Greenberg produced evidence to disconfirm the body image hypothesis.

Further support for the body image hypothesis was provided by a study of psoriatic patients (Leichtman, Burnett, & Robinson, 1981). Three groups, a mild psoriatic, severe psoriatic, and a dermatologic control group, were compared. It was found that the severe psoriatic patients included more body image concerns in their drawings, that is, omission of body parts, sexual overemphasis, and incompletely clothed figures.

Perhaps the most significant change in a woman's body image occurs during pregnancy. Hence, to assess the body image hypothesis, women's drawings at various points during their pregnancies should document dramatic differences in their bodily perceptions. Tolor and Digrazio (1977) had women in their first, second, and third trimester of pregnancy complete human figure drawings. Two additional groups, postpartum patients at a 6-week follow-up and a control group of 76 gynecological patients, also participated. No differences were found among the drawings of the women in their various stages of pregnancy and among the postpartum patients. Only a few differences were noted between the collapsed pregnancy groups and gynecological controls. Methodologically, it should be noted that subjects were told to draw a picture of a woman (not a person) to avoid a significant percentage of free choice male figures.

To summarize the trends among investigations addressing the body image hypothesis, the bulk of recent research is positive. This is in contrast to the conclusions of Roback (1968) and Swenson (1968) in their respective reviews of projective drawing research. Based on their independent reviews of research prior to 1968, they concluded that the evidence supporting the validity of the body image hypothesis was tentative. However, recent studies of obese, mentally retarded, physically handicapped, and psoriatic samples provide support for the body image hypothesis. It should be noted that disabilities may not be isomorphically represented in the drawing, that is, an obese individual drawing an overweight figure or a psoriatic patient adding skin abnormalities to the affected area. In these cases, the body image disturbance is typically revealed by more frequent omissions, and immature drawings relative to their levels of intellectual abilities. Research on the relationship of human figure drawings to sexual identification and self-concept provides additional evidence for judging the validity of the body image hypothesis.

Sex of First-Drawn Figure and Gender Identity

Machover (1949) hypothesized that when an individual draws a figure of the opposite sex as the first response, this reflects psychosexual maladjustment. Hence, if a male's first human figure drawing is female, this reflects information about his (maladjusted) sexual identity. Empirically, there are several trends apparent in investigations relating the sex of an individual's first-drawn figure and their gender identity. Approximately 23% of girls 9 years and older draw a figure of the opposite sex first (Brown, 1977, 1979; Fellows & Cerbus, 1969; Rierdan & Koff, 1981). The trend for males is to draw males; males draw the opposite sex first only about 5% of the time.

The trend for girls, age 9 and older, to draw male figures first may be interpreted in two different ways. It might be assumed that girls' sexual confusion increases at this point in time (Bieliauskas, 1960), or, as Tolor and Tolor (1974) suggest, the drawing choice might reflect a cultural influence (i.e., a male figure represents an appropriate initial identification in a male-dominated world). The latter hypothesis would conform to Denis's (1966) sociological perspective on drawings.

Additional evidence in support of the sociological perspective is provided by Teglasi (1980). He reported that undergraduate females with traditional sex role orientations were more likely to draw the opposite sex first. In a second study reported in the same article, he compared the drawings of members of the National Organization of Women (NOW) to a sample of married female nonmembers. None of the NOW members drew a male figure first, while 26% of the latter sample drew the opposite sex first.

Those with adjustment problems related to gender more frequently draw a figure of the opposite sex (Fraas, 1970; Gardner, 1969; Green, Fuller, & Rutley, 1972; Roback, Langevin, & Zajac, 1974; Skilbeck, Bates, & Bentler, 1975). Zucker, Finegan, Doering, and Bradley (1983) completed an interesting study with four groups of children: normal ($N = 30$), those referred for gender identity problems ($N = 36$), siblings of the gender-referred group ($N = 31$), and those with other psychiatric problems ($N = 23$). The children in the gender-referred group were identified using DSM-III diagnostic criteria; two-thirds of the group met all of the criteria for a diagnosis of gender-identity disorder, while the remaining one-third met a significant number of the criteria. Further information on these diagnostic issues is contained in Zucker (1972). The psychiatric group contained children referred for problems not associated with gender identity. The normal group approximated the gender-referred children in terms of age, intelligence, socioeconomic status, and family status. Results indicated that the gender-referred children drew an opposite-sex figure first 61% of the time, the sibling group 22% of the time, the psychiatric group 30% and the normal children drew the opposite-sex figure first only 10% of the time. Similar to the study by Skilbeck et al. (1975), there was also a trend that gender-referred children drew the opposite-sex figure taller than the same-sex figure. It was suggested that the taller figures may represent the more powerful parent or possibly the sex in which the individual had the most interest.

Fleming, Koocher, and Nathans (1979) investigated adults with gender-identity problems; all of the 14 females and 42 males were gender-dysphoric patients. This is an appropriate adult group to investigate because they wanted to assume the identity of their opposite-sex counterparts. A group of 43 males and 41 females in an evening undergraduate class in personality theory served as the control group. Results indicated that a total of 85% of the control males drew the same-sex figure first, while 33% of the dysphoric males drew the same-sex first. Of the female controls, 51% drew females first, while only 15% of the female dysphorics drew females first. Both of these differences were significant and in the expected direction. These findings were replicated by Fleming, Cohen, Salt, and Robinson (1982) with a sample of 19 transsexuals seeking sex reassignment surgery.

The reliability of this indicator definitely suggests that some caution be exercised when analyzing a child who has drawn the opposite sex first on a Draw-A-Person. Both M. Hammer and Kaplan (1964c) and Litt and Margoshes (1966) reported limited test-retest stability on this diagnostic sign. Thus, a child may draw a same-sex figure first in one administration and then in a subsequent testing draw the opposite-sex figure first.

Size of Drawing

The early writers (E. F. Hammer, 1958, 1959, 1960; Levy, 1950; Machover, 1949) in the area of projective drawings asserted that the size of the figure would provide insight into the examinee's self-concept. They believed that individuals with high levels of self-esteem drew large expansive figures, and those with low self-esteem drew small figures. This notion that self-concept and figure size were related developed from clinical observations rather than empirical investigations. In fact, most of the empirically based studies contain evidence that there is no systematic relation between figure size and level of self-esteem (Bennett, 1964, 1966; Dalby & Vale, 1977; Prytula, Phelps, & Morrissey, 1978; Prytula & Thompson, 1973).

The early writers also assumed that figure size was associated with depression. According to Machover (1949), deeply regressed or neurotically depressed persons were likely to draw small or diminutive figures. Lewinsohn (1964) compared the drawings of 50 depressed and nondepressed psychiatric patients. A significant difference between the heights of figures for the two groups was reported, and it was concluded that drawing height and depression are negatively related. Inspection of Lewinsohn's data, however, reveals that the average figure height for the depressed group was 14.6 centimeters, while the height for the nondepressed group was 16.7 centimeters. Although statistically significant, one must question the diagnostic utility of an absolute difference of 2.1 centimeters, especially when the standard deviations for both groups were approximately 5 centimeters. In another study, Roback and Webersinn (1966) failed to find a significant difference in the size of figures when comparing drawings for normals and depressed psychiatric patients.

Additional doubt is cast on the depression and drawing size hypothesis when one considers a recent study by Holmes and Wiederhold (1982). In this study, the MMPI (Depression scale T- score of 80–100) was used to classify 60 patients as depressed. A T- score of 46–60 on the Depression scale was used to define 6 nondepressed patients. Finally, the 21-item Beck Depression Inventory (Beck, Ward, Mendelson, Mock, & Erbaugh, 1961) was used to classify 77 hospital employees (the control) as nondepressed (7 were later eliminated because they scored 80 or higher on this depression scale). Holmes and Weiderhold reported no significant differences among the drawing heights of these three groups; that is, depressed individuals did not draw smaller figures.

In considering a different aspect of size, there is agreement among a number of investigations that no significant differences exist between the figure heights of males and females. This lack of significant sex differences has been reported for depressed and nondepressed psychiatric patients (Holmes & Wiederhold, 1982; Lewinsohn, 1964), psychiatric hospital employees (Holmes & Wiederhold, 1982), children from regular fifth-grade classes (Dalby & Vale, 1977), and for learning-disabled children from ages 6 to 12 (Black, 1976). Thus, it may be concluded that males and females draw comparably sized figures. Although there are no gender differences when mean drawing heights are compared, two investigations (Black, 1972; Cohen, Money, & Uhlenhuth, 1972) found that children's ages, actual heights, and perceived heights do influence the size of the drawing. As children get older, they tend to draw larger figures. Black reported that children's actual heights correlated with drawing size ($r = .67$), while the correlation of perceived heights with drawing size was $r = .24$.

Anxiety

In their review of the literature, Sims, Dana, and Bolton (1983) suggest that manifestations of anxiety in figure drawings have been the subject of a great deal of speculation and a moderate number of empirical investigations. The empirical studies may be separated into two types, those which experimentally induced anxiety and those of a correlational nature using a manifest anxiety scale as an anchor.

Handler and Reyher (1964) investigated the impact of experimentally manipulated stress on male college students' drawings. The stress condition was created by having subjects hooked up to polygraph machines with GSR electrodes attached to their hands. The experimental room was dimly lit, and the ambient noise level was relatively high. Of 21 anxiety indices (Handler, 1967; see Table 7-2), 15 significantly differentiated stress condition from nonstress condition drawings (a sign test was used for the statistical analysis). However, not all the differences were in the predicted directions; that is, some ran counter to Machover's (1949) hypotheses. For instance, shading, erasure, reinforcement, placement in the upper left corner, and emphasis lines were more frequently encountered in drawings

Table 7-2
Handler's Anxiety Indices for Human Figure Drawings

Shading	Cross-hatching or repetitive parallel lines on essential body part
Hair shading	Degree of shading on head
Erasure	Erasures on body areas
Reinforcement	Retracing lines
Light line/Heavy line	Thickness of predominant lines
Placement	Location of figure relative to four quadrants, in upper left, upper right, lower left, lower right
Omission	Omission(s) of essential body parts
Small size/Large size	Height of figure
Small head/Large head	Height of head measured from top to bottom
Head:body ratio	Proportion of head to body
Transparency	An area of the body shows through the clothing
Delineation line absence	Missing body lines, e.g., line between pants and shirt
Vertical imbalance	Midline of figure is not perpendicular to bottom of page
Emphasis line	Series of lines to emphasize a specific body part
Line discontinuity	Broken lines
Distortion	Abnormal size or oddly shaped body parts
Head simplification	Primitiveness of head (in a developmental sense)
Body simplification	Primitiveness of body (in a developmental sense)
Detail loss	Scored when two drawings have been administered, comparison of details lost on the second drawing relative to the first
Light line pressure/ Heavy line pressure	Pencil pressure on page, assessed by the use of carbon paper between multiple sheets

conducted under the nonstress conditions. The variables receiving support, that is, that were included more often in the stress condition drawings, were heavier lines, mechanical line breaks, line sketchiness, detached or omitted body parts, decreased size of figure, and distortions. With an automobile drawing used as a control measure, only 5 of the 17 anxiety measures differentiated the two experimental conditions. Hence, it was concluded that human figure drawings are more emotionally charged stimuli and that some drawing variables are sensitive to stressful conditions.

Handler and Reyher (1966) further explored their hypothesis that individuals would manifest less anxiety in an automobile drawing since it is a more "mental" drawing. Male college students' GSR responses to the automobile revealed that this drawing resulted in the least stress, while the drawing of a female resulted in the most stress, followed by a male drawing. The relationship of GSR and individual scoring variables were assessed with Pearson correlations; the magnitudes of these correlations were generally quite low ($r \cong .30$).

Doubros and Mascarenhas (1967) manipulated stress by having 14-year-old students complete drawings before and after a test. Following the test, stick figures were more commonly evident in drawings. This may have occurred because the students reduced their efforts after the test, or it may be interpreted that persons under stress tend to render more simplified figures. Regardless, eight of nine variables investigated by Doubros and Mascarenhas failed to reach statistical significance.

Sturner, Rothbaum, Visintainer, and Wolfer (1980) conducted an interesting study in which they manipulated the level of stress in 68 children admitted to a hospital for elective surgery (either tonsillectomy or myringotomy). All children completed two drawings separated by a 90-minute interval. During the interval, half the children received a stress condition (a blood test), while the other half received the blood test after they completed their second drawing (nonstress condition). Further, half of the children in the stress and nonstress groups received preparation for the venipuncture (information, rehearsal, and supportive care) while the other half received no preparation. Results indicated that the frequency of emotional indicators increased significantly from the first to the second drawing only for the stressed group that received the blood test without preparation. Thus, the study reveals that "state" variables may influence children's drawings.

Correlational studies have been the second major method used to investigate anxiety indicators in drawings. A manifest anxiety scale typically has been used as the anchor. The results of these studies have generally failed to support an interpretation that anxiety is manifested in and can be predicted from drawings (Craddick, Leipold, & Cacauas, 1962; Engle & Suppes, 1970; Hoyt & Baron, 1959; Handler, 1984; Handler & Reyher, 1965; J. H. Johnson, 1971a, 1971b; Lachmann, Bailey, & Berrick, 1961; Prytula & Hiland, 1975; Viney, Aitkin, & Floyd, 1974).

Artistic Quality

The influence of a child or adolescent's artistic ability on a practitioner's interpretations is an important question. E. F. Hammer (1958) dismisses the relevance of this dimension entirely. Further, both Roback's (1968) and Swenson's (1968) reviews of the projective drawing literature concluded that artistic quality was independent of projection; that is, more detailed and higher quality drawings did not provide more revealing projective insights. In other words, lower quality drawings had as many emotional indicators and signs of maladjustment as those of higher quality.

From a developmental perspective, art instruction has been shown to increase the quality of children's drawings. C. J. Burns and Velicer (1977) gave brief art lessons, two periods of 45 minutes, to fifth graders. A control group received art instruction, but not in the area of human figure drawing. After a pretest and two posttreatment human figure tests were administered, significant gains were evident between the groups after the first posttest using Harris's (1963) quantitative scoring method. It is interesting to note that the treatment group's performance declined from the first to the second posttest. Yet, while the decline was significant, it did not return the scores to pretest baseline levels. It seems safe to conclude that instruction impacts children's drawing behavior, yet the longevity of its impact is time-limited.

Psychometric Qualities

Interjudge Reliability

For the Draw-A-Person or Draw-A-Man techniques, interjudge reliability has typically been assessed in one of two ways. Some authors have used a percent agreement approach; that is, for each characteristic or indicator, the reliability statistic equals the number of scoring agreements, divided by the total possible agreements, multiplied by 100. Hence, in a 10-item scoring checklist, there would be 10 separate agreement percentages, one for each of the items. An alternative approach is to correlate the scores of two judges with a Phi coefficient for nominal data or a Pearson product–moment for interval level data. As can be seen by Table

7-3, the interjudge reliabilities for these techniques across a number of scoring conventions are generally adequate. In other words, there is substantial agreement between judges when they score the same drawing (Attkisson, Waidler, Jeffrey, & Lambert, 1974).

Test–Retest Stability

The test–retest stability of drawings is a relatively complex phenomenon to assess. For example, a child could draw a figure one way during a first-test administration and a very different way during a second administration. Assuming that the human figure drawing technique assesses state rather than trait characteristics, these different drawings could be very accurate and reliable measures of the child's state or mood at two different administration times. Simply stated, the child may have been quite happy while completing the first drawing and anxious during the second administration. Thus, it would be inappropriate to blindly conclude that the two drawings are unreliable, and thus invalid.

Another possible contribution to the apparent instability of human figure drawings involves the presence of different indicators of the same characteristic from one child's drawing to the next. For instance, in a first drawing, a highly anxious child may draw a small figure at the top of the page, while erasing frequently. In the second drawing, the same child might use excessive shading and overworked lines while drawing the figure. In both drawings, the child's anxiety is present, but a purely statistical approach to reliability would portray the drawing behavior of the child as unreliable.

The quantitative scoring approaches of Goodenough (1926) and Harris (1963) are not subject to either of the test–retest problems addressed above. In fact, Table 7-4 reveals that the complexity (i.e., the number of details) in a drawn figure remains relatively constant from one drawing to the next. The vast majority

Table 7-3
Illustrative Findings from Selected Studies on Interjudge Reliability of Human Figure Drawings

Scoring system	Researcher(s)	N	Reliability estimate
Harris (modified)	Brown (1977)	386	88%[a]
Harris	Evans, Ferguson, Davies, and Williams (1975)	90	.93
Harris	Pihl and Nimrod (1976)	44	.77
Koppitz	Eno, Elliot, and Woehlke (1981)	316	.75
Koppitz	Gayton, Tavormina, Evans, and Schuh (1974)	50	.97
Harris	Gayton et al. (1974)	50	.96
Handler			
McCarthy	Reynolds (1978)	322	.76
Koppitz	Sturner, Rothbaum, Visintainer, and Wolfer (1980)	68	.81
Harris	Sturner et al. (1980)	68	.86
Johnson and Greenburg	F. A. Johnson and Greenberg (1978)	64	.87
Koppitz	Koppitz (1968)	25	95%
McLachlan and Head	McLachlan and Head (1974)	80	.92[a]

[a]Reliability was calculated based on differences in the percentage of items scored by independent judges.

Table 7-4
Illustrative Findings from Selected Studies on the
Stability of Human Figure Drawings

Scoring system	Reference	N	Test-retest interval	Stability coefficient
Goodenough	Goodenough (1926)	194	1 day	.94
Goodenough	Brill (1935)	73	2½ weeks	.77
Goodenough	Smith (1937)	100[a]	Not specified	.91
Goodenough	McCarthy (1944)	386	1 week	.68
Goodenough	McCurdy (1947)	56	3 months	.69
Harris	Harris (1963)	104	1 week	NS[b]
Harris (modified)	Brown (1977)	386	2 weeks	96%[c]
Harris	Denson and May (1978)			
	Cerebral palsied	21	2 weeks	.80
	Controls	21	2 weeks	.77

[a]Smith calculated test–retest stabilities for 100 children at each age from 6 to 15. The coefficients exceed .91 for all age groups except age 15, for which $r = .84$.

[b]Harris used a repeated measures approach and found no significant difference between administrations.

[c]Brown calculated stability based on differences in the percentage of items included from the first to the second administration.

of studies have examined the stability of these quantitative approaches to scoring human figure drawings.

Brown's (1977) study is representative of a series of investigations which have examined the test-retest stability of quantitative scoring techniques for the Draw-A-Man test. Evaluating the stability of children's drawings, Brown had a total of 386 children ranging in age from 3 to 11 make two Draw-A-Man drawings, each separated by a 2-week interval. Five judges scored the drawings using a 105-item checklist based on the Goodenough–Harris Draw-A-Man Test (Harris, 1963). With interjudge reliability calculated at 88%, the findings revealed that, across the age groups, the children's drawings were stable between the first and second administrations. Using the Fattu Nomograph method, the difference between the percentage of children including a specific checklist item in their first drawing was compared with the percentage of those including that same item in their second drawing. Of the 105 items, less than 2 on the average differed between the administrations. Hence, it was concluded by Brown "that the drawings were reliable, at least over a 2-week period" (1977, p. 742).

Fewer researchers have investigated the stability of those interpretive or scoring approaches developed by Machover (1949) or others (Buck, 1948; E. F. Hammer, 1958). This could be a function of the problems noted above (i.e., drawings are subject to mood changes or a trait variable may be manifested by varying indicators) or due to the lack of objective scoring manuals. Starr and Marcuse (1959) and M. Hammer and Kaplan (1964a, 1964b, 1964c, 1966) have reported that the following indicators are stable across brief test-retest intervals: placement of figure on page, front profile orientation (figure facing to the right or left side of the page), completeness of drawing, omissions, shading, erasures, head-to-body ratio, and size of figure. M. Hammer and Kaplan (1964a) noted that children's front profile drawings were stable from the first to second administration, yet their side profile drawings, where the figures faced either to the left or right, were not stable. Children who drew right profiles were most likely to produce a front profile on the second administration. The same was true for those who first drew left profiles, but to a lesser extent. Thus, the left profiles were slightly more stable from one administration to the next.

M. Hammer and Kaplan (1964c) found that children who drew a same-sex figure first were highly likely to draw a same-sex figure first when readministered the Draw-A-Person. However, children who drew the opposite sex first were equally likely to draw either sex first on the second administration. This finding helped clarify Starr and Marcuse's (1959) observations that the sex of the first-drawn figure is stable for boys, but unreliable for girls. Since girls more frequently draw opposite-sex figures first, this variable would be more unstable among girls.

Factor Analytic Studies

Nichols and Strumpfer (1962) conducted one of the early factor analytic investigations with the human figure drawings. Their sample was heterogeneous and included male college students and Veterans Administration patients. The latter group included patients diagnosed as neurotic, patients diagnosed as psychotic, and patients admitted for nonpsychiatric reasons. A principal components method was used to factor analyze a variety of scoring variables for the drawings, for example, Albee and Hamlin's (1949) adjustment, Swenson's (1955) sexual differentiation, Dunn and Lorge's (1954) maturity, and Fischer's (1959) body image and 14 drawing detail variables. Four factors emerged from the analysis. Nichols and Strumpfer suggested that the first factor, which accounted for most of the variance, was related to artistic quality and level of adjustment. This was because the factor loadings of maturity, sexual differentiation, and artistic quality were high and positive (.80), while the loadings on the omission variables (e.g., lack of body parts, crude clothing) tended to be negative. The second factor represented a tendency to draw "big bosomy figures." The third factor was related to the size of the figures, while the aggression variables loaded highest on the fourth factor.

Eno, Elliot, and Woehlke (1981) investigated the factor structure of human figure drawings using Koppitz's (1968) scoring method. Children ($N = 316$) referred for school psychological services completed human figure drawings as part of their evaluations. A principal axes extraction with varimax and then promax rotations was used. Similar to Nichols and Strumpfer, a four factor solution was judged to best fit the data. The first factors in both studies were comparable; that is, it was related to the quality of the drawing and inclusion of such body details as eyes, nose, arms, legs, feet, and neck. The second factor loaded highly on variables which measured the inclusion of irrelevant details (e.g., clouds) and additional figures. The third and fourth factors were uninterpretable.

There are several differences between these two factor analytic studies. While Nichols and Strumpfer worked with adults and used multiple scoring systems, Eno *et al.* used children's drawings and limited their analysis to Koppitz's scoring system. It appears that the factor structure emerging from an investigation of this type is heavily dependent on the types of variables submitted for the analysis and possibly on the population selected as the sample.

Incremental Validity

In a review of research on clinical judgments, Goldberg (1968) concluded that the empirical evidence from research studies has failed to demonstrate a relationship between professional training and accuracy of diagnostic sorting. Schaeffer (1964) reported that clinical psychologists were unable to sort the human figure drawings of normal, neurotic, and psychotic individuals above the level of chance. Cressen (1975) found that clinical psychologists were unable to sort drawings of schizophrenic and normal adults above the chance level or to perform better than college graduates who lacked training in psychodiagnostic techniques. Murray and Delber (1958), however, reported higher than chance performances for diagnostic sorting accuracy when judges were given corrective feedback.

Wanderer (1969), using the assistance of experts in figure drawings, carefully designed a nomination procedure to select psychologists with outstanding skills in the interpretation of drawings. A group of 20 judges was asked to sort five pairs of drawings as coming from a psychotic, neurotic, mentally retarded, homosexual, or normal individual. The groups, with the exception of the mentally retarded, were matched on the basis of intelligence, age, marital status, socioeconomic class, and region of the country. Results indicated that the judges performed significantly better than chance. However, when the drawings from mentally retarded individuals were removed, the judges performed no better than chance with the four other groups.

E. F. Hammer (1969) vigorously criticized Wanderer's (1969) experiment. Hammer's comments may be generalized to the other studies investigating the incremental validity of drawings. These criticisms are as follows:

1. Diagnostic groups (e.g., neurotics, psychotics, homosexuals) are not mutually exclusive categories. The drawings of depressed neurotics and depressed psychotics may look quite similar, especially if only two drawings are sampled. It is naive to expect all persons in a given classification to be homogeneous and to produce comparable drawings.

2. It is inappropriate to interpret drawings in isolation. In clinical practice, other data are available, for example, case histories, interviews with clients and significant others, other projective test results, and objective measures of ability. Additionally, the judges are missing significant information which a clinician would have observed in administering the drawings, for example, spontaneous verbal associations, overt behaviors, and situational factors.

It is instructive to note that Chambers (1954) used a design similar to Wanderer's in order to investigate judges' diagnostic decision making. However, instead of figure drawings, the Rorschach was the instrument being scrutinized. Results indicated that the protocols of mentally retarded subjects were identified with the greatest level of accuracy. However, even with the protocols of these retarded subjects eliminated, the judges still performed significantly better than chance. Thus, contrary to Hammer's comment, it doesn't appear that Wanderer's results are a function of a poorly designed experiment. Rather, it appears that human figure drawings provide limited incremental validity.

The House–Tree–Person Technique

Administration

To administer the House–Tree–Person technique, Buck (1948) recommends using a 4-page booklet with pages that measure $7 \times 8\frac{1}{2}''$. On three of the pages are the words, "House," "Tree," and "Person." Most examiners, however, use standard $8\frac{1}{2}'' \times 11''$ white paper. When Bieliauskas and Farragher (1983) compared the two formats, no significant differences were found.

The house drawing is requested first. The examiner gives the following oral instructions: "Take one of these pencils please. I want you to draw me as good a picture of a house as you can. You may draw any kind of house you like, it will not be counted against you. And you may take as long as you wish. Just draw me as good a house as you can" (Buck, 1948, p. 327). Similar instructions are given for the tree and then the person drawings. For each drawing, the examiner notes how long the individual takes to finish.

After completion of the drawings, a series of questions constitute the postdrawing interrogation (see Table 7-5 for illustrative questions from Buck's postdrawing interrogation). According to Buck, the questions were not intended to be administered in a rigid, standardized fashion. Rather, the questions serve as stimuli to uncover additional data about the examinee's emotional reactions. During the postdrawing interrogation phase of the House–Tree–Person, the examinee is given the "opportunity to define, describe, and interpret the objects that he has just drawn and their respective environments, and to associate concerning them" (Buck, 1948, p. 328).

After the pencil version and postdrawing interrogation, the chromatic phase of the House–Tree–Person is administered. Buck suggests that this second phase be administered in a separate session. As would be expected, the chromatic phase is administered by giving the examinees crayons and asking them to successively draw a house, tree, and then a person. Following the color drawings, additional postdrawing interrogations are administered. These interrogations are comparable to the previous achromatic questionings.

Interpretation

Buck (1948) offered a step-by-step analysis of House–Tree–Person drawings. In Chapter III of his monograph, a quantitative scoring system is outlined. Similar to Goodenough's quantitative approach to the Draw-A-Man Test, details, proportions, and perspectives are scored for each of the three drawings. For instance, more credit is given for a complex two-dimensional roof than a one-dimensional or omitted roof.

Buck's notions regarding the qualitative interpretation of the House–Tree–Person are more frequently used in clinical practice than the quantitative approach noted above. Qualitative interpretation proceeds in three steps: (a) identification of omissions and unusual components, (b) synthesis of organization and interrelationship of items developed in the first phase, and (c) analysis and synthesis of a drawing relative to the examinee's personality and environment.

E. F. Hammer (1958) proposed the following symbolic interpretations for drawings of a house, tree, and person. He considered the house a dwelling which arouses feelings associated with home life and family relationships. For a child,

Table 7-5
Buck's (1948) Postdrawing Interrogation Items for the House–Tree–Person[a]

Person

P1.   Is that a man or a woman (or boy or girl)?
P2.   How old is he?
P3.   Who is he?
P4.   Is he a friend, relation, or what?
P5.   Whom were you thinking about while you were drawing?
P6.   What is he doing? (and where is he doing it?)
P7.   What is he thinking about?
P8.   How does he feel?
P9.   What does that person make you think of?
P10.   What does that person remind you of?
P11.   Is that person well?
P12.   What about that person gives you that impression?
P13.   Is that person happy?
P14.   What about him gives you that impression?
P15.   How do you feel about that person?
P16.   Do you feel that way about most people? Why?
P17.   What is the weather like in this picture?
P18.   Whom does that person remind you of? Why?
P19.   What does that person need most? Why?
P20.   What kind of clothing does this person have on?

Tree

T1.   What kind of tree is that?
T2.   Where is that tree actually located?
T3.   About how old is that tree?
T4.   Is that tree alive?
T5.   A. What is there about that tree that gives you the impression it's alive?
       B. Is any part of that tree dead? What part?
       C. What do you think caused it to die?
       D. When do you think it died?
T6.   Which does that tree look more like to you, a man or a woman?
T7.   What about it gives you that impression?
T8.   If that were a person instead of a tree, which way would the person be facing?
T9.   Is that tree by itself, or is it part of a group of trees?
T10.   As you look at the tree, do you get the impression that it's above you, below you, or about on a level with you?
T11.   What is the weather like in this picture?
T12.   Is there any wind blowing in this picture?
T13.   Show me what direction it is blowing.

(continued)

relationships between the self and parents or siblings may be manifested. With adults, the house drawings may reflect the current domestic milieu and the quality of the relationship with the spouse. E. F. Hammer (1958), however, notes that residual perceptions of and attitudes toward the parent may appear in drawings by adults.

E. F. Hammer speculates that the tree drawing uncovers the "deeper and more unconscious feelings" about the examinee (1958, p. 172). Unlike the drawing of a person, the tree drawing is further removed from what might be considered the drawing of a self-portrait. Hence, examinees might find it easier to project more negative and emotionally disturbing traits into the tree drawing.

In contrast, the person drawing is believed to capture a "closer-to-conscious"

**Table 7-5
(Continued)**

T14.	What sort of wind is it?
T15.	If you had drawn a sun in this picture, where would you have put it?
T16.	Do you see the sun as being in the north, east, west, or south?
T17.	What does that tree make you think of?
T18.	What does it remind you of?
T19.	Is that a healthy tree?
T20.	What is there about it that gives you that impression?
T21.	Is that a strong tree?
T22.	What is there about it that gives you that impression?
T23.	Whom does that tree remind you of? Why?
T24.	What does that tree need most? Why?
T25.	If this were a person instead of a bird (or other tree or other extra part of tree drawing), who might it be?

House

H1.	How many floors does that house have?
H2.	Is it a wood house, a brick house, or what?
H3.	Is that your own house?
H4.	Whose house were you thinking about while you were drawing?
H5.	Would you like to own that house yourself? Why?
H6.	If you did own that house and could do whatever you liked with it:
	A. Which room would you take for yourself? Why?
	B. Whom would you like to have live in the house with you? Why?
H7.	As you look at the house, does it seem to be close by or far away?
H8.	As you look at the house, does it appear to be above you, below you, or about on the same level?
H9.	What does that house make you think of?
H10.	What does it remind you of?
H11.	Is that a happy friendly sort of house?
H12.	What is there about it that gives you that impression?
H13.	Do you feel that way about most houses? Why?
H14.	What is the weather like in this picture?
H15.	Whom does that house make you think of? Why?
H16.	What does that house need most? Why?
H17.	To what does that chimney lead?
H18.	To what does that walkway lead?
H19.	Find out what room lies behind each door and window of the house, the use to which it is put, and who customarily occupies it. Also find same for any windows not visible in drawing (possible floor plan).

[a]These questions were abstracted from Buck's (1948) classic monograph on the House–Tree–Person.

view of the self. Thus, this drawing may manifest more state as opposed to trait characteristics. E. F. Hammer (1958) reports that the person drawing is more sensitive to changes during retesting whereas changes in the tree drawing occur only after intensive therapy or a significant alteration in a life situation.

Jollès (1971) reduced Buck's scoring system to a manageable outline form (see Table 7-6 for illustrative interpretations). In his monograph, Buck comments that individual sign interpretation is inappropriate, and thus, Jollès's outline must be used cautiously. Buck emphasized the critical importance of the examinee's spontaneous verbalizations. The examiner is instructed not only to record these statements verbatim, but also to record what the examinee was drawing at the time. Other behaviors are also recorded, for example, cooperation, stress symptoms, mannerisms, attention span, and reaction time.

Table 7-6
Illustrative Interpretations Abstracted from Jollès's (1971) Qualitative Guide to the House–Tree–Person[a]

General Interpretations
Erasure
  With redrawing
    If redrawing results in improvement, it is a favorable sign. Erasure with subsequent deterioration implies strong emotional reaction to the object being drawn or its symbolization.
  Without attempt at redrawing
    Detail arouses strong conflict over detail itself or what detail symbolizes.
Paper-basing
  Generalized insecurity. Depression of mood tone; the smaller the drawing and/or fainter the lines, the more marked the depression.
Paper-siding
  Implies space constriction with resultant heightened sensitivity and strong suggestion of aggressive-reactive tendencies, suppressed or not.
Paper-topping
  Tendency toward fixation on thinking and fantasy as sources of satisfaction. Satisfaction may or may not be obtainable by this mechanism.
Paper-turning
  Aggressive and/or negativistic tendencies. Pathoformic if occurring more than once. Perseveration indicated if paper-turning always in same direction.
Shading
  Pathoformic use of
    Anxiety.
  Unemphasized use of
    Sensitive, not necessarily unhappily sensitive, to relationships with others.
Sun
  Symbol of authoritative figure; often seen as source of power and/or warmth; frequently identified as father or mother.

House Interpretations
Chimney
  Phallic symbol of significance. Sensual maturity and balance. Symbol of warmth in intimate relationships.
  Absence of
    Feels home lacks psychological warmth. Difficulty dealing with male sex symbol.
  Almost completely hidden
    Reluctance to deal with emotion-producing stimuli. Castration fear.
  Emphasis upon
    Preoccupation with male sex symbol. May indicate preoccupation with chimney associations.
    Overconcern with warmth.
  Overly large
    Overconcern with sexual matters, with the need to demonstrate virility. Exhibitionist tendencies.
Gutters
  Heightened attitude to defensiveness and usually suspiciousness.
Roof
  Fantasy area. Intellectual area.
Room(s)
  Associations may be aroused by (1) person usually occupying room; (2) interpersonal relations experienced in room; (3) specific symbolism of room for the subject; (4) function usually associated with room per se or with room by the subject. Associations may result in positive or negative feelings regarding room. Room's significance needs to be checked by the manner drawn or implied by comments concerning room during drawing or the PDI.
  For functions of room, see Bathroom, Bedroom, Dining room, Kitchen, Living room.

(continued)

Table 7-6
(Continued)

Tree Interpretations
Bark
  Depicted by vine-like vertical lines well separated
    Suggests schizoid characteristics.
  Easily drawn
    Well-balanced interaction.
  Inconsistently or heavily drawn
    Anxiety.
  Meticulously drawn
    Compulsiveness, with overconcern about relationships with environment.
Branches
  Degree of flexibility of branches, number, size, and extent of interrelationship indicate view of adaptability and availability for deriving satisfactions in environment. Degree of ability to reach others or sustain growth in achievement.
  Absolute symmetry of
    Implies feelings of ambivalence; inability to grant dominance to emotional or intellectual course of action.
  Broken, bent, or dead
    Significant psychic or physical trauma. Castration feelings: psychosexual or psychosocial.
  Indicated by unshaded implication
    Oppositional tendencies.
  One-dimensional, not forming a system, and inadequately joined to a one-dimensional trunk
    Organicity. Impotence feelings, futility, lack of ego strength, with poor integration of satisfaction-seeking resources.
  Overemphasis to left
    Personality imbalance due to tendency to seek strenuously for immediate, frank emotional satisfaction: extratensivity.
  Overemphasis to right
    Personality imbalance produced by strong tendency to avoid or delay emotional satisfaction, or seek satisfaction through intellectual effort. If subject is of dull intelligence, further conflict is self-evident: intratensivity.
Roots
  Dead
    Intrapersonal imbalance of dissolution with suggested pathoformic loss of drive and grasp of reality. Obsessive-depressive feelings associated with early life.
Scars
  Psychic and/or physical experience regarded traumatically.

Person
Arms
  Tools to control or change environment.
  Absence of
    Strong feeling of inadequacy; cannot cope with problems presented by interpersonal relationships. Feeling of futility at continuing struggle; hence, suicidal tendencies may be present. Need for self-mutilation.
  Folded across chest
    Suspicious, hostile attitudes.
  Tense and held tight to body
    Rigidity.

---

[a]These illustrative interpretative statements were abstracted from Jollès (1971). It should be noted that Jollès developed his interpretations from Buck's (1948) monograph.

Psychometric Qualities: Reliability and Validity

Relative to the voluminous literature on the Draw-A-Person, there have been significantly fewer empirically based articles published on the House–Tree–Person technique. In the early 1970s, Marzolf and Kirchner (1970, 1971, 1972, 1973) conducted a series of analyses investigating the reliability of the House–Tree–Person and its relationship to the 16 PF. As Marzolf and Kirchner used only college students as participants in their studies, some caution is necessary in generalizing their findings to children and adolescents.

With respect to reliability, Marzolf and Kirchner (1970) found acceptable test–retest stability (4–6 weeks) in the drawings of 49 male and 87 female undergraduates. With the exception of a few individuals, there were not marked changes from the first to the second drawings. In analyzing color choice, Marzolf and Kirchner (1973) reported that selected colors were correlated with personality traits from the 16 PF. However, the correlations were low, and the authors questioned the practical significance of color choice.

Wildman, Wildman, and Smith (1967) investigated the drawings of patients who were judged as either extroverted or introverted. The hypothesis that extroverts would produce more expansive drawings was disconfirmed; there was no significant difference when drawings' mean areas were compared. It should be noted that Wildman *et al.* replicated this study and observed comparable results.

Blain, Bergner, Lewis, and Goldstein (1981) conducted a study of House–Tree–Person drawings from three groups of children: abused, nonabused but currently receiving therapy, and normal controls judged to be emotionally healthy by their elementary teachers. On the basis of a pilot study, 100 scoring variables were reduced to 15 potentially discriminating items. Of these 15 items, 5 of the ANOVAs for differences among the groups were significant beyond the $p < .05$ level. Post hoc tests revealed that when comparing the abused and nonabused clinical groups, only one item (smoke present in the chimney of the house) resulted in a significant difference. In general, the post hoc analyses revealed that the abused and nonabused clinical groups showed similar responses in the drawings, while the greatest differences were found in the comparisons of normal children's drawings versus those of the two clinical groups. Blain *et al.* concluded that the House–Tree–Person may be a valuable tool in the prediction of child abuse. However, their findings do not support this conclusion. For example, the most discriminating item of smoke present in the chimney occurred in 50% of the abused children's drawings, 22% of the nonabused clinical group, and 22% of the normal controls. The incremental validity of this item is obviously quite low, especially when one recognizes that the pilot study began with 100 items. By chance alone, one would expect an item to be more discriminating.

Davis and Hoopes (1975) administered the House–Tree–Person to prelingually deaf children and matched controls. For over 20 item comparisons, only 2 were statistically significant. First, hearing children were slightly more likely to shade the mouth; roughly 15% of the hearing and 4% of the deaf children manifested this sign. Second, there was a clear difference in the two groups' treatment of tree branches. The deaf children had a tendency to omit branches and drew a circle with foliage on top of a trunk. The most significant aspect of this study was the failure of the vast majority of items to achieve significance. The two groups represented ears, eyes, and (with the exception of mouth shading) mouths in the same way.

Finally, the season of the year has influence on the tree drawings. Pustel,

Sternlicht, and DeRespinis (1971) studied the drawings of adolescent and adult retarded samples. They found that leaves more frequently appear in achromatic drawings done in the spring, summer, and fall (i.e., less in the winter). Also, while retarded adolescents' chromatic drawings reflected the seasonal cycle, retarded adults' chromatic drawings were not influenced by the season. Researchers (Judson & MacCasland, 1960; Moll, 1962) have also documented that trees drawn during winter months are sparser and contain less foliage. These are important findings, because the absence of leaves and the relative size of the tree may be interpreted as a projection of an individual's personal dissatisfaction. Hence, alternative hypotheses, for example, seasonal influence, should be considered as competing explanations of drawing characteristics. Bluestein's (1978) alternative hypothesis for dead or broken tree branches reaffirms the importance of a comprehensive perspective on the drawing technique and interpretation. Based on clinical experience, Bluestein reported that dead or broken branches do not necessarily suggest severe emotional disturbance, but rather may reflect the loss of a loved one.

The Kinetic Drawing System

The Kinetic Drawing System is a recent integration of the Kinetic Family Drawing (R. C. Burns & Kaufman, 1970, 1972) and Kinetic School Drawing (Prout & Phillips, 1974) techniques. Recognizing their overlapping historical developments, their conceptual similarities, and their potential to provide more logical, integrated, and comprehensive data and analysis, Knoff and Prout (1985a, 1985b) combined these two kinetic drawing techniques. Before discussing the Kinetic Drawing System, a review and analysis of its two component parts will be presented.

The Kinetic Family Drawing

Administration

Comparable to other drawing techniques, the Kinetic Family Drawing is administered by giving the examinee a plain white sheet of 8½″ × 11″ paper and a #2 lead pencil with an eraser. The paper is presented ambiguously on the table so that the child can decide whether to hold it lengthwise or sideways. The examiner then gives the following verbal instructions: "Draw a picture of everyone in your family, including you, DOING something. Try to draw whole people, not cartoons or stick people. Remember, make everyone DOING something—some kind of actions" (R. C. Burns & Kaufman, 1972, p. 5). While the drawing is being completed, the examiner can observe the proceedings, recording verbalized statements and other behavioral observations. If the examinee does not wish to cooperate, he or she is encouraged to comply. As there is no specified time limit for the Kinetic Family Drawing, the examinee is given whatever time is necessary to complete the drawing. As with other drawing procedures, an examinee's questions are responded to noncommitally (i.e., the practitioner tells the examinee to do as he or she wishes, or to do the best that he or she can). Once finished, the examiner asks a series of postdrawing questions similar in content and rationale to the House–Tree–Person (see Table 7-7 for the Kinetic Drawing System inquiry questions).

Table 7-7
The Kinetic Drawing System Inquiry Process[a]

The Inquiry phase occurs after the child has completed the KFD or KSD and after the examiner has taken the child's pencil away. The Inquiry process attempts to clarify the child's drawing and investigate the overt and covert processes that affected its production. The ultimate goal is to elicit as much information and understanding about the drawing, the context, and the child as possible—within the bounds of time and examiner–child rapport.

The Inquiry questions below are *suggested* questions and can be adapted and extended as the situation dictates. The questions may be asked in any order, and may be expanded to comprise part of a psychological interview. Some clinicians follow their intuition and the discussion's direction and uncover clinical information that exceeds the actual drawings in significance and importance.

Suggested Questions for the Kinetic Drawing System Inquiry

1. Go through each figure in the drawing getting that person's name, relationship to the child, age, other meaningful characteristics or data.
2. Go through each figure in the drawing asking:
   "What is this person doing?"
   "What is good about this person?"
   "What is bad about this person?"
   "What does this person wish for?"
   "What is this person thinking?"
   "What is this person feeling?"
   "What happened to this person immediately before this picture?"
   "What will happen to this person immediately after this picture?"
   "What will happen to this person in the future?"
   "How does this person get along with other people?"
   "What does this person need most?"
   "What does that person make you think of?"
   "What does that person remind you of?"
   "How do you feel about that person?"
   "Do you feel that way about most people? Why?"
3. "What were you thinking about while you were drawing?"
4. "What does this drawing make you think of?"
5. Questions about the picture's weather:
   "What is the weather like in this picture?"
   "Is there any wind blowing in this picture?"
   "Show me the direction it is blowing?"
   "What sort of wind is it?"
   "If you had drawn a sun in this picture, where would you have put it?"
6. "What happened to this family/class in this picture immediately before this picture?"
7. "What will happen to this family/school in this picture immediately after this picture?"
8. "What will happen to this family/school in the future?"
9. "If you could change anything at all about this family/school picture, what would it be?"
10. "Is this the best picture that you could possibly make?"

[a]Reprinted and adapted with permission from Knoff and Prout (1985b).

Interpretation

R. C. Burns and Kaufman's (1970) Kinetic Family Drawing (KFD) was an outgrowth of Hulse's (1951) Family Drawing Test. Hulse, one of the more insightful writers in the area of projective drawings, emphasized the importance of observing the client's behavior (e.g., reactions and verbalizations) in conjunction to the analysis of the drawing. Working from a partially Freudian framework, R. C. Burns and Kaufman (1970, 1972) reviewed 10,000 KFDs from individual patients over a 12-year period. Using this case study approach, their interpretive system came into focus, resulting in the analysis of drawings' "actions," "styles," and "symbols."

Before looking at actions, styles, or symbols, the interpretation of a drawing begins by examining the characteristics of each figure. Characteristics are static qualities of the drawing: erasures, arm extensions, omissions of body parts, or elevations or omissions of family members from the KFD. The earlier works of Machover and Koppitz were used by Burns and Kaufman to discuss these characteristics.

Actions refer to the movement of energy between people. Thus, the total drawing rather than isolated figures must be reviewed to assess this area. Action may involve highly intense energy, as in competition, or low levels of energy, as represented by two people sitting and facing in opposite directions. Balls or other objects being passed between figures are also representative of action. According to Burns and Kaufman, such objects and occurrences are frequent in children's KFDs. They state that this energy being passed between figures may reflect anxiety, avoidance, or conflict. Specific to interpretation, Burns and Kaufman suggest that actions may be viewed from a variety of theoretical backgrounds, for example, from Lewin's positive and negative valences, Freud's conception of libido, or even Skinner's discriminative stimuli.

Style is another important variable when interpreting children's KFDs. Styles are most often associated with children's inabilities to effectively interact with significant family members. Styles are evident when children place barriers between figures. For example, members of a family may be separated by drawing lines and placing each figure in a box. Individuals may also be isolated when a child repeatedly folds the drawing paper, leaving each figure in its own box. This is known as folding compartmentalization. Another style which isolates family members is edging. This is evident when figures are positioned around the edges of the paper.

Burns and Kaufman are tentative when they discuss symbolic interpretation; they begin with a caution regarding the overinterpretation and misinterpretations of symbols. When assessing the meaning of a symbol, they state that "one must weigh the alternative and sometimes incompatible interpretation . . . (always) consider(ing) the totality of the individual" (R. C. Burns & Kaufman, 1972, p. 144). Sample symbols included in the interpretive guide include brooms, cats, clowns, fire, flowers, ironing boards, ladders, light bulbs, rain, and snakes. Symbols are suggested to be an expression of the unconscious (see Table 7-8 for the actions, styles, and symbol characteristics of the Kinetic Drawing System).

Psychometric Qualities: Reliability and Validity

In his review of the Kinetic Family Drawings, Harris (1978) harshly criticized the test because R. C. Burns and Kaufman's (1970, 1972) interpretive manual did not include information on psychometric reliability. Neither the reliability of interpreters nor the stability of children's drawing behaviors were addressed by Burns and Kaufman. Harris also criticized the manual for failing to precisely define the scoring variables, for example, encapsulation, edging, compartmentalization.

Other researchers have also recognized the subjectivity of the KFD's scoring system, and they have developed objective scoring methods (McPhee & Wegner, 1976; Meyers, 1978; Mostkoff & Lazarus, 1983; O'Brien & Patton, 1974). The mean interjudge reliabilities for these scoring systems, the ability for independent judges to agree that a variable is either present or absent in a drawing,

Table 7-8
Summary of Actions, Styles, and Symbols Characteristics
for the Kinetic Drawing System[a]

The Kinetic Family Drawing
  I. Actions between Figures
      A. Balls
      B. Hanging or falling figures
      C. Dirt themes
      D. Skin Diving
      E. Mother actions
      F. Father actions
      G. Position of figures
          with respect to safety
 II. Figure Characteristics
      A. Individual figure characteristics
          1. "Picasso eye"
          2. Jagged or sharp figures, toes, teeth
          3. Long or extended arm
          4. Shading or crosshatchings
          5. Occluded or cut-off body parts
          6. Omission of body parts
          7. Transparencies
      B. Global/comparative figure characteristics
          1. Number of household members
          2. Relative height of figures
          3. Similar treatment of figures
          4. Differential treatment of figures
          5. Idealized self-drawing
          6. Crossing out and redrawing entire
             figure
          7. Omission of figures
          8. Inclusion of extra figures
          9. Ordering of figures
          10. Stick figures
          11. Evasions
          12. Bizarre figures
III. Position, Distance, and Barriers
      A. Position characteristics
          1. Figure placement on the page
          2. Lack of interaction or integration of figures
          3. Rotated figures
      B. Distance characteristics
          1. Physical proximity of figures (general, close, distant)
      C. Barriers characteristics
          1. Fields of force
          2. The "A" syndrome
          3. The "X" syndrome
 IV. Style
      A. Line Quality
      B. Asymmetric drawing
      C. Excessive attention to details
      D. Transparencies
      E. Erasures
      F. Compartmentalization
      G. Encapsulation
      H. Folding compartmentalization
      I. Lining at the top
      J. Underlining at the bottom
      K. Underlining individual figures
      L. Edging
      M. Anchoring
      N. Figures on the back of the page
      O. Rejecting and redrawing an entire KFD
      P. Object perseveration
  V. Symbols
      A. Balloons
      B. Beds
      C. Bicycles
      S. Ladders
      T. Lawnmowers
      U. Leaves

(continued)

has been satisfactory, generally above .85. These four objective scoring methods are reviewed and discussed in greater detail by Knoff and Prout (1985a, 1985b).

Despite satisfactory levels of interjudge reliability, the McPhee and Wegner (1976), Meyers (1978), and O'Brien and Patton (1974) scoring methods have not attained adequate test-retest stability (Cummings, 1981). Cummings administered KFDs to a sample of 36 children from classes for the behaviorally disordered, to 36 learning disabled children, and to 37 children from regular classrooms. Each

Table 7-8
(Continued)

D. Brooms	V. Logs
E. Butterflies	W. The moon
F. Buttons	X. Motorcycles
G. Cats	Y. Paint brush
H. Circles	Z. Rain
I. Clowns	AA. Refrigerators
J. Cribs	BB. Snakes
K. Dangerous objects	CC. Snow
L. Drums	DD. Stars
M. Flowers	EE. Stop signs
N. Garbage	FF. Stoves
O. Heat/light/warmth	GG. The sun
P. Horses	HH. Trains
Q. Jump rope	II. Vacuum cleaners
R. Kites	JJ. Water themes

The Kinetic School Drawing
I. Actions of and between figures
   A. Self-figure engaged in academic behavior
   B. Self-figure engaged in undesirable behavior
   C. Recess activity/actions
II. Figure Characteristics
   Individual Figure Characteristics
   (see KFD interpretations)
   Global/Comparative Figure Characteristics
   A. Number of peers drawn
   B. Lack of people drawn
   C. Height of self-drawing
   D. Relative height of figures
   E. Characteristics of teacher drawing
   F. Excessively detailed teacher drawing
III. Position, Distance, and Barrier Characteristics (see KFD interpretations)
IV. Style
   A. Emphasis on physical features of a room
   B. Drawing viewpoints or perspectives
   C. Bird's-eye view of classroom/drawing
   D. Transparencies
   E. Outdoor pictures
V. Symbols
   A. Apples
   B. Chalkboard or bulletin board
   C. Clock
   D. Principal
   E. School bus

[a]Reprinted and adapted with permission from Knoff and Prout (1985b).

child was asked to complete two drawings, the second after a 4- to 6-week interval. None of the three scoring systems achieved a stability coefficient above a minimal level of .70. This indicates that children tend to change their drawings from one administration to another, and implies that *if* the KFDs are accurately assessing a child's feelings and perceptions of family interaction, then these feelings and perceptions are ephemeral. Comparable test-retest findings with the KFD were reported by Mostkoff and Lazarus (1983).

Achieving a consensus that certain attributes in KFD drawings indicate emotional disturbance has also been problematic, as illustrated in the validation studies with emotionally disturbed and "normal" children below. McPhee and Wegner (1976) compared the drawings of 102 emotionally disturbed children to the drawings of 162 normal children. A two-factor analysis of variance, with sex as the second factor, yielded a significant difference between the emotionally disturbed and control groups, but not between girls and boys. Specific results indicated that the normal children included more Burns and Kaufman "style" indicators than the emotionally disturbed children. According to R. C. Burns and Kaufman (1970), one would have predicted the opposite, that the emotionally disturbed children would include more style indicators in their drawings.

Meyers (1978) conducted a similar validation study by comparing emotionally disturbed children's drawings to those by a matched group of "well-adjusted" children from regular classrooms; both style *and* actions indicators were scored and analyzed. While a significant difference was found again, this time the emotionally disturbed children exhibited more style and action indicators.

Cummings (1981) reported that no significant KFD differences were observed between children drawn from regular classes and those from classes for the behaviorally disordered. Hence, one validation study reported significance contrary to the predicted direction, one study supported Burns and Kaufman's actions and style predictions, and a third validation effort turned up no significant differences.

KFDs have also been used to compare adolescent male delinquents with matched nondelinquent controls, resulting in a post hoc analysis and scoring system (Sobel & Sobel, 1976). Even with this methodological flaw, only three variables reached statistical significance. In their discussion section, the researchers questioned the diagnostic and discriminative value of the KFD technique.

The drawings of children from intact and divorced homes have also been compared. Cummings and Ingram (1980) used Meyers's (1978) objective scoring variables and the O'Brien and Patton (1974) scoring system. The authors predicted that children who had experienced a divorce would graphically represent their families differently than those from intact homes. In general, Cummings and Ingram's findings revealed that both scoring systems were not sensitive to the differences between the two groups of children.

To conclude, the empirical studies with the KFD technique provide limited support for Burns and Kaufman's interpretative method. As pointed out, the findings of the various studies have been mixed. Perhaps the greatest problem is related to the stability of the measure. If it is assumed that KFDs assess individuals' perceptions of family interactions (and that these perceptions are fairly stable over a 2- to 4-week interval), then the relative positions of figures on the drawing should not change dramatically from one drawing administration to another a few weeks later. For instance, if a child's first drawing has the self figure next to the mother inside the house and the father drawn a distance from the house in a shed (encapsulated), the interpretation might suggest some emotional distance between the individual and the father figure. If the child's second drawing has all of the family members placed together inside the house, a very different interpretation of the family interactions would likely be made. Due to the problem of stability, it would be inappropriate to rely heavily on the present version of the Burns and Kaufman scoring method.

The Kinetic School Drawing

Prout and Phillips (1974) were the first to publish a school adaptation for the KFD technique. They described the administration procedure and some interpretive guidelines. More recently, Sarbaugh (1983) has introduced another version of Kinetic School Drawings (KSD).

Administration

Prout and Phillips (1974) recommended the standard administration procedures for the KSD, that is, 8½″ × 11″ white paper and a #2 lead pencil. The oral instructions to the child are as follows: "I'd like you to draw a school picture. Put yourself, your teacher, and a friend or two in the picture. Make everyone doing something. Try to draw whole people and make the best drawing you can. Remember, draw yourself, your teacher, and a friend or two, and make everyone doing something." A postdrawing interrogation is conducted (see Table 7-7), in which the examiner asks the child to identify the people and their actions in the drawing. Objects in the drawing which are not readily identifiable should also be queried.

In contrast to Prout and Phillips, Sarbaugh (1983) recommends the following oral instruction for the examinee: "Draw a picture of people at school *doing something*" (p. 5). Sarbaugh suggests that the advantage of the open-ended instruction is to permit the child to project "attitudes, emphasis, and opinions." When the child asks for additional instructions, he or she is told to use his or her own ideas. Prout and Phillips (1974) note that the more specific instruction, "include a friend or two," was useful in eliciting spontaneous comments regarding relationships with peers. Based on the author's experiences in administering kinetic drawings, the Prout and Phillips instructions should be considered the more appropriate and useful because children frequently leave themselves out of drawings (sometimes even when told twice to include themselves). While one could argue that the greater specificity of Prout and Phillips's oral instruction reduces the ambiguity of the task, thus decreasing potential projective data, there are an unlimited number of ways and situations that the child may choose to depict the teacher, friends, and self figures.

Sarbaugh also recommends a second phase, a chromatic administration. Similar to the House–Tree–Person, crayons are used in the chromatic phase. However, Sarbaugh suggests the use of 24 crayons, with the possibility of substituting silver and gold for either the violet–blue, blue–green, or yellow–orange crayons.

Interpretation

Prout and Phillips's (1974) interpretation method parallels that outlined by R. C. Burns and Kaufman for the KFD procedure (1970, 1972). First, the characteristics associated with individual figures are analyzed using Machover's schema. Then the drawing is examined in terms of actions, styles, and symbols. Unlike the KFD, the child's perceptions of the teacher and school peers may be examined. Prout and Phillips did not present a detailed or empirically based method of interpretation; rather, several sample cases were briefly described.

Sarbaugh (1983) presented a much more comprehensive approach to the interpretation of KSDs. She suggests that school drawings' greatest values occur when they are interpreted from a "symbolic" perspective. She states that the interpretation of symbols does not necessarily require a specific psychological or philosophical background: "Children are constantly in the process of using already existing symbols. They may put their own individual stamp on these symbols. They also create new ones, or adopt them in response to life experiences such as movies or television programs" (Sarbaugh, 1983, p. 9).

Psychometric Qualities: Reliability and Validity

No data are presented by Prout and Phillips (1974) with respect to reliability or validity. Wise and Potkay (1983) and Peterson (1983) harshly criticized Sarbaugh's technique for also lacking the empirically based guidelines necessary for interpreting drawing responses. Similar to authors of other projective drawing techniques, Sarbaugh based her interpretive schema on years of clinical experience (work in public schools and child guidance and university reading clinics). The following is a sample interpretive hypothesis: "There can be an emphasis on the building, the classroom walls . . . or furniture. The emphasis on physical features of the room might suggest need for structure or an avoidance of social interaction. If there are no people present, or if the people are present only in such symbolic ways as desks, or name-cards, the avoidance of interaction is more probable" (Sarbaugh, 1983, p. 12). The only evidence to justify the above statement is Sarbaugh's clinical experience. Since empirically based evidence is not available, the KSD technique should be considered a tool needing research.

The Integration of the KFD and KSD

As noted above, the KFD and the KSD techniques share a conceptual base as well as similarities in administration, format, scoring, and interpretation. Their integration into the Kinetic Drawing System (Knoff & Prout, 1985b) seemed a logical direction to increase their clinical utility and interpretive depth, while emphasizing the need to administer *both* techniques for differential analysis (Knoff & Prout, 1985a). According to Knoff and Prout, the Kinetic Drawing System can investigate a child or adolescent's social–emotional difficulties across both home and school settings, identify home/family issues that explain school attitudes or behaviors or school/classroom issues that affect home behaviors (or both), and/or isolate setting-specific relationships or interactions which contribute to an individual's difficulty or which could become intervention resources.

The Kinetic Drawing System manual (Knoff & Prout, 1985b) comprehensively summarizes the research and literature from the KFD and KSD techniques while introducing the integrated system. Using R. C. Burns and Kaufman's (1970) KFD administration directions (above) and Prout and Phillips's (1974) KSD administration instructions (above), the Kinetic Drawing System is administered Family Drawing-first and School Drawing-second. The manual reviews all interpretive characteristics and hypotheses available in the literature, clearly identifying those which are based on empirical data versus clinical judgment. The Kinetic Drawing System is then presented as a heuristic system; that is, no additional or System-specific psychometric or other data are discussed; the authors are encouraging research in this unified system with the hope of facilitating a single, empirically based scoring and interpretive approach. Thus, the Kinetic Drawing System cannot be further analyzed at this time; it is a system for the future to use and evaluate.

A Case Study Using Drawing Techniques

This case study has been adapted from Knoff and Prout (1985b) with permission. The data presented below were extracted from a comprehensive personality assessment battery including an intellectual evaluation. Thus, the discussion below is provided to demonstrate some aspects of drawing techniques and their contributions to the entire battery. It is very difficult to separate one part of the battery from the entire battery, however. The reader is cautioned not to overgeneralize the potential, positive or negative, of projective drawings from this one case study.

Name: **Alan**
Chronological Age: **15-3**
Grade: **9**
The High School
Date of Testing: **November 13th**

Referral and Observations

Alan was referred to investigate his reasons and motivations for not participating in his classes this year and to evaluate some critical behavioral incidents which include bringing liquor to school, a number of detentions, and numerous in-school suspensions which are bringing him close to an exclusionary suspension. Alan entered his present school (The High School) from New York in the middle of last year and failed his math and science classes for the remainder of the year. A preevaluation conference last year determined that there were no academic reasons to necessitate a comprehensive assessment. This year, however, questions about Alan's social–emotional status and whether it is possible for him to function in the regular classroom prompted a formal referral.

An interview with Alan's mother revealed that Alan had had previous academic difficulties in the late elementary school years, and that Alan entered a parochial school in sixth grade to provide him more structure. While Alan didn't like the rigidity of the parochial school, he did do better academically, although he appeared to be an average C student. Alan's family moved because "they were ready for a move." Alan's father is self-employed, the move was not financially motivated, and the family discussed the move (in fact, Alan was looking forward to the move, according to his mother).

Since the move, Alan's mother reports that he has picked up the wrong type of friends, has had trouble with the police, talks about graduating from high school and returning to New York, and has had increasing conflicts with both parents and brothers. Alan has increased his requests to sleep over at friends' houses, but on a few occasions he has left the house in anger and stayed out the entire night. Academically, his mother feels that Alan can do the work when he studies, but is unsure of his motivation for grades. Last year, he did not appear "visibly" upset about his failures. In fact, he decided *not* to go to summer school to make these failures up.

An interview with Alan revealed that he didn't want to move, and that he does hope to graduate from high school. Many of Alan's detentions, according to him, are due to being late for class and fooling around in the hall. This quarter, Alan failed four subjects and gym, where he does not like to change into gym clothes and forgets them. Alan does not really know why he failed his subjects last year, and seemed to understand the consequences of bringing liquor into school this year. Socially, Alan doesn't see himself in a single peer group, but feels that he has friends. Out of school, he does admit to some liquor and drug involvement.

During the formal assessment, Alan seemed to work to his capacity with appropriate motivation. He understood directions well, took his time in answering questions, and generally reviewed his work. On many of the verbal tasks, Alan would repeat the question or problem aloud before answering. This may have been a compensatory strategy when material needed to be accessed from his long-term memory. At times, Alan would say that he didn't know answers. This appeared to be an evasive technique—that he didn't want to take the trouble to formulate an answer—and he would usually try when encouraged. Overall, Alan did appear to develop an acceptable rapport with me, and thus, these assessments do appear to validly reflect his current social–emotional status.

Alan's Spontaneous and Inquiry Responses

House

"I just drew a house. It's standing alone" . . . (Q) "It's 50 years old." (Q) "Old people live in the house—two grandparents—and the kids live far away." (Q) "It wishes it could be kept up more." (Q) (No response to question about how the house feels.) (Q) "It's wintertime."

Tree

"The tree is all alone, standing in the middle of a field with animals in the field." (Q) "It's 35 years old, a maple tree, and it's all alive." (Q) "It's a boy tree." (Q) "It's thinking, it wishes it could grow more." (Q) "It feels all alone—wishes he had some friends near him." (Q) "It's fall." (season)

Person

"I just drew a person." (Q) "It's a black person—he sells dope." (Q) "He's 22 years old and he dropped out of school. All his friends are druggies—he lives in a poor jurisdiction." (Q) "Thinking he just got stoned." (Q) "He's feeling high." (Q) "He wants to do something—steal something to eat. In 10 years he'll probably be arrested and sent to jail."

Kinetic Family Drawing

"We're all raking the leaves outside. The kids are not happy; they don't like to rake, but they were told to or they won't get no dinner." (Q) "Dad is saying, 'Get to work!' I don't like this—I'd rather be at a friend's house."

Kinetic School Drawing

"Everybody's playing basketball, but they won't let me play." (Q) "I'm sad and angry—if they don't want to play with me, I don't need them as friends. I'm going back to New York to live anyway."

Interpretive Hypotheses

House

Doesn't see his house as a place of/for psychological warmth.
Feelings of frustration due to a restricting environment.
Weak ego strength.
Fantasy satisfactions prominent.
Concern over interpersonal relationships.
Perceives home as prison-like.

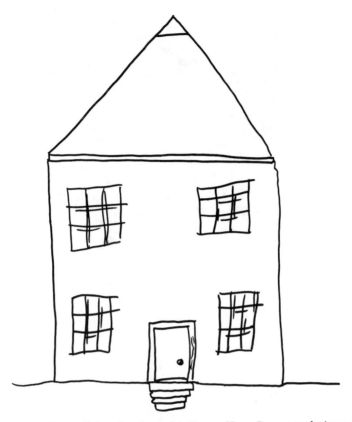

Figure 7-1. Alan's "house" drawing from the House–Tree–Person technique of the case study.

Tree
Feelings of isolation.
Self-centeredness.
Dissatisfaction with interpersonal relationships.
Impulsivity, emotional lability, inner tension.
Infantility.
Good contact with reality.
Feelings of insecurity and inadequacy.

Person
Aggressive tendencies.
Fantasy or escape used as a primary source of satisfaction.
Dependency needs and immature tendencies.
Feelings of inadequacy compensated by aggressive and socially
    dominant behavior.
Powerlessness; searching to regain power.
Suspicious of the environment.
Poor self-concept.
Out of touch with his environment.

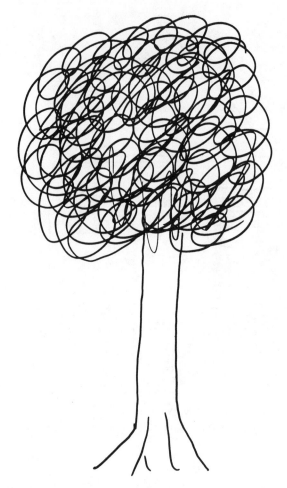

Figure 7-2. Alan's ''tree'' drawing from the House–Tree–Person technique of the case study.

Kinetic Family Drawing

Relative height of figures: Poor self-concept, feelings of insignificance, inadequacy feelings; perceptions of dominating parents, especially father; feelings of little influence within the family.

Stick figures: Defensiveness or resistance to the test setting; use of regression as a defense mechanism.

Figure placement on the page: Psychological identification with siblings over parents.

Physical proximity of figures: No relationship between distance between self and parent figures and psychological distancing.

''X'' Syndrome in drawings of children's bodies: Conflicts between parents and children; need to control aggressive tendencies and resistance toward parents.

Line quality: Tendency toward aggression; passive–aggressiveness.

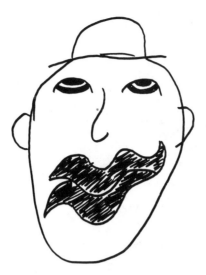

Figure 7-3. Alan's "person" drawing from the House–Tree–Person technique of the case study.

Kinetic School Drawing

Recess actions: Avoidance or anxiety around both academic and school achievement issues, and peer and socialization issues.

Number of peers drawn: Indications of academic achievement problems.

From Family Drawing Interpretations:

Presence of balls: Jealousy toward peer groups, feelings of rejection.

Stick figures: Use of regression as a defense mechanism.

Figure placements: Perceptions of being "left out" of the peer group, or desires to be left out or a loner.

Physical proximity of figures: No relationship between proximity and psychological distancing.

Line quality: Aggressive tendencies, anger (at being left out).

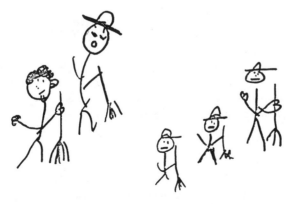

Figure 7-4. Alan's kinetic family drawing from the Kinetic Drawing System technique of the case study.

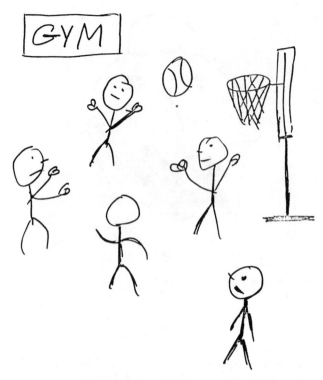

Figure 7-5. Alan's kinetic school drawing from the Kinetic Drawing System technique of the case study.

Summary of Analysis (Integrated from an Entire Personality Assessment Battery)

The personality assessment indicated a number of significant issues that are affecting Alan's social–emotional life, and may give some insights into some of his behaviors. Many of these issues revolve around his feelings of *powerlessness*. Alan is currently overreacting to a fairly typical adolescent concern that everyone in his life, except himself, is controlling his every move. This concern seems to have been present for a number of years, however (e.g., Alan was placed in parochial school when he was unable to academically achieve and structure himself). At this time, Alan is focusing on his "forced" move to his new community. Every bad thing that happens or that he does now can be blamed on that; Alan is absolving himself of any and all responsibility. Meanwhile, he is fighting this powerlessness in a passive–aggressive manner. His anger is not expressed overtly as much as in a passive way: by not working to his capacity in school, by bringing alcohol to school, troubles with the police, drug involvement. These passive–aggressive behaviors allow Alan to control his environment: No one can force him to change them if he doesn't want to.

Alan's academic difficulties pose another area of powerlessness. Alan *does* need academic support, and he does realize that he doesn't achieve like his peers. Yet, Alan does not have control of either the way that he learns, or the ways to get the help that he may need. Alan's reaction is to not try academically, to passively say that he doesn't know why he fails, and to state that he could achieve if he wanted to. (Incidently, his decision not to go to summer school was probably a good one; Alan most likely escaped another failure experience.)

Much of Alan's anger is more actively focused at home. When asked to draw his family doing something together, Alan said, "Huh? I don't want to do *that*." Alan is currently rejecting his family as a supportive unit. He rejects his parents as authority figures, expecting them to dominate and control his comings and goings. When too much pressure exists at home, Alan either asks to spend nights over at friends or takes control of his life by just leaving without permission.

Many of the current family/parental conflicts probably focus on things that Alan wants—whether tangible items or privileges. Alan has a distinct need to attain goals and privileges that *he* wants. This reflects his significant emotional immaturity and sometimes a lack of understanding and contact with his environment. While he wants these goals, Alan either does not know how to appropriately and/or independently attain them; or, he does not want to invest the physical and/or psychological energy necessary. Thus, Alan expects his environment to give him what he wants.

While he rejects his family as a support system, Alan has turned to peers to take up the slack. Unfortunately, this support system is less of an interpersonal support system and more of an escape mechanism due to its near-delinquent acts and drug involvement. Alan is currently using fantasy and drugs to not only escape from his perceived pressures, but again as a way that he can control his life. (He has not yet seen that drugs and peers control his life as much as parents and school.) Adult support systems are also rejected by Alan. He appears very suspicious of his environment; he is not willing to enter into another relationship that may require either an emotional investment or another possible loss of control.

Alan has no real plans or goals at this time. He is very caught up in the social–emotional issues that he perceives, and spends much of his time passively resisting his environment and its demands. He is not currently able to make decisions proactively on how to work with his environment or take responsibility—on a reality level—for changing and moving ahead.

Concluding Comments

Drawing advocates unanimously admonish mental health practitioners to avoid overgeneralizations based on a drawing's single sign or characteristic. For example, Hutt (1968) advocates the use of the clinical intuitive method of analysis. Using this method, the practitioner examines all aspects of a child's behavior, while remaining cognizant that graphic, verbal, and nonverbal behaviors are the result of a constellation of events in the child's history, for example, multiple determinism and contextualism (Mischel, 1977). Hutt suggests that a series of plausible hypotheses be formulated and then examined with data from other tests, life history, and behavioral observations. Hutt notes that the clinical intuitive method " . . . is an intricate, complex and time-consuming method—it requires considerable effort in generating appropriate hypotheses and testing them—and it has serious limitations since each analysis is like doing research with a single case" (1968, p. 407). It should be recognized that data from drawings should be used to generate hypotheses and not to provide evidence that a child is aggressive, emotionally disturbed, insecure, etc. One does not attempt to confirm or verify hypotheses generated from drawings. Hypotheses are tested, not confirmed. This is not a minor semantic point, but a statement that reflects a philosophy of assessment.

Given the conflicting nature of research on projective drawings, one is compelled to question whether or not drawings should be used to generate hypotheses. In other words, is the clinical intuitive method robust enough to avoid Type I errors, that is, detecting significance when it actually does not exist? If the practitioner operates with the null hypothesis and follows Hutt's admonition to conduct miniature research studies, the number of Type I errors should probably be within an acceptable range. Again, it must be stated that the practitioner must avoid an approach which solely seeks to confirm the speculative hypotheses generated from drawings. As is the case with scientific research, data should be collected to disconfirm or confirm a hypothesis.

Obviously, debates over the value of projective drawings have recurred periodically over the past three decades. A recent heated dialogue was started by Martin (1983) when he labeled the use of drawings as unethical. Martin's comments on drawings was an extreme instance of condemnation, and advocates for the clinical use of drawings responded (Paterson & Janzen, 1984; Saltzman, 1984). It is interesting that the pro arguments presented in 1984 were comparable to those made 15 years before by E. F. Hammer (1969) in his article entitled "DAP: Back against the Wall?"

It frequently has been noted that drawings are relatively unique in that they do not require verbal expression for a child to express feelings and attitudes. As Machover, Koppitz, and Hammer have stated, drawings provide a vehicle for the expression of nonverbal, symbolic messages. Cummings (1982) questioned whether practitioners are capable of decoding these messages. Based on a review of the research, it appears justifiable to state that there has been only partial success in breaking the code. Although drawings may appear to be simple acts, they are the result of complex interactions of eye–hand coordination, artistic ability, state and trait characteristics, and societal influences. It is very likely, as Harris (1963) has suggested, that there is no universal language of drawing symbols. There probably are multiple languages as well as various dialects. Researchers working in concert with experienced clinicians must collaboratively investigate the phenomenon of drawing behavior to unravel the code(s).

The author's impression is that too often the focus has been placed on the characteristics of the drawing, almost to the exclusion of the examinee's spontaneous verbalizations and test behaviors. This focus has been reinforced by instructional practices in assessment courses by having students bring in drawings for class discussion. By having students bring in the products, the emphasis is on the post hoc analysis of the drawing content rather than the interaction of the examinee with the task.

Perhaps the greatest value of drawings lies in the examinee's unique approach to the problem, that is, his or her affective responses when drawing family members, attributions regarding success and failure, and spontaneous comments which give insight into the reason for referral. It may be that the greatest value associated with projective drawings does not lie in the graphic symbols represented on the paper. Rather, the value of the technique may be the practitioner's opportunity to observe the examinee's behavior while drawing. Drawings and projective measures in general permit the child to engage in divergent problem solving. This is in contrast to a battery of psychological tests which require convergent production, for example, measures of cognitive and academic achievement functioning. Drawings provide a nonthreatening beginning point which should lead to an in-depth exploration of attitudes, feelings, and beliefs via the synthesis of direct interviews, third-party interviews, observations, and test data. As emphasized by Knoff (1983), the practitioner must operate from a theoretical yet flexible model of evaluation. A cautious and genuine hypothesis testing approach to the interpretation of a child's drawing behavior (not just a post hoc analysis of the drawing) will provide insight regarding both the reason for referral and potential interventions.

References

Albee, G. W., & Hamlin, R. (1949). An investigation of reliability and validity of judgements inferred from drawings. *Journal of Clinical Psychology, 5,* 389–392.

Apfeldorf, M., & Smith, W. (1966). The representation of the body self in human figure drawings. *Journal of Projective Techniques and Personality Assessment, 30,* 283–289.

Attkisson, C. C., Waidler, V. J., Jeffrey, P. M., & Lambert, E. W. (1974). Interrater reliability of the Handler Draw-A-Person scoring. *Perceptual and Motor Skills, 38,* 567–573.

Barnes, E. (1892). A study of children's drawings. *Pedagogical Seminary, 2,* 455–463.

Beck, A. T., Ward, C. H., Mendelson, M., Mock, J., & Erbaugh, J. (1961). An inventory for measuring depression. *Archives of General Psychiatry, 4,* 561–571.

Bennett, V. (1964). Does size of drawing reflect self concept? *Journal of Consulting Psychology, 28,* 285–286.

Bennett, V. (1966). Combinations of drawing characteristics related to the drawer's self concept. *Journal of Projective Techniques, 30,* 192–196.

Berger, L. (1968). Psychological testing: Treatment and research implications. *Journal of Consulting and Clinical Psychology, 32,* 176–181.

Bersoff, D. N. (1973). Silk purse in a sow's ear: The decline of psychological testing and a suggestion for its redemption. *American Psychologist, 28,* 822–899.

Bieliauskas, V. J. (1960). Sexual identification in children's drawings of the human figure. *Journal of Clinical Psychology, 16,* 42–44.

Bieliauskas, V. J., & Farragher, J. (1983). The effect of the drawing sheet on the H–T–P IQ scores. *Journal of Clinical Psychology, 39,* 1033–1034.

Black, F. W. (1972). Factors related to human figure-drawing size in children. *Perceptual and Motor Skills, 35,* 902.

Black, F. W. (1976). The size of human figure drawings of learning disabled children. *Journal of Clinical Psychology, 32,* 736–741.

Blain, G. H., Bergner, R. M., Lewis, M. L., & Goldstein, M. A. (1981). The use of objectively scorable House–Tree–Person indicators to establish child abuse. *Journal of Clinical Psychology, 37,* 667–673.

Bluestein, V. (1978). Loss of loved ones and the drawing of dead or broken branches on the HTP. *Psychology in the Schools, 15,* 364–366.

Brill, M. (1935). The reliability of the Goodenough drawing scale. *Journal of Abnormal Psychology, 26,* 701–708.

Brown, E. V. (1977). Reliability of children's drawings in the Goodenough-Harris "Draw-A-Man Test." *Perceptual and Motor Skills, 44,* 739–742.

Brown, E. V. (1979). Sexual self-identification as reflected in children's drawings when asked to "draw-a-person." *Perceptual and Motor Skills, 49,* 35–38.

Buck, J. N. (1948). The H–T–P technique, a qualitative and quantitative method. *Journal of Clinical Psychology, 4,* 317–396.

Burns, C. J., & Velicer, W. F. (1977). Art instruction and the Goodenough–Harris Drawing Test in fifth-grades. *Psychology in the Schools, 14,* 109–112.

Burns, R. C., & Kaufman, S. H. (1970). *Kinetic Family Drawings (K-F-D): An introduction to understanding children through kinetic drawings.* New York: Brunner/Mazel.

Burns, R. C., & Kaufman, S. H. (1972). *Actions, styles, and symbols in Kinetic Family Drawings (K-F-D).* New York: Brunner/Mazel.

Chambers, G. V. (1954). An investigation of the validity of judgments based on "blind" Rorschach records. *Dissertation Abstracts International, 14,* 2399–2400.

Cleveland, S. E. (1976). Reflections on the rise and fall of psychodiagnosis. *Professional Psychology, 7*, 309–318.

Cohen, S. M., Money, J., & Uhlenhuth, E. H. (1972). A computer study of selected features of self-and-other drawings by 385 children. *Journal of Learning Disabilities, 5*, 145–155.

Craddick, R. A., Leipold, W. D., & Cacauas, P. D. (1962). The relationship of shading on the Draw-A-Person test to manifest anxiety. *Journal of Consulting Psychology, 26*, 193.

Cressen, R. (1975). Artistic quality of drawings and judges' evaluation of DAP's. *Journal of Personality Assessment, 39*, 132–137.

Cummings, J. A. (1981). *An evaluation of Kinetic Family Drawings*. Paper presented at the annual meeting of the American Psychological Association, Los Angeles, CA.

Cummings, J. A. (1982). *Research on projective drawings: Implications for practice*. Paper presented at the annual meeting of the American Psychological Association, Washington, DC.

Cummings, J. A., & Ingram, R. (1980). *Kinetic Family Drawings of children from divorced and intact homes*. Paper presented at the annual meeting of the National Association of School Psychologists, Washington, DC.

Dalby, J. T., & Vale, H. L. (1977). Self esteem and children's human figure drawings. *Perceptual and Motor Skills, 44*, 1279–1282.

Davis, C. J., & Hoopes, J. L. (1975). Comparison of House–Tree–Person drawings of young deaf and hearing children. *Journal of Personality Assessment, 39*, 28–33.

Dennis, W. (1966). *Group values through children's drawings*. New York: Wiley.

Denson, T. A., & May, D. C. (1978). The reliability of children's drawings as indicators of brain damage. *Educational Research Quarterly, 3*, 45–48.

Doubros, S. G., & Mascarenhas, J. (1967). Effect of test produced anxiety on human figure drawings. *Perceptual and Motor Skills, 25*, 773–775.

Dunn, M., & Lorge, I. (1954). A gestalt scale for the appraisal of the human figure drawings. *American Psychologist, 9*, 357.

Eklund, S. J., Huebner, E. S., Groman, C., & Michael, R. (1980, April). *The modal assessment battery used by school psychologists in the United States: 1979–80*. Paper presented at the annual meeting of the National Association of School Psychologists, Washington, DC.

Engle, P. L., & Suppes, J. S. (1970). The relationship between human figure drawing and test anxiety in children. *Journal of Projective Techniques and Personality Assessment, 34*, 223–231.

Eno, L., Elliot, C., & Woehlke, P. (1981). Koppitz emotional indicators in the human-figure drawings of children with learning problems. *Journal of Special Education, 15*, 459–470.

Evans, R., Ferguson, N., Davies, P., & Williams, P. (1975). Reliability of the Draw-A-Man Test. *Educational Research, 18*, 32–36.

Fellows, R., & Cerbus, G. (1969). HTP and DCT indicators of sexual identification in children. *Journal of Projective Techniques and Personality Assessment, 33*, 376–379.

Fischer, C. T. (1959). Body activity gradients and figure drawing variables. *Journal of Consulting Psychology, 23*, 54–59.

Fleming, M., Cohen, D., Salt, P., & Robinson, L. (1982). The use of the Animal Drawing Test in the assessment and disposition of transsexualism. *Journal of Clinical Psychology, 38*, 420–424.

Fraas, L. A. (1970). Sex of figure drawing in identifying practicing male homosexuals. *Psychological Reports, 27*, 172–174.

Fuller, G. B., & Goh, D. S. (1983). Current practices in the assessment of personality and behavior by school psychologists. *School Psychology Review, 12*, 244–249.

Gardner, J. M. (1969). Indicators of homosexuality in the human figure drawings of heroin and pill-pushing addicts. *Perceptual and Motor Skill, 26*, 123–138.

Gayton, W. F., Tavormina, J., Evans, H. E., & Schuh, J. (1974). Comparative validity of Harris' and Koppitz' scoring systems for human figure drawings. *Perceptual and Motor Skills, 39*, 369–370.

Goh, D. S., Teslow, C. J., & Fuller, G. B. (1981). The practice of psychological assessment among school psychologists. *Professional Psychology, 12*, 696–706.

Goldberg, L. R. (1968). Simple models or simple process? Some research on clinical judgements. *American Psychologist, 23*, 483–496.

Goodenough, F. L. (1926). *Measurement of intelligence by drawings*. New York: Harcourt Brace & World.

Goodenough, F. L. (1931). Children's drawings. In C. Murchison (Ed.), *A handbook of child psychology* (pp. 480–514). Worcester, MA: University Press.

Green, R., Fuller, M., & Rutley, B. (1972). It-scale for children and Draw-A-Person test: 30 feminine vs. 25 masculine boys. *Journal of Personality Assessment, 33*, 349–352.

Hammer, E. F. (1954). Relationship between diagnosis of psychosexual pathology and the sex of the first drawn person. *Journal of Clinical Psychology, 10*, 168–170.

Hammer, E. F. (Ed.). (1958). *The clinical application of projective drawings*. Springfield, IL: Charles C. Thomas.

Hammer, E. F. (1959). Critique of Swenson's "Empirical evaluations of human figure drawings." *Journal of Projective Techniques, 23*, 30–32.

Hammer, E. F. (1960). The House–Tree–Person (H–T–P) drawings as a projective technique with children. In A. I. Rabin & M. R. Haworth (Eds.), *Projective techniques with children* (pp. 258–272). New York: Grune & Stratton.

Hammer, E. F. (1968). Projective drawings. In A. I. Rabin (Ed.), *Projective techniques in personality assessment* (pp. 366–393). New York: Springer.

Hammer, E. F. (1969). DAP: Back against the wall? *Journal of Consulting and Clinical Psychology, 33*, 151–156.

Hammer, E. F. (1981). Projective drawings: In A. I. Rabin (Ed.), *Assessment with projective techniques: A concise introduction* (pp. 151–185). New York: Springer.

Hammer, M., & Kaplan, A. M. (1964a). The reliability of profile and front facing directions in children's drawings. *Child Development, 35*, 973–977.

Hammer, M., & Kaplan, A. M. (1964b). The reliability of size of children's drawings. *Journal of Clinical Psychology, 20*, 121.

Hammer, M., & Kaplan, A. M. (1964c). The reliability of sex of first drawn figure by children. *Journal of Clinical Psychology, 20*, 251–252.

Hammer, M., & Kaplan, A. M. (1966). The reliability of children's drawings. *Journal of Clinical Psychology, 22*, 316–319.

Handler, L. (1967). Anxiety indexes in the Draw-A-Person test: A scoring manual. *Journal of Projective Techniques, 31*, 46–57.

Handler, L. (1984). Anxiety as measured by the Draw-A-Person test: A response to Sims, Dana, and Bolton. *Journal of Personality Assessment, 48*, 82–84.

Handler, L., & Reyher, J. (1964). The effects of stress on the Draw-A-Person test. *Journal of Consulting Psychology, 28*, 259–264.

Handler, L., & Reyher, J. (1965). Figure drawing anxiety indexes: A review of the literature. *Journal of Projective Techniques, 29*, 305–313.

Handler, L., & Reyher, J. (1966). Relationship between the GSR and anxiety indexes in projective drawings. *Journal of Personality Assessment, 36*, 263–267.

Harris, D. B. (1963). *Children's drawings as a measure of intellectual maturity*. New York: Harcourt Brace & World.

Harris, D. B. (1978). A review of Kinetic Family Drawings. In O. K. Buros (Ed.), *The eighth mental measurements yearbook* (Vol. 1, pp. 884–885). Highland Park, NJ: Gryphon Press.

Hogan, R., DeSota, C. B., & Solano, C. (1977). Traits, tests, and personality research. *American Psychologist, 32*, 255–264.

Holmes, C. B., & Wiederhold, J. (1982). Depression and figure size on the Draw-A-Person test. *Perceptual and Motor Skills, 55*, 825–826.

Hoyt, T. E., & Baron, M. R. (1959). Anxiety indices in same-sex drawings of psychiatric patients with high and low MAS scores. *Journal of Consulting Psychology, 23*, 448–452.

Hulse, W. C. (1951). The emotionally disturbed child draws his family. *Quarterly Journal of Child Behavior, 3*, 152–174.

Hulse, W. C. (1952). Childhood conflict expressed through family drawings. *Quarterly Journal of Child Behavior, 16*, 66–79.

Hutt, M. L. (1968). *The Hutt adaptation of the Bender–Gestalt Test* (2nd ed.). New York: Grune & Stratton.

Johnson, F. A. (1972). Figure drawings in subjects recovering from poliomyelitis. *Psychosomatic Medicine, 34*, 19–29.

Johnson, F. A., & Greenberg, R. P. (1978). Quality of drawing as a factor in the interpretation of figure drawings. *Journal of Personality Assessment, 42*, 489–495.

Johnson, J. H. (1971a). Note on the validity of Machover's indicators of anxiety. *Perceptual and Motor Skills, 33*, 126.

Johnson, J. H. (1971b). Upper left placement of human figure drawings as an indicator of anxiety. *Journal of Personality Assessment, 35*, 336–337.

Jollès, I. (1971). *A catalog for the qualitative interpretation of the House–Tree–Person (HTP)*. Los Angeles, CA: Western Psychological Services.

Judson, A. J., & MacCasland, B. W. (1960). A note on the influence of the season on tree drawings. *Journal of Clinical Psychology, 16*, 171–173.

Knoff, H. M. (1983). Personality assessment in the schools: Issues and procedures for school psychologists. *School Psychology Review, 12*, 391–398.

Knoff, H. M., & Prout, H. T. (1985a). The Kinetic Drawing System: A review and integration of the Kinetic Family and School Drawing techniques. *Psychology in the Schools, 22*, 50–59.

Knoff, H. M., & Prout, H. T. (1985b). *The Kinetic drawing system: Family and school.* Los Angeles, CA: Western Psychological Services.

Koppitz, E. M. (1966). Emotional indicators on Human Figure Drawings of young children. *Journal of Clinical Psychology, 22*, 313–315.

Koppitz, E. M. (1968). *Psychological evaluation of children's human figure drawings.* New York: Grune & Stratton.

Koppitz, E. M. (1983). Projective drawings with children and adolescents. *School Psychology Review, 12*, 421–427.

Lachmann, F. M., Bailey, M. A., & Berrick, M. E. (1961). The relationship between manifest anxiety and clinicians evaluation of projective test responses. *Journal of Clinical Psychology, 17*, 11–13.

Leichtman, S. R., Burnett, J. W., & Robinson, H. M. (1981). Body image concerns of psoriasis patients as reflected in human figure drawings. *Journal of Personality Assessment, 45*, 478–484.

Levy, S. (1950). Figure drawing as a projective test. In L. Abt & L. Bellack (Eds.), *Projective Psychology* (pp. 257–297). New York: Knopf.

Lewinsohn, P. M. (1964). Relationship between height of figure drawings and depression in psychiatric patients. *Journal of Consulting Psychology, 28*, 380–381.

Litt, S., & Margoshes, A. (1966). Sex changes in successive D–A–P tests. *Journal of Clinical Psychology, 22*, 471.

Loutitt, C. M., & Browne, C. G. (1947). The use of psychiatric instruments in psychological clinics. *Journal of Consulting Psychology, 11*, 49–54.

Lubin, B., Larsen, R. M., & Matarazzo, J. D. (1984). Patterns of psychological test usage in the United States: 1935–1982. *American Psychologist, 39*, 451–454.

Lubin, B., Wallis, R. R., & Paine, C. (1971). Patterns of psychological test usage in the United States: 1935–1969. *Professional Psychology, 2*, 70–74.

Machover, K. (1949). *Personality projection in the drawing of the human figure.* Springfield, IL: Charles C Thomas.

Martin, R. P. (1983). The ethical issues in the use and interpretation of the Draw-A-Person test and other similar projective procedures. *The School Psychologist, 38*(6), 8.

Marzolf, S. S., & Kirchner, J. H. (1970). Characteristics of House–Tree–Person drawings by college men and women. *Journal of Projective Techniques and Personality Assessment, 34*, 138–145.

Marzolf, S. S., & Kirchner, J. H. (1971). Color in House–Tree–Person drawings by college men and women. *Journal of Clinical Psychology, 27*, 504–509.

Marzolf, S. S., & Kirchner, J. H. (1972). House–Tree–Person Drawings and Personality Traits. *Journal of Personality Assessment, 36*, 148–165.

Marzolf, S. S., & Kirchner, J. H. (1973). Personality traits and color choices for House–Tree–Person drawings. *Journal of Clinical Psychology, 29*, 240–245.

McCarthy, D. (1944). A study of the reliability of the Goodenough drawing test of intelligence. *Journal of Psychology, 18*, 201–206.

McCurdy, H. G. (1947). Group and individual variability on the Goodenough Draw-A-Man Test. *Journal of Educational Psychology, 38*, 428–436.

McLachlan, J. F., & Head, V. B. (1974). An impairment rating scale. *Journal of Clinical Psychology, 30*, 405–407.

McPhee, J. P., & Wegner, K. W. (1976). Kinetic-Family-Drawing styles and emotionally disturbed childhood behavior. *Journal of Personality Assessment, 40*, 487–491.

Meyers, D. V. (1978). Toward an objective procedure evaluation of the Kinetic Family Drawings (KFD). *Journal of Personality Assessment, 42*, 358–365.

Mischel, W. (1977). On the future of personality measurement. *American Psychologist, 32*, 246–253.

Moll, R. P. (1962). Further evidence of seasonal influence on tree drawings. *Journal of Clinical Psychology, 18*, 109.

Mostkoff, D. L., & Lazarus, P. J. (1983). The Kinetic Family Drawing: The reliability of an objective scoring system. *Psychology in the Schools, 20*, 16–20.

Murray, D. C., & Delber, H. L. (1958). Drawings, diagnoses, and the clinicians learning curve. *Journal of Projective Technique, 22*, 415–420.

Nathan, S. (1973). Body image in chronically obese children as reflected in figure drawings. *Journal of Personality Assessment, 37*, 456–463.

Nichols, R. C., & Strumpfer, D. J. (1962). A factor analysis of Draw-A-Person test scores. *Journal of Consulting Psychology, 26*, 156–161.

O'Brien, R. P., & Patton, W. F. (1974). Development of an objective scoring method for the Kinetic Family Drawing. *Journal of Personality Assessment, 38*, 156–164.

Palmer, J. O. (1983). *The psychological assessment of children.* New York: Wiley.

Paterson, J. G., & Janzen, H. (1984). Another reply to Martin: Projective procedures an ethical dilemma. *The School Psychologist, 38*(6), 8–9.

Peterson, D. (1983). The Kinetic School-Drawing: A negative evaluation. *Illinois School Psychologists' Association Monograph Series, 1*, 76–82.

Pihl, R. O., & Nimrod, G. (1976). The reliability and validity of the Draw-A-Person Test in IQ and personality assessment. *Journal of Clinical Psychology, 32*, 470–472.

Piotrowski, C., & Keller, J. W. (1984). Psychodiagnostic testing in APA-approved clinical psychology programs. *Professional Psychology: Research and Practice, 15*, 450–456.

Prout, H. T. (1983). School psychologists and social–emotional assessment techniques: Patterns in training and use. *School Psychology Review, 12*, 35–38.

Prout, H. T., & Phillips, P. D. (1974). A clinical note: The kinetic school drawing. *Psychology in the Schools, 11*, 303–306.

Prytula, R. E., & Hiland, D. N. (1975). Analysis of general anxiety scale for children and Draw-A-Person measures of general anxiety level of elementary school children. *Perceptual and Motor Skills, 41*, 995–1007.

Prytula, R. E., Phelps, M. R., & Morrissey, E. F. (1978). Figure drawing size as a reflection of self-concept or self-esteem. *Journal of Clinical Psychology, 34*, 207–214.

Prytula, R. E., & Thompson, N. D. (1973). Analysis of emotional indicators in human figure drawings as related to self-esteem. *Perceptual and Motor Skills, 37*, 795–802.

Pustel, G., Sternlicht, M., & DeRespinis, M. (1971). Tree drawings of institutionalizational retardates: Seasonal and color effects. *Journal of Genetic Psychology, 118*, 217–222.

Reynolds, C. R. (1978). Teacher–psychologist interscorer reliability of the McCarthy Drawing Tests. *Perceptual and Motor Skills, 47*, 538.

Rierdan, J., & Koff, E. (1981). Sexual ambiguity in children's human figure drawings. *Journal of Personality, 45*, 256–257.

Roback, H. B. (1968). Human figure drawings: Their utility in the clinical psychologist's armamentarium for personality assessment. *Psychological Bulletin, 70*, 1–19.

Roback, H. B., Langevin, R., & Zajac, Y. (1974). Sex of free choice figure drawings by homosexual and heterosexual subjects. *Journal of Personality Assessment, 38*, 154–155.

Roback, H. B., & Webersinn, A. L. (1966). Size of figure drawings of depressed psychiatric patients. *Journal of Abnormal Psychology, 71*, 416.

Saltzman, C. (1984). Correlation coefficients and professional ethics: A reply to Martin. *School Psychologist, 38*(3), 6–7.

Sarbaugh, M. E. (1983). Kinetic Drawing-School (KS-D) technique. *Illinois School Psychologists' Association Monograph Series, 1*, 1–70.

Schaeffer, R. W. (1964). Clinical psychologist's ability to use the Draw-A-Person Test as an indicator of personality adjustment. *Journal of Consulting Psychology, 28*, 383.

Sims, J., Dana, R., & Bolton, B. (1983). The validity of the Draw-A-Person Test as an anxiety measure. *Journal of Personality Assessment, 47*, 250–257.

Skilbeck, W. M., Bates, J. E., & Bentler, P. M. (1975). Human figure drawings of gender-problem and school-problem boys. *Journal of Abnormal Child Psychology, 3*, 191–199.

Smith, F. O. (1937). What the Goodenough intelligence test measures. *Psychological Bulletin, 34*, 760–761.

Sobel, H., & Sobel, W. (1976). Discriminating adolescent male delinquents through the use of Kinetic Family Drawings. *Journal of Personality Assessment, 40*, 91–94.

Starr, S., & Marcuse, F. L. (1959). Reliability of the Draw-A-Person Test. *Journal of Projective Techniques, 23*, 83–86.

Sturner, R. A., Rothbaum, F., Visintainer, M., & Wolfer, J. (1980). The effects of stress on children's drawings. *Journal of Clinical Psychology, 36*, 325–331.

Sunberg, N. D. (1961). The practice of psychological testing in clinical services in the United States. *American Psychologist, 16*, 79–83.

Swenson, C. H. (1955). Sexual differentiation on the Draw-A-Person Test. *Journal of Clinical Psy-*

chology, *11*, 37–40.

Swenson, C. H. (1957). Empirical evaluations of human figure drawings. *Psychological Bulletin, 54*, 431–466.

Swenson, C. H. (1968). Empirical evaluation of human figure drawings: 1957–1966. *Psychological Bulletin, 70*, 20–44.

Teglasi, H. (1980). Acceptance of the traditional female role and sex of the first person drawn on the Draw-A-Person Test. *Perceptual and Motor Skills, 51*, 267–271.

Tolor, A., & Digrazio, P. V. (1977). The body image of pregnant women as reflected in their human figure drawings. *Journal of Clinical Psychology, 33*, 566–571.

Tolor, A., & Tolor, B. (1974). Children's figure drawings and changing attitudes toward sex roles. *Psychological Reports, 34*, 343–349.

Viney, L. L., Aitkin, M., & Floyd, J. (1974). Self-regard and size of human figure drawings: An interactional analysis. *Journal of Clinical Psychology, 30*, 581–586.

Vukovich, D. H. (1983). The use of projective assessment by school psychologists. *School Psychology Review, 12*, 358–364.

Wade, T. C., & Baker, T. B. (1977). Opinions and use of psychological tests. *American Psychologist, 32*, 874–882.

Wanderer, Z. E. (1969). Validity of clinical judgments based on human figure drawings. *Journal of Consulting and Clinical Psychology, 33*, 143–150.

Wildman, R. W., Wildman, R. W., II, & Smith, R. D. (1967). Expansive constriction of the H–T–P as measures of extraversion–introversion. *Journal of Clinical Psychology, 23*, 493–494.

Wise, P. S., & Potkay, C. R. (1983). The KS-D: A technique in need of validation. *Illinois School Psychologists' Association Monograph Series, 1*, 71–75.

Wysocki, B. A., & Whitney, E. (1965). Body-image of crippled children as seen in the D-A-P Test behavior. *Perceptual and Motor Skills, 21*, 494–504.

Wysocki, B. A., & Wysocki, A. C. (1973). The body-image of normal and retarded children. *Journal of Clinical Psychology, 29*, 7–10.

Zucker, K. J. (1972). Childhood gender disturbances: Diagnostic issues. *Journal of the American Academy of Child Psychiatry, 21*, 274–280.

Zucker, K. J., Finegan, J. K., Doering, R. W., & Bradley, S. J. (1983). Human figure drawings of gender-problem children: A comparison of sibling, psychiatric, and normal controls. *Journal of Abnormal Child Psychology, 11*, 287–298.

The Sentence Completion Techniques

Darrell H. Hart

Overview

Sentence completion techniques are among the most frequently used procedures for personality and attitude assessment. Lubin, Larsen, and Matarazzo (1984), in a recent survey evaluating the use of psychological tests, found that the sentence completion technique was among the 10 most frequently used tests, including those assessing intelligence. So popular is this procedure for eliciting psychodiagnostic information on individual's need states, attitudes, and personality dynamics, that it is rated as the third most frequently used projective tool in the psychological test battery. In addition to psychological treatment centers which use the method for diagnosis and patient care, school psychologists also find the technique useful in their psychoeducational and personality assessments with referred children and adolescents. Social scientists use the sentence completion technique as an assessment tool evaluating attitudinal and personality variables.

The sentence completion method consists of a number of incomplete sentence stems which an individual completes either orally or in writing. For example, the following sentence stems are taken from the Hart Sentence Completion Test for Children (HSCT; Hart, 1972):

1. *When mother and dad are together, they* . . .
2. *To the other kids, I* . . .
3. *The best thing about school* . . .
4. *I am the* . . .
5. *I wish* . . .
6. *My mother thinks* . . .

Responses to these sentence stems are voluntary and are limited only to the range of attitudes and feelings that they elicit from within the individual. A mental health practitioner or researcher then analyzes the responses to determine attitudes, per-

Darrell H. Hart. Educational Support Systems, Inc., Salt Lake City, Utah.

sonality styles and dynamics, and overall psychological adjustment (Goldberg, 1965).

There is some debate as to whether the sentence completion method should be classified as a projective, objective, or semiprojective technique. Campbell (1957), in his typology of testing procedures, considers the sentence completion method to be a direct, rather than an indirect, approach for eliciting personality attitudes and dynamics because, he believes, subjects are aware that they are revealing themselves in a very straightforward fashion. Rohde (1957), however, feels that the method obtains information about subjects' psychodynamics and personalized characteristics without an awareness that such aspects of personality are being revealed. The use of the sentence completion method as a projective technique to augment other projective data (e.g., from the Rorschach, the Thematic Apperception Test, and the Draw-A-Person) tends to support Rohde's perceptions.

Methods of scoring sentence completion tests have also caused debate. For example, unlimited response options make the development of structured scoring systems for some sentence completion tests difficult. Thus, many sentence completion tests do not formally evaluate their responses against standard criteria. In these cases, the practitioner gathers clinical impressions about the personality characteristics of a subject, integrating them with the other information generated through interviews, other projective instruments, and behavioral observations.

Some, however, are dissatisfied with this "impressions" approach of analyzing sentence completion responses. Primary concerns focus on examiner bias, the subjectivity of the process, and the heavy dependence on other sources of projective data. In response to these concerns, significant developmental efforts have resulted in sentence completion tests with established scoring criteria and guidelines, and the ability to evaluate responses according to (a) the types of content and affect, and (b) how typical they are for a given population (Rotter & Rafferty, 1950; Sacks & Levy, 1950).

Finally, the psychometric properties of sentence completion techniques are a last focus of controversy between researchers concerned with their lack of traditional measurement integrity and practitioners aware of their pragmatic utility (Anastasi, 1976). This controversy symbolizes the difficulties associated with the standardization of projective techniques and the tendency of practitioners to use sentence completion methods out of the context for which they were developed. Despite these differences, the popularity of this personality assessment technique has not diminished.

Among the different sentence completion tests available, there are notable similarities and differences. Besides their common formats, all of these tests typically include sentence stems related to self-image and emotions and perceptions of significant people and conditions in the environment. While subjects respond to these stems according to their own affective and cognitive processes, their different contents often stimulate thought and responses in diverse directions. Thus, these different tests vary with respect to content, as well as their length, complexity, and purpose.

Many sentence completion tests also have been devised to assess attitudes and personality dimensions specific to a particular theoretical model (Rohde, 1957). Others have been designed for specific populations or research uses (Hart, 1972; Holzberg, Teicher, & Taylor, 1947). The next section discusses a historical perspective of sentence completion test development, with a later emphasis on the present status of the technique.

Historical Perspectives of the Sentence Completion Technique

Historically, the sentence completion technique was developed to measure individuals' mental abilities as well as to gain insight into their attitudes and personalities. Two separate theoretical and experimental efforts, using words and sentences as stimuli to elicit free responses, were initiated around the turn of the century. Ebbinghaus (1897) hypothesized that different mental abilities could be identified through the analysis of incomplete sentence responses. The more complex responses were thought to reflect greater mental capacity, while simplistic and undeveloped answers were indicative of inferior mental abilities. Binet and Simon (1905) included sentence stems in their first intellectual assessment battery. Continuing efforts to use this technique to identify and predict intellectual capacity included the works of Trabue (1916) and Kelly (1917), and Piltz (1957) and West (1958) through the late 1950s. In the past 25 years, however, interest in using incomplete sentences to measure mental abilities has waned, primarily due to the complexities of test standardization, marginal predictive validities, and the presence of more reliable assessment measures.

From an attitude and personality assessment perspective, the word association technique appears to have been the forerunner of the sentence completion method. Jung (1904, 1906, 1907) was the first to explore in depth the relationship between stimulus words and elicited responses in a word association format. He was soon joined by other researchers who examined the process of determining attitudes from word associations (Kent & Rosanoff, 1910; Wells, 1911). In time, this research expanded to the use of multiple words and sentence stems. Basically, it was found that this expansion from one-word stimuli to incomplete sentence stems elicited responses of greater depth of feeling. Thus, more comprehensive information was available for the analysis of attitude and personality characteristics. Ultimately, sentence completion techniques were applied to the study of language and thought, as well as emotional states, guidance needs, and psychopathology.

Sentence completion techniques, as they are known today, evolved during World War II for the psychological evaluation and placement of American soldiers. The Office of Strategic Services, assigned the duty of personnel selection, included the method as a part of its psychological test battery (Murray & MacKinnon, 1946). A 100-item sentence completion test was developed to elicit responses in 12 different dimensions of personality: family, past, goals, drives, interstates, cathexis, optimism, pessimism, energy, reactions to frustration and failure, reaction to others, and reaction of others. The responses were evaluated according to (a) the rarity of responses when compared with other subjects, and (b) the frequency of similar response contents to different sentence stems. While the criteria were simple, the test screened different dimensions of personality that could be explored further in individual interviews. Of the many projective techniques included in the original military test battery, this sentence completion test was the only test retained as an integral part of the permanent battery.

The success of the sentence completion technique for military screening and guidance prompted the development of a 40-item sentence completion test by Rotter and Willerman (1947) for use in military hospitals. The test was later adapted for use with the general civilian population and was named the Incomplete Sentence Blank (ISB; Rotter, Rafferty, & Schachtitz, 1949). Not only is the ISB in use today, but it appears to serve as a general model for those developing sentence completion tests to meet their own particular clinical or research interests.

Of the numerous sentence completion tests that have been developed since the original one during World War II, those by Rohde (1946, 1947), Forer (1950), and Holsopple and Miale (1954) are among the most frequently referenced. Though developed more than 30 years ago, these three techniques are excellent illustrations of some of the distinguishing characteristics of the sentence completion tests being used and constructed today (see Watson, 1978, for a comprehensive review). Irrespective of history and time, these tests share similar formats of item structure and content, and, even though each has its own purpose, similar organizations of sentence stems and methods of evaluation. Specific to their own purposes, Rohde interprets her test using Murray's need–press theory; Forer structured sentence stems to elicit attitudes and perceptions in preselected content areas; and Holsopple and Miale developed their stems to allow subjects to project underlying psychological dynamics.

When contrasting the history of the sentence completion method with the current status of sentence completion tests, it is evident that the technological and statistical improvements in test construction over the past 30 years have not been applied to this method. There are few sentence completion tests today which have acceptable standards for test development, construction, and standardization. Other assessment tests (e.g., the MMPI, Wechsler Intelligence Scales, Quay–Peterson Behavior Rating Scales) *have* been maintained with up-to-date psychometric standards, and they have emerged as state-of-the-art instruments for use in research and psychodiagnostic testing. Even the Rorschach and the Thematic Apperception Tests, among other projective techniques, have received continued research and refinement in order to evaluate and enhance their validity, their scoring systems, and their practical applicability. These procedures have helped legitimize them as viable personality assessment measures.

Systematic efforts to construct better sentence completion tests have not occurred to any significant degree. Because the method was thought to be like a clinical interview with a wide range of possible responses and subjective interpretations, the rigors of quantifying and standardizing attitudinal and affective responses were not deemed necessary. Thus, mental health practitioners and researchers have chosen to proliferate more of the same for their own applications. There are dozens of sentence completion tests in use today, but most are loose iterations of earlier efforts. Thus, while the Rotter Incomplete Sentence Blank (and its imitations) is a frequently used sentence completion test, its technology is basically the same as when it was originally developed, and its continued use appears to be simply a matter of convenience and personal experience. The Rotter Incomplete Sentence Blank carries no more credibility in a psychodiagnostic battery or as a research tool than any other sentence completion test.

The lack of systematic research to improve the psychometric properties of sentence completion techniques has deterred their potential use as empirical predictors of human behavior. That is not to say that the method has not been considered useful in applied settings. The Goldberg (1965) and Murstein (1965) studies of the sentence completion method show that its "validity" as a testing technique has been demonstrated by its popular use, a kind of consensus validation. Those who used the method reported that their results related closely to other verbal data and behavioral observations, and that the method assessed personality dynamics which were of particular interest. The few empirically based studies evaluating the technique's potential for differential diagnosis have also been encouraging (Robyak, 1975; Rotter & Willerman, 1947; Sacks, 1949; Swanson, 1975; Wolkon & Haefner, 1961). Given all of these studies, there is reason to expect future sentence completion tests to have acceptable measurement properties and acceptable applied utility. For the present, however, practitioners must recognize that their conclusions and predictions from sentence completion techniques are only as good as their clinical skills in making subjective judgments.

A final observation, given the history of the sentence completion method, is that few sentence completion tests have been developed specifically for children and young adolescents. References in reviews of the sentence completion method indicate clinical use or research primarily with older adolescents and adults. Instability in the psychodynamic processes of children, inhibitions about making self-references to sentence stems, the ambiguity of the tasks to be completed, and the lack of ability to conceptualize and verbalize feelings and attitudes were some of the initial issues thought to interfere with the effective use of this technique with children. Actual experience in administering sentence completion tests to children lends some credence to these concerns; however, most child guidance clinics and schools have, over the past 15 years, found that the method is far more helpful than limiting. To adapt the method to young people, mental health practitioners have modified existing adult sentence completion tests or created new tests with more structured sentence stems and child-oriented content. Sentence stems containing references to parents, school, kids, and growing up have replaced adult stems referring to spouse, job, boss, and achievement needs.

Psychometrically, most of the child-oriented sentence completion tests have the same weaknesses as their adult counterparts with the absence of scoring systems, normative data, and appropriate reliability and validity data. Predictably, this has not deterred the sentence completion method's use with children. A notable exception to these tests is the Hart Sentence Completion Test for Children (HSCT; Hart, 1972), which is reviewed later in this chapter. The HSCT represents a concentrated effort to establish scoring criteria, reliability, and criterion-related validity, but it too lacks adequate normative standardization for comprehensive use. Thus, while the sentence completion technique is used regularly by practitioners in schools and child clinics, even less research and descriptive literature is available on this method's use with children than with adults. This is a critical need in the psychodiagnostic and clinical literature that should be addressed.

To summarize, although numerous sentence completion tests have been developed, research efforts have not systematically focused on such test-construction issues as their standardization procedures and their psychometric soundness. Thus, the full potential of the sentence completion process has not been realized. This method's use with children has also received limited attention, and most child-oriented sentence completion tests are based on their adult counterparts. Further understanding of this technique and ways to enhance their technological advancement are addressed below by examining how the key elements of sentence completion tests have been treated.

The Four Major Elements of Sentence Completion Tests

The process of developing sentence completion tests involves considerations of purpose, form, administration, and interpretation. These are the basic elements of the technique and are common to all sentence completion tests. The distinguishing characteristics of each sentence completion test are determined as the test developer makes the following decisions about these four elements:

1. What is the target population and what kind of information should the test provide about that population?
2. What diagnostic information is desired, and thus, what sentence stem content and structure should be used to elicit this information?
3. What test administration procedures should be developed to prepare and facilitate subjects' completion of the sentence stems?
4. How can the responses to the sentence stems be analyzed to ensure a valid assessment of the desired information and an appropriate understanding of the individual subject?

Operationalized, these decisions involve standardization and methodological procedures such as choosing and assessing appropriate population samples, establishing scoring and normative criteria and determining reliability and validity, and developing sentence completion tests with adequate interpretation capabilities. Given the historical discussion above describing the evolution of this technique, these procedures are necessary to update its psychometric qualities and clinical utility.

Purpose

Sentence completion tests have been designed primarily to obtain research or psychodiagnostic information. Social scientists use the technique because it provides information about attitudes which are thought to be difficult to obtain in direct questionnaire formats. This information has been used most often to analyze attitudes in relation to the environment, as well as for other diverse research applications. For example, Exner (1973) used the sentence completion technique to study egocentricity, and Aronoff (1972) and Wilson and Aronoff (1973) to study safety and esteem. MacBrayer (1960) compared perceptions of the opposite sex held by males and females with this technique, and Harris and Tseng (1957) looked at the attitudes of parents and peers. Finally, McKinney (1967) studied the relationships among personality, school behavior, and potential for self-actualization, while Ulman (1972) and Robyak (1975) compared the response contents of handicapped and normal children.

The frequency and use of the sentence completion technique as a psychodiagnostic tool were highlighted in the Overview and Historical Perspectives sections above. Examples, from this discussion, of three specific sentence completion test purposes illustrate its range of clinical application. Rotter and Rafferty (1950) wanted their sentence completion test to serve as a diagnostic screening device for practitioners engaged in interviewing and treatment planning. Their test was not designed to expose fundamental personality functioning. The Rohde Sentence Completion Method (1957), however, was developed to explore the dynamics of neurotic personality disorder and to better understand schizophrenic patients. Finally, the Sacks Sentence Completion Test (Sacks & Levy, 1950) was prepared to obtain conscious, preconscious, and even unconscious thoughts and feelings which might support and augment similar data obtained through other projective techniques.

Form

The purposes for developing a test dictate its form. For this discussion, form refers to the content and structure of the sentence stems. The content of the stimulus stem is designed to increase the propensity of the subject to reveal conscious and/or unconscious attitudes and dynamic constructs of personality. If a practitioner were exploring children's hidden conflicts, the content of the sentence stem might refer to mother, sex, or fears. A researcher, studying students' perceptions of school, might include the words "math," "recess," or "teachers" in the content of the stem.

Structure in the sentence stem refers to the detail and specificity of the content. A multiword stem with content that focuses on a specific topic indicates a test developed to structure or direct the subject's thinking and responses. An unstructured test, meanwhile, has stimuli which are ambiguous, allowing the subject to respond with a wide array of possible responses. To illustrate, a structured stimulus might be, "When mother and father are together, they . . . "; an unstructured stimulus might be, "I . . . . " Following the hypothesis that there are varying levels of personality (Coleman, 1969), it might be predicted that unstructured stimuli evoke responses which reveal deeper and more inaccessible personality dynamics than more structured stimuli. Indeed, the most ambiguous of the unstructured stimuli would access the deepest levels of personality. It would follow, therefore, that subjects' conscious control over their responses is dictated by stimulus structure. By varying the structure of the sentence stems, subjects' awareness or unawareness of the psychological meanings of their responses will vary.

The use of first- and third-person referents has also been an important form consideration when constructing sentence stems. Studies by Sacks (1949) and Cromwell and Lundy (1954) concluded that the first-person stems produce more clinically useful information than third-person stems. However, Stricker and Dawson (1966) found that first- and third-person forms were equally important when evaluating anxiety, dependency, and hostility. Finally, Wood's (1969) data suggest that subjects project more psychopathological responses when referents are not in the first person. Considering the absence of definitive research, the tendency of most authors over the past 10 years has been to include a mix of first, third, and nonperson referents in their sentence stems.

From a test construction perspective, the form of the sentence stems is the heart of the development process. Decisions that must be made, as the content and structure of the stems are composed, are based on (a) what content best reflects the author's predetermined purposes and theoretical orientation, (b) the desired amount of conscious control that the subjects will have over their responses, and (c) the importance of first and/or third-person referents in the sentence stems.

Administration

Variations in the administration of different sentence completion tests generally occur due to their differing (a) formats, (b) instructions or directions given to subjects, and/or (c) provisions for inquiry or behavioral observations to obtain additional diagnostic information. Researchers often prefer a cost-efficient administration format consisting of, for example, inviting subjects to complete the sentence stems while in small group settings, counseling groups, or classrooms. In these cases, a group leader explains the purpose of the sentence completion technique, the subjects read the printed instructions (with the leader's help or clarification if needed), and the subjects independently complete the sentence stems. Some community-based agencies or clinics use a self-administered procedure where the sentence completion test is part of a larger diagnostic screening battery, complete with other self-administered questionnaires, given to incoming clients. This process is later followed by more complex testing and, eventually, treatment if needed.

For psychodiagnostic assessment, a frequently used administration format has the practitioner read the sentence stem to a child or adolescent and encourage him or her to verbally complete the stem with whatever comes to mind. The practitioner records the response verbatim and the next sentence stem is provided. While this individual administration is time-intensive, the secondary benefits of observing subjects' general behaviors under the pressure of the testing process and specific behavioral reactions to individual items or formats usually outweigh the inefficiency.

While authors' primary intentions are to elicit sentence responses which accurately reflect the psychological dynamics of their subjects, test instructions from test to test still vary. Some authors believe that the speed of the elicited response influences the spontaneity and unguarded revelation of emotion and perception. "Complete the items as quickly as possible, write or say the very first thing that comes into your mind" are directions designed to emphasize speed in the hope of avoiding excessive conscious control. Other authors use an alternative strategy informing their subject to complete each sentence in whatever way desired, that the purpose of the test is to share "real feelings." Responses generated by this "careful thought" process are often judged to be excellent clues to ego processes. How particular content is avoided as well as how responses are stated also provide information for analysis.

A few researchers have investigated the relationship between the type of instruction and the kind of responses generated. Stricker and Dawson (1966), Wood (1969), and Flynn (1974) all found no differences between instructions emphasizing verbal speed and instructions calling for real feelings and no concern for speed. The dependent variables were general maladjustment, dependency, anxiety, and hostility. Only Siipola (1968) found differences due to variations in instructions. In that study, time pressure was judged to produce more ego-alien and conflicted responses.

From the above discussion and a review of actual psychometric practice, it is safe to conclude that the kind of instructions used with sentence completion tests is determined primarily by the theoretical orientation of the practitioner. Certainly, the test authors' intentions implied in the printed directions can be overridden by a practitioner's administration directions and personal preference, unless a standardized scoring process is available and used.

The inquiry process is an administration activity that is most dependent upon the practitioner's clinical expertise. Using a one-on-one administration format, the practitioner has the option of (a) following a subject's response with an inquiry which clarifies the meaning of the response, (b) seeking reasons why the subject feels a particular way, or (c) tracking feelings or perceptions to deeper levels and causes. The option to collect more information is not possible with group and self-administration formats unless the practitioner pursues selected items with individual subjects after the test's completion. At that point, the context in which the response was given and the spontaneity of the perception are usually obscured with other thoughts and experiences. The need to review or clarify a response later may also cue the subject to become cautious and protective about additional self-disclosure.

Practitioners often find the inquiry process necessary and useful for responses that are unusual, ambiguous, or diagnostically sensitive. An out-of-context or unusual response may indicate fragmented thought processing, thought blocking, loss of attention, perseveration, or overt defensiveness. The practitioner's query, "I'm not sure what you mean, tell me some more" usually elicits both content and process information which helps to analyze and evaluate these many hypotheses. For ambiguous responses, questions prompting additional information often generate explanations from subjects which facilitate accurate interpretation and conclusions. Finally, when subjects make self-referenced responses or those with exaggerated emotional content, inquiries into these diagnostically sensitive issues are important. "Tell me how it is that you feel that way—how come?" is an effective query which can uncover the underlying causes of those feelings and contents as well as their pervasiveness and roles in the structure of the personality.

Sometimes subjects respond hesitantly to certain sentence stems; this can indicate cognitive or emotional blocking or loss of attention. If no response is given after a sufficient amount of time, the practitioner might restate the stem and follow with encouragement like, "Just say whatever comes to your mind." Or, the practitioner might return at the end of the test to an item that appeared difficult for the subject to discuss the feelings that that item's content seemed to elicit. Blocking on stems that have some similarity of content may be particularly helpful to identify subjects' underlying fears and conflicts which seem to need defense systems for control.

To summarize, inquiry strategies generally are not part of the formal administration procedures developed by sentence completion test authors; rather, they are clinical procedures many practitioners use to maximize the data and diagnostic interpretations obtained from these techniques. Ultimately, the inquiry process will depend on (a) whether the analysis and evaluation process follows a standardized or unstandardized administration and scoring process, (b) whether the test administration follows a group or individual format, and (c) whether a particular theoretical orientation guides or dictates the analysis.

Interpretation

The process of interpreting sentence completion tests is influenced initially by their use in either research or psychodiagnostic assessment. As a technique to research attitudes of a selected population, the interpretation process may focus on specific perceptions, expressed in the test responses, without concern for their underlying causes or their implications for future behavior. In a clinical setting, however, interpretation might involve the use of specific personality theories which guide analyses into important personality dynamics. This is possible given the generally accepted classification of sentence completion tests as projective or semiprojective tools. Regardless, the purpose and the form of a sentence completion test are the characteristics that most govern its interpretation and potential use with a specific theoretical orientation. More pragmatically, however, responses to incomplete sentences are most frequently analyzed by one or a combination of four strategies.

The most common interpretation approach with sentence completion tests involves a review of each item's content to obtain clinical impressions about personality dynamics. This becomes a search for patterns, clues, and thought processes that generate hypotheses consistent with the test author's or practitioner's view of human behavior. Rohde (1957) proposes Murray's need–press theoretical system as the conceptual framework for the analysis of the Sentence Completion Method. To operationalize, a practitioner using Murray's theoretical orientation might interpret children or adolescents' sentence responses as representing their general dynamic functioning and their specific inner states, personality traits, need systems, and environmental presses. Those who focus on these intrapersonal conditions, which the clinical impression approach provides, find little need for criterion-based scoring systems. In fact, these systems are thought to reduce sentence completion data to sterile interpersonal comparisons of responses which are analyzed in broad content categories.

The second interpretation strategy is to cluster sentence items with similar contents, thereby focusing on the specific perceptions of those content areas. This is a modification of the item-by-item analysis used in the clinical impressions approach; however, this approach assumes that the preselected, clustered items have enough commonality in content and structure that similar psychological information should be elicited. The clusters might be theoretically based or reflections of a practitioner or researcher's particular interests. For example, Forer (1950) designed a checksheet for the Forer Structured Sentence Completion Test to help organize responses into seven major content areas which reveal specific attitudes and motivations. The added structure inherent in this approach often leads to a more "surface" or conscious analysis of personality attitudes and behaviors in the predetermined areas. Thus, interpretations seem to be more easily supported by behavioral observations and other testing data. This clearly contrasts the clinical impressions approach which analyzes each item for the semiconscious and unconscious interplay of all possible personality dynamics.

The Rotter Incomplete Sentence Blank (ISB; Rotter & Rafferty, 1950) includes an interpretation strategy that represents the third approach to evaluating sentence responses, a simple rating approach. For the ISB, a child's response to each sentence stem is rated according to the degree of apparent conflict. The severity of conflict ratings range from negative to neutral to positive. A weighted score is assigned to each response, and their summation provides an overall adjustment score, which improves the understanding of personality and personality dynamics (Rotter & Willerman, 1947). These rating scores could also be used to create standardized local norms such that individuals could be compared with criterion groups and for possible differential diagnosis. While the rating approach, in general, has insufficient research support to justify individual diagnosis, it is commonly used to screen for psychopathology. Again, the practitioner's theoretical orientation is important. The practitioner may choose, for example, to screen the sentence responses for conflict, negativism, or thought distortion, and then to carefully examine each item's content for theoretically consistent indications of positive or maladaptive personality dynamics.

The most structured of the four general interpretation approaches involves formal and/or standardized scoring systems which compare responses to item criteria. One example of this approach matches sentence responses to predetermined anchor points along a continuum, resulting in specific numerical scores. An example of a structured scoring system using item criteria is provided later in this chapter with an in-depth analysis of the development and application of a sentence completion test for children.

In summary, responses to sentence completion stems are analyzed and interpreted using one or a combination of four systems:

1. The interpretation of each item of a test resulting in clinical impressions of the psychodynamics of personality,
2. The interpretation of items which are clustered into predetermined content areas resulting in focused perceptions of attitudes and needs,
3. The rating of each item or group of items according to a simple scale, usually negative to positive, and
4. The comparison of items or clusters of items to establish criteria based on the similarities of response contents.

These four approaches provide different degrees of interpretation, structure and guidance. For example, the clinical impression approach focuses more on unconscious and theoretical processes, while the rating and scoring approaches focus more on identifying response deviation from a population or local sample mean. All four interpretation approaches provide information according to the content and structure of the sentence stems, and some practitioners use a combination of these approaches to ensure comprehensive interpretation.

Moving from Concepts to Practice

A working understanding of the elements (i.e., purpose, form, administration, and interpretation) of sentence completion techniques is most effectively obtained by tracking the development of one specific test from its theoretical bases to its clinic applications. Below, the sentence completion techniques previously discussed will be reviewed briefly, and then the HSCT will be used to demonstrate this theory to application process. In addition, the enhancement of the interpretation element will be explored through criteria-based scoring strategies and efforts to establish interscorer reliability and criterion-related validity.

The Rotter Incomplete Sentence Blanks (RISB)

The RISB (Rotter & Rafferty, 1950) was designed primarily as a screening device. A 40-item test available in three forms, the RISB is scored quantitatively, and it provides an overall adjustment index score which can be evaluated against published norms. As discussed in the manual, the RISB can be used as a more clinical tool, since the diagnostic information obtained can structure subsequent interviews and possibly help in the development of specific treatment strategies. When utilized in these more qualitative ways the RISB's scoring and interpretation, as Rotter and Rafferty note, become more dependent on practitioners' experience and theoretical orientations.

The Rohde Sentence Completion Method (RSCM)

This sentence completion method (Rohde, 1957) uses Murray's (1938) conceptual scheme of needs and presses to assess specific personality dynamics. By evaluating how subjects organize their response material, Rohde generates diagnostic and personality-related hypotheses that are based primarily on individuals' psychological motivations. Operationally, the RSCM assesses these individual personality dynamics by interpreting sentence completion responses at three separate levels: (a) at the overt content level, which reveals attitudes and values that structure one's inner or private world; (b) at the latent content level, which infers particular underlying personality dynamics; and (c) at the global level where aspects of the entire protocol, including the actual structure and grammatical format of the responses, may indicate organic mental dysfunctions or, for example, schizophrenia. Rohde does not provide formal scoring criteria in the RSCM manual, but does give myriad examples and case presentations applying Murray's conceptual scheme to personality interpretation.

The Sacks Sentence Completion Test (SSCT)

Sacks and Levy (1950) present a more structured sentence completion test that organizes its sentence stems to evaluate specific subject attitudes. The SSCT uses four sentence stems to assess each of 15 separate attitudes (e.g., toward mother, friends, fears, future goals). Responses to each attitude's four sentence stems are grouped and, using a nonobjective scoring system, individually rated on 3-point scale designed to determine the degree of disturbance present. This allows the identification of specific areas of disturbance as well as an overview of interrelationships among the various attitudes.

The Forer Structured Sentence Completion Test

This sentence completion test (Forer, 1950) consists of 100 highly structured sentence stems and is available for both male and female subjects. As a "structured" test, the Forer "forces" individuals to respond to material in seven major areas (e.g., affective level, aggressive tendencies). While there is no formal scoring system, the authors suggest that this form and administration format assists the systematic interpretation of the protocol and the development of interventions which address individuals' specific personality and social–emotional issues and conflicts.

The Miale–Holsopple Sentence Completion Test (M-HSCT)

This sentence completion test (Holsopple & Miale, 1954) is global and unstructured, attempting to elicit information that is less well defended. The M-HSCT is completed without a time limit, because the authors feel that unconscious defense mechanisms may be more active in time-limited situations. This tends to contaminate subjects' responses and to decrease the potential utility of the diagnostic data. Holsopple and Miale do not provide any formal scoring information for the M-HSCT, suggesting instead a more global and qualitative analysis. Nine types of response phrasing are presented (e.g., passive or active response, amount of verbalization) to assist in this interpretation process. Like the other unstructured sentence completion tests above, the interpretation of the M-HSCT is highly dependent on the skill and experience of the practitioner. According to the authors, however, this technique may facilitate a more predictive means of inferring personality dynamics than those sentence completion tests that use more objective analyses. This statement, nonetheless, has not been supported in the literature.

The Hart Sentence Completion Test for Children (HSCT)

The HSCT was developed for two reasons. The first was to develop a test specifically for children rather than modifying an existing test designed for adults. This would allow the test's form and interpretation to be generated from and be consistent with child development principles instead of general personality theory and adult psychopathology. The need for such a test was heightened by the passage of Public Law 94-142 (Education of All Handicapped Children's Act) in 1975 which mandated the psychoeducational support of all behaviorally disordered children. Schools and other educational and psychological service centers were therefore in need of an effective social–emotional screening instrument which (*a*) had predictive value and (*b*) would suggest appropriate educational and psychological intervention strategies.

The second reason for developing the HSCT was that other child-oriented sentence completion tests had poorly developed scoring systems or no standardized scoring systems at all and little documentation of any reliability and validity data. The HSCT was developed to begin to meet these important test construction and psychometric needs and qualities.

A Pragmatic Theory for Assessing Children's Emotional Adjustment

Based on extensive experience in child assessment, the HSCT is theoretically founded on four dimensions of the world of children which are considered important to their social and emotional adjustment. The four dimensions include children's (*a*) family environments, (*b*) social environments, (*c*) school environments, and (*d*) intrapersonal or internal conditions. Children's behavior is most easily understood by examining their perceptions of each of the three environmental dimensions and their personal interactions with each of these environments. The fourth dimension, children's self-perceptions, is most easily assessed by examining children's need orientations and their self-evaluations. Assessments that shed light on these four dimensions provide practitioners with important information which can be analyzed and used to develop useful educational and therapeutic interventions. Briefly, these analyses of individual children can:

1. Identify distorted, conflicting, and out-of-context thought processes,
2. Identify inaccurate, inhibiting, overgeneralized, and defensive perceptions,
3. Identify self-defeating and maladaptive behaviors,
4. Identify causal links between environmental presses, perceptions, and behaviors, and
5. Identify ego strengths, positive self-perceptions, and adaptive behavior.

Planning the HSCT Test Construction Activities from the Assessment Objectives

The objectives guiding the development of the HSCT significantly directed its test construction and research activities. The first task was to develop and organize sentence stems according to the four dimensions of children's lives hypothesized to have educational and clinical relevance. The forms of the sentence stems were designed to elicit children's perceptions of family, peers, school, and self, as well as their perceptions of their interactions with family, peers, and school. Since children often struggle with ambiguous test directions and item stimuli, the stems were moderately structured. In addition, the first-person reference was used frequently to uncover information about conscious and semiconscious thought processes, rather than material deeply repressed in children's psyches. For example, the stem "I don't like people who . . . " was used to direct children's thinking toward social contexts that call for responses for which they must consciously be aware.

The second development task was to determine effective ways to interpret the HSCT sentence responses. Subjective analysis of the sentence stems by practitioners, based on their clinical experience and the theoretical orientations, would require no scoring system. Yet, one of the primary objectives for the HSCT was to have scores that could be used for different criterion groups. Thus, a system for quantifying children's responses to the sentence stems assessing the four life dimensions was developed. A scale-rating system that provided a "gestalt" summary of children's perceptions of each life dimension received the first attention. Second, an item-by-item comparison of the responses, with predetermined scoring criteria, was completed. With either of these two scoring strategies, the responses were quantified, thereby allowing comparisons between different criterion groups when needed by the practitioner.

Determining the administration procedures was the next task. To allow for maximum flexibility, easily understood instructions were included at the top of the test so it could be self-administered or practitioner directed. Because the test, theoretically, was to collect perceptions available to children's conscious thought, no speed conditions were included in the instructions. Psychodynamics below the level of consciousness could still be explored, however, by sensitizing practitioners to content and behavioral cues leading to children's unconscious thought and emotional processes. Those cues could then be investigated through in-depth inquiry procedures.

Determining the HSCT's psychometric properties was the fourth task. First, interscorer reliabilities for the HSCT were determined. Once these were at appropriate levels, the development of criterion-related validity proceeded. Since criterion keying is the easiest way to demonstrate validity, the ability of the two scoring systems to discriminate between different criterion groups with preestablished conditions and characteristics was tested. The target criterion groups, consistent with the reasons for developing the HSCT, were school-age children with various known handicapping conditions and school-age children judged to be free from significant personal adjustment problems.

Operationalizing the HSCT

Items

A pool of 200 sentence stems was generated to be the resource base for the HSCT. This pool was eventually reduced to 40 stems which comprise the HSCT. Some stems were created to fit specific content areas and others were taken from existing sentence completion tests. All of the stems were eventually organized by their content into four groups designed to elicit perceptions about the four dominant life dimensions. Face and content validity were the sole criteria used by a clinical psychologist and two school psychologists to place the stems into the four categories.

For the three dimensions representing the external environment, 24 sentence stems were selected, 8 for each dimension. Half of the items (four) for each dimension focused on children's perceptions of that particular environment, while the other four items assessed their self-perceived interactions with that environment.

The fourth dimension assessing children's "selves" does not elicit perceptions about the external environment. The 12 final items like "The best thing about me . . . ," and "I can't . . . " are internally directed even though their origins may be in environmental settings. To obtain a broad perspective of this dimension, sentence stems to elicit responses about children's needs orientations and self-concepts were included. Four relatively unstructured items related to children's needs, and, therefore, their dominant presses (or motivating forces) were written to sample reactions to achievement, security, aggression, materialism, affiliation, and isolation. Eight personal evaluation or self-concept items were written to elicit perceptions of physical abilities, physical attributes, personal adequacies, and general self-worth.

Scales

The conceptual scheme of the HSCT is presented in Table 8-1. Identified in the table are eight scales or groupings of items that reflect the four theoretical dimensions, and two additional scales that were added during the pretesting process. During the HSCT's planning, it was thought that assessments of the four life dimensions would provide a comprehensive understanding of all children. During the pretesting process, however, a number of child psychologists suggested a ninth scale to assess the future orientations and psychosexual awarenesses of latency-aged children and adolescents. Thus, four items were added to the test to assess these areas, even though the conceptual model was somewhat sidestepped and the length and complexity of the test was increased. The four items

Table 8-1
Conceptual Scheme of the Hart Sentence Completion Test[a]

Four dimensions of a child's world	Areas of assessment	Scales	Number of items
Family	External environment	1. Perception of family	4
		2. Interaction with family	4
Social		3. Perception of peers	4
		4. Interaction with peers	4
School		5. Perception of school	4
		6. Interaction with school	4
Self	Self-perception	7. Need orientation	4
		8. Personal evaluation	8
	Intrapersonal functioning	9. Psychosexual awareness and future orientation	4
		10. General mental health	A gestalt analysis of all 40 items

[a]Adapted from Hart, Kehle, and Davies (1983).

are not included in the scoring system, but they do provide qualitative information which can be pursued if needed or desired through in-depth interviewing or additional testing.

A tenth scale was added to synthesize the information obtained from all 40 HSCT items. It has no specific sentence stems and, therefore, allows the mental health practitioner to be sensitive to clinical symptoms like confused thought patterns, negativism, perseveration, and poor reality testing without being encumbered by a forced scale analysis. When all 40 items are analyzed without categorical separation, it is subjectively believed that the total score and summary conclusions represent the best statements about the general mental health of children.

Administration Instructions

Since the HSCT was designed for use with children ages 6–18, the administration directions were kept simple and are aided by an example. The words in the parentheses below are for use with children under the age of 8: "I'm going to say part of a sentence (some words) and I want you to finish it (them) with the first things you think of. If I say the words, "I like . . . ," you should finish the sentence (words) in any way you want by saying "[Put example in here]." . . . Good. Now here are some more."

The instructions are printed on the top of the sentence completion form so that the practitioner can read them to the child as a model for the 40 items to come. With the instructions printed on the form, there is little cause for misunderstanding or for differences in test administration procedures when the test is administered in a group setting.

Scoring

A scale rating system and an item-by-item rating system comprise the HSCT's two scoring approaches which provide quantitative scores for each content area. In the former, the practitioner reads the responses to all of the items within a specific scale and then makes a single gestalt summary rating along a 5-point negative-to-positive continuum (1 equals negative, 3 equals neutral, and 5 equals positive). No guidelines or criteria are provided, thus each scale's rating reflects the practitioner's subjective judgment, averaging the responses to the four individual items. The scale rating approach quickly focuses the practitioner's attention to a cluster of items representing a specific life dimension. The rating summarizing the scale can be used for intratest, cross-scale comparisons or for intertest comparisons with the scores of other children. In short, the scale rating scoring process attempts to quantify subjective judgments about sentence responses without the use of reference criteria.

The item-by-item rating system, developed by Swanson (1975) and modified by Hart (1980), provides judgment criteria for each sentence stem. For each item, 250 responses were reviewed by five school psychologists and rated as negative, neutral, or positive. From those responses placed in each rating category, four to six responses were identified as most representative and were selected to become criteria for that category. A scoring template identifies each scale's items and provides the practitioner with negative, neutral, and positive scoring criteria. A composite rating score for each scale is determined by combining the individual item ratings. Finally, the composite ratings from all of the scales can be profiled for interscale comparisons.

One strength of the item-by-item scoring system is its ability to reduce practitioners' subjective and variable ratings through the criterion-referenced analysis of each scale's sentence stems. Practitioners who employ "gut feeling" analyses of the sentence stems based on quick rundowns of each scale's responses will find the time and effort of item scoring excessive unless they require the precision necessary to compare children's scale profiles to the standard referent or norm groups. Naturally, the practitioner's diagnostic needs and purposes will dictate the analysis process. The availability of criteria-based intraperson comparisons also increases the potential of the item scoring process to pinpoint individual differences needing specific remedial intervention. Finally, the criteria-based scores permit the assessment of the HSCT's reliability and validity and the derivation of comparative norms to assist in psychodiagnostic classification.

Reliability and Validity

Ulman (1972) completed the first reliability study with the HSCT's scale rating system by examining the interscorer reliabilities of three school psychologists' scoring judgments. Each psychologist independently scored 60 HSCT protocols completed by 30 children diagnosed as mild to moderately emotionally handicapped and 30 children who were from the general school population. Ulman found that the average reliabilities on the eight family, social, school, and self-perception scales ranged from a low of .50 to a high of .86, with each being statistically significant at the .01 level. The scales with the highest interrater reliabilities were interaction with peers (.86), personal evaluation (.78), interaction with school (.74), and interaction with family (.72). The judges differed most on evaluating the responses to the perception of school scale (.50). When age (7–14) and sex of the child were considered, no statistical differences were found among the average interscorer reliabilities across the eight scales.

In a departure from the original eight scales, Ulman also redistributed the HSCT items to reflect specific needs and clinical symptoms or syndromes. He found, however, that the interrater reliabilities for these new scales only ranged from .02 to .56. He concluded that the items in the eight major HSCT scales elicit responses which can be scored consistently, and that reorganization of items into scales designed to reflect children's needs and symptom patterns was not successful. This might have occurred because (a) the new constructs were not valid for children or (b) the items in the new scales were not sufficiently homogeneous in content to elicit consistent responses and, therefore, scorings.

Given Ulman's (1972) demonstration of the HSCT's scoring reliability, Robyak (1975) tested its psychometric validity. Using a sample similar to Ulman's and reaffirming the HSCT's interrater reliability, Robyak demonstrated that five of eight HSCT scales could distinguish between emotionally handicapped school children and typical school children regardless of their ages or sex. Further, the scales were discrete, and there were no significant interaction effects. Robyak's emotionally disturbed school children sample revealed more negative perceptions of their family, school, and social world as well as more negative interactions within their school and social worlds than the typical children. The two self-perception scales and the scale measuring interaction with family did not distinguish between the emotionally disturbed and typical students. Thus, the HSCT and its scale rating scoring system *was* sufficiently sensitive to elicit and discriminate, respectively, responses from significantly different groups of children attending the same public schools. Parenthetically, while the children's emotional handicaps were not severe, they were still detected by the HSCT scoring system.

An evaluation of the alternative item-by-item scoring system, based on the specific scoring criteria, was completed by Swanson (1975). Her primary research purpose was to examine the HSCT's utility as a screening instrument for children with emotional problems.

Swanson first determined if the HSCT item-by-item scoring system produced reliable results using a random sample of 32 students selected from a pool of 247 school children (89 with mild to moderate emotional problems, 72 with learning disabilities, and 96 judged to be free from emotional or learning difficulties). The HSCT protocols of these students were scored by two regular classroom teachers and one school psychologist. The scoring criteria for the scales measuring family, social, school, and self-perception were carefully followed, and the resulting interscorer reliabilities ranged from .90 to .99. Clearly, the scoring structure provided the scorers with a reference base that produced consistent and replicable scoring results. With this kind of scoring consistency, the development of norms for different populations becomes defensible and quite feasible.

Swanson then investigated the HSCT's power to discriminate among the 247 emotionally disturbed, learning disabled, and normal subjects categorized by age and handicapping condition. Collapsing the eight scales into the four HSCT dimensions using the item-by-item scoring system, Swanson computed scores for each dimension as well as a total score across all four dimensions. The results indicated that the HSCT data significantly differed among the emotionally handicapped, learning disabled, and nonhandicapped students for all scales. Not only did the scores differ across categories, but a review of profiled scores revealed pattern differences among the three groups. A final result indicated that negative responses increased with age across all groups, particularly on the family and school scales.

To summarize, Hart, Kehle, and Davies (1983), in their review of the effectiveness of sentence completion techniques, stated:

> . . . research on the HSCT reveals that the two scoring systems are effective. The scale rating scoring system had moderate interscorer reliability on the eight major HSCT scales. And, the item-by-item rating scoring system had very high interscorer reliability on all HSCT scales. Both scoring systems effectively distinguished among various school-age populations including emotionally disturbed, learning disabled, and non-handicapped or typical children. However, no effective scoring system quantitatively identified students' need states or the existence of clinical symptoms such as confused thought or perseveration. (p. 433)

Decisions for Use

There are other considerations for selecting a particular test besides its ease in administration, its scoring options, and its reliability and validity. The amount of time required to give a particular test, for example, is critical. It takes between 15 and 30 minutes to administer the HSCT, depending on the age of the child and the interest of the practitioner in pursuing and follow-up on responses. At an extreme, practitioners have used the test to structure hour-long clinical interviews. The median time, however, is estimated to be 20 minutes. Thus, practitioners must decide which diagnostic tools are processes provide the most useful data for the kind of analyses desired.

Work with the HSCT indicates that responses provided by children ages 6 and 7 are often impoverished and repetitive. Thus, a child's comfort with verbal expression is also a variable to be considered when choosing a test. For example, native American high school students appear much more at ease with the Performance Scale of the Wechsler Intelligence Scale for Children-Revised (WISC-R) than with the verbal subtests of that scale or with the HSCT.

Finally, the presence of norm groups to compare response patterns across different ages and clinical/educational populations is also an important consideration when choosing particular tests. The HSCT's normative data are presently being compiled and are not yet available for various classification groups beyond those cited in the reliability and validity studies above. Depending on their assessment goals, practitioners may choose not to use this test due to this specific limitation. In fact, if a practitioner desires more referents for comparisons of particular population subgroups, then it would be unwise to use the sentence completion technique in its present state of development.

Case Studies Using the HSCT

Below, examples of the HSCT illustrate its possible uses in research, school, and clinical settings. The flexibility provided by the HSCT's quantitative scoring systems is highlighted, but the qualitative clinical analysis typically used with most sentence completion tests is also recognized.

Research Uses

Those who are engaged in research need to select measures of dependent variables which provide numerical data for statistical analysis and which also are reliable and valid. The following research questions illustrate possible uses of the HSCT and its criteria-based scoring system.

1. What are the pre–post treatment differences in delinquent adolescents' perceptions about family, society, and self?
2. What is the relationship between behavior as recorded on a behavioral rating scale and perceptions of self and peers as determined by the HSCT for latency-aged children? Are there sex differences?
3. What diagnostically relevant differences are there among learning disabled and nonhandicapped school-age children's perceptions of school, family, peers, and self? What are these differences' implications with respect to curriculum planning?
4. What cutoff score on a sentence completion test has a high probability (85%) of predicting emotional disturbance before additional psychological testing is conducted?
5. Do children of abusive parents change their perceptions of family and self due to their parents' participation in group psychotherapy?

In these examples, the researcher would not be interested in making subjective appraisals of the personality dynamics of the subjects. Rather, quantitative data that summarize subjects' perceptions and allow for accurate comparisons are needed and emphasized. This need, along with appropriate item content, administration and scoring ease, and sound psychometric properties make sentence completion tests viable and important tools for research purposes.

Educational Uses

School practitioners frequently use the sentence completion technique when an individual assessment of a child's emotional or social adjustment is needed. Often, this assessment requires tests that are useful in determining handicapping

classifications for placement or providing intervention directions for school programming. Sentence completion responses can be organized into logical content
groupings, and they can be scored and compared with normative data, thereby
greatly enhancing the classification process. Or, sentence completion responses
can be reviewed by school practitioners, given their theoretical perspectives and
clinical experiences, in order to gain insight into children's psychological functioning. This also has important classification implications.

From a programming perspective, school practitioners can use sentence completion tests to identify individual variables and characteristics which are critical
to the development of appropriate educational programs for special needs or
handicapped students. While a sentence completion test is helpful in making intraindividual comparisons of clusters of content-related items, many school practitioners find the qualitative analysis of responses to be most useful for programming. Looking for indications of children's values, fears, social perceptions, and
self-appraisals (as well as the psychological dynamics these conditions imply),
practitioners can integrate sentence completion and other test results into sensitive and comprehensive pictures of these children's social–emotional and intervention or programming needs.

To illustrate the utility of the HSCT and its quantitative scoring system, a
sample of sentence stems from a 12-year-old boy's test protocol appears in Table
8-2. A qualitative analysis of the same sentence stems is also presented to demonstrate the value of using these two analysis procedures together. Brent was referred for a psychoeducational evaluation by his seventh-grade teacher because
of his poor social skills and withdrawn behavior. The HSCT was administered verbally by a school psychologist who recorded his responses verbatim. The psychologist pursued unclear, contradictory, atypical, and out-of-content responses during the test administration.

Table 8-2 contains four items from the HSCT that illustrate the sentence
stems, the scales from which they came, Brent's responses, examples of the scoring
criteria, and the response ratings given by the school psychologist. The criteria-
based ratings for the four items show Brent's negative perceptions of his family
and his interactions with peers. His personal evaluation is also negative. His
perception of school, however, is neutral. While his responses to the other HSCT
items are not reported here, the complete profile showing the results of the item-
by-item scoring is reproduced in Figure 8-1.

A quick review of this profile shows Brent's very negative perceptions of
his social world (Scales 3 and 4) and his other negative perceptions about his family
environment (Scales 1 and 2) and himself (Scales 7 and 8). Additional information will help in understanding Brent's item rating process. Brent's score on Scale
1, Perception of Family, produced a total rating score of 1 based on his negative
responses to the four sentence stems in that scale. This is consistent with the
HSCT's guidelines which call for a scale score of 1 when there are three or four
negative responses out of the four sentence stems in that scale. In Scale 2, the one
neutral, one positive, and two negative responses about relationships in the family
resulted in a score of 2. Brent scored in the typical range only on the school scales.
His total adjustment score of 15 is average for the emotionally handicapped
students who participated in two separate research projects described above.

If a qualitative or clinical analysis is to accompany a criteria-based scoring
system, then an effective written record of the test responses and administration
is very important. A review of the first response to Item 3 in Table 8-2 will il-

Table 8-2
Illustrations of Four Sentence Stems, the Responses of a 12-Year-Old Boy,
Brent, Examples of the Scoring Criteria for the Stems, and the
Rating Applied to the Responses[a]

Scale 1: Perception of family

Item 15   Sentence stem: *When mother and dad are together, they* . . . .
          Response of Brent: . . . *fight—he doesn't come home very much.*
          Scoring criteria: Positive—go out; have fun; kiss.
                              Neutral—talk; sleep; don't fight.
                              Negative—talk about how bad I am; fight; cuss my brother out.
          Rating: Negative (Perception of family)

Scale 4: Interaction with peers

Item 22   Sentence stem: *To the other kids, I* . . . .
          Response of Brent: . . . *am alone* (Q) *They leave me alone—I don't care.*
          Scoring criteria: Positive—I am nice; am fun to be around; am a good friend; like
                              to play.
                              Neutral—talk a lot; am shy sometimes; am another person.
                              Negative—am stupid; fool around too much; look ugly.
          Rating: Negative (Interaction with peers)

Scale 5: Perception of school

Item 3   Sentence stem: *The best thing about school* . . . .
          Response of Brent: . . . *getting out* (Q) *I can do school okay, but I don't like it* (Q) *I*
                              hate the kids.
          Scoring criteria: Positive—any school subject including gym; school-sponsored
                              activities.
                              Neutral—recess; lunch; friends.
                              Negative—nothing; when it's over; summer vacation.
          Rating: Neutral (Perception of school)
                        Negative (Interaction with peers)

Scale 8: Personal evaluation

Item 24   Sentence stem: *I am the* . . . .
          Response of Brent: . . . *one who is too fat.*
          Scoring criteria: Positive—greatest; person people tell their problems to; a good
                              runner.
                              Neutral—youngest; smallest guy; one who takes care of the yard.
                              Negative—worst reader; dumbest in my class; one who gets
                              forgotten.
          Rating: Negative (Personal evaluation)

[a]This table was originally published in Hart, D. H., Kehle, T. J., & Davies, M. V. (1983). Effectiveness of sentence completion techniques: A review of the Hart Sentence Completion Test for Children. *School Psychology Review, 12,* 432.

lustrate this point. The response, "getting out," called for two follow-up questions (Q) by the school psychologist to clarify Brent's perception of school. Brent's additional responses, drawn out by the follow-up requests "Tell me some more," and "Can you tell me what you mean?" indicate that he feels all right about schoolwork, but dislikes his school peers. Had the test been self-administered or administered without these clarifying questions, interpretation would likely have been difficult, inadequate, or incorrect.

A qualitative analysis of Brent's responses to the three other stems in Table 8-2 provides additional clinical data. Along with Brent's social difficulties, the analysis suggests two additional stresses, (*a*) a negative body image which could be causing his social withdrawal and peer rejection, and (*b*) a family support system that is in conflict and possibly disruptive.

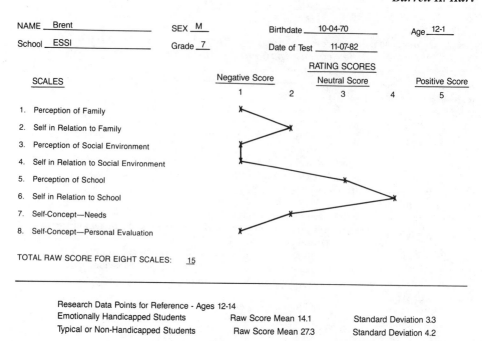

NAME __Brent__   SEX _M_   Birthdate __10-04-70__   Age _12-1_

School __ESSI__   Grade _7_   Date of Test __11-07-82__

Figure 8-1. Item Rating Profile of the Hart Sentence Completion Test.

An integration of Brent's quantitative HSCT score profile and the qualitative analysis of his HSCT responses seems to provide the most useful diagnostic data for both classification and the understanding of his particular personality dynamics. Certainly, other evaluation tools and procedures are essential to expand and validate sentence completion hypotheses before classification and intervention. Yet, the knowledgeable use of a good sentence completion test may provide a screening that identifies the need for additional psychodiagnostic assessment and a framework for further clinical evaluation.

Agency Uses

Mental health agencies also use the sentence completion method to assist with evaluation, treatment, and research programs. Each clinic, juvenile court, hospital, or mental health center utilizes the test for its own purposes; screening for possible psychopathology, developing treatment strategies, assessing the effects of therapy, predicting responsiveness to treatment, and developing diagnostic profiles are just some of the possible clinical applications. Whatever the purpose, the administration process is the same as in educational settings, although the analysis strategies may differ. This may be due, in part, to the severity of cases often referred to community or private mental health agencies and the corresponding degree of pathology evidenced in sentence completion responses. Given these more serious (when compared to those typically referred to school practitioners) cases, agency practitioners have reported that the HSCT's scoring system is mechanical and somewhat superficial for an adequate understanding of the child.

Two brief qualitative evaluations of the HSCT responses made by an 8-year-old male clinic patient are presented to illustrate different interpretative approaches that agency practitioners might take during a sentence completion test analysis. The first involves a systematic content and process analysis where insight is sought concerning the dominant themes, needs, behaviors, and response styles (process) that characterize the child. This is somewhat similar to the qualitative analysis made by school practitioners in conjunction with the criteria-based scoring analysis. The second clinical approach relies heavily on understanding the psychodynamics of the child within the context of personality development theory. Background information obtained about the boy is useful in both analysis processes, but imperative for the latter.

Scott was taken from his natural mother at birth and lived with foster parents until he was legally adopted at 15 months. He was brought to a child psychologist when he was 8 years old with symptoms of alternating withdrawal and aggression toward his mother, narcissistic ideation, and social ineptness. The HSCT was administered to Scott as part of an evaluation battery. The four sentence stems referenced earlier plus two additional ones are reproduced in Table 8-3 along with Scott's responses and their criteria-based ratings.

The content and process approach analyzing Scott's six responses looks for patterns, inconsistencies, and repeated themes. While there are no obvious common themes in the content of these six items, it is notable that Scott was hesitant to respond to half of these items. Two of Scott's responses conflict with background information. On Scale 1, Item 15, Scott indicated that his parents "aren't together," yet the marriage is intact with both parents involved in his care. On

Table 8-3
Illustrations of Six Sentence Stems, the Responses of an 8-Year-Old Boy, Scott, and the Rating Applied to Each Response from the Item Rating Scoring Criteria

Scale 5: Perception of school

Item 3　Sentence stem:　*The best thing about school . . . .*

　　　Response of Scott:　. . . (no response) (Q) *When is this test going to be over?* (Q) (no response)

　　　Rating:　Negative

Scale 7: Need orientation

Item 6　Sentence stem:　*I wish . . . .*

　　　Response of Scott:　. . . *for all the gold in the world.*

　　　Rating:　Neutral

Scale 1: Perception of family

Item 15　Sentence stem:　*When mother and dad are together, they . . . .*

　　　Response of Scott:　. . . (pause) . . . *They aren't together.*

　　　Rating:　Neutral

Scale 4: Interaction with peers

Item 22　Sentence stem:　*To the other kids, I . . . .*

　　　Response of Scott:　. . . *I'm really bitchen* (Q) *Oh, they think I'm real cool.*

　　　Rating:　Positive

Scale 8: Personal Evaluation

Item 24　Sentence stem:　*I am the . . . .*

　　　Response of Scott:　. . . (pause) . . . *one . . . I don't know.* (Q) (silence).

　　　Rating:　Neutral

Scale 2: Interaction with family

Item 30　Sentence stem:　*My mother thinks I . . . .*

　　　Response of Scott:　. . . *I'm really bad* (Q) *'Cause she's always yelling at me.*

　　　Rating:　Negative

Scale 4, Item 22, Scott implied that he is positively perceived by his peers, but the initial parent interview suggested that he has difficulty getting along with his friends. No other clues seem to be available from the content and process analysis of the six items; the criteria-based ratings provide no additional help. With one positive, three neutral, and two negative responses, no red flags are raised that Scott's responses are significantly atypical from those of most 8-year-old boys.

Obviously, the responses to the other 34 items of the HSCT would validate the usefulness of the six items above and present a more comprehensive picture of Scott. A review of the 40 responses organized into the 10 scales would also probably reveal dominant content themes about Scott's perception of his environment and personal adjustment. Finally, the scoring system could provide references for inter- and intraindividual comparisons.

The second interpretation strategy used by agency practitioners analyzes item responses (*a*) in the context of other information that has already been collected, and (*b*) according to a theoretical notion about child development that is suggested from that other information. While it is true that some practitioners analyze all information through one theoretical position, others choose from a number of developmental theories, seeking to logically integrate sentence completion test responses and other psychological data into a conceptual whole.

In the case of Scott, the responses might be examined through object-relation development constructs which have their foundation in psychoanalytic theory. The separation/individuation phase of development typically occurs for children between 18 and 36 months, resulting in the psychological birth of the child. During that time, a sense of self as separate from others emerges and allows the development of children's individual identities. Scott's adoption at 15 months pulled him away from foster parents to whom he belonged. His perceived abandonment triggered the early rise of separation anxiety which inhibited a clear passage to individuation. Instead of having the security bond between mother and child which brings safety in reaching out for an identity and sense of self, Scott's anxiety restricted the new relationship through denial, silence, and withdrawal. Further, his sense of abandonment prevented him from forming meaningful relationships as he continued to grow. While he acquired skills to mechanically adjust to his home, neighborhood, and school, his emergence as a legitimate psychological entity did not occur. Scott's emotional responses are often similar to those of a 15-month-old child, and much of his 8-year-old behavior involves compensating for his feelings as he attempts to justify and validate his oneness.

Scott's responses now might be analyzed from a new perspective. His hesitancy to respond to three items is consistent with an angry withdrawal, particularly when he had to think about the family and self issues raised in Items 15 and 24. His refusal to respond to Item 3 reflects a defensiveness toward cooperative relationships. Those kinds of behaviors elicit responses from others that confirm his badness and abandonment. His Item 6 response of wanting "all of the gold in the world" might be interpreted as his desire to make everything good and to restore the sense of oneness experienced with his foster mother, but not yet attained with his adoptive mother. Scott's message on Item 15, that his mother and father are not together, reflects his love–hate conflict with his mother. In denying that she is together with his father, he again demonstrates his longing for oneness without intrusion by his father. In theory, resolution of total acceptance in oneness must precede chosen separateness. For Scott, he has been forced out prematurely. The bravado on Item 22 about his peers perceiving him as "cool" is a defensive longing to be adequate. Scott's hesitancy on Item 24 ("I am the . . . ") gives further support to his withdrawal tendencies when confronted with identity issues. It's as though he might be saying, "If I don't hear or see, then I don't have to know or deal with it." His response, "I am the . . . one . . . I don't know" clearly indicates this identity struggle. Finally, Scott's response to Item 30, which describes his mother perceiving him as bad, is likely the result of (a) his self-perceived excessive anger and demandingness coming from resentment over his abandonment and (b) his self-fulfilling expectations that he has no legitimate individual worth and identity.

A Statement of Caution

It is important to conclude this chapter on the sentence completion method with cautions on two of its major limitations: deficiencies within the tests themselves, and inappropriate use of the tests by practitioners. Insufficient work has been done to bring sentence completion tests to the higher psychometric standards of the testing community. Most applied mental health practitioners use the method for its intuitive value in understanding personality characteristics without concern for reliability and validity. Standardized evaluation procedures and norm-reference groups are not available or are seldom used, and inferences are made about human behavior which depend solely on the subjective impressions and theoretical orientations of the practitioners.

The HSCT was used to illustrate the application of an appropriate test construction methodology because it utilizes technological advances toward better psychometric properties and increased test versatility. The present limitations of the HSCT highlight its upcoming research directions: Subject reliability must be determined and replicated, norms according to age groupings have not yet been established, the scoring system must evolve from raw score comparisons to standard scores and percentiles, profiles for different clinical populations and ages are needed, and other methods for determining criteria-related validity must be followed to support the findings of the criterion keying process. Finally, sufficient research must be completed to show adequate replicability and cross-validation of all of the above efforts.

Most practitioners in clinical practice know the importance of using a number of assessment tools and procedures in their diagnostic assessment work. However, practitioners must take care to practice this knowledge. Information from other projective tests, behavioral observations, clinical interviews, and developmental histories should all be assimilated into a complete picture of a child or adolescent's personality. An interpretation of personality characteristics that leads to a diagnosis or remedial action without multiple sources of collaborative data is unethical.

Two additional cautions should be noted:

1. Atypical responses to sentence stems may reflect atypical developmental levels, inadequate understanding of the testing process, lack of motivation, or poor examiner–examinee rapport. Responses should not be interpreted out of context and viewed as representative of a maladaptive personality condition when, in fact, they are situation-specific and actually developmentally appropriate. Iden-

tifying misleading external and internal responses during the testing process prevents the misinterpretation of the sentence completion responses.

2. The practitioner must constantly guard against the incorrect interpretation of sentence completion responses. Deficiencies in analysis occur most often when practitioners force responses into inflexible theoretical models of personality, or when "the clinician" within the practitioner fails to put responses into the contexts of the individuals' real worlds. It is sometimes forgotten that many useful interpretations of a child's attitudes and feelings are within the child's awareness and do *not* need the practitioner's projective analysis.

Summary

This chapter has highlighted the historical development of the sentence completion method, evaluated the present status of the technology, and reviewed the four major elements of sentence completion tests. The Hart Sentence Completion Test for Children was selected to illustrate the present state of the technology by tracking its theoretical conceptualization, through its stages of development, and on to its clinical use. The following statements summarize the sentence completion method and its application.

1. The sentence completion technique had its origin in the early 1900s with efforts to determine mental abilities through incomplete sentences and the desire to examine the relationship of word associations to personality.

2. With the use of the sentence completion technique in World War II for the evaluation and placement of military personnel, the method gained in popularity, and numerous sentence completion tests were constructed to assess attitudes and personality in diverse clinical settings.

3. Sentence completion techniques were relatively easy to construct and there was no pressure from the professional community to require the rigorous psychometric data typically expected of other psychological and educational tests.

4. The anatomy of a sentence completion test reveals four elements: (*a*) purpose; (*b*) form, which includes its item structure and content; (*c*) administration; and (*d*) interpretation, which includes its psychometric properties and support.

5. Many sentence completion tests do not have a theoretical base that directs the item structure and content; most are without scoring systems that are criterion related.

6. Four dimensions of a child's world—family, school, social, and self— underlie the 40-item HSCT and are hypothesized to be the fundamental data sources for understanding a child's social–emotional development.

7. Two scoring systems, scale rating and criterion-based item-by-item rating, were shown to be sufficiently reliable and valid such that they could correctly discriminate between groups of emotionally handicapped and non-handicapped children.

8. Comparisons between quantitative and qualitative analyses illustrated the HSCT's diagnostic flexibility and interpretative value when the practitioner has access to both evaluation processes.

9. Interpretation of responses to sentence completion stems requires (*a*) an awareness of the psychometric limitations of the test, (*b*) supporting information from other data sources (e.g., other tests, interviews, observations), and (*c*) sensitive mental health practitioners who are aware of extraneous variables unique to the referred individual and the testing setting, and their own theoretical biases that might lead to inappropriate interpretations and intervention recommendations.

References

Anastasi, A. (1976). *Psychological testing* (4th ed.). New York: Macmillan.

Aronoff, J. (1972). *A manual to score safety, love and belongingness, and esteem motives* (Tech. Rep.). Unpublished manuscript.

Binet, A., & Simon, T. (1905). Methodes nouvelles pour le diagnostic du niveau intellectuel des anormaux. *Annee Psychologique, 11*, 191–244.

Campbell, D. T. (1957). A typology of tests, projective and otherwise. *Journal of Consulting Psychology, 21*, 207–210.

Coleman, J. C. (1969). The levels hypothesis: A re-examination and reorientation. *Journal of Projective Techniques and Personality Assessment, 33*, 118–122.

Cromwell, R. L., & Lundy, R. M. (1954). Productivity of clinical hypotheses on a sentence completion test. *Journal of Consulting Psychology, 18*, 421–424.

Ebbinghaus, H. (1897). A new method to examine intellectual abilities and their utilization in school children. *Zeitschrift Psychologia Physiologica Sinnesorga, 13*, 401–459.

Exner, J. E. (1973). The self focus sentence completion: A study of egocentricity. *Journal of Personality Assessment, 37*, 437–455.

Flynn, W. (1974). Oral vs. written administration of the Incomplete Sentences Blank. *Newsletter for Research in Mental Health and the Behavioral Sciences, 16*, 19–20.

Forer, B. R. (1950). A structured sentence completion test. *Journal of Projective Techniques, 14*, 15–30.

Goldberg, P. A. (1965). A review of sentence completion methods in personality assessment. *Journal of Projective Techniques and Personality Assessment, 29*, 12–45.

Harris, D. B., & Tseng, S. C. (1957). Children's attitudes toward peers and parents as revealed by sentence completions. *Child Development, 28*, 201–211.

Hart, D. H. (1972). *The Hart Sentence Completion Test for Children*. Unpublished manuscript, Salt Lake City, UT: Educational Support Systems, Inc.

Hart, D. H. (1980). *A quantitative scoring system for the Hart Sentence Completion Test for Children*. Unpublished manuscript, Salt Lake City, UT: Educational Support Systems, Inc.

Hart, D. H., Kehle, T. J., & Davies, M. V. (1983). Effectiveness of sentence completion techniques: A review of the Hart Sentence Completion Test for Children. *School Psychology Review, 12*, 428–434.

Holsopple, J. Q., & Miale, F. (1954). *Sentence completion*. Springfield, IL: Charles C Thomas.

Holzberg, J., Teicher, A., & Taylor, J. L. (1947). Contributions of clinical psychology to military neuropsychiatry in an Army psychiatric hospital. *Journal of Clinical Psychology, 3*, 84–95.

Jung, C. G. (1904). *Diagnostische assoziationsstudien*. Leipzig: Barth.

Jung, C. G. (1906). Diagnostische assoziationsstudien. *Jahrbuch fur Psychologie and Neurologie, 8*, 25–60.

Jung, C. G. (1907). Diagnostische assoziationsstudien. *Jahrbuch fur Psychologie and Neurologie, 9*, 188–197.

Kelly, T. J. (1917). Individual testing with completion test exercises. *Teacher's College Record, 18*, 371–382.

Kent, G. H., & Rosanoff, A. (1910). A study of association in insanity. *American Journal of Insanity, 67*, 37–96, 317–390.

Lubin, B., Larsen, R. M., & Matarazzo, J. D. (1984). Patterns of psychological test usage in the United States: 1935–1982. *American Psychologist, 39*, 451–453.

MacBrayer, C. T. (1960). Differences in perception of the opposite sex by males and females. *Journal of Social Psychology, 52*, 309–314.

McKinney, F. (1967). The sentence completion blank in assessing student self-actualization. *Personnel and Guidance Journal, 45*, 709–713.

Murray, H. A. (1938). *Explorations in personality; a clinical and experimental study of 50 men of college age, by the workers of the Harvard Psychological Clinic.* Oxford University Press, NY/London.

Murray, H. A., & MacKinnon, D. W. (1946). Assessment of OSS personnel. *Journal of Consulting Psychology, 10*, 76–80.

Murstein, B. I. (Ed.). (1965). *Handbook of projective techniques.* New York: Basic Books.

Piltz, R. J. (1957). Problems in validity for the Copple Sentence Completion Test as a measure of "effective intelligence" with Air Force personnel. *Dissertation Abstracts International, 17*, 1914–1915.

Robyak, S. L. (1975). *A validation study of the Hart Sentence Completion Test.* Unpublished master's thesis, University of Utah, Salt Lake City.

Rohde, A. R. (1946). Explorations in personality by the sentence completion method. *Journal of Applied Psychology, 30*, 169–181.

Rohde, A. R. (1947). *Sentence completions test manual.* Beverly Hills, CA: Western Psychological Services.

Rohde, A. R. (1957). *The sentence completion method: Its diagnostic and clinical application to mental disorders.* New York: Ronald Press.

Rotter, J. B., & Rafferty, J. E. (1950). *Manual: The Rotter Incomplete Sentences Blank.* New York: Psychological Corporation.

Rotter, J. B., Rafferty, J. E., & Schachtitz, E. (1949). Validation of the Rotter Incomplete Sentences Blank for college screening. *Journal of Consulting Psychology, 13*, 348–366.

Rotter, J. B., & Willerman, B. (1947). The incomplete sentences test as a method of studying personality. *Journal of Consulting Psychology, 11*, 43–48.

Sacks, J. M. (1949). The relative effect upon projective responses of stimuli referring to the subject and of stimuli referring to other persons. Journal of Consulting Psychology, 13, 12–20.

Sacks, J. M., & Levy, S. (1950). The sentence completion test. In L. E. Abt & L. Bellak (Eds.), *Projective psychology* (pp. 357–402). New York: Knopf.

Siipola, E. M. (1968). Incongruence of sentence completions under time pressure and freedom. *Journal of Projective Techniques and Personality Assessment, 32*, 562–571.

Stricker, G., & Dawson, D. D. (1966). The effects of first person and third person instruction and stems on sentence completion responses. *Journal of Projective Techniques and Personality Assessment, 30*, 169–171.

Swanson, C. H. (1975). *A validation study of the Hart Sentence Completion Test.* Unpublished master's thesis, University of Utah, Salt Lake City.

Trabue, M. R. (1916). *Completion test language scales.* New York: Columbia University Press.

Ulman, J. E. (1972). *Inter-scores reliability on the scoring system for the Hart Sentence Completion Test.* Unpublished master's thesis, University of Utah, Salt Lake City.

Watson, R. I., Jr. (1978). The sentence completion method in clinical diagnosis of mental disorders. In B. B. Wolman (Ed.), *Clinical diagnosis of mental disorders: A handbook* (pp. 255–280). New York: Plenum Press.

Wells, F. L. (1911). Practice effects in free association. *American Journal of Psychology, 22*, 1–13.

West, J. T. (1958). An investigation of the constructs "effective intelligence" and "social competence" with the Copple Sentence Completion Test utilizing a school of social work population. *Dissertation Abstracts International, 19*, 1121.

Wilson, J. P., & Aronoff, J. (1973). A sentence completion test assessing safety and esteem motives. *Journal of Personality Assessment, 37*, 351–354.

Wolkon, G. H., & Haefner, D. P. (1961). Change in ego strength of improved and unimproved psychiatric patients. *Journal of Clinical Psychology, 17*, 352–355.

Wood, F. A. (1969). An investigation of methods of presenting incomplete sentence stimuli. *Journal of Abnormal Psychology, 74*, 71–74.

9

The Personality Inventory for Children: Approaches to Actuarial Interpretation in Clinic and School Settings

David Lachar
Rex B. Kline
David C. Boersma

Introduction

The Personality Inventory for Children (PIC) is an objective multidimensional measure of behavior, affect, ability, and family function used to assess children from preschool ages through adolescence. The PIC is completed by an adult informant (usually the mother of the referred child or adolescent), and scale scores are derived from that adult's responses to brief inventory items. The objective format of the PIC requires limited professional time for administration and scoring, and interpretive guidelines are available to clarify its application and interpretation (Lachar, 1982; Lachar & Gdowski, 1979; Wirt, Lachar, Klinedinst, & Seat, 1984). The same item pool can be successfully applied from age 3 through adolescence, and family socioeconomic status and cultural background have minimal influence on test interpretation (Lachar & Gdowski, 1979; Wirt *et al.*, 1984).

PIC scales may be integrated into a traditional psychometric evaluation, may form the first stage of a sequential assessment process, or may serve to identify children in need of a psychological evaluation. Each PIC scale is standardized to a *T* score with a mean of 50 and a standard deviation of 10. For each scale, a higher *T*-score elevation (i.e., increasingly positive deviations from the mean) represents a reduced probability of occurrence among nonreferred children and an increased probability of psychopathology or deficit.

PIC informants answer "True" or "False" to the first 131, 280, or 420 items of the Revised Format Administration Booklet and record these answers on a hand-scoreable or optically scannable answer sheet, or respond to inventory items presented directly to them by a microcomputer program. In contrast to the 1977 administration booklet in which all 600 inventory items must be completed in order to score all of the scales on the PIC profile, the items of the 1981 Revised Format

David Lachar. Institute of Behavioral Medicine, Good Samaritan Medical Center, Phoenix, Arizona.
Rex B. Kline. Department of Psychology, University of Saskatchewan, Saskatoon, Saskatchewan, Canada.
David C. Boersma. Center for Forensic Psychiatry, Ann Arbor, Michigan.

Administration Booklet have been rearranged so that scoring and interpretation options increase with the number of items completed. Responses to the first 131 items generate scores for the Lie scale, a measure of respondent defensiveness and four broad-band scales derived through factor analysis: I: Undisciplined/Poor Self-Control; II: Social Incompetence; III: Internalization/Somatic Symptoms; and IV: Cognitive Development (Lachar, 1982; Lachar, Gdowski, & Snyder, 1982). This five-scale format is most useful in research projects when time is extremely limited, as a brief screening device to determine the need for a more detailed evaluation, or when respondent ability to complete a greater number of items is limited.

Response to the first 280 items of the Revised Format Administration Booklet (less than 50% of the 600 items comprising the PIC item pool) provides the 20 scales of the Revised Format Profile Form: the 4 factor scales, 3 measures of informant response style, a general screening scale, and 12 scales that measure child ability, behavior, affect, and family status. The relative efficiency of the 280-item format was obtained through item rearrangement and by a process which shortened 14 of the 20 scales by removing an average of 18% of each scale's items. These shortened scales proved comparable to their full-length equivalents (Lachar, 1982). The 14 shortened scales are designated with a ''-S'' suffix that is also added to each scale's abbreviation. Figure 9-1 presents the Revised Format Profile Form that is used when responses to the first 280 inventory items are scored.

Completion of the first 420 inventory items provides scores for all 20 scales in their full-length format as well as responses to a critical item list composed of 162 items that are assigned to 14 mutually exclusive categories: Depression and Poor Self-Concept; Worry and Anxiety; Reality Distortion; Peer Relations; Unsocialized Aggression; Conscience Development; Poor Judgment; Atypical Development; Distractibility, Activity Level, and Coordination; Speech and Language; Somatic Complaints/Current Health; School Adjustment; Family Discord; and Other. The final 180 items of the Revised Format Administration Booklet include those that are not included on any profile scale, although they may appear on one or more of the 17 experimental scales currently available (see Wirt *et al.*, 1984).

The dimensions represented by scales selected for the PIC profile do not reflect a specific theoretical perspective in regard to personality, psychopathology, or child development, but rather reflect those dimensions routinely assessed by clinicians regardless of theoretical preference or bias. Scale construction methodology has also varied as a function of the characteristics to be measured and the variety of applications envisaged. Practical issues, such as the availability of appropriate criterion groups, also influenced choice of scale construction methodology. Factor analysis, empirical keying, and rational/content methodologies have been applied to scale item selection in the construction of narrow- and broad-band scales. Characteristic of all the profile scales, however constructed, is their ability to successfully predict non-PIC measures of child adjustment and ability. It is this established actuarial character of the PIC that will be explored in some detail later in this chapter.

Selection of the mother as the primary PIC informant overcomes two of the major obstacles that commonly occur when a referred child or adolescent is asked to respond to numerous self-report descriptions in order to obtain a multiple-scale objective evaluation. First, the majority of children seen by mental health practitioners appear for such evaluations because of noncompliant behavior and/or documented problems in academic achievement, most notably in the development of reading skills. It therefore seems quite unlikely that a technique requir-

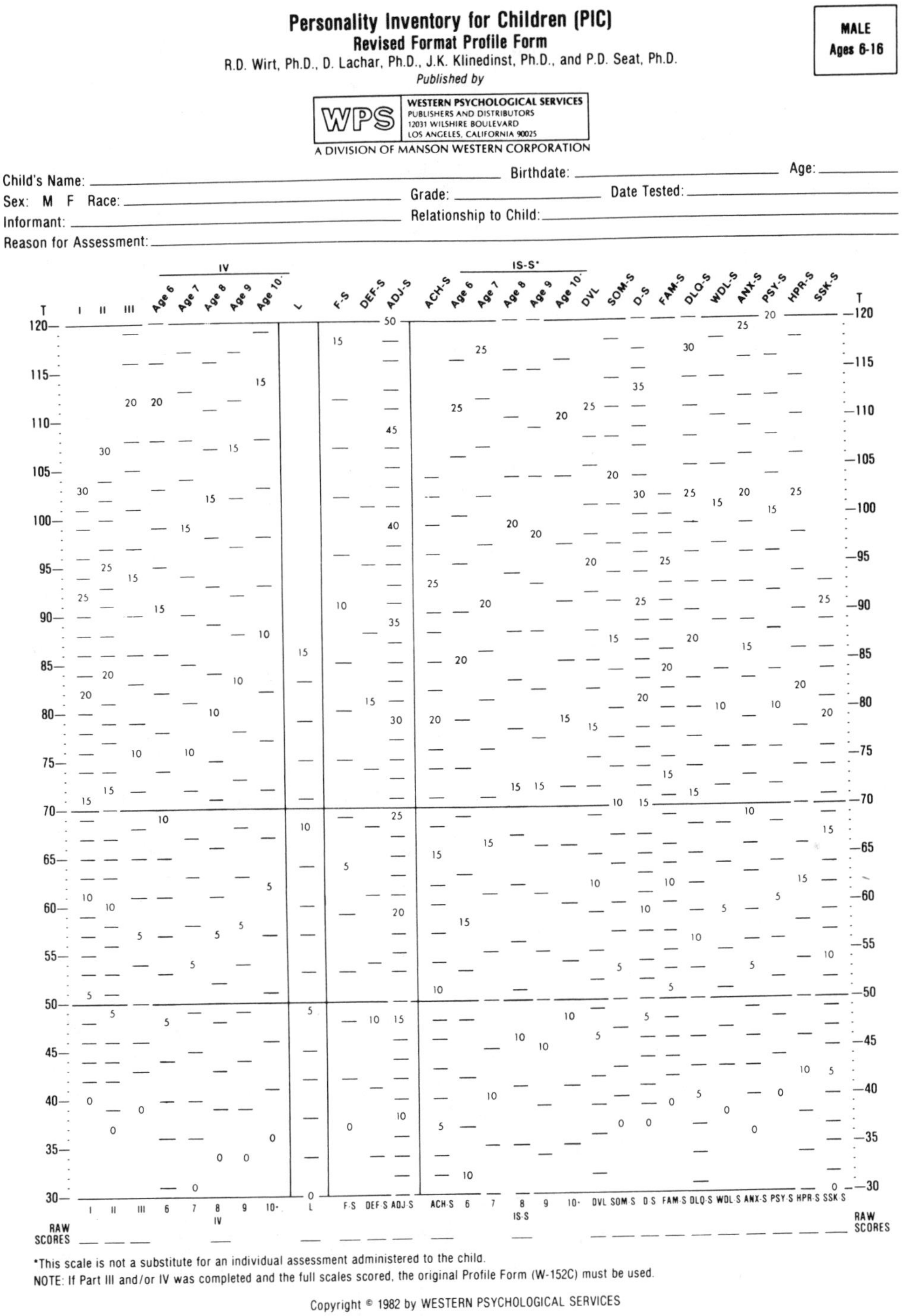

Figure 9-1. Personality Inventory for Children (PIC): Revised Format Profile Form.

ing such children to read and reliably respond to a large set of self-descriptions will find broad acceptance in routine clinical practice. Second, self-report inventories must be able to apply their methodologies to children with wide differences in verbal comprehension. If one assumes that the effectiveness of self-report personality descriptors is related to their richness and variety of language, restrictions of those descriptors to second- or third-grade reading vocabularies would severely limit the item writer's expression of more subtle aspects of child affect and family interaction. In fact, it appears that several child self-report measures are further retricted in their application by requiring reading levels that are actually higher than those stated by the test authors (Harrington & Follett, 1984).

Using adult respondents to PIC items is advantageous in several other ways. When both parents independently complete the PIC, a comparison of the profiles generated may identify areas of agreement and disagreement, thereby providing additional information useful within a family- or systems-oriented perspective. Incidentally, involving parents in their child's assessment may not only increase their later commitment to recommendations and intervention programs, but also fulfills a requirement of Public Law 94-142 which establishes guidelines for the psychological evaluation of children in need of special education services.

Adult response to PIC items may make the assessment of linguistic and culturally different referred children more valid and reliable. Occasionally, these children's linguistic and cultural differences obscure their need for special education placements and make direct assessments of their needs at best difficult. In these cases, it is possible to use translations of the PIC, which have been established and validated, with a child's parent. Thus, a Spanish translation of the PIC might be used by a monolingual mental health practitioner to determine whether a child with limited English language competence will be optimally served by intensive language training, or if current problems also reflect behavioral, emotional, or family characteristics, or deficits in cognitive functioning. Such translations (currently completed in Italian, French, Norwegian, and Spanish) also facilitate cross-cultural study of child adjustment and personality development.

Finally, as mothers are often invited to preassessment conferences in the schools or actually accompany their children to community or private agency testing sessions, the PIC can be given to them for independent completion, thus not increasing the professional time needed to complete an additional evaluation in the assessment battery. The 280-item length PIC can easily be completed while a child is assessed with an intelligence scale, an achievement test, and a visual-motor screening tool. The only additional costs to the clinician are the cost of a reusable administration booklet, an answer sheet, a profile form, and the few minutes needed to score the answer sheet to obtain scale raw scores. Parents not only see this task as reasonable and are often not only pleased, but actually relieved to have the opportunity to detail their concerns.

The fact that PIC responses are obtained from parents instead of the child or adolescent has also been perceived as a disadvantage in that observer distortion could have the opportunity to compromise scale accuracy. Prominent professionals in assessment research and evaluation have expressed their concern that PIC results may represent a mother's intentional distortion (Cronbach, 1984) or actually reflect the respondent's personality (Achenbach, 1981). It appears that potential users of informant-derived child evaluation measures are often unable to move beyond their initial reactions to the sources of questionnaire responses. This reaction appears to limit their appreciation of the psychometric process by which these responses are transformed into measures that allow the generation of actuarial predictions.

The psychometric performance of the PIC scales has been offered as evidence of the absence of problematic bias and distortion (Lachar & Wirt, 1981; Wirt & Lachar, 1981). Indeed, evidence of scale validity has been generated in samples in which the profile scales that measure potential response distortion, such as respondent defensiveness or exaggeration, have not been applied to restrict analyses to those profiles least likely to be affected by respondent distortion. In addition, some data are available that address the relation between respondent personality or level of adjustment as measured via self-report and PIC scale performance.

Lachar and Sharp (1979) correlated maternal respondent MMPI scales with the PIC descriptions of their children seen for a child guidance evaluation. No consistent relation was obtained across PIC scales, although considerable evidence was obtained to associate respondent psychopathology with the elevation of the PIC Family Relations scale, a measure of parental adjustment. Several of the PIC scales were essentially uncorrelated with respondent MMPI variance, and significant MMPI–PIC correlations were obtained twice as often when PICs described daughters than when they described sons.

The demonstration of a relationship between maternal and child description would not necessarily provide evidence that respondent characteristics compromise PIC scale accuracy. For example, when a mother describes both herself on the MMPI and her daughter on the PIC as depressed, this observed psychometric relationship may represent a variety of processes, including the following: (a) Mothers who tend to describe themselves in negative terms (whether or not accurate) describe others in similar terms; (b) depressed mothers view others as depressed when they are not; (c) depressed mothers serve as salient role models for their daughters and/or generate an interpersonal environment conducive to child maladjustment; and (d) depressed daughters may have a negative influence on maternal adjustment. A more direct assessment of the hypothesis that respondent character or adjustment compromises PIC scale validity would be to evaluate PIC scale performance in samples varying in respondent adjustment or personality. In a recent study, the authors constructed two study samples: one of mothers with elevated MMPI profiles, the other of mothers who generated within-normal-limits MMPI profiles. Each mother completed a PIC on a child or adolescent for whom ratings were available from parents, teachers, and clinicians. The expectation that the greater psychopathology present in the sample with elevated MMPI profiles would compromise PIC predictive validity was not supported. The same or similar PIC scales predicted the majority of the external rating dimensions to the same degree. Contrary to expectation, group trends suggestive of differential validity supported the position of better PIC scale performance within the sample of respondents with elevated MMPI profiles.

The Profile Scales

Informant Response Style

Lie Scale (L)

This rationally developed scale was constructed to identify an informant's defensive response set demonstrated by his or her tendency to ascribe the most virtuous of behaviors and to deny minor, commonly occurring behavior problems in the referred child. Scale items include "My child sometimes disobeys his (her) parents," and "Sometimes my child will put off doing a chore." Correlations with other PIC scales and ratings of the child suggest that L reflects the absence or denial of behavior problems, especially those classified as delinquent and asocial, as well as the absence or denial of family problems and psychological discomfort. L elevation increases when the respondent intentionally attempts to portray the child as having fewer problems than is actually the case (Daldin, 1985; McVaugh & Grow, 1983). Daldin (1985) found that $L > 59T$ increased from 4% to 92% when mothers were asked to complete the PIC as though their children did not have the problems that brought them to a child guidance clinic.

Frequency Scale (F)

This scale consists of items that were seldom endorsed in the normative sample's scored direction ($M = 5\%$) or in a sample of preadolescent boys evaluated at child guidance clinics ($M = 14\%$). Scale items include "My child is afraid of animals," "My child thinks others are plotting against him (her)," and "My child doesn't seem to care for fun." Item content was varied so that a single pattern of severe disturbance could not account for an extreme scale elevation. The F scale obtains extreme elevations ($120T$) for profiles when inventory items are completed without regard for item content (Wirt *et al.*, 1984). When parents were asked to describe their normal children through the PIC in such a manner to convince a practitioner of the presence of psychological disturbances, F increased from $55T$ to $115T$ (McVaugh & Grow, 1983). Similarly, when mothers of children being evaluated at a child guidance clinic were asked to answer PIC items a second time, exaggerating the difficulties and problems that brought them to the clinic, F-S increased from $67T$ to $118T$ (Daldin, 1985). Finally, a recent study has suggested that F elevation may be strongly influenced by parental perception of disturbance that need not be corroborated by systematic school or clinic observation (Lachar, Gdowski, & Snyder, 1984). In a large child guidance sample high F elevations were fairly frequent: 10% for $100–109T$, and 10% for $> 109T$ (Lachar & Gdowski, 1979).

Defensiveness Scale (DEF)

This empirically constructed scale is composed of a heterogeneous set of inventory items that separated mothers judged to be high-defensive from mothers judged to be low-defensive based upon a diagnostic interview about the referred child. Although a cutting score of $> 59T$ correctly identified 93% of the low-defensive and 88% of the high-defensive protocols, recent application found an increase in DEF $> 59T$ from 0% to only 40% under fake-good instructions (Daldin, 1985).

General Adjustment

Adjustment Scale (ADJ)

Item endorsement rates for 600 normal boys from 7 to 12 years of age were compared to the item endorsement rates for 200 maladjusted boys from 7 to 12 years of age to develop a screening measure to identify children in need of a psychological evaluation, and as a general measure of poor psychological adjustment. Scale item content reflects both internalizing and externalizing characteristics. Application of a cutting score of $>59T$ correctly classified 86% of normal and 89% of clinic protocols. These classification rates have remained stable through subsequent analyses.

The Cognitive Triad

The first 3 of the 12 substantive scales reflect the cognitive status of the referred child. Although clinicians may resist a procedure that evaluates a child's ability without directly assessing the child, the value of such measures on the profile is considerable. These scales may be applied to determine probable need for individual assessment of ability and achievement, and they play a central role in defining relatively homogeneous subgroups of disturbed children through classification of total profile configurations.

Achievement Scale (ACH)

The item endorsement rates for second- and third-grade boys who evidenced serious retardation in the development of reading ability were compared with the item endorsement rates of those children whose reading ability was grade-appropriate to construct a scale to assist in the identification of children whose academic achievement is significantly below age expectation regardless of intellectual capacity. A cutting score of $>59T$ correctly identified 97% of construction and 92% of cross-validation protocols. Factor analysis of scale items suggested that ACH not only measures limited academic abilities and poor achievement ["My child could do better in school if he (she) tried"], but also reflects a dimension of poor psychological adjustment characterized by impulsivity, limited concentration, over- or underassertiveness with peers. ["My child will do anything on a dare," "My child can't seem to keep attention on anything"], and disregard for parental expectations ["My child will never clean his (or her) room"] (Wirt *et al.*, 1984).

Intellectual Screening Scale (IS)

This scale was constructed to identify children whose difficulties may be related to impaired intellectual functioning or specific cognitive deficits, and for whom an individually administered intellectual assessment would be indicated. Items were identified by contrasting the protocols of retarded children with normal, nonretarded disturbed, and psychotic children.

Development Scale (DVL)

These items, selected through the consensus of experts, primarily reflect retarded development in motor coordination, poor school performance, and lack of any special skill or abilities. Other factors reflect limited motivation to achieve in school, clumsiness and weakness, limited reading skills, and deficient pragmatic skills (e.g., counting change).

Several investigators have established the relationship between a variety of ability and achievement measures, as well as special education classification, and ACH, IS, and DVL (cf. Bennett & Welsh, 1981; Clark, 1982; DeKrey & Ehly, 1981; DeMoor-Peal & Handal, 1983; Dollinger, Goh, & Cody, 1984; Durrant, 1983; Kelly, 1982; Schnel, 1982). Studies by these authors suggest that child sex, age, and race do not moderate the relationship between scale T-score elevation and measured ability and achievement (Kline, Lachar, & Sprague, 1985). ACH, IS, and DVL T scores may be interpreted by reference to the replicated external correlates associated with normal, mild, moderate, and severe *T*-score elevation ranges (Lachar & Gdowski, 1979), as well as through a composite Cognitive Index. Both actuarial approaches will be discussed below.

Other Clinical Scales

Somatic Concern Scale (SOM)

This scale is composed of items selected by judges to measure various health-related variables: frequency and seriousness of somatic complaints and illness, adjustment to illness, appetite and eating habits, sleep patterns, energy and strength, headaches and stomachaches, as well as the physical basis for symptoms. SOM items include "My child often has headaches," "My child takes illness harder than most children," and "My child seldom complains of stomachaches." This scale represents a unique and rather small factor when a large number of PIC scales are subjected to factor analysis (Wirt *et al.*, 1984). Two study groups to date have obtained a mean SOM elevation above 60*T*: boys exhibiting physical symptoms considered by a physician to be related to experienced stress (Stewart, 1971) and boys and girls with cancer (Armstrong, Wirt, Nesbit, & Martinson, 1982). Pipp (1979) found SOM correlated with only one MMPI scale for both male and female adolescent psychiatric patients: Hypochondriasis. Kelly (1982) found that only one Child Behavior Checklist scale correlated with SOM: Somatic Complaints. Lachar and Gdowski (1979) found limited but highly appropriate correlates for SOM: fatigue, aches and pains, insomnia, somatic response to stress, and malingering.

Depression Scale (D)

These inventory items were judged by experienced clinicians to reflect childhood depression. Factor analysis of scale items yielded dimensions labeled Brooding/Moodiness, Social Isolation, Crying Spells, Lack of Energy, Pessimism/Anhedonia, Concern with Death and Separation, Serious Attitude, Sensitivity to Criticism, Indecisiveness/Poor Self-Concept, and Uncommunicativeness. Scale items include "My child hardly ever smiles," "My child has little self-confidence," "My child tends to pity him (her) self," and "My child is as happy as ever." Leon, Kendall, and Garber (1980) found D to significantly correlate with the Child Depression Inventory in a sample of elementary school children. Children designated as "depressed" by their D *T* scores attributed positive events to external causes significantly more often than did children not so identified. Kelly (1982) found D to be most strongly correlated with Child Behavior Checklist scales of Social Withdrawal, Depressed, Uncommunicative, and Social. Pipp (1979) found that D was significantly correlated with the MMPI Social Introversion scale for both male and female adolescent psychiatric patients, but significantly correlated with the MMPI Depression scale for only female adolescents. D has also significantly separated children independently labeled depressed according to DSM-III criteria, on the basis of maternal interview (*M* = 85*T*) from children who did not meet this criteria (*M* = 61*T*); comparable classification performance of the Children's Depression Inventory was no better than that of D applied without the potential incremental validity of other PIC profile scales (Lobovits & Handal, 1985).

Family Relations Scale (FAM)

This scale assists in determining the role that family and parental factors play in the development of child psychopathology and also evaluates the need for in-depth assessment of family and parental characteristics. Scale items were selected from the nominations of experts to assess the following dimensions: parental role effectiveness, ability to cooperate in making family decisions, family involvement in community affairs, presence of feelings of love and happiness in the home, parental emotional adjustment, appropriateness of discipline, and concern for the rights of the child. FAM items include "Our family seems to enjoy each other more than most families," "The child's parents frequently quarrel," "The child's parents disagree a lot about rearing the child," and "The child's father is hardly ever home." Lachar and Sharp (1979) found that FAM was the only PIC profile scale that consistently correlated with a broad range of maternal MMPI scales. FAM elevations are higher for children from divorced than from nondivorced parents (Schreiber, 1982), and FAM obtained the highest mean scale elevation in profiles of children who had a parent in treatment for alcoholism (Anderson & Quast, 1983). Snyder and Gdowski (1980) compared the scores of the Marital Satisfaction Inventory (MSI) from parents when FAM was $>59T$ to the MSI scores when FAM was $<46T$. High FAM parents obtained significantly higher elevations on 9 of the 11 MSI profile scales. It is also interesting to note that the 1984 manual presents only one criterion group with an elevated mean FAM: adjudicated delinquents.

Delinquency Scale (DLQ)

Item response rates of adjudicated and nonadjudicated adolescents were compared to develop a scale designed to be a concurrent measure of the behavioral characteristics manifested by delinquents and as a diagnostic aid in the identification of delinquent children. DLQ obtained a scale score-to-criterion validity of .89 in a cross-validation sample in which a cutting score correctly identified 95% of delinquents and normals. Adjudicated delinquents obtained very high T-score elevations, with 58% obtaining $DLQ>99T$. Factor analysis of scale items yielded two substantial factors labeled Disregard for Limits/Interpersonal Insensitivity and Antisocial Tendencies, and several small factors labeled Irritability/Limited Tolerance, Sadness, Lack of Interest/Impulsivity, Interpersonal Hostility, and Disrespect for Parents. DLQ includes items such as "My child often disobeys me," "My child doesn't seem to learn from mistakes," "My child seems bored with school," "Several times my child has been in trouble for stealing," and "My child plays with friends who are often in trouble." Pipp (1979) found DLQ to correlate significantly with the MMPI scales Psychopathic Deviate and Hypomania for both male and female adolescents. Kelly (1982) found that DLQ correlated the most highly with Child Behavior Checklist scales Delinquent and Aggressive. Lachar et al. (1984) found DLQ to correlate significantly with parent, teacher, and clinician rating form dimensions of externalization, impulsivity, antisocial character, and hostility/emotional lability. McAuliffe and Handal (1984) suggest that DLQ may reflect meaningful variance at much lower T-score elevations. When students attending parochial high school were divided into two groups at $50T$ (the "elevated" sample scoring in the majority between 50 and $70T$), the elevated DLQ sample scored significantly lower on the Socialization scale of the California Psychological Inventory and higher on a self-report measure of delinquent acts.

Withdrawal Scale (WDL)

These items were nominated to measure withdrawal from social contact. Factor analysis of WDL items resulted in content dimensions labeled Social and Physical Isolation, Shyness/Fear of Strangers, Isolation from Peers/Uncommunicativeness, Emotional Distance, Intentional Withdrawal/Distrust, and Isolative Intellectual Pursuits. WDL items include "I often wonder if my child is lonely," "My child is usually afraid to meet new people," "My child doesn't seem to care to be with others," and "My child usually doesn't trust others." Psychotic children obtain mean WDL elevation above 69T (Wirt *et al.*, 1984). Kelly (1982) obtained significant correlations between WDL and Child Behavior Checklist scales Social Withdrawal, Uncommunicativeness, and Social. Pipp (1979) found that WDL correlated significantly with MMPI scale Social Introversion for both male and female adolescents.

Anxiety Scale (ANX)

These items were nominated as measuring the various manifestations of anxiety. Factor analysis of scale items resulted in content dimensions labeled Brooding/Moodiness, Fearfulness, Worry, Fear of the Dark, Specific Fears/Crying Spells, Poor Self-Concept, Insecurity/Fearfulness, and Sensitivity to Criticism/Pessimism. ANX items include "My child worries about things that usually only adults worry about," "Often my child is afraid of little things," and "My child will worry a lot before starting something new."

Psychosis Scale (PSY)

This empirically keyed scale was constructed to discriminate children with psychotic symptomatology from normal, behaviorally disturbed nonpsychotic, and retarded children. Scale score-to-criterion validity was .88 in construction and .84 in cross-validation samples. Psychotic children obtain very high PSY elevations: 84% of the scale construction protocols scored above 99T. Pipp (1979) found that PSY correlated significantly with the MMPI scales Schizophrenia and Social Introversion for both male and female adolescents. PSY was the only PIC scale to correlate significantly with a clinician rating dimension labeled Disorganization/Limited Reality Testing (Lachar *et al.*, 1984). PSY items include "My child is liable to scream if disturbed," "My child gets lost easily," "My child needs protection from everyday dangers," "Other children make fun of my child's different ideas," and "Often my child will laugh for no apparent reason."

Hyperactivity Scale (HPR)

These scale items were empirically selected so as to separate children seen at guidance clinics who were described by their teachers as hyperactive (DSM-III: Attention Deficit Disorder with Hyperactivity) from children also evaluated at child guidance clinics who were not seen as hyperactive by their teachers. HPR items include "Others think my child is mean," "My child loses most friends because of his (or her) temper," "My child tends to brag," "My child can't seem to keep attention on anything," and "School teachers complain that my child can't sit still." HPR obtained a scale score-to-criterion validity of .78, and a cutting score of 59T correctly classified 90% of hyperactive and 94% of maladjusted nonhyperactive samples. Breen and Barkley (1983) obtained similar classification rates, and Voelker, Lachar, and Gdowski (1983) found HPR elevation to be related to treatment with stimulants and favorable response to such treatment. Kelly (1982) obtained significant correlations between HPR and Child Behavior Checklist scales Hyperactive, Aggressive, and Delinquent. Clark, Wanous, and Pompa (1982) obtained a considerable number of significant correlations between HPR and teacher ratings of special education students on such rating scale items as "Does not conform to limits," "Easily distracted," "Poor achievement due to distractibility," and "Poor achievement due to impulsivity."

Social Skills Scale (SSK)

This scale is composed of items selected by judges to measure the various characteristics that reflect effective social relations in childhood. SSK item content dimensions reflected in factor groupings suggest that this scale measures both the lack of success in social activities (lack of friends, peer rejection, absence of club membership, adults as only social contacts) and the reasons for this lack of success (aggressive behavior with peers, absence of leadership qualities or social influence, social behavior suggesting poor sportsmanship, egocentrism, and obstinacy). SSK items include "My child has very few friends," "Other children don't seem to listen to or notice my child much," "My child is usually rejected by other children," "Other children look up to my child as a leader," and "Others have said my child has a lot of 'personality.'" SSK has been found to significantly relate to measures of moral judgment and cognitive perspective-taking (Kurdek, 1980), a self-report measure of social competence (Kurdek & Krile, 1983), and a peer acceptance rating (Kurdek, 1982). SSK has been found to significantly correlate with the Peer Support scale of the self-report Children's Perception of Social Support Inventory as well as with parental and self-report measures of the quality of peer support (Schreiber, 1982).

The Factor Scales

I: Undisciplined/Poor Self-Control (I)

The majority of the items of this scale remained constant in factor membership across solutions in which 12, 10, 8, and 6 factors were extracted. Factor I items appear primarily on scales ADJ, DLQ, and HPR. A factor analysis of scale items resulted in content dimensions labeled Ineffective Discipline, Impulsivity, Problematic Anger, Poor Peer Relationships, Limited Conscience Development, and Poor School Behavior. Correlation with parent, teacher, and clinician ratings provides independent evidence that Factor I reflects hostility/emotional lability, impulsivity, and antisocial behavior (Lachar et al., 1984).

II: Social Incompetence (II)

This scale is the combination of two item dimensions: at the 8-factor solution labeled Friendships, and Shyness at the 10-factor solution. The majority of Factor II scale items are also found on ADJ, D, WDL, ANX, PSY, and SSK. A factor analysis of scale items resulted in content dimensions labeled Sadness, Shyness, Peer Rejection, Lack of Leadership Qualities, Social Isolation, Lack of Friends, and Adjustment. Factor II correlates with teacher and clinician ratings of social withdrawal and a parent rating dimension labeled Depressive/Somatic symptoms (Lachar et al., 1984). The obtained relationship between dysphoric affect and deficient social skills and lack of positive peer relations in children and adolescents is not surprising (Costello, 1981).

III: Internalization/Somatic Symptoms (III)

The majority of these items remained stable in their factor membership for solutions in which 12, 10, 8, and 6 factors were extracted. Factor III items appear primarily on SOM, D, and ANX. A factor analysis of scale items resulted in content dimensions labeled Worry/Poor Self-Concept, Somatization, Crying Spells, Insecurity/Fearfulness, Vision Problems, Psychotic Behavior, and Body Temperature. Factor III significantly correlated with parent and clinician dimensions labeled Depressive/Somatic Symptoms (Lachar *et al.*, 1984).

IV: Cognitive Development (IV)

This scale is composed of two dimensions (Development of Abilities and Comprehension) that remained stable through 12-, 10-, and 8-factor solutions and merged into one factor at the 6-factor solution. The majority of Factor IV items are also found on ACH, IS, DVL, and PSY. Factor IV significantly correlates with the parent rating dimensions Developmental Delay and Cognitive/Attentional Deficits, the teacher rating dimension Academic Delay, and the clinician rating dimension Language/Motor Deficits (Lachar *et al.*, 1984). Factor IV has also been found to correlate $-.53$ with the McCarthy General Cognitive Index and $-.63$ with the Peabody Picture Vocabulary IQ (Durrant, 1983).

Actuarial Interpretation

Actuarial interpretation is that process by which test data are transformed into categories that have been found to be statistically related to meaningful nontest data. In this manner specific scale values, test indices, or profile scale patterns reliably predict characteristics of the client being evaluated. The meaning of test indices is thereby statistically determined, rather than extrapolated by the clinical process in which a psychologist integrates a personal understanding of a test's ability and performance with theoretical and empirical preferences regarding child development and personality structure to determine the meaning of test results. (An excellent discussion of the process of actuarial interpretation may be found in a chapter by Marks, Seeman, and Haller, 1974.) Discussion of a hypothetical case clarifies the value of actuarial assessment in the interpretation of the PIC profile.

A Case Study: "Little Melissa"

"Little Melissa" is brought to the clinic by her parents. This 8-year-old appears quite different from the majority of children evaluated at this urban child guidance facility. She is friendly, appears happy, and is quite cooperative during the entire assessment process. The PIC profile obtained through maternal report, in contrast, is notable due to an apparent, considerable elevation of the Delinquency scale (85T). An initial impulse to classify these test results as inaccurate is neither supported by an extreme elevation on the Frequency scale, nor by review of initial performance of DLQ that is presented in the 1977 PIC Manual.

What can be said of a DLQ performance of 85T when it is obtained by an 8-year-old girl? Although such a scale elevation reliably separates adjudicated adolescent delinquents from normal adolescents (while being somewhat low for the average criterion delinquent), can the clinician accurately infer that characteristics frequently displayed by this criterion group describe this preadolescent girl being evaluated by a child guidance agency? Should the clinician predict that Little Melissa is known to the police because of her antisocial behavior? Does she belong to a gang, participate in auto theft, or exhibit substance abuse and its related behaviors? Quite unlikely—even for young participants in our urban clinics!

The task of the clinician, then, is to determine what this scale elevation means when obtained by younger children being evaluated in settings other than juvenile justice clinics; that is, the clinician must determine the child characteristics that are reliably related to DLQ elevation, as well as the minimum T-score elevation or T-score range in which each description is likely to be accurate. The clinician could infer what these characteristics are by the idiosyncratic integration of the clinician's knowledge about the PIC, child development, personality theory, and accumulated clinical experience. Or, better, he or she could consult an actuarial guide, constructed through the statistical analysis of data, that would describe the relationship between PIC scale elevations and a variety of meaningful characteristics and behaviors of children evaluated at child guidance clinics; that is, the clinician wishes to know in this case the child characteristics that are reliably related to DLQ elevation, as well as the minimum T-score elevation or T-score range in which each description is likely to be accurate. Lachar and Gdowski (1979) and Lachar (1982) document the process through which individual scale's T scores are correlated with ratings from parents, teachers, and clinicians. Rated child characteristics that reliably relate to a specific PIC scale are said to be *correlates* of that scale.

Returning to the interpretation of the DLQ scale, Lachar and Gdowski (1979) report 24 parent, 19 teacher, and 30 clinician correlates for this scale (Lachar & Gdowski, 1979, p. 27). Parent correlates include "Often skips school, Hangs around with a 'bad crowd,' Disobeys parents, Can't be trusted, Steals"; teacher correlates include "Habitually rejects the school experience through actions or comments, Reacts with defiance to instructions or commands, Doesn't conform to limits on his/her own without control from others, Poor class attendance, Steals things from other children"; and clinician correlates include "Truancy, Involved with the police, Running away from home, Stealing, Disobediance to parents, Displays irresponsible behavior, Lying."

Scale correlates are transformed into actuarial interpretation through the process of relating test categories to nontest data. To develop guidelines for interpretation of individual PIC scales, each scale was divided into T-score ranges of 10 points, and the incidence of established scale correlates was tabulated for these T-score ranges to determine the minimum scale elevation necessary for a correlate to become descriptive. Figure 6-1 of Lachar and Gdowski (1979) and Tables 3-11, 4-8, and 5-10 of that monograph document that DLQ correlates begin to become descriptive of children and adolescents evaluated at child guidance agencies at 80T. Correlates descriptive for 80–89T range (returning specifically to our case study of "Little Melissa") include "Has a 'chip on the shoulder,' Disobeys parents, Lies, Talks back to grown-ups, Won't obey school rules, Can't be trusted, Steals" from parent ratings, "Complains about others' unfairness and/or discrimination toward him/her, Distorts the truth by making statements contrary to fact, Doesn't obey until threatened with punishment, Argues and must have the last word in verbal exchanges" from teacher ratings, and "Impulsive behavior, Blames others for his/her problems, Displays irresponsible behavior, Lying, Poor judgment/needs much supervision" from clinican ratings.

The DLQ elevation of 85 *T* does not suggest that Little Melissa is a delinquent; rather, it suggests that her problems center around an unwillingness to conform to limits requested by adults, impulsivity, and poorly modulated hostility. Lachar and Gdowski (1979) suggest the following DLQ interpretation for this *T*-score range:

> Resistance to the requests of adults at home and in school is often indicated. Similar children are frequently described as impulsive by mental health professionals who may note irresponsible behavior, poor judgment, or an established tendency to blame others for current problems. A hostile, unsocialized orientation may be suggested by argumentativeness, lying, or theft. (p. 94).

Actuarial Interpretation of Individual Profile Scales

Lachar and Gdowski (1979) established interpretive *T*-score ranges and provided a set of 37 interpretive paragraphs for the basic 16 profile scales. An important finding of this study was that the minimum scale elevation necessary to signify clinically meaningful maladjustment differed across these scales. For some scales a *T* score of 60 was significant (L, ADJ, ACH, DVL, FAM, HPR), while for other scales a *T* score greater than the traditionally assigned value of 70 was necessary to predict clinically meaningful characteristics (F, DLQ, PSY).

The following review of the correlates of a few of the profile scales and their *T*-score placements suggests the considerable value of the actuarial approach to test interpretation. For example, Achievement scale correlates form three interpretive bands. Scores about 59 *T* uniformly suggest problematic performance in a variety of academic subjects. When ACH is elevated above 69 *T*, teachers are likely to observe deficiencies in basic abilities that are prerequisite to appropriate achievement, such as verbal comprehension for reading. ACH values above 79 *T* suggest a problematic adjustment, reflecting the effects of either severe and/or chronic academic failure, that signals the need for professional intervention. Teacher correlates for this *T*-score range suggest the presence of a negative self-image: "Frequent daydreaming, Approaches new tasks and situations with an 'I can't do it' response, Gives up easily/expects failure."

Correlates of the Depression scale are placed within two *T*-score ranges. Scale values greater than 69 *T* reflect manifestations of dysphoric affect, while scores greater than 79 *T* suggest associated disturbances of eating and sleep, as well as suicidal thought and behavior for adolescents. It is interesting to note that D elevations above 79 *T* are related to clinicians' assessment of suicidal content, while D elevations above 89 *T* are related to parents' concern about their child's potential for self-destruction. As clinicians routinely discuss this topic during an evaluation and parents often become concerned about the potential for suicide when their child either threatens or attempts such action, an additional hypothesis suggested by these data is that suicidal ideation is more likely to be associated with threats or attempts within higher Depression scale elevations. Finally, Family Relations correlates appear to fall within three *T*-score ranges: scores above 59 *T* reflect family conflict and parental inconsistency, scores above 69 *T* suggest parental emotional disturbance and the possibility of parental alcoholism or substance abuse, while scores above 79 *T* suggest parental rejection and criticism, as well as other behaviors that may justify the label of child abuse.

The actuarial data presented in Lachar and Gdowski (1979) support a conservative interpretation of both the Delinquency and Psychosis scales. Antisocial behaviors and substance abuse were found to be descriptive of DLQ elevations >109T, and symptoms clearly related to defective reality testing were associated with PSY elevations >109T. Hyperactivity scale values appear to predict two subsets of correlates. HPR values greater than 59T reflect difficulties in classroom adjustment associated with impulsivity, restlessness, distractibility, and an excessive or perhaps undercontrolled sociability. HPR>69T suggests, in addition, the presence of limited frustration tolerance, undercontrolled hostility, and manipulative and perhaps antisocial behaviors that are likely to be associated with poor relationships with peers.

Lachar (1982) presented actuarially determined interpretive paragraphs for each of the four factor scales. The factor scales become clinically meaningful at 70T, and each scale is associated with two to four T-score interpretive ranges. Based on an expanded study sample, Lachar provides 12 interpretive paragraphs for these four broad-band factor scales.

The Cognitive Index

The Cognitive Index is a measure of cognitive deficit that reflects the actuarially determined T-score ranges of the three scales of the Cognitive Triad: ACH, IS, and DVL. The Index is merely a number from 3 to 12; each scale contributes a value from 1 (normal limits) to 4 (extreme elevation). The scale T-score ranges associated with each weight are presented in Table 9-1. This index is easily calculated and helps determine whether individually administered assessments of intellectual functioning and academic achievement are likely to be useful. Table 9-1 represents the relation between Full Scale IQ and the Cognitive Index within a diverse sample of 329 children and adolescents evaluated at a psychiatric facility.

Table 9-1
Distribution (%) of Full Scale IQs within Five Cognitive Index Score Ranges

Cognitive Index	Full Scale IQ					(Σ)	χ^2 (4)
	<70	70–84	85–99	100–114	>114		
3/4	4.2	16.0	31.9	34.0	13.9	(144)	40.68**
5/6	14.9	25.7	40.5	14.9	4.0	(74)	3.58
7/8	21.2	36.5	32.7	7.7	1.9	(52)	9.49*
9/10	28.6	42.9	25.7	2.8	0.0	(35)	16.15**
11/12	54.2	33.3	12.5	0.0	0.0	(24)	35.37**
Expected	15	26	32	20	7		
(Σ)	(51)	(84)	(105)	(65)	(24)	(329)	

Rules for the Computation of the PIC Cognitive Index

Weight	Achievement (T)	Intellectual screening (T)	Development (T)
1	<60	<70	<60
2	60–69	70–79	60–69
3	70–79	80–89	70–79
4	≥80	≥90	≥80

*$p \leq .05$.
**$p \leq .01$.

The values in the row labeled "expected" provide the actual frequencies of each IQ classification within the entire sample. (For example, only 15% of this sample has Full Scale IQs less than 70, and only 7% had Full Scale IQs greater than 114.) When this sample is classified within five Cognitive Index categories, four significantly deviate from total sample expectations. As would be expected, low values (3/4) suggest a higher incidence of average and above-average IQs and a below-average incidence of IQs less than 85. Cognitive Index values 7/8, 9/10, and 11/12 obtained progressively greater proportions of lower IQ values and progressively fewer average or above-average IQs.

Table 9-1 is presented to demonstrate the potential value of such an index as well as the ease in which such a table could be constructed to predict any cognitive or achievement variable, given a reasonable sample of PICs and scale scores obtained by individual assessment of the child. Many guidance clinics and school systems currently have the data base of PIC profiles and individually administered tests to construct such tables. The tests to be predicted and the ranges of score values from these tests can be determined by local and state guidelines, and the relationships obtained will then reflect local base rates as well as clinical and classification preference and practice.

Classification of Special Education Needs

Actuarial approaches to the interpretation of the PIC have been employed in recent research efforts in both clinic and school settings. The potential value of actuarial assessment in the school setting is perhaps most readily apparent in the classification and placement of children, especially the educably mentally retarded, the emotionally disturbed, and the learning disabled into special education.

The process whereby these students are declared eligible for special education services and placed in programs for specialized instruction has been criticized in recent years for the lack of clear, consistent relationships between the classification categories and the assessment information used to place children into these categories. Classification and placement decisions in special education have traditionally relied on the school psychologist's (and child study team's) integration of information and data from several sources. There is little indication, however, that school psychologists agree on which assessment tests and techniques to select, which information to sample, and what data to integrate to make these decisions for specific referrals or circumstances (Sinclair, 1983).

Although some have criticized the current classification system in special education, namely, Public Law (PL) 94-142 (Education of All Handicapped Children's Act of 1975), for its imprecision (Duffey, Salvia, Tucker, & Ysseldyke, 1981; Forness, 1976; Hallahan & Kauffman, 1976, 1977), others have attributed the lack of consistency in special education classifications to inadequate assessment and classification practices (Helton, Workman, & Matuszek, 1982; McDermott, 1982; Ysseldyke, 1983). In this regard, classification practices have been cited for their overreliance on parental reports (McCoy, 1976), teacher observations (Ysseldyke, 1983), technically inadequate tests (Helton *et al.*, 1982), including projective techniques (Peterson & Batsche, 1983), and other potential biasing factors (McDermott, 1982).

To improve classification consistency in special education, McDermott (1982) has proposed more widespread use of actuarial assessment procedures and has recently developed an actuarial assessment process for differential diagnosis in the schools that provides decision rules, based on relevant assessment information, for various decision points in a branching decision tree format. Recent research using the PIC has also suggested the value of actuarial assessment in the classification of special education needs. Three doctoral dissertations have used the PIC in multiple discriminant function analyses to place children into various educational classifications (Clark, 1982; DeKrey, 1982; Schnel, 1982). The results of these studies revealed conceptually meaningful differences among the PIC profiles of children in regular education classes and in programs for the learning disabled, emotionally disturbed, and educably mentally retarded. In addition, substantial percentages of these children were correctly classified by PIC-based discriminant function rules.

Development of an Actuarial Classification System

A more recent study (Boersma, 1984) has employed the PIC in the construction of an actuarially based classification system for special education. Two groups of subjects were included: a derivation sample of 248 public school children (ages 6–13) attending regular and/or special education classes in suburban Detroit, Michigan schools, and the three validation samples from the Clark (1982), DeKrey (1982), and Schnel (1982) investigations in Michigan, Iowa, and California, respectively. Validation samples were included in this investigation in order to evaluate the generalizability of the proposed PIC-based classification system across school districts in different states.

Derivation sample subjects received special services within six special education placements: Learning Disabled–Self-Contained Classroom (LDSC; $N = 30$), Learning Disabled–Teacher Consultant Support Services (LDTC; $N = 38$), Trainable Mentally Impaired (TMI; $N = 29$), Educable Mentally Impaired (EMI; $N = 30$), Emotionally Impaired (EI; $N = 24$), and School Social Work Services (SSW; $N = 41$). The learning-disabled, mentally impaired, and emotionally impaired placements required certification as educationally handicapped according to criteria established by the Michigan State Board of Education (1980) for this purpose. The school social work classification is not a special education category; it represents a common placement option for children who are referred for emotional and/or behavioral problems, but are not eligible for special education services under the EI designation. These six special services placements were included in this investigation because (a) they represent the most common placement options considered by school psychologists in the assessment process, (b) they rely most often on assessment information typically provided by school psychologists, and (c) they are therefore most amenable to the exploration of actuarially based relationships with test data. A seventh sample consisted of 56 regular education students who had never received special education services and who did not currently require such services according to their teachers. These students were matched as closely as possible to the age, grade, and sex distributions of the special education subjects.

Validation samples included the following: 111 students in regular education classes (grades 2–5) and 83 students in programs for the learning disabled (Schnel, 1982); 32 students in regular education classes and 63 special education students (ages 6–13) in programs for the learning disabled ($N = 23$), emotionally disturbed ($N = 20$), and mentally disabled ($N = 20$) (DeKrey, 1982); and 134 students (ages 6–16) in programs for the learning disabled ($N = 70$), emotionally impaired ($N = 47$), and educably mentally impaired ($N = 17$) (Clark, 1982). Special education students in these three samples were not classified as to their type of placement (self-contained classroom vs. teacher consultant services).

Like McDermott's (1982), this investigation sought to develop decision rules that could be applied in a branching decision tree format to identify children who would benefit from inclusion in one classification category as opposed to others. Unlike McDermott, the assessment information used in the construction of these decision rules consisted entirely of PIC scale scores. The PIC is ideally suited for this task because it is multidimensional and assesses many areas relevant to the cognitive and social–emotional problems presented by children who are referred for consideration of a special education placement. It was not intended that the resulting PIC-based classification system would serve as a substitute for traditional assessment practice in the schools; rather, it was hoped that PIC-based actuarial predictions might be used to augment the psychoeducational assessment process by suggesting areas in need of further assessment.

Figure 9-2 presents the branching decision tree that summarizes the conceptual model used in the construction of these profile classification rules. The classification task was defined as a series of successive decisions that allows progressively finer distinctions to be made about the classification category or placement in which the student would most likely benefit. The first decision is whether a student would need special education services or would best be served by continued regular education programming. An actuarially based decision rule corresponding to this decision could be applied practically in a screening program such as the "child find" programs currently mandated by PL 94-142 which identify preschoolers who might be candidates for later special education programming. Such a rule might also be applied to screen children in regular classes whose problems suggest the possible need for special education services.

The second level of this decision tree is applied to the PIC results of children classified as likely to need special education services. This level determines whether a child's presenting problems are primarily cognitive or primarily emotional/behavioral in nature. If the child's problems are considered to be primarily cognitive, the next decision is whether these problems are more similar to those presented by mentally impaired children or learning-disabled children. A final discrimination determines the type of learning-disability program or the level of mental impairment. If, on the other hand, the child's problems are predicted to be primarily emotional/behavioral, a final decision recommends either school social work services or classification as emotionally impaired, with the special classroom or support services that typically are provided for such children.

Figure 9-2 also presents the rules for each decision within this classification system. Each rule is a linear combination of PIC profile scale T scores and is easily calculated for an individual student once scale raw scores are transformed into T-score units. Each rule was constructed on the basis of a discriminant function analysis of the two categories or groups of derivation sample students relevant to that decision in the classification system. In the analysis corresponding to Rule 1, the discriminated groups were regular education students versus all special education students, ignoring specific placement category. The scales included in this rule reflect the multiple cognitive and emotional–behavioral problem dimensions that typically distinguish students in special education from their peers in regular education classrooms.

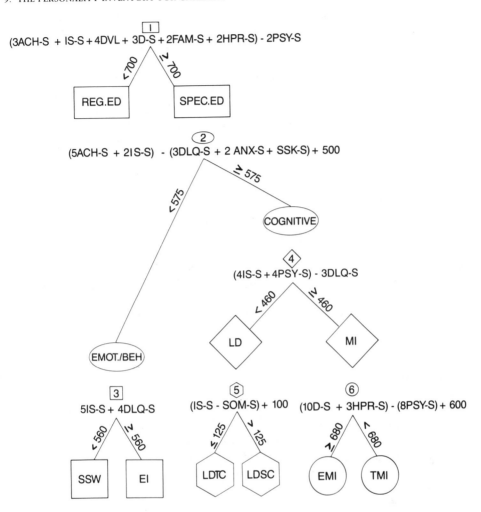

Note: REG.ED. = Regular Educational Programming; SPEC ED. = Special
Educational Programming; COGNITIVE = Primary Cognitive Impairment;
EMOT./BEH = Primary Emotional/Behavioral Impairment; LD = Learning
Disabled; MI = Mentally Impaired; SSW = School Social Work Services'
EI = Emotionally Impaired; LDTC = Learning Disabled Teacher Consultant
Services; LDSC = Learning Disabled Self-Contained Classroom;
EMI = Educable Mentally Impaired; TMI = Trainable Mentally Impaired

Figure 9-2. Proposed rules for a PIC-based educational classification system.

Rule 2 was derived by contrasting all learning-disabled and mentally impaired
students from all students either certified as emotionally impaired or supported
by school social work services. The PIC dimensions reflected in Rule 2 are consistent with the decision to be made at this level of the decision tree, as high scores
reflect the preponderance of cognitive deficit characteristics and low scores indicate a preponderance of emotional/behavioral problem characteristics.

The two groups discriminated in the derivation of Rule 4 were all learning-
disabled versus all mentally impaired students. The dimensions included in Rule
4 reflect the intellectual and adaptive behavior deficits that are commonly assessed
in the differential diagnosis of learning-disabled and mentally impaired students.

The derivation of Rules 3, 5, and 6 was dependent on discriminations of the two groups within each of the three general impairment categories—emotionally/behaviorally impaired, learning disabled, and mentally impaired. The composition of each of these rules likewise conceptually reflects the discriminations made at each of these points on the decision tree. For example, Rule 3 dimensions assess the relative severity of cognitive and behavioral impairments required for certification as emotionally impaired. Scores for Rule 5 reflect, in part, differences in the level or breadth of cognitive impairments between children receiving services in special classes for learning disabilities versus those receiving services in support programs. Rule 6 dimensions reflect differences in adaptive behavior and emotional/behavioral problem characteristics that have been reported for TMI- and EMI-classified students (Cole, 1976).

The scales in each classification equation are weighted to reflect the relative importance of each variable's contribution to the decision process. Constants were added to three of the rules to avoid the possibility of negative values. Inclusion of the suffix "-S" to the scale abbreviations in these rules indicates that they are based upon the 12 substantive scales (ACH–SSK) available when the first 280 items of the Revised Format Administration Booklet are completed. Three scale subsets had been applied to these classification tasks: 12 full-length profile scales, 12 shortened profile scales, and 4 broad-band factor scales. Because the shortened version's clinical profile scales performed with equal or superior effectiveness in the initial discriminant function analysis, they were chosen for use in the final rule development. The advantage of using a scale subset that requires completion of only a part of the inventory item pool is obvious given the psychoeducational process where time pressures and/or parental resistance may preclude completion of the entire inventory.

Once the classification rules had been constructed, cutting scores were established for each rule by examining the distribution of scores obtained in each pair of groups studied. These cutting scores are placed in Figure 9-2 on the branches of the decision tree model. In order to evaluate the effectiveness of the rules system for classifying individual students according to their educational placement, all derivation sample and validation sample subjects were processed through the system in two stages. The first stage evaluated the PIC as a screening instrument, that is, its ability to separate regular education from special education students. The second stage evaluated the PIC as a classification/placement instrument within special education in terms of its ability to classify known groups of students receiving various types of special education services. The accuracy of the derivation and validation samples' placements was assessed at both the level representing the type of major handicap (emotional/behavioral, learning disabled, mentally impaired) and at the six end points that represent the much more narrow specific placements.

Screening and Classification Accuracy

Application of the PIC-based classification rules in both the derivation and validation samples suggested considerable value for this actuarial approach to assessing special education needs. Rule 1 accomplished its screening purpose with considerable effectiveness as better than 90% of derivation sample subjects (96% of regular education and 89% of special education) were correctly predicted to be members of either regular or special education programs. When misclassifications did occur, examination of actual group membership indicated that most of these misclassifications were for students in the least impaired special education placement groups (LDTC and SSW) for which service delivery does not involve special class placements. Similarly, impressive classification results were obtained for Rule 1 predictions in the three validation samples (85–90% correct classifications), suggesting considerable generalizability for this rule in assessing the need for special education services.

How might Rule 1 be practically applied in psychoeducational assessment and classification? This study suggests that the assessment practitioner can be reasonably confident (by virture of the obtained statistical relationship between Rule 1 scores and the classifications of regular and special education students) that an individual student obtaining a Rule 1 value above the cutting score should be considered for special education services. The practitioner may then choose to continue the assessment process with traditional assessment methods or through application of subsequent rules in this PIC-based classification system. It is suggested that Rule 1 will require validation in preschool and secondary populations before it can be applied with confidence to individual students in these age groups.

Application of Rules 2–6 in both the derivation and validation samples, although less impressive than the results for Rule 1, nevertheless suggest the value of an actuarial approach to the classification of special educational needs. Table 9-2 presents the results of the application of Rules 2 and 4 to derivation sample special education students to predict general impairment category. Table 9-3 summarizes the additional application of Rules 3, 5, and 6 to this sample. Examination of these two tables documents that these rules were considerably more effective in predicting the intermediate impairment categories than the more specific special education placements. These rules were most effective in classifying mentally impaired students at both levels of classification, as 90% of Trainable Mentally Impaired (TMI) and 80% of Educable Mentally Impaired (EMI) students were correctly classified when processed through the entire PIC decision tree. Although it is reasonable to conclude that these students would be more accurately classified using a traditional individual assessment, these results which distinguished mentally impaired students from children with other educational handicaps provide rather impressive evidence for classifications based solely on maternal-derived revised format PIC profile scales.

Table 9-2
Intermediate Special Education Program Classifications for Derivation Sample Special Education Subjects

		Predicted group membership		
Actual group	N	Learning disabled	Mentally impaired	Emotionally/ Behaviorally impaired
Learning disabled:	68	41 (60.3%)	13 (19.1%)	14 (20.6%)
Mentally impaired:	59	2 (3.4%)	57 (96.6%)	0
Emotionally/Behaviorally impaired:	65	9 (13.8%)	1 (1.5%)	55 (84.6%)

Percentage of cases correctly classified: 79.7%

Table 9-3
Final Special Education Program Classifications for
Derivation Sample Special Education Subjects

Actual group[a]	N	Predicted group membership					
		LDSC	LDTC	TMI	EMI	EI	SSW
LDSC:	30	14 (46.7%)	4 (13.3%)	1 (3.3%)	7 (23.3%)	2 (6.7%)	2 (6.7%)
LDTC:	38	3 (7.9%)	20 (52.6%)	1 (2.6%)	4 (10.5%)	4 (10.5%)	6 (15.8%)
TMI:	29	0	1 (3.4%)	26 (89.7%)	2 (6.9%)	0	0
EMI:	30	0	1 (3.3%)	5 (16.7%)	24 (80.0%)	0	0
EI:	24	4 (16.7%)	1 (4.2%)	1 (4.2%)	0	12 (50.0%)	6 (25.0%)
SSW:	41	1 (2.4%)	3 (7.3%)	0	0	10 (24.4%)	27 (65.9%)

Percentage of cases correctly classified: 64.1%

[a]LDSC, Learning disabled–self-contained classroom; LDTC, learning disabled–teacher consultant support service; TMI, trainable mentally impaired; EMI, educable mentally impaired; EI, emotionally impaired; SSW, school social work services.

This branching rules system also impressively classified students whose emotional/behavioral characteristics were assumed to underlie the primary handicapping condition (EI and SSW). Although classification accuracy was substantially reduced when predictions were extended to the level which identified a specific placement category, the majority of misclassifications for these students were within the same general impairment category. This suggests the value of the actuarial approach at the intermediate level of classification for students presenting these emotional/behavioral characteristics.

Learning-disabled students were the most difficult to classify at both levels using these rules. The 60% correct classification rate at the intermediate level indicates that a significant proportion of PIC-predicted learning-disabled students received final placement classifications outside of the two learning disability options. For example, the majority of PIC prediction errors for LDSC students were identifications as EMI placements, a result that likely reflects the below-average IQs of many of these students (LDSC mean IQ derivation sample = 85). This finding may also reflect the suggestion in the literature that increasing societal pressures and changing classification standards have allowed many EMI students to obtain special education services for the learning disabled (Goldstein, Arkell, Ashcroft, Hurley, & Lilly, 1975; Gottlieb, Alter, & Gottlieb, 1983). The majority of misclassifications for LDTC students, on the other hand, were predicted by this PIC-based classification system to receive either EI or SSW services. This finding likely reflects a frequent observation that emotional/behavioral difficulties are associated with learning disabilities (Porter & Rourke, 1985; Ross, 1976, 1977) as well as the fact that nearly one-third of those students also received school social work services.

Classification of special education students in the three validation samples revealed, in most cases, the reduction in classification accuracy expected on cross-validation. Interestingly, learning-disabled students in the three samples were actually classified more accurately by Rules 2 and 4 than were learning-disabled students in the derivation sample (64% to 87% correct classifications). It was not possible to further classify these students into specific placement categories as these students had not been identified by type of placement (self-contained vs. teacher consultant) in these studies. An unexpected finding was that two of the validation sample groups showed substantial reductions in classification accuracy when compared with their counterparts in the derivation sample. Only 25% of Clark's (1982) emotionally impaired (EI) subjects were correctly classified by the rules, the majority being misclassified as learning disabled. Similarly, only 55% of DeKrey's (1982) mentally disabled subjects were correctly classified by the rules, with a substantial percentage being misclassified as LDSC. Because sample-specific characteristics may account in large part for these findings (e.g., a majority of DeKrey's mentally disabled students obtained IQs between 70 and 85, reflecting Iowa state guidelines), the important effects of differences in sample characteristics for similarly classified students across different school districts and states demonstrate the inherent difficulties with actuarially based classification using a system of mutually exclusive categories.

Future Applications in Special Education

The difficulties encountered by this system in correctly classifying learning-disabled students in the derivation sample and emotionally impaired and mentally disabled students in the Clark (1982) and DeKrey (1982) samples, respectively, suggest an important limitation of this approach to actuarial classification of special education needs. One characteristic of branching classification rules is that referred students cannot be compared to every possible handicapping category and placement group the individualized psychoeducational assessment process allows; that is, once a student's scores place him or her within one branch of the decision tree, classifications positioned on alternative branches cannot be considered. Based upon the PIC profile scale T scores, each student, in effect, is identified as similar to only one general handicap category and to only one placement group. This approach would be quite satisfactory if each handicap category and each special education placement represented an orthogonal set of child characteristics. The school psychology literature stongly suggests that this is not the case (Forness, 1976; Hallahan & Kauffman, 1976, 1977), particularly with regard to the classifications of learning disabled and emotionally impaired. Therefore, these current classification rules may not accurately capture the characteristics of students who present problems in more than one area. In addition, this classification approach fails to appreciate the heterogeneity of characteristics that has been demonstrated for children similarly classified both within and across school districts (Hallahan & Kauffman, 1977; McDermott, 1982; Wepman, Cruickshank, Deutsch, Morency, & Strother, 1975).

Future classification efforts might improve upon this system by employing one of two alternative strategies. The first strategy, currently being pursued by the authors, compares students' profiles with a series of mean profiles, each representing a special education handicapping condition or specific placement to generate an index of similarity to each mean profile. In this manner, students with multiple problems might appear equally similar to two or more mean profiles. The second approach might apply cluster analyses to large heterogeneous samples of children receiving special education services. The resulting stable empirically validated clusters would supplement or replace traditional handicapping categories. This approach has recently been applied to the classification of children and adolescents evaluated in a guidance setting, resulting in a diagnostic system that could serve as an alternative to traditional classification nosologies. This project is presented below.

PIC Interpretation through
Profile Classification

The development of an actuarial interpretive system for the individual PIC profile scales has facilitated a descriptive understanding of child behavior at home and in the classroom. In this manner, information about an individual child is obtained for several substantive problem behavior areas (Lachar, 1982; Lachar & Gdowski, 1979). In fact, the wealth of child behavior information provided by multidimensional instruments such as the PIC has stimulated serious consideration that such measures could form the basis of a classification system that would represent an alternative to traditional psychiatric diagnostic categories (cf. Lessing, Williams, & Gil, 1982). As discussed in Chapter 1 of this volume, the available psychiatric diagnostic systems used with children and adolescents, such as the 3rd edition Diagnostic and Statistical Manual, (DSM-III; American Psychiatric Association, 1980), and the Group for the Advancement of Psychiatry (GAP) (1966), have problems due to their unreliability (cf. Mattison, Cantwell, Russell, & Will, 1979; Werry, Methven, Fitzpatrick, & Dixon, 1983) and their questionable validity (cf. Garmezy, 1978; Rutter, 1978). Further, single diagnostic labels (such as Attention Deficit Disorder with Hyperactivity) typically describe a single dimension of behavior for an individual child. Realistically, children who receive the same global diagnostic label are likely to vary on a significant number of other behavioral dimensions (e.g., problem-solving ability, social skills, internalization symptomatology) that are also related to their overall adjustment and prognosis (cf. Breen & Barkley, 1983).

Despite the common knowledge regarding the weaknesses of psychiatric diagnostic labels for children and adolescents, there has been relatively little research until very recently which has explored the usefulness and ability of objective, parent-informant measures such as the PIC to assign children within a classification system. While the actuarial systems of Lachar (1982) and Lachar and Gdowski (1979) provide relatively comprehensive descriptions of individual children, these systems do not conveniently classify children into separate groups, each with its own unique pattern of problem behavior. The primary goal of any classification typology (which psychiatric diagnostic categories have not yet achieved) is to partition a population of children referred for mental health services into a discrete number of "types" or groups, each with their own characteristic features and systems. Thus, children with similar overall ability levels, degree of impulse control, external stressors, and areas of poor adjustment should be classified together and separately from children with other behavioral and social–emotional patterns. Further, if children with varying patterns of assets and problems require distinctly different types of intervention for optimal outcome (e.g., outpatient vs. inpatient treatment, medication, family participation in therapy), a reliable and valid classification system should be capable of making these distinctions.

Identification of PIC Profile Types

Recent research has used the PIC profile scales as the basis for an empirically derived typology that may offer an alternative to the current psychiatric diagnostic labels. Gdowski, Lachar, and Kline (1985) used the classification procedure of cluster analysis within a sample of almost 1,800 children and adolescents who were referred for mental health services to construct such a typology. The total sample included 1,226 evaluations at one child psychiatry facility (67% male; 56% white, 44% black; M age = 11.6) and six "marker" samples, including psychotic ($N = 79$), mentally retarded ($N = 138$), adjudicated delinquent ($N = 151$), hyperactive ($N = 80$), neurologically impaired ($N = 73$), and somatizing ($N = 35$) children. These six samples are fully described in Wirt et al. (1984). These marker samples were included to determine whether the resulting PIC profile typology classified the cases in a conceptually meaningful way (e.g., the PIC profiles of hyperactive children should not have been randomly assigned across profile clusters, nor should the profiles of psychotic children have appeared in the same clusters with adjudicated delinquent children).

Cluster analysis is a multivariate statistical technique that forms groups of subjects based upon their similarity across several measures such that cases within each group are more similar to each other than to members of other groups. In this study, "similarity" was determined by computer comparisons among the PIC profiles of all children in this large sample. Gdowski et al. (1985) also partitioned this sample into separate halves (split 1, $N = 889$; split 2, $N = 893$) to ensure that profile groups identified by cluster analysis were stable and replicated across these independent samples. A total of 11 PIC profile types formed by the cluster analysis replicated across the Split 1 and 2 samples and classified over 80% of all cases. Subsequent analyses demonstrated that these PIC clusters differed significantly in subject age, sex, and the proportion of the six marker samples classified into each cluster.

Table 9-4 presents the mean PIC scale T scores in both study samples for the 11 replicated clusters. In order to more clearly present the pattern of PIC scale elevations most characteristic of these 11 profile types, mean T scores are reported only for those scales with mean elevations within the clinical range ($T > 59$ for L, ADJ, ACH, DVL, FAM, and HPR; $T > 69$ for DEF, IS, SOM, D, WDL, ANX, and SSK; $T > 79$ for DLQ and PSY; $T > 99$ for F).

Table 9-5 presents the marker sample composition of each cluster and the proportion of the heterogeneous child guidance profiles classified within each cluster for both split 1 and split 2 samples. Goodness-of-fit chi-square analyses are presented for clusters that classified at least 10 marker sample profiles to test whether the composition of each cluster differed significantly from sample base rates.

Characteristics of Profile Clusters

Inspection of Tables 9-4 and 9-5 reveals that these 11 PIC profile types had distinct mean profiles and that the marker sample protocols were not randomly assigned to these groups by the cluster analysis algorithm. PIC profile types included a within-normal-limits (WNL) mean group (Cluster 1) and clusters with mean elevations suggestive of cognitive impairment (see mean elevations of ACH, IS, and DVL: Clusters 3, 4, 5, and 6), behavioral dyscontrol (see mean elevations of DLQ and HPR: Clusters 4, 7, 10, and 11), depression and anxiety (see mean

Table 9-4
Mean PIC Profiles for Replicated Clusters

PIC scale	Split sample		Replicated PIC cluster										
			1	3	4	5	6	7	8	9	10	11	12
	1	(N)	137	41	62	42	81	38	27	42	102	74	80
	2	(N)	158	51	50	47	65	44	25	43	82	77	89
L	1		—a	—	—	—	—	—	—	—	—	—	—
	2		—	—	—	—	—	—	—	—	—	—	—
F	1		—	—	—	—	—	—	—	—	—	—	—
	2		—	102	—	—	—	107	—	—	—	—	—
DEF	1		—	—	—	—	—	—	—	—	—	—	—
	2		—	—	—	—	—	—	—	—	—	—	—
ADJ	1		63	93	101	86	72	99	82	98	87	82	75
	2		67	102	99	92	73	104	77	89	85	90	78
ACH	1		—	79	80	77	71	64	—	66	61	—	71
	2		—	82	80	79	75	67	62	—	60	—	71
IS	1		—	89	88	114	111	—	—	—	—	—	—
	2		—	98	85	114	118	—	—	—	—	—	—
DVL	1		—	81	76	86	76	61	60	62	—	—	69
	2		—	86	77	90	83	61	69	—	—	—	69
SOM	1		—	—	—	—	—	—	—	—	—	—	—
	2		—	70	—	—	—	73	—	71	—	—	—
D	1		—	83	70	—	—	85	—	84	—	—	—
	2		—	88	—	—	—	88	—	86	—	—	—
FAM	1		—	—	62	—	—	70	—	67	69	—	—
	2		—	65	—	—	—	68	—	64	69	62	—
DLQ	1		—	—	96	—	—	105	—	85	114	—	—
	2		—	83	101	—	—	115	—	81	109	89	—
WDL	1		—	89	—	—	—	79	71	—	—	—	—
	2		—	83	—	—	—	80	—	—	—	—	—
ANX	1		—	70	—	—	—	—	—	83	—	—	—
	2		—	78	—	—	—	76	—	84	—	—	—
PSY	1		—	111	81	109	—	87	100	83	—	—	—
	2		—	113	—	112	—	96	117	—	—	—	—
HPR	1		—	—	78	—	—	—	—	77	61	80	—
	2		—	—	81	—	—	72	—	—	—	79	61
SSK	1		—	77	79	75	—	83	76	77	—	68	61
	2		—	84	74	78	—	78	71	72	—	76	—

aMeans are reported for those scales with elevations above their respective interpretive T-score cutoffs.

elevations of D and ANX: Clusters 3, 7, and 9), family conflict (see mean elevation of FAM: Clusters 7 and 10), and social skills deficits (see mean elevation of SSK: Clusters 3, 4, 5, 7, and 8). Consistent with the problem behavior areas suggested by their mean PIC profiles, Clusters 3, 5, and 8 classified above base rate proportions of psychotic children; Clusters 5 and 6 represented high proportions of retarded children; Clusters 7 and 10 contained high proportions of adjudicated delinquents; and Clusters 11 and 12 included relatively high proportions of hyperactive children. The mean ages of Clusters 5 and 6 (characterized by cognitive impairment) were significantly younger than sample base rate, while the two clusters containing high proportions of adjudicated delinquents (Clusters 7 and 10) were significantly older than base rate. These 11 profile types did not differ with regard to their racial or socioeconomic composition.

Development of Classification Rules

While these initial results appeared very promising, the actual use of this classification system with individual children was problematic. These PIC profiles were classified into cluster groups by a very complex computer program which evaluated the degree of similarity between individual profiles and the mean profiles of all clusters. This is hardly an activity that clinicians could reasonably hope to duplicate without computer access and expertise. In order to facilitate classification of individual PIC profiles into this typology, a series of objective and easy-to-use rules were developed by Kline, Lachar, and Gdowski (in press). These rules specify the T-score elevations most characteristic of each cluster and are presented in a flowchart in Figure 9-3.

These rules correspond to the identically numbered clusters previously described. To classify in individual profile, the clinician scans down the flowchart until a complete match between the T-score specifications and individual profile is obtained. Thus, these rules are sequentially applied and a profile is classified by the first rule for which all specifications are met. Rule 1 identifies all within-normal-limits (WNL) PIC profiles which have all 12 PIC substantive profile scales below clinically significant elevations. Rule 2 classifies all profiles having a single significantly elevated PIC scale and thus identifies all "spike" profiles. Rules 3–6 identify "cognitive-deficit" types which all have at least two significant elevations on the scales of the PIC Cognitive Triad (ACH, IS, DVL). Rules 7–12 classify "noncognitive-deficit" types which include IS scores within the normal range. An individual child's profile could be left unclassified at two points in this decision tree; these options are designated by the "exit" points in Figure 9-3.

Table 9-5
Proportion (%) of Criterion Marker Samples within Replicated PIC Clusters

Marker	Split	\multicolumn{11}{c}{Replicated PIC cluster}

Marker	Split	1	3	4	5	6	7	8	9	10	11	12
Hyperactive	1	10	0	0	0	4	0	0	75	0	64	41
(14%)[a]	2	22	0	25	4	0	0	0	20	0	67	50
Delinquent	1	43	0	25	0	2	100	0	0	97	4	19
(27%)	2	13	14	42	0	0	100	0	20	97	11	23
Cerebral dys-	1	20	0	38	4	13	0	0	25	0	21	22
function	2	24	7	8	4	19	0	0	40	0	17	23
(13%)												
Psychoso-	1	20	8	0	0	0	0	7	0	0	4	7
matic (6%)	2	19	0	0	0	2	0	0	20	3	6	5
Retarded	1	6	23	38	53	75	0	21	0	3	7	7
(25%)	2	2	29	17	46	74	0	7	0	0	0	0
Psychotic	1	0	69	0	43	6	0	71	0	0	0	4
(14%)	2	0	50	8	46	5	0	93	0	0	0	0
χ^2	1	.01	.01	—[b]	.01	.01	—[b]	.01	—[b]	.01	.01	.01
	2	.01	.01	ns	.01	.01	—[b]	.01	—[b]	.01	.01	.01
General	1	14[c]	5	9	2	5	6	2	6	11	8	9
Clinic	2	17	6	6	3	4	6	2	6	8	10	11

[a]Percentage of total criterion profiles ($N = 556$),
[b]$p < .10$.
[c]Percentage of sample 1 or 2 general clinic profiles (each $N = 613$).

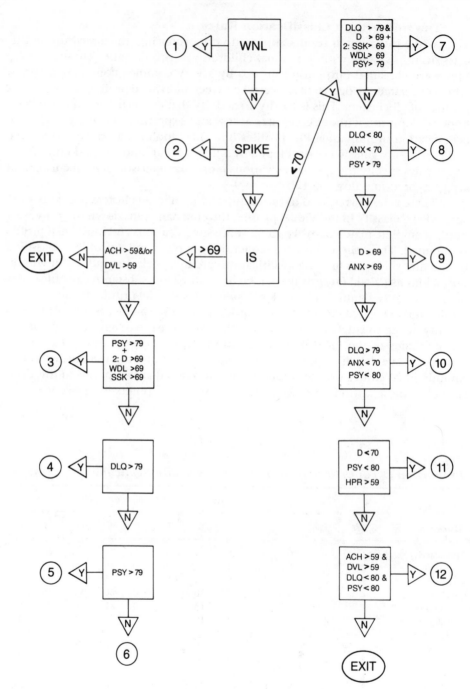

Figure 9-3. PIC profile type classification rules.

Kline *et al.* (in press) demonstrated that the groups generated by the application of the rules presented in Figure 9-3 correspond very closely with their original cluster counterparts. These rules also classified over 90% of the Gdowski *et al.* (1985) samples.

Interpretation of Profile Types

The Kline *et al.* (in press) and Gdowski *et al.* (1985) studies demonstrate that PIC profile types identified by the cluster analysis replicated across independent samples and classified meaningful proportions of marker sample children. Further, individual children were easily classified into one of these profile types upon the application of a set of sequential rules. The major issue for a typology, however, was yet to be addressed: Is this PIC typology valid? Does membership in this profile typology have any relationship to independent and external information about child and adolescent adjustment?

This critical issue was evaluated by Kline, Lachar, and Gdowski (1984) as 1,333 children and adolescents who obtained psychiatric evaluations were classified into 12 PIC profile types as defined in Figure 9-3. External information was available for each case in the form of behavior rating forms completed by each child's mother or other female guardian, classroom teacher, and interviewing clinician. The parent rating form was completed at home prior to the first clinic appointment and contained 102 items which yielded information about the child's problem behaviors and their chronicity and medical, pregnancy, and developmental history. The teacher rating form contained 95 items descriptive of classroom behavior and academic achievement. The clinician rating form included 168 items reflecting the child's affective state, cognitive status, interview behavior, and family characteristics. All items were in the form of a true–false format, and endorsement of any item indicated the presence of some particular problem behavior. These three forms are reproduced in Lachar and Gdowski (1979).

In order to summarize the information presented by these numerous rating form items, the items of each form were separately subjected to factor analyses (Lachar *et al.*, 1984). Factor analysis of the parent checklist yielded five dimensions that incorporated 52 items; factor analysis of the teacher form yielded seven dimensions that incorporated 74 items; and factor analysis of the clinician form yielded seven dimensions that incorporated 72 items. The specific items that loaded on each of these 19 dimensions are entirely reproduced in Lachar *et al.* (1984). Simple unit weights (1 for present, 0 for absent) were assigned for each item, and the rating dimension scores for each case were the total number of endorsements within each of these dimensions.

The rating form dimensions and the number of items represented by each dimension were as follows: Parent Dimensions: Hostility/Dyscontrol (16), Depressive/Somatic Symptoms (16), Antisocial Behavior (11), Developmental Delay (12), and Cognitive/Attentional Deficits (9); Teacher Dimensions: Hostility/Impulsivity (24), Poor Study Skills (12), Academic Delay (11), Poor Classroom Adjustment (12), Poor Self-Concept/Depressive Symptoms (11), Social Withdrawal (8), and Distractible/Motor Restlessness (9); and Clinician Dimensions: Hostility/Dyscontrol (14), Language/Motor Deficits (11), Emotional Lability/Impulsivity (13), Disorganization/Limited Reality Testing (8), Depressive/Somatic Symptoms (11), Antisocial Behavior (7), and Social Withdrawal (8).

Table 9-6 presents the mean scores for these 19 problem behavior dimen-

Table 9-6
PIC Rule Group Means across All Problem Behavior Factors[a]

Problem behavior dimension	WNL	Spikes	IS>69			IS<70							Whole sample	F(10, 1,199)
	1	2	3	4	5	6	7	8	9	10	11	12		
(N)	24	64	156	149	36	75	153	51	161	204	79	28	1,333	
Parent informant factors														
I. H/D	3.7	6.3	9.5	10.9	7.5	7.2	10.5	7.5	8.1	9.5	8.8	5.0	8.8	19.40**
II. D/SS	3.2	3.4	7.1	5.5	5.1	3.9	7.5	4.9	7.9	4.6	3.6	4.4	5.7	28.19**
III. AB	2.1	3.3	4.4	5.4	2.4	2.8	6.2	2.8	4.2	6.1	3.5	2.4	4.5	29.77**
IV. DD	1.0	1.0	2.6	2.3	3.4	2.0	1.6	1.9	1.0	1.2	1.2	0.9	1.7	12.56**
V. C/AD	2.1	3.1	6.2	5.9	6.2	5.0	5.3	4.8	4.5	4.2	4.7	4.5	4.8	18.39**
Teacher informant factors														
I. H/I	6.2	8.5	10.6	13.5	8.0	10.1	9.7	9.3	8.3	11.5	12.0	6.5	10.2	8.22**
II. PSS	2.5	3.6	4.5	5.5	4.3	4.9	4.4	4.1	3.3	4.1	4.0	5.0	4.2	4.29**
III. AD	1.7	2.9	5.2	5.7	5.0	5.7	3.1	3.3	2.6	3.2	3.1	5.3	3.8	15.85**
IV. PCA	4.0	4.9	6.3	6.9	5.8	5.9	5.6	5.0	4.8	6.4	5.8	5.1	5.7	5.35**
V. PSC/DS	1.9	2.1	2.7	2.8	1.5	2.2	2.7	2.4	2.5	2.2	2.0	2.2	2.4	1.78
VI. SW	1.2	2.0	2.7	2.3	2.5	2.1	2.3	2.8	2.3	1.8	1.7	2.8	2.2	3.35**
VII. D/MR	2.1	2.9	3.6	3.7	4.4	3.6	2.7	3.9	2.8	2.9	3.6	3.2	3.2	5.56**
Clinician informant factors														
I. H/D	2.2	3.4	4.8	6.2	3.6	4.5	5.9	4.5	3.8	5.6	4.5	3.4	4.9	8.60**
II. L/MD	0.6	1.4	3.6	2.5	4.8	3.0	1.5	1.7	1.3	1.5	1.7	2.3	2.0	27.72**
III. EL/I	2.9	4.6	6.7	7.6	6.1	4.9	6.9	5.8	5.1	6.1	5.8	3.9	6.0	12.19**
IV. D/LRT	0.4	0.6	0.9	0.3	1.3	0.4	0.4	1.1	0.5	0.3	0.3	0.1	0.5	7.97**
V. D/SS	2.4	2.3	2.9	2.5	1.7	2.6	2.8	2.9	3.9	1.9	1.9	2.4	2.6	10.82**
VI. AB	0.6	0.9	1.3	1.5	0.4	0.8	2.1	0.7	1.1	2.3	0.8	0.9	1.4	17.23**
VII. SW	1.1	1.7	3.2	2.4	2.7	2.4	2.8	2.7	2.3	2.0	1.7	2.0	2.4	7.48**

PIC rule groups

**p < .01.

[a]H/D, Hostility/Dyscontrol; D/SS, Depressive/Somatic Symptoms; AB, Antisocial Behavior; DD, Developmental Delay; C/AD, Cognitive/Attentional Deficits; H/I, Hostility/Impulsivity; PSS, Poor Study Skills; AD, Academic Delay; PCA, Poor Classroom Adjustment; PSC/DS, Poor Self-Concept/Depressive Symptoms; SW, Social Withdrawal; D/MR, Distractibility/Motor Restlessness; L/MD, Language/Motor Deficits; EL/I, Emotional Lability/Impulsivity; D/LRT, Disorganized/Limited Reality Testing.

sions from the three informant sources for each of the 12 PIC profile types. Results of analysis of variance tests for each rating dimension across profile types are also reported in Table 9-6. Of the 19 dimensions, 18 differed significantly across the 12 PIC profile types, suggesting strong correspondence between membership in this typology and ratings of home and school behavior. Post hoc comparisons conducted between all pairs of PIC profile types for each rating dimension demonstrated a wealth of differences among these profile types. In fact, these intergroup differences were so abundant that it was difficult to delineate the problem behavior patterns characteristic of each profile type.

Table 9-7 presents an alternative analysis in which the mean dimension score for each profile was contrasted with a mean score derived from the remainder of the sample. Scanning down each column of Table 9-7 quickly identifies those characteristics descriptive (+ and + + for means significantly above base rate) and not descriptive (– and – – for means significantly below base rate) of each PIC type. For example, relatively less symptomatology was associated with the WNL (Rule 1) and ''spike'' (Rule 2) profile groups, while the Rule 3–6 types were all associated with greater than base rate attributions of cognitive and attentional deficits by parents, assignment of academic delay and distractibility/motor restlessness by teachers, and observation of language and motor deficits by clinicians. The Rule 7 group, characterized by elevations on DLQ, D, and at least two of scales WDL, PSY, and SSK, evidenced greater than base rate internalization and externalization symptomatology, while the Rule 11 group (with an elevation of HPR) received above base rate levels of teacher descriptions in the areas of hostility and impulsivity. The Rule 9 group, characterized by ANX and D elevations, was associated with above base rate parental and clinician description of depression/ somatic symptomatology. Also, the Rule 10 type, with a single significant elevation on DLQ, was associated with higher than base rate levels of hostility, impulsivity, and antisocial behavior by all rating sources, as well as with significantly lower than base rate levels of internalization symptoms and emotional distress.

Future Developments

These preliminary findings for this profile-based classification system appear very encouraging. The authors are currently completing several studies that expand the base of validation data for this typology. For example, a series of analyses have been conducted which have determined the specific behavior correlates for each profile type, much in the same way that the correlates for the individual profile scales were identified. These analyses have attempted to discover the more molecular behaviors that are associated with each profile type to supplement the information conveyed by these 19 rating dimensions. In addition, we have begun to examine the case histories and course of treatment information of individual children and adolescents from each type who have been evaluated and received treatment. It is hoped that these analyses will outline specific etiologies or treatment outcomes characteristic of each profile type.

Summary

The Personality Inventory for Children (PIC) is an objective, multiscale instrument completed by an adult informant, usually the child's or adolescent's mother. The PIC can be completed in 15 to 60 minutes, depending upon the in-

Table 9-7
Problem Behavior Patterns of the 12 PIC Rule Groups[a]

	WNL	Spikes		IS>69					IS<70			
Problem behavior dimension	1	2	3	4	5	6	7	8	9	10	11	12
Parent informant factors												
I. Hostility/Dyscontrol	--	--	+	++	ns[b]	--	++	-	-	++	ns	--
II. Depressive/Somatic Symptoms	--	--	++	ns	ns	--	++	ns	++	--	--	ns
III. Antisocial Behavior	--	--	ns	++	--	--	++	ns	ns	++	--	--
IV. Developmental Delay	--	--	++	++	++	ns	ns	--	ns	--	-	--
V. Cognitive/Attentional Deficits	--	--	++	++	++	ns	++	ns	-	--	ns	ns
Teacher informant factors												
I. Hostility/Impulsivity	--	-	ns	++	ns	ns	ns	ns	--	++	+	--
II. Poor Study Skills	--	ns	ns	++	ns	ns	ns	ns	--	ns	ns	ns
III. Academic Delay	--	-	++	++	++	++	-	ns	--	--	ns	+
IV. Poor Classroom Adjustment	--	ns	+	++	++	++	-	ns	--	++	ns	ns
V. Poor Self-Concept/Depressive Symptoms	--			++	++	ns	ns	ns	--	++	ns	ns
VI. Social Withdrawal	--	ns	++	ns	ns	ns	ns	+	ns	--	-	ns
VII. Distractibility/Motor Restlessness	--	ns	+	++	++	ns	--	ns	-	--	ns	ns
Clinician factors												
I. Hostility/Dyscontrol	--	--	ns	++	-	ns	++	ns	--	++	ns	-
II. Language/Motor Deficits	--	--	++	++	++	++	--	ns	--	--	ns	ns
III. Emotional Lability/Impulsivity	--	--	++	++	ns	--	++	ns	--	ns	ns	--
IV. Disorganized/Limited Reality Testing	ns	ns	++	-	++	ns	ns	++	ns	--	ns	ns
V. Depressive/Somatic Symptoms	--	--	ns	ns	--	--	++	--	++	--	--	ns
VI. Antisocial Behavior	--	--	ns	ns	--	--	++	--	-	++	--	ns
VII. Social Withdrawal	--	--	++	ns	ns	ns	++	ns	ns	--	--	ns

—(not conducted)—

[a] +, -, $p<.05$; ++, --, $p<.01$.
[b] ns, Not significant.

ventory length selected (131, 180, 420 items). Scales have been constructed using a variety of item selection procedures, although the demonstration of external validity has been an integral part of this process. Scales measure cognitive ability, behavioral and emotional dimensions, and family character, as well as provide estimates of inventory validity. These dimensions represent a relatively comprehensive description of current status and appear appropriate in the clinical assessment of children and adolescents within child guidance/child psychiatry, special education, pediatrics, and juvenile justice populations. A unique characteristic of the PIC is the availability of actuarially based interpretive systems for individual scales, scale patterns, and profile types. This chapter has surveyed PIC scales and presented some evidence of their validity. Four actuarially based interpretive systems are briefly presented. Although the PIC appears straightforward and relatively simplistic in its application, accurate interpretation of profiled scores requires a rather sophisticated comprehension of the interpretive guidelines presented in current technical manuals (Lachar, 1982; Lachar & Gdowski, 1979; Wirt *et al.*, 1984).

References

Achenbach, T. M. (1981). A junior MMPI? [Review of *Multidimensional description of child personality. A manual for the Personality Inventory for Children and Actuarial assessment of child and adolescent personality: An interpretive guide for the Personality Inventory for Children profile*]. *Journal of Personality Assessment, 45*, 332–333.

American Psychiatric Association. (1980). *Diagnostic and statistical manual of mental disorders* (3rd ed.). Washington, DC: Author.

Anderson, E. E., & Quast, W. (1983). Young children in alcoholic families: A mental health needs-assessment and an intervention/prevention strategy. *Journal of Primary Prevention, 3*, 174–187.

Armstrong, G. D., Wirt, R. D., Nesbit, M. E., & Martinson, I. M. (1982). Multidimensional assessment of psychological problems in children with cancer. *Research in Nursing and Health, 5*, 205–211.

Bennett, T. S., & Welsh, M. C. (1981). Validity of a configural interpretation of the intellectual screening and achievement scales of the Personality Inventory for Children. *Educational and Psychological Measurement, 41*, 863–868.

Boersma, D. C. (1984). *Objective assessment of special needs among elementary students: Applications of the Personality Inventory for Children*. Doctoral dissertation, Wayne State University, Detroit, MI.

Breen, M. J., & Barkley, R. A. (1983). The Personality Inventory for Children (PIC): Its clinical utility with hyperactive children. *Journal of Pediatric Psychology, 8*, 359–366.

Clark, E. (1982). *Construct validity and diagnostic potential of the Personality Inventory for Children (PIC) with emotionally disturbed, learning disabled, and educable mentally retarded children*. Doctoral dissertation, Michigan State University, East Lansing.

Clark, E., Wanous, D. S., & Pompa, J. L. (1982, August). *Construct validation of the Personality Inventory for Children (PIC)*. Paper presented at the 90th annual convention of the American Psychological Association, Washington, DC.

Cole, L. J. (1976). *Adaptive behavior of the educable mentally retarded child in the home and school environment*. Doctoral dissertation, University of California, Berkeley.

Costello, C. G. (1981). Childhood depression. In E. J. Mash & L. G. Terdal (Eds.), *Behavioral assessment of childhood disorders* (pp. 305–346). New York: Guilford Press.

Cronbach, L. J. (1984). *Essentials of psychological testing* (4th ed.). New York: Harper & Row.

Daldin, H. (1985). Faking good and faking bad on the Personality Inventory for Children–Revised, shortened format. *Journal of Consulting and Clinical Psychology, 53*, 561–563.

DeKrey, S. J. (1982). *Construct validity and educational applications of the Personality Inventory for Children (PIC) - shortened form version*. Doctoral dissertation, University of Iowa, Iowa City.

DeKrey, S. J., & Ehly, S. W. (1981). Factor/cluster classification of profiles from Personality Inventory for Children in a school setting. *Psychological Reports, 48*, 843–846.

DeMoor-Peal, R., & Handal, P. J. (1983). Validity of the Personality Inventory for Children with four-year-old males and females: A caution. *Journal of Pediatric Psychology, 8,* 261–271.

Dollinger, S. J., Goh, D. S., & Cody, J. J. (1984). A note on the congruence of the WISC-R and the cognitive development scales of the Personality Inventory for Children. *Journal of Consulting and Clinical Psychology, 52,* 315–316.

Duffey, J. B., Salvia, J., Tucker, J., & Ysseldyke, J. (1981). Non-biased assessment: A need for operationalism. *Exceptional Children, 47,* 427–434.

Durrant, J. E. (1983). *Concurrent validity of the narrow-band and broad-band intellectual scales of the Personality Inventory for Children within a preschool population.* Unpublished master's thesis, University of Windsor, Windsor, Canada.

Education of All Handicapped Children's Act of 1975. Public Law 94-142. November, 1975. 20 USC 1401.

Forness, S. R. (1976). Behavioristic orientation to categorical labels. *Journal of School Psychology, 14,* 90–96.

Garmezy, N. (1978). DSM-III: Never mind the psychologists: Is it good for the children? *Clinical Psychologist, 31,* 4–9.

Gdowski, C. L., Lachar, D., & Kline, R. B. (1985). A PIC profile typology of children and adolescents: I. An empirically-derived alternative to traditional diagnosis. *Journal of Abnormal Psychology, 94,* 346–361.

Goldstein, H., Arkell, C., Ashcroft, S. C., Hurley, O. L., & Lilly, M. S. (1975). Schools. In N. Hobbs (Ed.), *Issues in the classification of children* (Vol. 2, pp. 4–61). San Francisco, CA: Jossey-Bass.

Gottlieb, J., Alter, M., & Gottlieb, B. W. (1983). Mainstreaming mentally retarded children. In J. L. Matson & J. A. Mulick (Eds.), *Handbook of mental retardation* (pp. 67–77). Oxford: Pergamon Press.

Group for the Advancement of Psychiatry (GAP). (1966). *Psychopathological disorders in childhood: Theoretical considerations and a proposed classification.* New York: Author.

Hallahan, D. P., & Kauffman, J. M. (1976). *Introduction to learning disabilities.* Englewood Cliffs, NJ: Prentice-Hall.

Hallahan, D. P., & Kauffman, J. M. (1977). Labels, categories, behaviors: ED, LD, and EMR reconsidered. *Journal of Special Education, 11,* 139–149.

Harrington, R. G., & Follett, G. M. (1984). The readability of child personality assessment instruments. *Journal of Psychoeducational Assessment, 2,* 37–48.

Helton, G. B., Workman, E. A., & Matuszek, P. A. (1982). *Psychoeducational assessment.* New York: Grune & Stratton.

Kelly, G. T. (1982). *A comparison of the Personality Inventory for Children (PIC) and the Child Behavior Checklist (CBCL) with an independent behavior checklist completed by clinicians.* Doctoral dissertation, Duke University, Durham, NC.

Kline, R. B., Lachar, D., & Gdowski, C. L. (1984, August). *A Personality Inventory for Children (PIC) typology: Comparison with psychiatric diagnosis.* Paper presented at the 92nd annual convention, American Psychological Association, Toronto, Canada.

Kline, R. B., Lachar, D., & Gdowski, C. L. (in press). *A Personality Inventory for Children (PIC) profile typology of children and adolescents: II. Classification rules and specific behavior correlates,* manuscript submitted for publication.

Kline, R. B., Lachar, D., & Sprague, D. J. (1985). The Personality Inventory for Children (PIC): An unbiased predictor of cognitive and academic status. *Journal of Pediatric Psychology, 10,* 461–477.

Kurdek, L. A. (1980). Developmental relations among children's perspective taking, moral judgment, and parent-rated behaviors. *Merrill-Palmer Quarterly, 26,* 103–121.

Kurdek, L. A. (1982). Long-term predictive validity of children's social-cognitive assessments. *Merrill-Palmer Quarterly, 28,* 511–521.

Kurdek, L. A., & Krile, D. (1983). The relation between third-through eighth-grade children's social cognition and parents' ratings of social skills and general adjustment. *Journal of Genetic Psychology, 143,* 201–206.

Lachar, D. (1982). *Personality Inventory for Children (PIC) revised format manual supplement.* Los Angeles, CA: Western Psychological Services.

Lachar, D., & Gdowski, C. L. (1979). *Actuarial assessment of child and adolescent personality: An interpretive guide for the Personality Inventory for Children profile.* Los Angeles, CA: Western Psychological Services.

Lachar, D., Gdowski, C. L., & Snyder, D. K. (1982). Broad-band dimensions of psychopathology: Factor scales for the Personality Inventory for Children. *Journal of Consulting and Clinical Psychology, 50,* 634–642.

Lachar, D., Gdowski, C. L., & Snyder, D. K. (1984). External validation of the Personality Inventory for Children profile and factor scales: Parent, teacher, and clinician ratings. *Journal of Consulting and Clinical Psychology, 52,* 155–164.

Lachar, D., & Sharp, J. R. (1979). Use of parents' MMPIs in the research and evaluation of children: A review of the literature and some new data. In J. N. Butcher (Ed.), *New developments in the use of the MMPI* (pp. 203–240). Minneapolis: University of Minnesota Press.

Lachar, D., & Wirt, R. D. (1981). A data-based analysis of the psychometric performance of the Personality Inventory for Children (PIC): An alternative to the Achenbach review. *Journal of Personality Assessment, 45,* 614–616.

Leon, G. R., Kendall, P. C., & Garber, J. (1980). Depression in children: Parent, teacher, and child perspectives. *Journal of Abnormal Child Psychology, 8,* 221–235.

Lessing, E. E., Williams, V., & Gill, E. (1982). A cluster-analytically derived typology: Feasible alternative to clinical diagnostic classification of children? *Journal of Abnormal Child Psychology, 10,* 451–482.

Lobovits, D. A., & Handal, P. J. (1985). Childhood depression: Prevalence using DSM-III criterion and validity of parent and child depression scales. *Journal of Pediatric Psychology, 10,* 45–54.

Marks, P. A., Seeman, W., & Haller, D. L. (1974). *The actuarial use of the MMPI with adolescents and adults.* Baltimore, MD: Williams & Wilkins.

Mattison, M., Cantwell, D. P., Russell, A. T., & Will, L. (1979). A comparison of DSM-II and DSM-III in the diagnosis of childhood psychiatric disorders: II. Interrater agreement. *Archives of General Psychiatry, 36,* 1217–1222.

McAuliffe, T. M., & Handal, P. J. (1984). PIC delinquency scale: Validity in relation to self-reported delinquent acts. *Criminal Justice and Behavior, 11,* 35–46.

McCoy, S. A. (1976). Clinical judgments of normal childhood behavior. *Journal of Consulting and Clinical Psychology, 44,* 710–714.

McDermott, P. A. (1982). Actuarial assessment systems for the grouping and classification of school children. In C. R. Reynolds & T. B. Gutkin (Eds.), *The handbook of school psychology* (pp. 243–272). New York: Wiley.

McVaugh, W. H., & Grow, R. T. (1983). Detection of faking on the Personality Inventory for Children. *Journal of Clinical Psychology, 39,* 567–573.

Michigan State Board of Education. (1980). *Michigan special education rules as amended August 13, 1980.* Lansing, MI: Author.

Peterson, D. W., & Batsche, G. M. (1983). School psychology and projective assessment: A growing incompatibility. *School Psychology Review, 12,* 440–445.

Pipp, F. D. (1979). *Actuarial analysis of adolescent personality: Self-report correlates for the Personality Inventory for Children profile scales.* Unpublished master's thesis, Wayne State University, Detroit, MI.

Porter, J. E., & Rourke, B. P. (1985). Socioemotional functioning: A subtypal analysis of personality patterns. In B. P. Rourke (Ed.), *Neuropsychology of learning disabilities: Essentials of subtype analysis* (pp. 257–280). New York: Guilford Press.

Ross, A. O. (1976). *Psychological aspects of learning disabilities and reading disorders.* New York: McGraw-Hill.

Ross, A. O. (1977). *Learning disability: The unrealized potential.* New York: McGraw-Hill.

Rutter, M. (1978). Diagnostic validity in child psychiatry. *Advances in Biological Psychiatry, 2,* 2–22.

Schnel, J. (1982). *The utility of the Student Behavior Checklist and the Personality Inventory for Children to assess affective and academic needs of students with learning disabilities.* Doctoral dissertation, University of San Francisco, CA.

Schreiber, M. D. (1982). *The relationship between extra-familial support networks and coping in children of divorced and non-divorced families.* Doctoral dissertation, Ohio State University, Columbus.

Sinclair, E. (1983). Educational assessment. In J. L. Matson & J. A. Mulick (Eds.), *Handbook of mental retardation* (pp. 245–255). Oxford: Pergamon Press.

Snyder, D. K., & Gdowski, C. L. (1980, October). *The relationship of marital dysfunction to psychiatric disturbance in children: An empirical analysis using the MSI and PIC.* Panel discussion: *New developments in the actuarial assessment of marital and family interaction.* Paper presented at the annual meeting of the National Council of Family Relations, Portland, OR.

Stewart, D. (1971). The construction of a somatizing scale for the Personality Inventory for Children (Doctoral dissertation, University of Minnesota, 1970). *Dissertation Abstracts International, 32*, 572B. (University Microfilm No. 71-18, 824).

Voelker, S., Lachar, D., & Gdowski, C. L. (1983). The Personality Inventory for Children and response to methylphenidate: Preliminary evidence for predictive utility. *Journal of Pediatric Psychology, 8*, 161–169.

Wepman, J. M., Cruickshank, W. M., Deutsch, C. P., Morency, A., & Strother, C. R. (1975). Learning disabilities. In N. Hobbs (Ed.), *Issues in the classification of children* (Vol. 1, pp. 300–317). San Francisco, CA: Jossey-Bass.

Werry, J. S., Methven, R. J., Fitzpatrick, J., & Dixon, H. (1983). The interrater reliability of DSM-III in children. *Journal of Abnormal Child Psychology, 11*, 341–354.

Wirt, R. D., & Lachar, D. (1981). The Personality Inventory for Children: Development and clinical applications. In P. McReynolds (Ed.), *Advances in psychological assessment* (Vol. 5, pp. 353–392). San Francisco, CA: Jossey-Bass.

Wirt, R. D., Lachar, D., Klinedinst, J. K., & Seat, P. D. (1984). *Multidimensional description of child personality: A manual for the Personality Inventory for Children*, (1984 revision by David Lachar). Los Angeles, CA: Western Psychological Services.

Ysseldyke, J. E. (1983). Current practices in making psychoeducational decisions about learning disabled students. *Journal of Learning Disabilities, 16*, 226–233.

10

Behavior Rating Scale Approaches to Personality Assessment in Children and Adolescents

Roy P. Martin
Stephen Hooper
Jeffrey Snow

Introduction

This chapter is concerned with rating scales as they are used to assess normal personality and the presence or absence of behavioral abnormality in children and adolescents. The term "rating scale" is used in a more general way here than in some other contexts. For purposes of this discussion, a rating scale is any paper and pencil device whereby one (usually a caretaker such as a parent or teacher, though not excluding peers) assesses the behavior of that individual based on his or her observation of the child or adolescent over an extended period of time (usually more than a month). Further, this discussion will be limited to devices that generate summative scores from a number of items or stimuli.

Behavior rating scale approaches come in a variety of formats. Some utilize a checklist format in which the presence or absence of a behavioral characteristic is indicated (e.g., *Behavior Problem Checklist*; Quay & Peterson, 1975). In such cases, the score generated represents the number of behaviors of a certain type that the child is felt to manifest. Other devices provide a Likert response format in which a statement is followed by a continuum on which three to seven anchoring points are indicated. The continuum may be based on how well the item describes the child to be rated, for example, "very much like him," "somewhat like him," "not at all like him" (Behavior Rating Profile; L. L. Brown & Hammill, 1978), or the frequency that the item occurs, for example, "almost always," "often," "never" (Temperament Assessment Battery; Martin, 1984).

Devices utilizing these response formats also vary greatly in the extent to which the items are stated in behavioral terms; that is, some call for greater conceptual leaps by the rater and some for ratings of more generalized behavioral

Roy P. Martin. Department of Educational Psychology, University of Georgia, Athens, Georgia.
Stephen Hooper. Department of Psychiatry, Vanderbilt University School of Medicine, Nashville, Tennessee.
Jeffrey Snow. Department of Counseling and Educational Psychology, University of Missouri, Columbia, Missouri.

styles than others. For example, the item, "Is self-centered egocentric," is much more general than "Violates curfew," or "Steals in company of others." Thus, this chapter is not limited to those few scales that maintain a strong behavioral orientation. Rating scales that vary in this way are discussed because (*a*) some of the most widely used rating scales would have been eliminated from consideration if very stringent behavioral criteria were utilized, and (*b*) substantial research shows that ratings of more abstract items on more general dimensions can contribute to predictions of real world behaviors under specified conditions, while ratings of behavioral items on concrete behavioral dimensions may provide other advantages in this prediction process. Thus, the authors advocate an empiricist, actuarial perspective: If a device works in making predictions, then it should not be eliminated from consideration.

Advantages of Rating Technology

Rating scales are the techniques of choice for many personality assessment referrals because they are the only technology that can be practically applied. Consider the practitioner who is concerned about the behavioral effects on a 6-month-old infant of a difficult forceps delivery. The infant obviously cannot read or write, so self-report scales or interviews are ruled out. The child cannot speak or draw with a pencil on paper, so expressive projectives are ruled out. Physiological measurements (e.g., heart rate) could be taken, but measurements must be made by technically trained personnel over a number of days. Even then, the resulting data would provide only a limited glimpse of the effects of the difficult delivery on the infant. Direct behavioral observation is an option, but suffers many of the same difficulties that occur with electromechanical recording of physiological or behavioral medical data. It also is expensive because trained personnel must do the observations (even training mothers can be expensive), and observations must be done over long periods of time and in a variety of situations. The technology best suited to the practitioner in this example is the rating scale—an opportunity to ask the mother and/or father an organized set of questions about the behavior of the child since the delivery. These questions should be presented in a standardized manner with normative data from other mothers of infants using the same set of questions, available for comparison purposes. Thus, the most practical technology available is a norm-referenced rating scale.

Rating scales are used with preschoolers, children of elementary school age, and adolescents for similar reasons. It is a low-cost assessment method that can be used as long as the rater has sufficient knowledge of the person to be rated in a specific setting and is capable of responding to the rating instrument. Of course, as the child increases in age and skill, a variety of other technologies (e.g., self-report instruments, projective techniques) can be used in addition to, or in place of, rating scales. The cost of observation or direct electromechanical measurement becomes even more prohibitive in older children. For example, it is possible to attach electrical sensing equipment to a newborn, but this becomes very difficult for adolescents due to their ability to move from place to place and the intrusion that such a device, even if portable, would make on the normal life of the adolescent.

Even among low-cost assessment alternatives, rating scales maintain their advantages. For example, compared to self-report instruments where a person rates his or her own behavior (rather than being rated by another person), rating scales have distinct advantages. First, many young children and some handicapped children do not have the cognitive and conceptual abilities needed to respond to a self-report device. These processes include the ability (a) to read or to comprehend the questions asked by the examiner (or device), (b) to self-monitor a variety of social–emotional behaviors, (c) to maintain behavioral incidents in long-term memory, (d) to assign weights to these incidents and aggregate them, thereby formulating a generalized description, and (e) to verbalize or in some other way communicate responses to the questions asked. (As will be seen in a later discussion, this is only a partial list of the mental processes utilized in making ratings.) Second, the practitioner often is as interested in the observations and reactions of a caretaker to the child's behavior as he or she is to the child's reaction to his or her own behavior. Third, rating scales are often less biased than an individual's self-ratings. If unbiased observations were available from caretakers and from the child, then it wouldn't matter who provided the observation. However, since raters (self or other) bias all observations in various ways, practitioners use procedures and techniques that best minimize this bias.

Teachers often are excellent raters of the behavior of children. Their educational role demands observations of children of similar age on a daily basis under relatively consistent environmental circumstances. Further, teachers are trained observers and have some ideas about the behaviors that most concern mental health practitioners and parents. Thus, a rating scale completed by a teacher is likely to be less biased due to the teacher's expertise and educational role than an individual's self-rating where that individual may be experiencing significant social–emotional stress.

Disregarding the issue of relative bias, many clinicians are interested in the viewpoints of different persons in the child's or adolescent's environment. Investigating differences in mothers' ratings versus those of fathers, teachers, and clinicians can be useful in determining factors influencing referred problems and remedial strategies. In a recent study, Pfeffer and Martin (1983) calculated the interrater reliabilities between mothers' and fathers' temperament ratings for two groups of children—those who were referred for psychological evaluations due to behavior problems and those who had never been referred. The interrater reliability for the referred group was near zero across the eight scales rated, while it was in the .30 to .60 range for the nonreferred group. While the implication of this finding is not absolutely clear, it is evident that parents' views of referred children were almost completely unrelated. Should two parents' ratings significantly differ, the practitioner should explore whether the discrepancy is symbolic of broader parental differences which may then explain the child's problem or the referral situation.

Ratings capitalize on observations carried out by observers in the child's normal environment. Thus, they have three advantages not yet mentioned. First, observers often have observed the target child for extended periods of time. Parents, of course, have been observing their children since the moment of birth. They have seen their behavior in a wider range of settings and circumstances than any other observer. Even allowing for biases in perception (presenting their child in the best or the worst possible light) and selective memory, parents' observations are important and useful to personality assessment. Second, caretakers are intensely motivated to observe children. If carried out properly, ratings summarize these highly motivated observations. Third, the caretaker or peer observer is a natural part of the environment of the child or adolescent observed. Thus, the child does not inhibit his or her natural behavioral style during observation due to the presence of a stranger in the setting.

Finally, it has become clear that rating scales yield more objective and reliable data than projective techniques and clinical interviews (Edelbrock, 1983). The reasons for this superiority are clear. Most clinicians do not utilize standardized questioning techniques in interviews or in projective assessment. Data are aggregated idiosyncratically across clinicians, and normative comparison data are usually not available. For these reasons and others, a great deal of clinical variance (clinician subjectivity) influences the responses elicited from the client and their analysis and interpretation. Thus, the reliability of interviews and projective assessments tends to be low (Anastasi, 1976), thereby lowering the maximum possible validity of the data. In light of these comparative data, it is interesting that projective techniques and interviews are far more frequently utilized by school psychologists than rating scales (Fuller & Goh, 1983).

Disadvantages of Rating Scale Technology

While rating scales are among the most widely used measurement devices by all types of applied psychologists (industrial/organizational, clinical, counseling, and school psychologists), there remains a pervasive feeling that they are second-class measurement tools: "Most reservations, regardless of how elegantly phrased, reflect fears that rating scale data are subjective (emphasizing, of course, the undesirable connotations of subjectivity), biased, and at worst, purposefully distorted" (Saal, Downey, & Lahey, 1980, p. 413).

Misgivings about rating scales are often warranted. Many school practitioners have had experience with teachers who, in interacting with a particular child who is difficult to deal with, have negatively biased their ratings of the child to facilitate his or her removal from the classroom. Similarly, parents of children referred for gifted placements often positively bias behavior rating data solicited from them to enhance the chances of their children's placement in the program. Purposeful or inadvertent biasing of ratings can occur in all situations in which this type of data are collected.

Eliminating deliberate bias from our discussion momentarily, there are a number of reasons why rating scales are subject to inadvertent biases. These reasons are a function of the complexity of the mental and emotional processes that occur when a rating is made. The mental processes in operation when one person rates the behavior of another have been discussed by Cooper (1981) and involve the following:

1. Observation of action
2. Observation encoding, aggregation, and storage in short-term memory
3. Short-term memory decay
4. Transfer to long-term storage and aggregation
5. Long-term memory decay
6. Presentation of categories to be rated
7. Observation and impression retrieval from long-term storage
8. Recognition of observations and impressions relevant to rating category

9. Comparison of observations and impressions to raters standards
10. Incorporation of extraneous considerations
11. Making the rating

Well-motivated raters can produce different descriptions of a target child's behavior due to idiosyncratic processes operating at each stage of this process. For example, individual differences in attending to the child's behavior can affect the actions that are observed in step 1. Further, as different raters observe the child in different settings and at different times, the observed behavior will probably change and, thus, the raters' observations (and eventual ratings) will differ.

Expectations concerning a child's behavior can affect steps 2–5. Consider, for example, a fifth-grade teacher who has been told by a child's fourth-grade teacher that the child has a tendency to behave aggressively. As a result, the current teacher becomes hypervigilant about aggressive behavior from the student. This results in encoding this behavior into a mental schema of the child as an aggressive person. The teacher also may give much heavier weight to one or two incidents of aggressive behavior, when considering all observations of the child, than to the occurrences of nonaggressive behavior. Finally, because the aggressive incidents fit the schema "aggressive child," they will be held in short-term memory longer and more clearly than nonaggressive incidents.

The processes influenced by a biasing communication may affect short-term memory decay, ease of transfer to long-term memory, and long-term memory decay. Thus, several steps in the cognitive process of making ratings can be affected by raters' expectations. Similarly, stereotypes based on race, sex, ethnicity, and socioeconomic class may affect the rating process.

Other factors that affect many steps in Cooper's (1981) process include reading ability, receptive vocabulary, and general cognitive ability. Ratings work best with relatively bright, well-educated raters. For example, in some areas, the use of parent rating scales of any kind presents serious problems, since 30–40% of the population cannot read at a fifth-grade level.

Types of Response Bias

While there are many types of specific biases, those most often discussed and researched in the literature include (a) halo effects, (b) leniency or severity, and (c) central tendency or range restriction (Saal et al., 1980).

Halo effects have been defined in various ways, but they are generally thought of as a rater's failure to discriminate among distinct and independent aspects of a ratee's behavior (Saal et al., 1980). The teacher who rates all of his or her brightest students as having socially desirable characteristics (e.g., low anxiety, high sociability, low impulsivity, long attention span) and his or her less able students as having less desirable characteristics is probably manifesting a halo bias. The presence of this bias would be validated if the characteristics mentioned above are not truly correlated with scholastic ability and/or if other observers disagree with the teacher's perceptions and observations.

The leniency or severity bias is easily understood. It occurs when ratings are consistently higher or lower than are warranted. Sometimes leniency or severity is inferred when a rater predominantly uses one extreme or the other of the rating scale. It is also inferred when one rater gives more severe or more lenient ratings of his or her ratees than other raters give different ratees; for example, when one teacher rates *all* his or her pupils more severely than another teacher who rates his or her pupils. Neither of these situations, of course, presents strong support for the severity or leniency bias. Thus, the presence of this bias is accurately diagnosed only when an acceptable external criterion is obtained. Such a situation is diagnosed with more certainty when a father, teacher, teacher aide, and clinician rate a child as being very active, and the mother rates the child's activity in the average range.

The third response bias occurs when raters predominantly utilize the central range of a rating scale. This type of error is referred to as a restriction of range or as a central tendency error (Saal *et al.*, 1980). This type of error may occur when a practitioner asks a teacher in a private school to rate a child's behavior. Fearing that the parents will be upset with the teacher and remove the child from the school (with the resulting loss of tuition revenue), the teacher restricts the range of all ratings to the average or positive range of the scale. (In the latter case, the restriction of range is also a leniency bias.)

Summarizing and Overcoming the Disadvantages of Rating Scales

There are four important sources of variation on assessment data which summarize the disadvantages of rating scales—source variance, setting variance, temporal variance, and instrument variance. Source variance was discussed above as the subjectivity of rater; it is the primary source of error in rating scale data.

Setting variance occurs because all organisms are, to greater or lesser extents, affected differently by the various environments in which they find themselves. Most adolescents behave differently in a classroom where their behavior is monitored versus in a car with friends cruising around town. Often, mental health professionals collect and analyze data that generalize behavioral tendencies across settings. In such cases, setting variance contributes to measurement error as an extraneous source of variance. If an adolescent appeared anxious to peers, parents, and teachers, then interventions which work across settings or in spite of a particular setting would be appropriate. If anxiety were rated high only by teachers and only in the educational setting, then a school-based treatment might be in order.

A related source of variance, temporal variance, explains variability in behavior produced by the passage of time. Most parents recognize that their children are very difficult on some days, while they are easily managed, delightful companions on others. The rating scale process tends to average out short-range variability of this type, since the assessment devices usually are designed to measure raters' impressions summed over a period of a few months. However, children and adolescents change dramatically in behavior over longer periods of months or years. Often, multiple ratings taken over these periods are sensitive to such changes. Nonetheless, such developmental processes as well as day-to-day fluctuations in behavior create temporal variance in rating scale measurements.

One final problem to be overcome through an appropriate assessment design is instrument variance. Measurement-oriented practitioners have known for many years that different measurement devices designed to assess the same trait produce different scores. Thus, this score variability occurs, in part, due to qualitative (e.g., how the trait was defined and operationalized) and quantitative (e.g., how the standardization data were compiled and normed) differences between the two devices or instruments. D. T. Campbell and Fiske (1959) discussed a now classic method for assessing this type of problem (a design that results in a multitrait, multimethod data matrix), and many applications of the technique have produced sizable estimates of instrument or method variance. Parenthetically, if two rating scales are used to measure a construct, the resulting difference in outcome from the two measures would be referred to as instrument variance. If the same construct (e.g., anxiety) was measured with a rating scale and a projective device, then the differences in scores would be most properly referred to as method variance, since entirely different types or methods of measurement were used.

These four sources of variation in assessment data—source variance, setting variance, temporal variance, and instrument variance—are present in most assessment situations, regardless of the assessment device used. Most clinicians pay little systematic attention to these sources of variance. For example, private or community-based practitioners often make the implicit assumption that setting effects are small. They assume that children's behavior in the office is typical or in some way representative of their behavior elsewhere. Similarly, when practitioners use one device to measure different domains (cognitive, perceptual-motor, emotional, social), they assume that instrument or method variance is negligible. Even behaviorally oriented practitioners are often insensitive to setting and instrument variance when interpreting their behavioral observations. If rating technology is understood and used appropriately, it can help sensitize the practitioner to these effects.

The Aggregation Principle

If utilized appropriately, one general principle, the aggregation principle, can help to account for and control all four of these sources of variance. Most mental health practitioners are aware of this principle in one context, but have not traditionally applied it in others. Simply stated, the aggregation principle points out that the data from any observation or measurement reflect two classes of phenomena: the behavior the assessor intends to measure and the characteristics of the persons, situation, time, instruments, or observer that the assessor did not intend to measure. To maximize the measurement of the desired behaviors, two or more observations or measurements of the same characteristic (assuming that they are correlated) are added together, resulting in an aggregated measure which is more reliable than the individual component observations or measurements. This occurs because the part of the measurement that assesses the desired behavior accumulates additively, while the error part of the measurement does not accumulate because the error from the two measurements is theorized to be uncorrelated. Ghiselli, Campbell, and Zedeck (1981) provide an extended discussion of this important principle.

While this principle sounds a little complicated, it is the primary reason why assessment instruments are more than one item long. We all know that as a test gets longer, it becomes more reliable. We also know that 2 hours of behavior observation is more reliable than 2 minutes. The Spearman–Brown formula states explicitly in mathematical terms the nature of the relationship between test length and reliability. The principle is also involved when researchers apply experimental conditions to a large number of subjects instead of to one. All graduate-trained practitioners are aware of these applications of aggregation, but often have not seen them applied to personality assessment and design.

In a recent series of articles, Epstein (1979a, 1979b, 1980, 1983) and others (Eaton, 1983) have documented the place of aggregation in personality research and clinical assessment. Epstein (1980) points out that we can expect the same gains in reliability that are obtained from lengthening a test, if we (*a*) test over several time periods and settings (instead of one), (*b*) use several assessment methods (instead of one), and (*c*) use several raters (instead of one). He notes, " . . . the same amount of aggregation, no matter what the form, should produce the same increase in reliability" (Epstein, 1980, p. 797).

The type of aggregation, however, determines the type of reliability gain we obtain. If we assess a child over three sessions instead of one, we gain in the temporal stability of the data collected (test–retest reliability increases). If we have a child rated by more than one rater, we reduce the subjectivity of the ratings and increase interrater reliability. Aggregation across instruments increases the reliability of the data in much the same way that lengthening a test does. This increase is most related to internal consistency reliability. There is no traditional reliability index associated with cross-situational stability, but gains accruing from aggregation across setting may be related to test-retest reliability and will broaden the measurement of the construct measured. This will consequently result in enhanced validity.

The Multisetting, Multisource, Multi-instrument Design

In order to apply the aggregation principle to control the problems of rating scale assessment (and other types of assessment), an assessment design must be constructed (see Figure 10-1).

This design, referred to as the multisetting, multisource, multi-instrument design, has several important characteristics. First, assessments are made in three settings—home, school, and clinic. These three settings were chosen because practitioners can often obtain ratings from persons who have observed the child's behavior in these settings. The choice of settings is somewhat arbitrary. The settings chosen should include settings of importance to the child and settings that have different characteristics which affect the behavior of the child.

The second feature of the design is that at least two raters provide data in each setting. This allows for aggregation across raters within settings as well as across settings. Thus, if setting effects are of interest, they can be studied without relying on one rater in that setting. When only one rater is used in each setting, setting and rater are confounded, so that a relatively low or high rating might result from setting effects or rater effects (setting variance or source variance, respectively).

The third feature of the design is that two or more measurement devices are used to assess the same constructs for each rater in each setting. Such redundancy aids in the control of instrument variance. An important requirement of the design is that the same measurement devices or parallel devices are used in each setting by each rater. This allows for direct comparison from setting to setting.

Although this aspect of the design is not illustrated in Figure 10-1, another important design procedure is the collection of data from all raters on more than

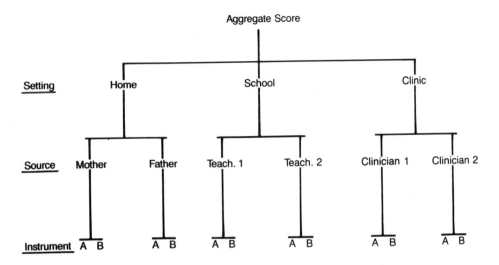

Figure 10-1. The Multisetting, Multisource, Multi-Instrument Design.

one occasion. This allows for control of temporal variance as the data are aggregated across occasions.

The advantages of this design can be demonstrated through an example. Suppose a second-grade teacher refers a student because of a short attention span. An interview between the school psychologist and the teacher suggests that overactivity, distractibility, short attention span, and poor perseverance are all present when the student is faced with difficult learning tasks. The psychologist then selects two rating scales. He asks the referring teacher *and* the child's parents to complete both scales. Further, *he* completes the two scales based on observations in the classroom and during a formal assessment. (Realistically, some scales contain items that would have a low probability of occurrence during brief observation periods, so it may be difficult to find two scales that can be used by clinicians.) For this example, let's assume that the psychologist has no other professionals available to provide ratings in the assessment situation.

Based on the resulting data, the psychologist has the following options. First, if completely aggregated data are desired, he can simply sum the scores across all raters and all settings for each scale. Since the resulting data are an aggregate of four or five ratings, it is much more reliable than data from the separate measures. If both measurement devices produce elevated scores on activity, impulsivity, and short attention span, then support for the teacher referral has been obtained and the psychologist has a reliable behavioral description of the referral problem.

If important disagreements in ratings occur, then the possibility that the referred behaviors are situation-specific should be investigated. For purposes of illustration, let us assume that both parents and the psychologist saw no significant signs of abnormally high activity level, impulsivity, or short attention span. However, both teachers did. Source variance can be momentarily ruled out unless the ratings were not made independently; that is, since both raters in the school setting agree, we cannot attribute the differences between their ratings and those of the parents and psychologist to the individual response styles or sets of the individual teachers. Thus, the best hypothesis for the measurement variance present is a setting effect; that is, the child seems to be behaving differently in school than in other settings. Thus, a search for the "causative" factor(s) in the school setting can begin. Perhaps the child is bored with the academic work presented or is overwhelmed by it. Perhaps it is a response to the social content of the classroom. A variety of hypotheses could be entertained and would be checked out through other types of assessment and data collection.

The hypothesis and problem-solving process generated when using this design is very different from that which would occur if only the one referring teacher rated the child as active, distractible, and impulsive. In that case, the first hypothesis to be ruled out would be that of a teacher–child mismatch (e.g., teacher bias, poor teacher–child communication). A maturational problem and other child-specific types of hypotheses could not be ruled out, of course, without further data.

The model design proposed here cannot always be attained. It may be impossible to obtain father ratings or to burden all raters with two instruments. However, to the extent that the assessor's design falls short of this model, the conclusions drawn from the assessment process are weakened. In such cases, the practitioner should qualify the conclusions made by talking about the various hypotheses that are supported by the data.

A Review of Four Rating Scales

In this portion of the chapter, four rating scales are reviewed. The scales were selected from the large number of rating scales available based on two criteria. First, all four scales provide data that help the practitioner determine if a child's behavior is typical or atypical, and they classify the nature of atypical behavior if present. Since most mental health practitioners often are asked to make decisions about the presence of atypical behavior exhibited by children and adolescents, scales that focus in this area were selected over scales that deal with the measurement of normal behavior traits. The second criterion used in selecting the four scales was that each scale had to have been evaluated and utilized in a sizable number of published research studies. It was also considered advantageous if the devices could be used by parents *and* teachers to allow for use in a multisource, multisetting assessment design. The devices selected for review are the Child Behavior Checklist (Achenbach & Edelbrock, 1983), the Conners Rating Scales (Conners, 1982), the Missouri Children's Behavior Checklist (Thompson & Curry, 1983), and the Behavior Problem Checklist (Quay & Peterson, 1975).

These four instruments represent only a portion of the instruments that meet the criteria listed above. For a more complete listing of other rating scales which briefly describes each scale, see Table 10-1. The four instruments reviewed are new instruments that are not widely used to date (e.g., the Achenbach Child Behavior Checklist), or are instruments for which no manual exists to summarize their psychometric properties. In the latter case, the authors' purpose was to bring together in one place a summary of the reliability and validity data available on these instruments.

The Achenbach Child Behavior Checklist

Description

The Child Behavior Checklist (CBCL) is a well-standardized behavior rating scale designed to be completed by parents for their children ages 4–16. The CBCL requires the parent to have a fifth-grade reading level, or it can be read to the parent by the practitioner. The CBCL usually can be completed in 15 to 17 minutes.

The CBCL was developed as an extension of Achenbach's (1966) behavior problem checklist whose items were drawn from a survey of the existing literature and case histories of 1,000 child psychiatric patients. The original checklist was completed by raters who reviewed these case histories and chose whether specific behaviors were present or absent. Subsequently, the checklist was modified for use by a child's parents by simplifying terminology, adding new items, and expanding the response alternatives from the two-choice response format to a three-choice response format (0 = not true, 1 = somewhat true, 2 = very true). Finer differentiations of behavior, such as a 5-point response format indicating frequency (1 = hardly ever, to 5 = often), were not attempted because increased gradations in behavior were thought to be difficult to determine by the rating scale method (Achenbach & Edelbrock, 1978).

In the construction of the behavior problem scales, Achenbach and Edelbrock (1978, 1979) utilized clinical samples. Clinically referred children from 42 mental health agencies (e.g., community mental health centers, child guidance clinics, family services) located in the eastern United States formed the basis of the clinical sample. Parents completed the CBCL at the various agencies during their intake procedures to secure services. In an effort to control for the variables of age and sex, separate principal component factor analyses were performed for males and females at ages 4–5, 6–11, and 12–16. These age ranges were selected because they reflected important transitional periods in the cognitive, physical, educational, and social–emotional development of children (Achenbach & Edelbrock, 1983). A total of 2,300 completed CBCLs were obtained from the mental health facilities, with stable sampling distributions for each sex in the various age groupings. Socioeconomic status was taken into account by having the parents list their occupation. The racial distribution included approximately 81% white, 17% black, and 2% other. For the clinical sample, the CBCL was completed by mothers for 83% of the children, fathers for 11.5%, and other guardians for about 5.5% of the children.

Normative data on the CBCL are impressive. The criterion for inclusion in the normative sample was that a child could not have received mental health agency services during the previous year. Interviewers were sent to randomly selected homes in the Washington, D.C., Maryland, and northern Virginia area. Using 1970 census tract data on age, race, and socioeconomic distributions, samples were randomly selected so as to approximate the SES and racial distributions in the clinical sample. Interviews with the CBCL were conducted with 1,442 parents during the last 4 months of 1976 by five female interviewers. Achenbach and colleagues then extracted samples of 50 children of each sex at each age having SES and racial distributions consistent with the clinical samples. The overall racial distribution was 80.5% white, 18% black, and 1.5% other. The CBCL was completed by mothers in 83% of the cases, fathers in 13.5% of the cases, and other guardians in 3.5% of the cases (Achenbach & Edelbrock, 1983).

Table 10-1
Assessment Instruments Designed to Differentiate between Normal and Pathological Behavior Exhibited by Children

Title:	Behavior Problem Checklist (Original and Revised)	Behavior Rating Profile	Bristol Social Adjustment Guides	Burk's Behavior Rating Scales
Author:	H. C. Quay D. R. Peterson	L. L. Brown D. D. Hammill	D. H. Stott	H. F. Burks
Publisher:	Privately printed by the developers	Pro-Ed Publishers 5341 Industrial Oaks Blvd Austin, Texas 78735	Educational and Industrial Testing Service P.O. Box 7234 San Diego, California 92107	Western Psychological Services 12031 Wilshire Blvd. Los Angeles, California 90025
Age:	5–16	6–13	6–15	6–15 3–6 (Preschool kindergarten version)
Rater:	Parent, Teacher	Parent, Teacher, Self	Teacher	Teacher, Parent
Scales:	Conduct Problems Personality Problems Inadequacy-Immaturity Socialized Delinquency Psychotic Signs (Revised edition includes: Conduct Problems Socialized Aggression Attention Problem-Immaturity Anxiety-Withdrawal Psychotic Behavior Motor Excess)	General Adjustment as seen in Home, School, and with Peers	Overaction Underreaction Unforthcomingness Withdrawal Depression Inconsequence Hostility Peer Maladaptiveness	Excessive Self-Blame Excessive Anxiety Excessive Withdrawal Excessive Dependency Poor Ego Strength Poor Physical Strength Poor Coordination Poor Intellectuality Poor Attention Poor Impulse Control Poor Reality Contact Poor Sense of Identity Excessive Suffering Poor Anger Control Excessive Sense of Persecution Excessive Aggressiveness Excessive Resistance Poor Social Conformity
Manual:	Yes	Yes	Yes	Yes
Evaluation of Manual[a]	Fair	Adequate	Fair	Good

[a]Manual evaluated on a 5-point scale: poor, fair, adequate, good, very good.

Table 10-1
(Continued)

Child Behavior Checklist	Personality Inventory for Children	School Behavior Checklist	Walker Problem Behavior Identification Checklist
T. M. Achenbach C. S. Edelbrock	R. D. Wirt D. Lachar J. K. Klinedinst P. D. Seat	L. C. Miller	H. M. Walker
Psychiatric Associates	Western Psychological Services 12031 Wilshire Blvd. Los Angeles, California 90025	Western Psychological Services 12031 Wilshire Blvd. Los Angeles, California 90025	Western Psychological Services 12031 Wilshire Blvd. Los Angeles, California 90025
4–16	3–16	4–6 (Form A1) 7–13 (Form A2)	9–13
Parent (Parent Form) Teacher (Teacher Form)	Mother	Teacher	Teacher
Internalizing Externalizing Social Withdrawal Depression Immature Somatic Complaints Sex Problems Delinquency Aggressive Schizoid Hyperactive Obesity Social Competency School Competency Activities (Teacher form taps somewhat different variables)	General Adjustment Intellectual Screening Development Somatic Concern Depression Family Relations Delinquency Withdrawal Anxiety Psychosis Hyperactivity Social Skills	Low Need Achievement Aggression Anxiety Cognitive Deficit (Form A1 only) Hostile Isolation Extraversion Normal Irritability (Form A1 only) School Disturbance (Form A1 only) Total Disability	Acting-Out Withdrawal Distractibility Disturbed Peer Relations Immaturity
Yes	Yes	Yes	Yes
Very good	Good	Adequate	Adequate

The final edition of the CBCL includes 118 behavior problems (e.g., threatens people, sulks a lot, sets fires, shy or timid) (Achenbach & Edelbrock, 1983). Within the 118 items are several open-ended responses for which parents can add other physical problems with no known medical cause and other problems not included in the CBCL.

The CBCL is exemplary in its design to investigate profiles of behavior problem children (Achenbach & Edelbrock, 1978). Primary-order (or broad-band) factors, derived empirically from responses to individual items, fell into two major areas, Internalizing Syndromes and Externalizing Syndromes. Although these primary-order factors are consistent across the 4–16 age range of the CBCL as well as the male–female dichotomy, second-order (or narrow-band) factors do vary somewhat between the age ranges and the sexes. For example, for boys age 4–5 years, the narrow-band syndromes include social withdrawal, depressed, immature, somatic complaints, sex problems, delinquency, aggressive, schizoid. For girls in this age range the scales are the same except that delinquency and immaturity are omitted, and obesity and hyperactivity are added.

Along with the behavior problems listed, assessments of a child's positive behavioral characteristics were developed in several formats with parents. These items comprise the CBCL Social Competency Dimension and fall into three areas: the Activities scale, the Social scale, and the School scale.

The Activities scale uses parental ratings to evaluate the quality and quantity of the child's participation in sports, nonsports, hobbies, activities and games, and jobs. The parent is asked to report which sport the child likes best (up to three), and then how much time the child spends in the sports listed and how well the child performs relative to his or her age-mates. Parents choose among the ratings "Don't Know," "Below Average," "Average," and "Above Average." This same format is followed for the nonsports activities and jobs items. Scores are assigned on a 0 to 2-point basis for the number of activities in which the child is involved and for each of the peer comparison ratings.

The Social scale is used to rate the child's membership and participation in organizations, the number of friends and contacts with friends, and behavior with others and alone. Points are assigned in a fashion similar to that of the Activity scale.

The third scale, the School scale, consists of ratings based on the child's average performance in academic subject areas, placement in a regular or special education class, being promoted or retained in a particular grade, and the presence or absence of a school problem. For each area, parental ratings range across "Failing," "Below Average," "Average," and "Above Average." The School scale is not scored for 4- to 5-year olds.

Once parents complete their ratings, the CBCL data can be entered on the Child Behavior Profile (CBP). The CBP displays the child's standings as rated by the parents across the narrow- and broad-band syndromes. Using either a hand-scored or computerized version of the CBP, the clinician or researcher can review the behavioral syndromes manifested by the child, the specific items rated by the parents, and how the child compares to typical children of the same age and sex. The CBP is organized according to the primary- and secondary-order factors, with the profile being constructed with percentiles and *T* scores. Diagnostically, Achenbach and Edelbrock (1983) cautioned that although many of the second-order factors have labels similar to DSM-III categories, they should be interpreted as descriptive statements and not as diagnostic entities. Further, they suggest that a child should not be described as an Internalizer or an Externalizer unless the Total Behavior Problem score is above the 40th percentile for their age/sex group *and* there exists a difference of at least 10 *T*-score points between the primary factors.

Reliability

Item selection procedures for the CBCL and its various factors were discussed earlier. Internal consistency of the CBCL appears more than adequate.

In an effort to determine the consistency of the rank ordering of the items of the CBCL over time (temporal stability), as well as to account for the magnitude of differences between ratings of an item, Achenbach utilized the interclass correlation coefficient (ICC). The ICC can be affected by differences in the rank orderings of the correlated scores and differences in their magnitude. Item test-retest reliabilities were computed from CBCLs obtained by a single interviewer of 72 mothers of nonreferred children at a 1-week interval. The overall ICC was .95 for the 118 behavior problems and .996 for the 20 social competence items. Over a 3-month interval with 12 mothers of nonreferred children, the ICCs remained high, with $r = .84$ for the behavior problems and $r = .97$ for the social competence items (Achenbach & Edelbrock, 1983).

With respect to the temporal stability of the scale scores, the average median correlation over a 1-week interval for nonreferred males and females of all ages across all scales was $r = .89$ (Achenbach & Edelbrock, 1983). Specifically, the mean of the Pearson correlations between test 1 and test 2 scores on the social competence scales, narrow- and broad-band behavior problem scales, and Total Score for behavior problems was $r = .83$ for 4- to 5-year-old boys, $r = .89$ for 6- to 11-year-old boys, $r = .82$ for the 12- to 16-year-old boys, $r = .81$ for 4- to 5-year-old females (Achenbach & Edelbrock, 1983), $r = .88$ for 6- to 11-year-old females, and $r = .90$ for 12- to 16-year-old females (Achenbach & Edelbrock, 1979). These reliability coefficients provide the foundation for calculating the Standard Error of Measurement for each of the behavior problem and social competence scales.

For a sample of 6- to 11-year-old boys ($N = 14$) in residential treatment for behavioral difficulties, significant test-retest correlations of parent ratings of the CBCL ranged from $r = .48$ for the Hyperactive dimension to $r = .86$ for the Schizoid or Anxious factor over a 3-month period. Over the same time period, child-care workers' ratings on the CBCL ranged from $r = .51$ (not significant) on the Schizoid or Anxious factor to $r = .84$ on the Aggressive factor. In addition, it was noted on retest that the parents' ratings significantly decreased upon retesting. This might suggest that children's behavior improved during home visits more than in the treatment setting (Achenbach & Edelbrock, 1983). Generally, the average correlations for parent and child-care workers were similar over the 3-month period ($r = .74$ for parents, $r = .73$ for child-care workers). Test-retest scores on the social competence scales were not available.

Achenbach and Edelbrock (1983) reported interparent agreement on item scores to be extraordinarily high for clinically referred children, ranging from $r = .978$ for the social competence items to $r = .985$ for the 118 behavior problems ($N = 168$). In another sample of 107 clinically referred children divided by age groupings and sex, interparent correlations on the behavior problems scale range from $r = .30$ on the Aggressive scale for 6- to 11-year-old girls ($N = 21$), to $r = .88$ on the Schizoid or Anxious factor for 4- to 5-year-old girls ($N = 11$). For the combined sample, the correlations between parents ranged from $r = .53$ on the Schizoid or Anxious factor to $r = .78$ for the Delinquent factor. On the Social Competence scales, overall interparent correlations ranged from $r = .44$ on the Activities scale to $r = .81$ on the School scale.

From the normative data sampling, Achenbach and Edelbrock (1983) compared the CBCL data obtained by three different interviewers on 241 children who were matched for age, sex, race, and socioeconomic status to 241 children whose parents were interviewed by each of the two other interviewers ($N = 723$). Achenbach and Edelbrock (1983) found significant ICCs of .959 for the 118 behavior problems and .927 for the social competence items, thus providing support for the interscorer reliability of the CBCL.

Validity

Convergent validity was demonstrated by correlations between raw scores of the CBCL and raw scores on the Conners Parent Questionnaire (Conners, 1973) and the Quay–Peterson Revised Behavior Problem Checklist (Quay & Peterson, 1983). Parents of 51 clinically referred children ages 6–11 years were asked to complete the three instruments in succession. The sequence of administration was counterbalanced across the sample to control for response sets. Results indicated that for boys, all Conners Parent Questionnaire scales significantly correlated with scales of similar content on the CBCL ranging from $r = .85$ for the CBCL Somatic scale and the Conners Psychosomatic scale to $r = .45$ for the CBCL Externalizing factor and Impulsive-Hyperactive scale of the Conners. For girls, the correlations were all significant except for two. The significant correlations ranged from $r = .44$ between the CBCL Somatic Complaints scale and the Conners Psychosomatic scale, to $r = .91$ between the CBCL Externalizing factor and the Impulsive-Hyperactive scale of the Conners. Similar findings also were evidenced between the CBCL and the Quay–Peterson Revised Behavior Problem Checklist. Correlational coefficients ranged from $r = .34$ (CBCL Social Withdrawal and BCP Anxiety Withdrawal) to $r = .88$ (CBCL Aggressive and BCL Conduct Disorder) for males; and $r = .45$ (CBCL Internalizing and BCP Psychotic) to $r = .92$ (CBCL Externalizing and BCP Motor Excess; CBCL and BCP Total Scores) for girls (Achenbach & Edelbrock, 1983). Similar findings were presented when T scores on the narrow-band factors were correlated with Conners Parent Questionnaire for mother ratings of 34 boys, ages 6–11, referred for hyperactivity concerns (Achenbach & Edelbrock, 1978), and 28 children, ages 6–17, referred for various mental health concerns (Weissman, Orvaschel, & Padian, 1980). Mash and Johnston (1983) also reported significant correlations between T scores for the Externalizing and Internalizing factors and the Conners Abbreviated Rating scale and the Werry–Weis–Peters Activity scale for nine hyperactive and normal children. Generally, the convergent validity of the CBCL appears adequate.

Discriminant validity of the CBCL has received support in that it has been able to discriminate between clinical and nonclinical samples on all Social Competence and Behavior Problem scales (Achenbach, 1978; Achenbach & Edelbrock, 1979). Race, sex, and age have been found to have minimal effects on scale scores (Achenbach & Edelbrock, 1983).

In differentiating clinical from nonclinical samples, Achenbach and Edelbrock (1983) discussed the use of cutoff scores for the CBCL. In establishing a cutoff score, the Total Score of the behavior problem items and the total score of the social competence items were employed, as they remain the best indices of the CBCL. The authors recommended the use of the 90th percentile for the behavior problem scores and the 10th percentile of the social competence scores as the cutoff criteria (Achenbach & Edelbrock, 1981). Behavior problem scores falling above the 90th percentile or social competence scores falling below the 10th percentile should be considered in the clinically significant range. The criteria for the behavioral problem scales classified an average of 90% of six non-referred samples as typical and 75% of the six referred samples as falling in the clinically significant range, with an overall misclassification rate of about 18%. For the social competence scales, the cutoff scores classified 90% of the nonreferred children as typical and 57% of the referred children as falling in this significant range. The total misclassification rate was approximately 16%. A discriminant analysis procedure produced similar findings with respect to correct classification rates (Achenbach & Edelbrock, 1983).

Summary

The CBCL is a rating scale designed to be completed by the parents of children ages 4–16. It requires the parents to have a fifth-grade reading level and can be completed in 15 to 17 minutes. Parents are asked to respond to items directed toward behavior problems as well as behavioral assets. The data derived from the CBCL can then be profiled on the Child Behavior Profile. This profile reports the individual items checked and the standardized scores for each of the narrow-band scales. Normative data are well founded, with reliability and validity questions adequately addressed. A comprehensive manual recently has been written and is easy to follow. In general, the CBCL appears to be a useful instrument which could be used in school as well as clinic settings. The CBCL also has been complemented by a Teacher Version, further adding to its diagnostic utility.

The CBCL has not been in wide use for a sufficient length of time for its weaknesses to become apparent. The only weakness that is currently obvious is that it is a complex set of instruments that requires more practitioner study than most checklists in order to be used appropriately. Further, hand scoring is somewhat laborious. A computer program is available for some microcomputers, yet given its price (approximately $100.00) and the fact that separate programs are needed for the parent and teacher forms, the cost may be a limiting factor for some users.

Teacher Version of the Achenbach Child Behavior Checklist

Description

The Teacher Report Form (TRF) is a questionnaire designed to parallel the Child Behavior Checklist as completed by the parents (Edelbrock & Achenbach, in press). It is a four-page questionnaire designed to address behavioral symptomology in the school setting and is completed by teachers or teacher aides. The TRF consists of 118 specific behavior problems derived directly from the parent form of the CBCL, with 25 items modified to be more applicable for teacher ratings. These 25 items originated from a pilot study with the TRF as well as from previously existing teacher behavior rating scales (Conners, 1969; Miller, 1972). Teachers are asked to respond to an item along a 3-point scale regarding how well it describes a student's behavior over the past 2-month period (0 = not true, 1 = somewhat true, 2 = very true or often true). This differs with the instruction to parents who are asked to include behaviors evident in the past 6 months; however, the authors state that these time periods can be modified as necessary by the clinician. The TRF can be completed by teachers in approximately 15 minutes and yields scores on multidimensional behavior problems, adaptive functioning, and school performance. Raw scores are plotted on the Teacher Profile and transformed into *T* scores and percentile ranks. Presently, the TRF is normed for boys, ages 6–11, with subsequent normative data for other age groupings in process.

The behavior problem scales of the teacher profile were derived in a fashion similar to the parent CBCL. Teachers completed TRFs on 450 boys referred to 18 mental health agencies in the eastern, midwestern, and southern parts of the country. The sample consisted of about 80% white, 19% black, and 1% other. The sample maintained approximately equal numbers of boys for each age level from 6 to 11 and was differentiated according to SES utilizing Hollingshead's (1957, 1975) scales of parent occupations, resulting in 22% falling in the upper SES, 39% in the middle SES, and 39% in the low SES. Normative data for the TRF were obtained from 300 completed TRFs of nonreferred boys, 50 at each age from 6 to 11. Racial composition and socioeconomic differentiation were similar to those characteristics of the referred group of boys.

After excluding items that were too rare (reported by less than 5% of teachers) or too common (reported by more than 95% of teachers), a principal components factor analysis was performed with a varimax rotation. Although this procedure produced 14 factors, six were eliminated because they had no more than five items with loading greater than .30. The remaining eight factors each had at least seven items with factor loadings of .30, and the largest factor, the Aggressive factor, included items with loading greater than .40. These eight second-order factors included Anxious, Social Withdrawal, Unpopular, Self-Destructive, Obsessive-Compulsive, Aggressive, Nervous-Overacting, and Inattentive. A factor analysis produced two factors similar to the Internalizing and Externalizing factors of the parent CBCL, as well as a mixed dimension containing second-order factors equally loading on both primary factors (Edelbrock, Costello, & Kessler, in press).

School Performance and Adaptive Functioning are rated by the teacher, then transformed into *T* scores. The school performance section simply consists of a space for listings of subject areas (to be provided by the teacher) and a 5-point scale after each on which to indicate if the child is "far below grade level" (rated 1), "somewhat below grade level" (rated 2), up to "far above grade level" (rated 5). The adaptive functioning section consists of four items rated on a 7-point scale (much less = 1; much more = 7). For example, "Compared to typical pupils of the same age, how hard is he or she working?" A mean rating for school performance is obtained by averaging the raw scores for each academic subject rated. A separate, total adaptive functioning score ranging from 4 to 28 can be obtained by adding teacher ratings on all four adaptive functioning items (Edelbrock *et al.*, in press). Normalized *T* scores were constructed on the basis of the normative sample (*N* = 300) for both areas.

Reliability
The items selected for the TRF and the inclusion of particular items for the derived factors are consistent with procedures used with the parent version of the CBCL. Consequently, internal consistency was deemed adequate.

No interrater reliability or interscorer reliability studies have been reported at this time.

Test–retest estimates of the TRF occurred over intervals of 1 week, 2 months, and 4 months. Utilizing a sample of 21 boys, ages 6–11, attending a special school for disturbed children, Edelbrock *et al.* (in press) reported 1-week average test-retest coefficients of $r = .89$ for the behavior problem scales, $r = .93$ for teacher ratings of school performance, and $r = .86$ for total adaptive functioning scores.

On a separate sample of 21 boys, ages 6–11, referred for special services due to behavioral or emotional problems, Edelbrock *et al.* (in press) reported a 2-month test-retest coefficient of $r = .77$ and a 4-month test-retest coefficient of $r = .64$ for the behavior problem scales. Generally, temporal stability of the TRF appears encouraging over the short term; however, these data should be interpreted cautiously in light of the small sample sizes.

Validity

Edelbrock *et al.* (in press) present evidence for the content validity of the TRF merely by deriving this instrument from the parent CBCL format. Support for discriminative validity of the TRF was provided by the authors as they found the TRF to effectively discriminate between clinically referred boys and non-referred boys across all eight narrow-band factors, the two broad-band factors, and the total score of the TRF. In addition, the school performance and adaptive functioning scales produced significantly lower scores for clinically referred boys as compared to their nonreferred counterparts.

Convergent and discriminant validity also have been demonstrated with the TRF. Edelbrock and Reed (1983) demonstrated that the teacher ratings of the Internalizing factor correlated significantly with observational ratings of Internalizing, but not with observational ratings of the Externalizing factor. In a related study, Reed and Edelbrock (1983) found that the total behavior score derived from the TRF correlated positively with observational assessments of problem behavior in the classroom and negatively with on-task behaviors. They also found that the Adaptive Functioning and School Performance scales correlated in a negative direction with observational ratings of problem behavior and in a positive manner with on-task ratings. Further refining the differential diagnosis potential of the TRF, Edelbrock *et al.* (in press) compared a heterogeneously comprised clinic control group to boys diagnosed with attention-deficit disorder (ADD). Specifically, boys diagnosed ADD obtained significantly higher scores on the Inattentive scale, and boys diagnosed ADD with hyperactivity obtained significantly higher scores on the Nervous-Overactive scale than boys diagnosed ADD without hyperactivity. These data provide preliminary support for the use of the TRF as a diagnostic tool in the school setting.

Summary

The Teacher Version of the Child Behavior Checklist was designed to closely parallel its parent instrument. Most of the items were directly extracted from the CBCL and, consequently, its factor structure aligns with the two primary- and eight secondary-order factors identified on the CBCL. Internal consistency and temporal stability of the TRF appear adequate, as does its validity, although little work has been done with this scale as yet. Nonetheless, the TRF is well normed for males, ages 6–11, and should prove at least comparable to other teacher behavior rating scales in assessment uses consistent with this population. Normative data for males younger than 6 and older than 11 as well as for females at all age levels should be forthcoming in the near future.

The Conners Parent Rating Scales

The Conners Parent and Teacher Rating Scales are perhaps the most widely used rating scales in clinical, school, and research settings, particularly with respect to identifying hyperkinetic behavior (Barkley, 1981). However, each of these scales yields multiple dimensions of childhood psychopathology, in addition to a hyperkinetic factor, thus lending themselves to screening for other specific child behavior problems. Both of these instruments have been adopted by the National Institute of Mental Health as part of its standardized assessment battery for childhood psychopharmacology (U.S. Department of Health, Education and Welfare, 1976).

Description

The Parent Rating Scale (PRS) is a 48-item instrument based on a listing of behavior problems compiled by Cytryn, Gilbert, and Eisenberg (1960). The PRS produces scores across five primary factors including Conduct Problems, Learning Problems, Psychosomatic, Impulsive-Hyperactive, and Anxiety (Conners, 1982). These five factors comprise a shortened version of the original PRS which consisted of 93 items grouped into 25 major headings (Conners, 1969, 1973). These clinical groupings were then factor analyzed into eight major factors for 683 children between the ages of 6 and 14. These factors included Conduct Disorder, Fearful-Anxious, Restless-Disorganized, Learning Problem-Immature, Psychosomatic, Obsessional, Antisocial, and Hyperactive-Immature (Conners & Blouin, 1980). Glow (1979), using a sample of 1,919 school children in South Australia, obtained 13 factors; and O'Conner, Foch, Sherry, and Plomin (1980) found 12 factors with a sample of 216 children.

The shortened version was devised in an attempt to simplify administration and interpretation. Items not loading in previous factor analyses were dropped, redundant items deleted, and other items reworded to increase clarity. Each item is answered "Not at All," "Just a Little," "Pretty Much," or "Very Much," and the number of points assigned to each answer is 0, 1, 2, or 3, respectively.

In both the original and revised versions of the PRS, there are 10 key items which comprise a Hyperactivity Index, although only four of these items load on the Impulsive-Hyperactive factor (Barkley, 1981). Scores for the Hyperactivity Index, as well as each of the empirically derived factors, are obtained by simply adding the raw scores gained from the parent ratings, with higher scores reflecting greater symptomology. The composite factor score is then divided by the number of items to obtain a mean factor score which is then transformed into a standardized T score. T scores greater than 70 (two standard deviations above the mean) should be used as the cutoff score for identifying significant behavior problems.

Normative data on the Revised Conners Parent Rating Scale were obtained from parents of 570 children in Pittsburgh, Pennsylvania. Target households were selected from the telephone book. Parents were asked to complete a questionnaire for each child between the ages of 3 and 17. The average age of the children in the normative sample was 9.9 years, with males comprising 55% and fe-males 45% of the sample. The sample included 98% white children, 1% black, and 1% other (Goyette, Conners, & Ulrich, 1978).

Reliability

Goyette *et al.* (1978) produced significant item-total correlations (one aspect of internal consistency reliability) on the 48-item PRS ranging from $r = .13$ on item 44 (vomiting or nausea) to $r = .65$ on item 6 (sucks or chews thumb, clothing, blanket), with an analysis of their normative data. Corrected for length, the 10-item Hyperactivity Index generated an alpha coefficient of .92 for a sample of 716 children (Sandberg, Wieselberg, & Shaffer, 1980).

At the item level, Goyette *et al.* (1978) found stability on 43 of the 48 items between mother and father ratings; however, for five of the items, mothers reported more observed problems than fathers. With respect to the factor structure of the PRS, product-moment correlations between mother and father scores were computed for 362 children. Correlations ranged from $r = .46$ on the Psychosomatic factor to $r = .57$ on the Conduct Problem factor, with a mean correlation of $r = .51$. In comparison, teacher–parent rating correlations ranged from $r = .33$ on the Conduct Problem factor to $r = .49$ on the Hyperkinesis Index. This is somewhat lower than the parent–parent comparison and provides support for investigating the context in which a behavior occurs. Glow (1979) provided additional support for the lower teacher–parent correlations with similar findings.

No interscorer reliability is reported, but it is probably high due to the simplicity of the scoring procedures.

Test-retest reliability of the PRS is adequate; however, the study typically reported employs a modification of the PRS. Using the Adelaide version of the PRS, Glow, Glow, and Rump (1982) obtained parental ratings of 254 children, ages 5–12, attending a small private government school in Australia. Over a 1-year period, test-retest correlational coefficients ranged from $r = .09$ on the Antisocial factor to $r = .71$ for Miscellaneous Factor for all subjects. For 5- to 6-year-olds the test-retest coefficients ranged from $r = .02$ (Antisocial) to $r = .77$ (Sleeping Difficulties); for 7- to 8-year-olds, $r = -.04$ (Antisocial) to $r = .74$ (Immature-Inattentive); and for 9- to 11-year-olds, $r = .38$ (Antisocial) to $r = .76$ (Hyperactive-Impulsive). In another modification of the PRS, O'Conner *et al.* (1980) produced 12 factors based on the original items of the PRS. Over a 2-month period, test-retest reliabilities for 28 children ranged from $r = -.08$ for Steals to $r = .95$ for School Problem. Although the stability of the PRS appears adequate over time, to date there have been no documented test–retest studies specifically with the 48-item PRS.

Validity

Much of the PRS's validation has focused on the number of factors produced by the PRS and the interest in the Hyperkinesis Index. With respect to the number of factors, there have been numerous studies (Conners, 1973; Glow, 1979; Goyette *et al.*, 1978; O'Conner *et al.*, 1980). The most popular factor structure, based on its use in the field, appears to be the revision of the original PRS by Goyette *et al.* (1978). Generally, of the eight factors that Conners (1973) produced, Goyette and colleagues obtained the first five (conduct problem, learning problem, psychosomatic, impulsive-hyperactive, anxiety). Although not necessarily statistically superior to the O'Conner *et al.* and Glow *et al.* versions, Goyette *et al.*'s PRS does lend itself more easily to administration and scoring. Further, its factor structure appears to provide the PRS with satisfactory convergent validity.

S. B. Campbell and Steinert (1978) had mothers of 45 normal children and 35 clinic children complete the Quay–Peterson Behavior Problem Checklist. They found that ratings by mothers of clinic children on the Conduct Problems, Learning Problems, and Hyperactivity scales all significantly intercorrelated, suggesting an externalizing dimension, while the Immaturity, Anxiety, and Personality Problem scales significantly intercorrelated, suggesting an internalizing dimension. Mothers of the control group rated their children similarly. Generally, the work of Campbell *et al.* provided support for the convergent validity of the PRS. The PRS Hyperactivity factor also has been found to relate significantly to the Werry–Weiss–Peters Activity Rating Scale (Barkley, 1981).

The Hyperkinesis Index has received much attention in the validity realm and has been useful in assessing drug-induced treatments with hyperactive children (Sprague & Sleater, 1973). However, Werry and Sprague (1974) do caution that this measure can be unstable across time, particularly due to a practice effect which lowers scores most generally from the first to the second administrations of the Index. In fact, this finding is relevant to all the factor scores on the Conners.

Sex differences have been noted on the PRS, with boys receiving more pathological ratings than girls, and mothers rating their children more harshly than fathers. Scores on the PRS also tend to decline as children grow older (Barkley, 1981). Barkley (1981) reported that the hyperactivity score and the total score of the 48-item PRS do not correlate significantly with objective measures of activity or attention; however, he does report that these measures do positively correlate with measures of child noncompliance to parental commands. Conners (1970), using the longer version of the PRS and a discriminant analysis function, presented discriminant validity for the PRS. Specifically, he found that the PRS factor scores correctly identified 77% of neurotic children, 70% of clinic-referred children, 83% of normal children, and 74% of hyperactive children.

Summary

The Conners Parent Rating Scale is a multidimensional instrument that has encouraged a vast amount of research. Nonetheless, a major problem in interpreting the results occurs due to the many versions of the scale which have been used; this severely limits study-to-study comparisons. Nonetheless, data collected across scales have been similar, suggesting adequate reliability and validity of the PRS components. The PRS maintains a wide age range of application (ages 3–17), and good normative data exist, particularly for the shortened version. The PRS also maintains the advantage of having a complementary Teacher Rating Scale and Hyperactivity Index, which were normed on the same populations as the PRS (Goyette *et al.*, 1978). The lack of a published manual for the PRS is a critical shortcoming.

The Conners Teacher Rating Scale

Description

The Conners Teacher Rating Scale (TRS) is a 39-item instrument structured in a format similar to the PRS (Conners, 1969). As previously described, the items are based on work done by Cytryn *et al.* (1960). The original 39-item TRS has been involved in four major factor analytical studies in four different countries. These include Conner's (1969) original analysis with a clinical sample of American children; Werry, Sprague, and Cohen's (1975) analysis with New Zealand children; Glow's (1979) work with South Australian children; and Trites, Blouin, and La-Prade's (1979) study with Canadian children. The results of these studies have been relatively similar. For example, the factor analytic procedures used by Trites *et al.* generated six factors which accounted for over 63% of the total variance of the TRS. These factors included Hyperactivity, Conduct Disorder, Emotional-Overindulgent, Anxious-Passive, Asocial, and Daydreams/Problem Attendance. Children in this normative sample ranged in age from 4 to 12 and included one-quarter of the elementary school population of Ottawa, Canada.

A revised 28-item TRS has been described by Goyette *et al.* (1978) which produced three factors: Conduct Problems, Hyperactivity, and Inattentive-Passive. These factors accounted for about 62% of the total variance within a normative group of 383 children ranging in age from 3 to 17.

Reliability

Trites, Blouin, and LaPrade (1979) generated mean interitem correlations for each of the six derived TRS factors (an index of internal consistency). These correlations ranged from $r = .27$ on Factor 6 (Daydreams/Problem Attendance) to $r = .52$ on Factor 2 (Conduct Disorder). Alpha coefficients for each of the scales fell into a moderate range of .61 on Daydreams/Attendance Problems to .95 on Hyperactivity. Similar alpha coefficients were generated by Glow (1979) using the Adelaide version of the TRS. Further support for the internal consistency of the scale was provided by coefficients of congruence calculated between factors derived from analyses of the whole sample and factors calculated on random half samples of the data. Although the order of emergence of the factors was slightly altered for the randomly selected half samples, the coefficients were quite adequate, ranging from $r = .86$ to $r = .99$. Using a five-factor solution, Lahey, Green, and Forehand (1980) found moderate correlations between the Conduct Problem, Hyperactivity, Inattentive-Passive, and Sociability scales. None of these scales was correlated with the Tension-Anxiety scale except for Inattentive-Passive. Generally, the internal consistency of the 39-item TRS appears adequate.

Glow (1979), using the Adelaide version of the TRS, reported teacher–teacher agreements (interrater reliability) ranging from $r = .38$ for Anxious to Please to $r = .75$ for Antisocial. Trites, Dugas, Lynch, and Ferguson (1979) provided further support for interrater agreement of the TRS by examining the percentage of children exceeding cutoff scores on ratings by two different teachers ($N = 1,154$). Generally, with the exception of the Tension-Anxiety factor, all factors were found to be stable as rated by the teachers.

No interscorer reliabilities have been reported, but the simplicity of the TRS suggests minimal difficulty in this regard.

In the original TRS, Conners (1973) reported adequate test-retest reliability ranging from about $r = .70$ to $r = .90$ over a 1-month interval. Over a 1-year period, the reliability coefficient generally remained significant, but it decreased slightly. Specifically, Glow *et al.* (1982) with the Adelaide version of the TRS found that test-retest correlations ranged from $r = -.01$ for Anxious to Please to $r = .57$ for Socially Rejected over a 1-year period. With respect to specific age ranges, Glow *et al.* reported ranges of $r = -.14$ for Anxious to Please to $r = .49$ for Hyperactive-Inattentive in 5- to 6-year-old children; $r = .12$ on Anxious to Please to $r = .66$ on Hyperactive-Inattentive for 7- to 8-year-olds; and $r = .14$ for Anxious to Please and Conduct Problems to $r = .57$ for Socially Rejected.

Validity

The content validity of the TRS appears to have a rich history simply in terms of its item selection procedures. The various factor structures do provide support for the construct validity of the TRS, although these vary somewhat from study to study. To date, the large normative sample collected by Trites, Dugas, Lynch, and Ferguson (1979) appears to provide a firm foundation for six basic factors comprising the TRS.

Criterion-related validity also appears adequate. Specifically, the TRS has been shown to discriminate between normal and hyperactive children (Kupietz, Bialer, & Winsberg, 1972; Sprague, Christensen, & Werry, 1974), and appears sensitive to drug treatment and behavior therapy (Conners, Taylor, Meo, Kurtz, & Fournier, 1972; Gittelman-Klein *et al.*, 1976; Werry & Sprague, 1974). Glow *et al.*'s (1982) multimethod factor matrix of the TRS also provided evidence for most of the TRS factors. Specifically, the TRS scales of Hyperactive-Inattentive, Unforthcoming-Unassertive, Socially Rejected, and Depressed Mood provided good discriminant validity over a 1-year period. The three other scales in their seven-factor solution of the TRS were indistinguishable from each other over that time interval.

The effects of age, sex, and socioeconomic status within the TRS also have been investigated. In the Goyette *et al.* (1978) study, males presented significantly more problems on the dimensions of Conduct Problem and Learning Problem than their female counterparts. The age of the child was found to account for a significant portion of the variance on the Psychosomatic and Impulsive-Hyperactive factors, with younger children having fewer psychosomatic problems and an increased number of impulsive-hyperactive problems. Both age and sex were found to be significant for the Hyperkinesis Index, with younger male children demonstrating the most problems on this dimension. Despite these results, Trites, Dugas, Lynch, and Ferguson (1979) found similar results with respect to age and sex, yet presented evidence to indicate that the proportion of variance accounted for by age and sex was small. The only effect of any significance, according to their measure of association (eta), was the variable sex on the Hyperactivity factor, with boys demonstrating significantly more hyperactive qualities than girls.

Aside from the major factor analytic studies with the Conners TRS, much of the literature relevant to the TRS has been directed toward its use as a measure of hyperactivity, and consequently, to its convergent validity in this diagnostic area. Specifically, the Conners TRS has been found to correlate significantly with the (*a*) Quay–Peterson Behavior Problem Checklist and the David's Hyperkinetic Rating Scale (Davids, 1971) with normal public school first-grade students (Arnold, Barneby, & Smeltzer, 1981); (*b*) the Quay–Peterson Scale and Devereux Elementary School Behavior Scale with emotionally disturbed children (von Isser, Quay, & Love, 1980); (*c*) peer evaluation, direct behavioral observations, and standardized academic achievement scores (Lahey *et al.*, 1980); and (*d*) teacher-reported hyperactivity on the Behavior and Temperament Survey and School Behavior Survey (Sandoval, 1981). In contrast, the TRS has not been found to correlate well with behavioral measures of activity such as teacher behavioral observations, actometer, stabilimeter, or structured freeplay observations (Kivlahan, Siegel, & Ullman, 1982). This finding has been supported by Rapoport, Abramson, Alexander, and Lott (1971) in a sample of children referred to hyperactivity concerns.

Kendall and Brophy (1981), however, found evidence to suggest that the Conners Scale may be more directed toward the activity component of hyperactivity than to the attentional component, despite an earlier TRS study (R. Brown & Wynne, 1982) which suggested that it could be sensitive to attentional deficits. Based on teacher and peer perceptions, King and Young (1982) found the TRS to be useful in sorting out the DSM-III diagnosis of Attention Deficit Disorder with and without hyperactivity. From this diagnostic perspective, the TRS also has been utilized with children manifesting depressed mood. Specifically, Jacobsen, Lahey, and Strauss (1983) found that for boys there was a significant correlation between three measures of depression and Unpopularity and Conduct Problem ratings on the TRS; for females, there was a significant relationship between the TRS total score and teacher ratings of depression.

Summary

The Conners Teacher Rating Scale is a short rating scale designed to be used in the school setting. It yields scores across numerous factors as well as a Hyperactivity Index, and it has been normed cross-culturally. The TRS seems to maintain adequate reliability and validity; however, as with its parent counterpart, there are several versions of the TRS upon which these psychometric properties have been based. The Goyette *et al.* (1978) version does provide the advantage of having the same normative population as the PRS, while the Trites, Dugas, Lynch, and Ferguson (1979) investigation provided an extremely large standardization sample. Generally, both Conners rating scales appear useful in contributing to school and clinic functioning. The need for an organized manual detailing the various forms of the TRS and PRS as well as the psychometric properties of each version has become acute, particularly in light of the continued popularity of these instruments.

Missouri Children's Behavior Checklist

Description

The Missouri Children's Behavior Checklist (MCBC) is a 70-item instrument designed to contribute to the differential diagnosis of behavioral pathology in children ages 5–16. Parents are asked to indicate whether their child has shown the behavior described during the past 6 months. The Missouri can be completed by a child's mother or father in approximately 15 to 20 minutes and yields ratings across six dimensions. These dimensions include Aggression, Inhibition, Activity Level, Sleep Disturbance, Somatization, and Sociability (Sines, Pauker, Sines, & Owen, 1969). An additional scale, the Sex scale, was added by Thompson and McAdoo (1973) in a minor modification of the MCBC; however, Curry and Thompson (1982) have found this scale to be infrequently endorsed, with an average score of less than 1. Finally, a Total Pathology Score, comprised of the scores on all the scales except Sex and Socialization, has been suggested by DeFilippis (1979).

The Missouri items, which require a yes or no response, describe (with only one exception) different types of children's pathological behavior. These items were selected from an initial pool of 95 behavioral descriptions drawn from the literature to create six factors. This selection process was guided by four criteria:

1. No item could contribute to more than one dimension.
2. An item on a reported factor had to have a factor loading of .30 or greater.
3. The behavioral dimension projected for an item had to be consistent with its use in the research.
4. An item had to appear in the same factor in more than one study (Sines *et al.*, 1969).

Items were retained in the final checklist and assigned to a specific dimension if the point-biserial correlation between the item and the total dimension score was at least .30 and the square of the point-biserial correlation was at least two times as large as the square of the correlation between that item and any of the other five dimensions (Sines *et al.*, 1969). Ultimately, factor analytic studies demonstrated the existence of the desired six factors. Three of the behavioral clusters—aggression, inhibition, and activity level—are statistically consistent and represent orthogonal clusters of the relevant behavioral characteristics. The three other clusters, although somewhat less stable and consistent in existence, involve sleep disturbance, somatization, and sociability.

Standardization data for the Missouri were collected from a wide array of settings in the United States and Canada, including child psychiatry, pediatric, and mental health clinics. Most of the children were seen for psychological evaluation. The sample consisted of 404 boys and 250 girls, ages 5–19; however, the Missouri's psychometric properties were constructed from the sample of males (Sines *et al.*, 1969). The final number of subjects in each age group varied extensively, ranging from 7 males for age 16 to 69 males for age 9. The effects of age, sex, and SES were not tested.

Ten years later, DeFilippis (1979) presented additional normative data on the six-dimension form of the MCBC. After randomly selecting their names from the public school files of a midwestern community, 302 mothers of children ages 7–9 completed the MCBC. While few minority group members were included in the sample, sex, SES, and IQ variables were tested for their effects on the MCBC scores. In addition to normative data for males and females, results of the study suggested that males significantly differed from females as they received higher scores on the Aggression scale, the Activity Level scale, and the Total Pathology scale, and lower scores on the Sociability scale. No effects of SES or IQ were obtained, with the exception of low IQ males having lower Sociability scores than their higher IQ counterparts. Following Miller, Hampe, Barrett, and Noble's (1971) lead, DeFilippis (1979) suggested a cutoff point of one standard deviation above the mean for the Total Pathology scale in defining groups of disturbed children, and further supported this cutoff score criterion by correctly identifying 89% of children recommended for treatment.

In a sample of average functioning, southern black children ($N = 437$), Kelly and King (1980) generated normative data for ages 5–16 on the MCBC. Males and females were combined to produce means and standard deviations for each of the six scales. Each sample ranged from $N = 9$ for age 5 to $N = 61$ for age 10. Significant age effects for the Aggression and Somatization scales were found, with these characteristics diminishing with age, as well as significant sex effects for the

Inhibition and Somatization scales, with females being rated higher than males on each scale.

The MCBC has a relatively easy scoring system whereby a child receives one point for each item reported in the pathological direction. Consequently, the higher a child's total score on any of the factors, the greater the possibility of that child exhibiting the deviant behavior described by the factor. This convention differs for the Sociability dimension where a higher score indicates more positive behavior.

Reliability

Internal consistency reliability was assessed on each of the six MCBC factors by the split-half (odd–even) method. Utilizing the Spearman–Brown correction formula to correct for the shortened factor length, Sines *et al.* (1969) produced internal consistency correlations ranging from $r = .67$ on the Sociability dimension to $r = .86$ on the Aggression dimension. Sines *et al.* (1969) also investigated the internal consistency of the Missouri by correlating the six dimensions. They stated that the dimensions are relatively independent, although nearly all of the intercorrelations were significant beyond the .01 level. The correlations ranged from $r = .01$ between the Somatization and Sociability dimensions, to $r = .43$ between the Aggression and Activity Level dimensions. This latter intercorrelation accounted for approximately 18.5% of the shared variance between the two dimensions.

The authors contend that high scoring reliability can be regularly achieved, although no data were presented to support this claim. However, the simplicity of the "yes/no" response format clearly would facilitate scoring of the Missouri.

During the initial data collection process, Sines *et al.* (1969) collected behavior checklists from both parents of 47 children. On individual items, the agreement between mothers and fathers (interrater reliability) ranged from 53% to 94%. For each dimension, the agreement percentage was slightly more restricted, ranging from 69% to 93%. In a subsequent study, Thompson, Curry, and Yancy (1979) also found a high degree of consistency between mothers' and fathers' behavior checklist ratings, particularly with female children. However, there was a tendency for mothers to rate their sons as significantly higher on Aggression, Inhibition, Somatization, and Sleep Disturbance than did fathers.

No temporal stability data for the MCBC have been reported.

Validity

Most of the studies using the MCBC to date have investigated its ability to identify different populations of children. In the initial development of the Missouri, Sines *et al.* (1969) demonstrated significant differences on four of the six dimensions between referred and typical boys. Specifically, MCBCs of 24 boys seen in a child psychiatry clinic were compared to checklist scores of 24 normal boys matched for age and IQ scores. Boys in each of the groups ranged in age from 6 to 14 years old ($\chi = .988$, $SD = 2.21$), while IQ scores for the clinic group averaged 103.67 as compared to 104.04 for the nonclinic boys. The clinic boys obtained significantly higher ratings on the Aggression, Inhibition, Activity Level, and Sociability dimensions, with no differences between the two groups on the Sleep Disturbance and Somatization dimensions. The lack of statistically significant differences on these latter dimensions was attributed to the selectivity of the children referred to child psychiatry clinics. The authors speculated that children whose primary complaints included somatic problems and/or sleep disturbances would not typically be referred to child psychiatry clinics. Although these findings supported the construct validation of the MCBC, Sines *et al.* (1969) did caution that they reflect descriptive characteristics of the MCBC rather than validity characteristics.

Using a similar paradigm, Curry and Thompson (1979) obtained Revised Missouri Behavior Checklists from mothers of 50 children referred to a child psychiatry clinic, 50 children referred to a developmental disabilities clinic, and 50 nonreferred control children. The subjects in the three groups were individually matched on age, sex, and socioeconomic status. No participants had an IQ of less than 80. Each group of 50 children included 30 males and 20 females. Hypothesizing that differences would exist between the two clinic groups and between each of the clinic groups and the normal controls, Curry and Thompson found that children referred to the psychiatric clinic were rated higher on the dimensions of Aggression, Activity Level, and Sleep Disturbance than were children referred to the developmental disabilities clinic. Both clinical groups were rated higher on these dimensions than were the nonreferred children. Further, the psychiatrically referred children were rated higher on the dimensions of Somatization and Sex than the developmental disabilities-referred children; however, there was no difference between the normal and developmental disabilities children on these two dimensions. Interestingly, the Sociability dimension did not differentiate between psychiatric and control group children, but both of these groups were rated higher in Sociability than their developmentally disabled counterparts. The Inhibition dimension, although rated higher for the clinic groups when compared to the control group, did not discriminate between the two clinic samples.

Similar findings have been produced between controls and mental health clinic-referred children (Thompson & McAdoo, 1973) and children referred for evaluation to two separate clinics for developmental disabilities (Thompson, Curry, & Yancy, 1979). Generally, results with the MCBC indicate that children referred for developmental disabilities evaluation have higher ratings of behavioral disturbance than normals, but lower ratings (less severe) than children referred for psychiatric services (Curry & Thompson, 1979). Further, although children referred to developmental disability clinics exhibited homogeneous group MCBC ratings, their areas of behavioral disturbance differed on the basis of their presenting problems (Thompson *et al.*, 1979).

Curry and Thompson (1979) also investigated individual sex differences in this three-sample study, although cross-sex differences were not described. Males in the psychiatry-referred sample were rated highest in the Activity Level dimension, and they significantly differed from males in the other two groups, while the developmentally delayed males were rated higher than the control group males on this dimension. Psychiatrically referred males were rated higher on the dimensions of Sleep Disturbance, Somatic Complaints, and Sex than the other two groups, while no differences on these scales were noted for the control and developmental disabilities-referred males. Both male clinic groups received significantly higher scores on the Aggression and Inhibition dimensions than the control group males, but the scores between the clinic groups did not differ. No differences were observed on the Sociability dimension between any of the samples.

Female children in the psychiatry-referred sample were rated higher on the

Aggressive dimension than the other two groups of females; no differences between the latter two groups were demonstrated on this dimension. Consistent with the overall findings on the Sociability scale, developmental disability-referred females were rated as significantly less sociable than child psychiatry-referred females, who also did not differ from control group females. Differences were demonstrated on the Inhibition, Activity Level, and Sleep Disturbance scales between the clinic and control groups, but not between the two clinic groups. No differences occurred on the Somatization and Sex dimensions for any of the groups.

Thompson *et al.* (1979) found no sex differences for any of the seven MCBC scales with two separate developmental disabilities clinic samples. Obtaining MCBCs on 126 males and 47 females referred to separate clinics and on 27 male and 32 female normal controls from pediatrician offices, Thompson *et al.* (1979) found remarkable consistency across settings for the seven dimensions. These results were presented as evidence for the homogeneity of behavioral problems in children.

Employing cluster analysis techniques, Curry and Thompson (1982) further explored this contention by determining if the MCBC could provide information pertaining to broad-band syndromes (e.g., undercontrolled vs. overcontrolled) and narrow-band syndromes as represented by the seven dimensions. In a well-designed study, they found four reliable behavioral clusters in a population of children referred to developmental evaluation centers. These clusters included Aggressive-Action, Inhibited, Mixed Disturbance, and Normal. Based on the inspection of the replicated cluster profiles, classification rules were developed for each of the clusters. Applying these rules to the two separate developmental evaluation clinic samples resulted in correct classification rates of 74% and 78% ($N = 126$), with the majority being classified in the normal cluster. When the same classification rules were applied to 105 children referred to a community guidance clinic, over half of the children were unclassified, further supporting previous results where children referred for developmental disabilities were quantitatively and qualitatively different than their child psychiatry-referred peers (Curry & Thompson, 1979).

These results require a careful inspection of MCBC's broad-band interpretation across different samples of children. Although two of the clusters appear to align with Achenbach's (1966) broad-band patterns of Externalization (Aggressive-Active) and Internalization (Inhibition), the third cluster (Mixed Disturbance Group) presents a more heterogeneous pattern of disturbance. Thus, this latter group may be more difficult to interpret and less practical in its application. Construct validity for this classification scheme and the behavioral dimensions was obtained later with developmentally delayed children by comparing MCBC profiles to specific clinical findings and recommendations obtained through independent interdisciplinary evaluations (Thompson & Curry, 1983).

Utilizing the classification scheme and the dimensions of the MCBC described above, Thompson, Curry, Sturner, Green, and Funk (1982) investigated preschool children for their "at-risk" potential in developmental and learning areas. Children ($N = 105$) participating in a prekindergarten health screening program completed the McCarthy Scales of Children's Abilities (McCarthy, 1972), while their parents completed the MCBC. Based on the McCarthy results, the children were divided into two groups: an at-risk group ($N = 42$) defined as those preschoolers who obtained a General Cognitive Index (GCI) greater than 1 standard deviation below the mean (GCI = 84), and a nonrisk group ($N = 63$) which scored 84 or above on the GCI. An additional comparison group ($N = 20$) of children referred to a developmental evaluation center also was obtained. All groups were similar with respect to race, sex, and SES. On the six scales of the MCBC, the at-risk children received significantly higher ratings on the Inhibition and Activity Level scales, and significantly lower ratings on the Sociability scale than the nonrisk children. The developmentally disabled group received significantly higher ratings on the dimensions of Aggression, Inhibition, and Activity Level than the nonrisk children, and significantly higher ratings on Aggression and Inhibition than their at-risk counterparts. Across the MCBC's behavioral clusters, the developmentally disabled preschoolers evidenced the most Aggressive-Active, Inhibited, Mixed, and Unclassified profiles as well as the lowest number of normal profiles. The nonrisk group had the highest percentage of normal profiles. On all of the profiles, the at-risk preschool group percentages fell between the developmentally disabled and nonrisk groups. The Sleep Disturbance and Somatization scales as well as the mixed profile did not differentiate among the three groups.

Although the MCBC was based on items from homogeneous factors found in the literature, a formal factor analysis of the MCBC has never been published. Thus, the empirical structure of the variables of the MCBC is somewhat suspect. McMahon, Kunce, and Salomak (1979) partially addressed this issue; however, they employed the original 95-item version of the Missouri in their analysis. Using a conservative approach in factor delineation, McMahon *et al.* obtained three orthogonal factors in a sample of 120 males, ages 9–11, referred to a midwestern university hospital setting. These three factors accounted for 43%, 30%, and 27% of the total variance, respectively. All items of each factor had factor loadings above .40; however, because the third factor consisted of only eight items, the authors considered it statistically limited and deleted it. No further discussion of this third factor was presented. The two remaining factors were labeled Aggression, consisting of 21 items, and Social Responsibility, consisting of 18 items. Utilizing these two factors in identifying children with behavior problems, the authors found that the factors correlated significantly with interdisciplinary staff diagnosis of behavior disorder and hyperkinesis. These results also suggested the utility of maternal ratings on the MCBC as a potential resource in the multidisciplinary evaluation and diagnosis of children.

Summary

The Missouri Children's Behavior Checklist is an interesting rating scale designed to be completed by parents and assist in the clinical differentiation of psychopathology in children ages 5–16. The MCBC yields scores across six or seven dimensions, as well as a Total Score, and has been useful in identifying clusters of behavioral symptomology across different populations of children. Reliability and validity of the MCBC appear adequate; however, these data must be tempered by recognizing that the normative base of the MCBC is less than adequate. Further, in the original test construction, only males were included to form the psychometric properties of the scale, and the items were grouped into their respective scales by a clinical review of the literature. Unfortunately, the only formal factor analytic procedure reported to date employed the original version of the MCBC. Interestingly, this factor analysis produced two large band factors similar to Achenbach's (1966) broad-band factors. Support for the specific scales was not provided by this factorial procedure, prompting serious questions about the uniqueness of the MCBC dimensions. Another liability, the MCBC's lack of a teacher counterpart scale, also limits its applicability to the home setting. Further research with this instrument, particularly with respect to its psychometric foundation, multirater–multisetting use, and clinical utility, is needed before the MCBC can be used routinely in a school or clinic setting. An organized test manual also would prove useful.

The Quay–Peterson Behavior Problem Checklist

Description
The Behavior Problem Checklist (BPC) is comprised of 55 items investigating children's and adolescents' behavior traits. Each item of the scale is scored on a 3-point system. A score of "0" indicates no problem for that particular behavior or item, a score of "1" represents a mild problem in that area, and a score of "2" suggests a severe problem. The BPC is comprised of three primary scales (Conduct Problem, Personality Problem, and Inadequacy-Immaturity) and one secondary scale (Socialized Delinquency). The Conduct Problem scale has 17 items, the Personality Problem scale 14 items, the Inadequacy-Immaturity scale 8 items, and the Socialized Delinquency scale 6 items. Additionally, the BPC contains four items designed to alert the rater to possibly more severe behavior problems (autism and childhood psychosis) as well as six items which are not scored. A total score for each of the three primary scales and the secondary scale is obtained by summing each item's raw score ("1" or "2") for that scale.

A major strength of the BPC is that it was developed based largely on empirical data. Initial items were compiled by reviewing case folders from a child guidance clinic and noting referral problems for each child. A total of 58 item-behavior descriptions were selected and a checklist was formulated. This checklist was then completed by teachers for a sample of 831 kindergarten through sixth-grade students and the item scores were factor analyzed. The results indicated a two-factor solution, with one factor called Conduct Problem and the other factor called Personality Problem. Further research with a group of seventh and eighth graders yielded a third factor called Inadequacy-Immaturity. These are the three primary scales of the BPC. Those items that consistently had high factor loadings on a particular scale across the different studies were retained in the BPC. The Socialized Delinquency subscale was derived from separate but similar research concerned with behavior problems of juvenile delinquents. In essence, then, the BPC represents an instrument developed through the compilation of factor analytic data.

The BPC has been one of the more widely used behavior checklists in research studies. The next sections focus on reviewing empirical evidence on the BPC. Because of previous reviews, the present discussion will focus on articles published after 1979. Readers interested in reviews prior to 1979 should see Quay and Peterson (1975, 1979).

Reliability
The reliability of the BPC has been the focus of a number of different studies. In general, the results indicate adequate reliability for the scales. Internal consistency coefficients have ranged from .26 to .89 (Mack, 1969; Quay & Parsons, 1972). Test-retest reliability coefficients ranged from .74 to .91 with a 2-week in-

terval, and from .21 to .58 with a 1-year interval (Eaves, 1975; Quay & Peterson, 1967). The primary focus of more current literature is on interrater reliability (Jacob, Grounds, & Haley, 1982; Lindholm & Touliatos, 1982; Touliatos & Lindholm, 1981).

The degree of interrater agreement on the BPC has been somewhat variable, depending on the specific comparison made (i.e., parent–parent, parent–teacher). In general, there tends to be a moderate to fairly high correspondence between ratings of parents. Lindholm and Touliatos (1981b) reported coefficients ranging from .68 to .77 between ratings of mothers and fathers, with a sample of elementary and middle school children receiving counseling. Jacobs *et al.* (1982) found a higher correlation between parental ratings on the Conduct Problem scale ($r = .73$) than on the Personality Problem scale ($r = .43$). The interrater agreements between parents and teachers tend to be somewhat lower than do ratings between parents. Touliatos and Lindholm (1981) reported correlations between mothers and teachers to range from .13 to .45 and from .17 to .38 for ratings between fathers and teachers. Lindholm and Touliatos (1982) found correlations between parents and teachers to range from .16 to .52. Interparent agreement also tended to be somewhat higher than parent–counselor ratings and teacher–counselor ratings.

Validity

Firestone, Kelly, and Fike (1980) utilized the BPC in examining the effectiveness of parent training groups in modifying behavior problems with children. The sample consisted of 18 parents of children 3–11 years of age. All of the children had been referred by physicians who reported behavior problems such as aggressiveness or noncompliance. Three groups were then formed: Group 1 consisted of six sets of parents who received training in a behavioral–social learning program; Group 2 consisted of six mothers who received the same training; and Group 3 was a control group. All of the parents completed the BPC before and after the intervention program. The results indicated that both treatment groups showed improvement on the Conduct Problem scale when compared to the controls; however, a significant decline in problem behaviors occurred only within the parents of Group 1. Specific to the Personality Problem scale, the two treatment groups again showed improvement when compared with the control group; however, the Group 2 mothers also showed a significant improvement in scores over Group 1.

Lindholm and Touliatos (1981a, 1981b) reported findings supporting the BPC's sensitivity to developmental changes in behavior problems. One study used a large sample ($N = 2,991$) of white boys and girls enrolled in kindergarten through eighth grade (Lindholm & Touliatos, 1981a). Teacher ratings were completed using the BPC resulting in two general developmental patterns. The first was that Conduct Problem, Personality Problem, Inadequacy-Immaturity, and Psychotic signs tended to increase from kindergarten to about third grade, decline from third to sixth grade, and then stabilize from sixth through eighth grade. In the second pattern, the Socialized Delinquency scale increased from kindergarten to third grade, and then stabilized through the eighth grade. Similar developmental patterns were reported in the second study (Lindholm & Touliatos, 1981b).

Differences also have been reported among teacher ratings on the BPC for children from different family structures (Touliatos & Lindholm, 1980). Touliatos and Lindholm (1980) compared the teacher ratings for children living with both parents ($N = 2,991$), children living with mothers only ($N = 34$), children living with their mother and stepfather ($N = 264$), and children living with their father and stepmother ($N = 341$). The primary analyses consisted of a comparison of those children living with both parents and with those children from the other conditions. In general, the results suggest that the BPC is sensitive to differences among the groups. For example, the children living with mothers only scored significantly higher than the children from intact homes on all of the scales. Results for the other groups indicated significant differences on only the Socialized Delinquency and Conduct Problem scales.

The relationship between the BPC and measures of marital hostility and marital adjustment was investigated by Porter and O'Leary (1980). The ratings were obtained from parents of 64 children, referred to a child psychological clinic, who completed the BPC, the Short Marital Adjustment Test (SMAT), and the O'Leary–Porter Scale (OPS). The SMAT is a measure of marital adjustment which helps to discriminate distressed from nondistressed marriages. The OPS was apparently designed for this study to index the frequency with which a child observed various forms of marital hostility. The children for this study ranged in age from 5 to 16 years. In order to determine the relationship between sex, age, and marital problems, the children were divided into four groups: boys and girls 10 years old and younger ($N = 13$) and boys and girls 11 years old and older ($N = 17$), respectively. The results indicated a significant correlation between the Conduct Problem scale and the OPS for the younger boys. In addition, significant correlations were found between the Personality Problem, Inadequacy-Immaturity, and the Socialized Delinquency scales and the OPS for the older boys. There were no significant correlations for either group of girls between any of the BPC scales and the other two tests. The authors discussed numerous possible interpretations of these findings, including that the behavior problems manifested by girls are less salient for parental distress.

Lueger (1980) examined differences on the BPC between transgressor (those that cheated on a task) and nontransgressor behavior-problem adolescents. The sample consisted of 60 adolescent males who were in either group-care homes or short-term diagnostic facilities. The subjects participated in one of two experimental conditions (arousal-inducing or arousal-reducing situations), and the rate of transgressor behavior was obtained using a picture arrangement task. Across both experimental conditions, 34 of the 60 subjects exhibited some degree (i.e., changing of at least one answer) of transgressor behavior. Comparisons were then made among the scales of the BPC between the transgressor and nontransgressor groups. The results indicated significant differences between the groups on the Conduct Problem scale and the Socialized Delinquency scale with the transgressors scoring higher.

The BPC, as discussed earlier, was originally formulated by examining the factor structure of ratings on a number of different behaviors. In this sense, it can be argued that the instrument has demonstrated adequate construct validity, since factor analysis is a primary means of providing such evidence. However, there is the question as to the generalizability of these results to other populations not included in the original standardization studies. Two recent studies have examined the factor structure of the BPC with different samples (Arnold *et al.*, 1981; Gajar & Hale, 1982).

Arnold *et al.* (1981) factor analyzed the BPC using a random sample ($N = 225$) of first graders. The authors indicated the importance of these data, arguing that Quay and Peterson's (1967) repeated factor analyses used only clinical and nonrandomly selected typical children. Their analysis for this study yielded the same four factors reported by Quay and Peterson (1967), but a pattern of item loadings which varied somewhat. The first factor was very similar to the Conduct Problem scale except for the significant loadings of several additional items which they characterized as measures of distrust. Arnold *et al.* (1981) called this a "Hyperkinetic" factor. The second factor was similar to Quay and Peterson's Personality Problem factor except several additional items also significantly loaded here. Arnold *et al.* (1981) called this a "Shy-inept" factor. The third factor was quite different from Quay and Peterson's and reflected what Arnold *et al.* (1981) felt was a "Depressed" dimension. The fourth factor was similar across the studies reflecting "Dyssocial" behavior.

Gajar and Hale (1982) examined the factor structure of the BPC across different racial groups. The BPC was factor analyzed separately with a sample of white and black exceptional children. The results for the white sample indicated that three factors accounted for 81.4% of the common variance. The first factor was considered conduct disorder, the second personality problem, and the third immaturity-inadequacy. The analysis for the black sample indicated that four factors accounted for 78.8% of the common variance. For this sample, the first factor was considered conduct disorder, the second immaturity-inadequacy, the third personality problem, and the fourth racially specific factor was suggested to indicate resistance by black children to expectations within white academic settings.

The relationship of the BPC with other measures designed to assess the same or similar constructs also provides information concerning the validity of the test. Von Isser *et al.* (1980) intercorrelated the BPC with the Conners' Teacher Questionnaire (CTQ) for a sample of 93 elementary and junior high students enrolled in emotional disability classes. The results indicated a significant correlation between the Conduct Problem scales for both tests. The Conduct Problem scale of the BPC also showed a significant relationship with the Hyperactivity scale of the CTQ and a negative correlation with the CTQ's Inattentive-Passive scale. The BPC Personality Problem scale was negatively correlated with the Conduct Problem and Hyperactivity scales and positively correlated with the Tension-Anxiety scale. The Inadequacy-Immaturity scale of the BPC correlated significantly with the CTQ's Inattentive-Passive and Tension-Anxiety scales.

Summary

The BPC appears to be a useful behavioral checklist. One of its primary strengths is its development through an empirical, factor analytic procedure. The BPC appears to be sensitive to differences between groups, developmental changes with behavior problems, and intervention strategies. The factor structure of the BPC is fairly consistent across groups, and the scales appear to have adequate reliability. In general, the research suggests that the BPC can contribute meaningful information to a clinical assessment with children.

The Revised Behavior Problem Checklist

Quay (1983) outlined the development of the Revised Behavior Problem Checklist (RBPC). The item pool for the RBPC was expanded from 55 to 150 items and was administered to four samples of deviant children. Items that were endorsed by less than 15% or more than 85% of the raters within each sample were not included for further analysis. The revised items were then factor analyzed for each of the samples. Item retention was based on consistency across analyses as well as nondetrimental effects to a scale's reliability coefficient. The RBPC contains four major scales and two minor scales. The major scales of the checklist are Conduct Disorder, Socialized Aggression, Attention, Problem-Immaturity, and Anxiety-Withdrawal. The two minor scales are Psychotic Behavior and the Motor Excess scale.

Quay (1983) reported some reliability and validity data for the RBPC. Internal reliability coefficients for the scales range from .72 to .94. Interrater reliability coefficients range from .52 to .85. The scales of the RBPC appear to discriminate normal from clinical samples as well as differentiate among different clinical groups. The data suggest the clinical utility of the RBPC, although further research is needed.

Case Study

The case study material that follows was selected because it exemplifies the multisetting, multisource design presented earlier in this chapter. Unfortunately, case material that is collected in a manner consistent with this design is rare. Therefore, the authors did not have access to cases that utilized the four devices just reviewed. The case chosen does utilize an experimental preschool version of the Revised Behavior Problem Checklist (Quay, 1983) and the Temperament Assessment Battery (TAB; Martin, 1984).

The TAB is a battery of three rating scales consisting of a parent form, a teacher form, and a clinician form. It is designed for children aged 3–7. Each form was designed to measure six social–emotional variables believed to have some genetic component of temperament (see Buss & Plomin, 1975, for a detailed discussion). The scales are designed to measure activity level, adaptability (ease and speed of adjustment to new environments), approach/withdrawal tendency in new social situations, emotional intensity, distractibility, and persistence (attention span and perseverance when faced with difficult learning tasks).

The reader will find that the processes of data aggregation and data reporting demonstrated here can be generalized to any case in which rating scale data are obtained. The case material presented is factual, with only minor changes made in background data in order to protect the anonymity of the child and his family. All names have been changed to further protect client anonymity.

Reason for Referral

Donald was referred to a university-based preschool clinic by his mother because she wanted to know if his social/emotional and cognitive development were progressing at an appropriate rate.

Background

Donald is a 5-year-old white male who lives with his mother, a stepfather, and a younger brother (age 2) in a small, southern college town. Donald's biological parents were divorced when he was 1 year of age, and his mother remarried within 6 months. Donald's brother, Billy, was the product of the second marriage.

Donald's stepfather, David, is an advanced graduate student in pharmacy at a major state university. His mother, Anne, is a mathematics teacher in a public junior high school. Anne provides the majority of the financial support for the family; David has a small assistantship which covers most of his educational expenses. The family is struggling a bit financially, but they are optimistic about their economic future when David graduates. He plans to become a research pharmacist for a pharmaceutical company.

The family has faced several significant stresses during Donald's life that the mother feels may have had some adverse psychological effects on him. First, the separation and divorce from her first husband created a great deal of stress for Anne, which she fears may have been transferred in some way to Donald. Second, Donald has had to adjust to a new father, and more recently, to a new baby brother. Third, Anne and David's work schedule is such that Donald and Billy are left in the care of a day-care, preschool center 5 days per week, 7 hours per day. Both Anne and David worry about the effects of this child-care arrangement and the effects of being away from their sons so much.

Regarding David's general developmental progress, his mother reports that he attained the major gross-motor milestones somewhat earlier than other children in their neighborhood. His speech development and language acquisition have seemed to progress at about an average rate. As an infant, Donald was "colicky," had sleep problems (frequently had trouble falling asleep, awakening during the night), and seemed to cry more than other infants. However, these problems seem to have decreased as he has matured. Toilet training and weaning progressed at appropriate times without incident.

Assessment Design

Donald first came to the preschool clinic at age 3 years, 2 months. He was administered a battery of cognitive assessment instruments consisting of the Stanford-Binet Intelligence Scale, the Peabody Picture Vocabulary Test-Revised, and the Developmental Test of Visual-Motor Integration. His mother, father, and nursery school teacher completed the parent and teacher forms of the Temperament Assessment Battery (TAB; Martin, 1984). His mother was extensively interviewed about background data and Donald's cognitive and social–emotional development. The graduate student assessor in the clinic also completed the clinician form of the TAB immediately after the assessment of Donald.

Donald was assessed on two subsequent occasions, at age 4 years, 1 month, and at age 5 years, 2 months, with the same instruments used during the first assessment, with some exceptions. During the second assessment, the McCarthy Scales-Mental scale was administered instead of the Stanford-Binet, the Peabody Picture Vocabulary Test-Revised was not administered, and the Revised Behavior Problem Checklist-Preschool Version was completed by the mother. During the third assessment, the Revised Behavior Problem Checklist was again completed by the mother, and the teacher was asked to complete the Bristol Social Adjustment Guide (BSAG) (Stott, 1970). The BSAG is a teacher rating instrument designed to determine the presence of pathological social–emotional tendencies. Like the Achenbach Child Behavior Checklist, the device produces data on two broad factors—Overreaction and Underreaction. Subscales then provide measures of variables under each of the broad categories. Under the Underreaction category, the subscales are Unforthcomingness, Depression, Withdrawal. Under the Overreaction category, the subscales are Hostility and Inconsequence.

Assessment Results

The results of the cognitive assessment across the three assessment periods are presented in Table 10-2. It can be seen that IQ scores increased across the assessment periods, with the overall mean being approximately 108. Results from the Peabody Picture Vocabulary Test-Revised and the Developmental Test of Visual-Motor Integration followed the same pattern and were at approximately the same level. The importance of three assessments can be seen in these results. Even for the generally reliable measures in the cognitive domain, significant differences in scores across time and trends across time are evident.

The results across the three assessment periods for the TAB can be seen in Tables 10-3 and 10-4. Table 10-3 presents raw scores for each rater at each assessment. Also,

Table 10-2
Results of Donald's Cognitive Assessment at Three Preschool Ages

Type of test	Age at assessment		
	3 years, 2 months	4 years, 1 month	5 years, 2 months
Scholastic Aptitude			
IQ	100	109	116
	(Binet)	(McCarthy)	(Binet)
Peabody Picture Vocabulary Test			
Standard score	83	No data	102
Percentile	11		55
Developmental Test of Visual-Motor Integration			
Age equivalent	3 years, 0 months	4 years, 6 months	5 years, 7 months
Developmental rate	98	108	110

Table 10-3
Raw Scores for Ratings of Donald on the
Temperament Assessment Battery at Three Preschool Ages

Rater scale	Age at assessment			Mean	Setting mean
	3 years, 2 months	4 years, 1 month	5 years, 2 months		
Mother					(Home)
Activity	27	36	39	34.0	32.2
Adaptability	42	34	39	38.3	36.2
Approach	19	23	21	21.0	23.9
Intensity	24	23	19	22.0	24.4
Distractibility	33	31	30	31.3	33.0
Persistence	28	32	34	31.3	33.9
Father					
Activity	23	35	33	30.3	
Adaptability	32	36	34	34.0	
Approach	37	20	23	26.7	
Intensity	20	31	29	26.7	
Distractibility	43	31	30	34.7	
Persistence	36	35	39	36.7	
Teacher					(School)
Activity	40	17	15	24.0	24.0
Adaptability	29	54	48	43.7	43.7
Approach	26	36	44	35.3	35.3
Intensity	40	24	27	30.3	30.3
Distractibility	34	25	19	26.0	26.0
Persistence	28	45	55	42.7	42.7
Clinician					(Clinic)
Activity	5.6	2.6	3.8	4.0	4.0
Adaptability	4.7	3.8	5.7	4.7	4.7
Approach	3.0	2.6	4.0	3.2	3.2
Intensity	5.4	2.8	2.6	3.6	3.6
Distractibility	4.0	4.0	3.8	3.7	3.9
Persistence	3.2	1.8	4.2	3.1	3.1

Table 10-4
Three-Year Summary Scores and Grand Mean
for Ratings of Donald on the Temperament Assessment
Battery (in T-Score Form)

	Setting			
Scale	Home	School	Clinic	Grand mean
Activity	50.5	42.8	50.0	47.8
Adaptability	38.6	55.9	43.0	45.8
Approach	37.6	50.5	44.7	44.3
Intensity	48.4	46.7	47.4	47.5
Distractibility	(41.4)	34.2	49.3	41.8
Persistence	40.8	58.7	44.0	47.8

mean raw scores aggregated across assessment periods are presented for each rater. Finally, mean raw score ratings for each setting are also presented. For school and clinic settings, the mean setting ratings are the same as the teacher and clinician ratings, respectively, because only one type of rater contributed to the setting rating. For the home setting, the aggregate is composed of the mean of the mother and father ratings.

Note that while the assessments carried out using the TAB approximated the multisource, multisetting design, and the assessments were available on three occasions, the design fell short of the model in several areas. First, only one teacher was used during each assessment period. This shortcoming is not serious in the present case, since different teachers made the ratings across occasions. If an analysis of setting effects on one occasion was desired, then these data could be misleading in that source and setting are confounded. Second, only one clinician rated the child during each assessment period. Again, if we aggregate across periods, it is not a serious limitation, since different raters were used at each period. Third, only one device was used to measure the variables in question at each assessment period. This problem is more serious, although interview data and data from the Revised Behavior Problem Checklist were used as a rough second measure.

The first analysis a psychologist should carry out using multisource, multisetting data is to create a grand mean for all variables aggregated across all raters. This can only be done if the measures produce scores on the same metric. Since the raw scores from each of the TAB forms have different means and standard deviations, all setting means were transformed to *T*-score form (mean of 50, standard deviation of 10), then an average was calculated. The results of this process appear in Table 10-4. (For reasons peculiar to the TAB, the grand mean for distractibility was calculated from clinician and school ratings only. Parent data are not comparable to clinician and teacher ratings on this dimension.)

From these data we can see that the child was less than one-half of one standard deviation from the mean on activity, adaptability, emotional intensity, and persistence. Thus, he can be tentatively described as average on these dimensions. He was more than one-half of one standard deviation from the mean on approach/withdrawal (his score indicates a mild withdrawal pattern) and on distractibility. Thus, he can be tentatively described as being mildly shy in new situations and marginally less distractible than his peers.

The second step in the analysis is to look for setting effects. A glance at the *T* scores in Table 10-4 reveals that he is rated more negatively at home than in any other setting (i.e., more active, less adaptable, less approaching, more intense, less persistent). Since we have two raters from the home setting, an attempt can be made to determine if the lower ratings are due to source effects (the mother or father rates the child very harshly) or to setting effects (this could be inferred if there were little difference between the raters). Looking back on Table 10-3, we can see that both mother and father rate Donald in much the same way. Therefore, Donald either behaves more negatively at home than at the school or clinic, or his parents share a stricter view of what is appropriate than other raters. The psychologist should explore with the parents both these hypotheses, come to a tentative decision, and plan the consultation with the parents accordingly.

A glance at the teacher and clinician ratings across occasions shows far greater variability than exists for the parents.This is to be expected, since parents share their views of the child with one another, while teachers and clinicians across a period of 1 year may not have the opportunity to do so.

A final kind of analysis possible with these data is to look for trends across time. This is important with children and adolescents, since maturation is progressing at such a rapid pace during these years. In the present example, Donald's mother sees him as becoming more persistent, less distractible, less intense, and more active over time. Some similar trends can be seen in the teacher data. The assessor can use such data to point out normal developmental progress and idiosyncratic patterns. For example, it is normal for 5-year-old children to be less intense and more persistent than 3-year-olds. If the reverse pattern occurred, a red flag should go up in the psychologist's mind.

Table 10-5 presents data from the Revised Behavior Problem Checklist, mother interviews, and teacher ratings on the Bristol Social Adjustment Guide. We can see that the mother has expressed concern about shyness, fearfulness, and activity level in the interviews and in response to the Revised Behavior Problem Checklist. However, the teacher sees no problem at age 5 years, 2 months, except that Donald has a mild tendency toward shyness. The data in Table 10-5 are very consistent with the summary data analyzed by setting from the TAB.

Table 10-5
Assessments of Presence/Absence of Psychopathology for Donald at Three Preschool Ages

	Age at assessment		
Information source	3 years, 2 months	4 years, 1 month	5 years 2 months
Behavior Problem Checklist-Revised (Preschool Experimental Version)	No data	Restless[a] Short attention span Generally fearful Distractible Resists leaving mother	Restless[a] Short attention span Generally fearful Distractible Has temper tantrums Self-conscious Hyperactive
Mother interview	Shy Fearful Highly active Sensitive to criticism	Shy Fearful Highly active	Shy Fearful Highly active
Teacher	No data	No data	(Bristol Social Adjustment Guide) No significant score Mild tendency toward shyness

[a]All problems checked were indicated to be mild, not severe.

Summary

The data presented in this case lead us to describe Donald as being an average to bright average 5-year-old whose receptive vocabulary and visual-motor integration is at a level commensurate with his scholastic ability. His social–emotional development is progressing normally. Specifically, he appears to be a typical child in terms of activity level, adaptability, emotional intensity, and persistence. He has a mild tendency toward shyness and may be less distractible than other children his age. There is no current indication of serious social–emotional problems. He is viewed somewhat more negatively by parents than by others. This may result from more stringent expectations for behavior on the part of the parents or from the fact that Donald behaves more inappropriately at home than at school or in the clinic. Further information is needed to help make a decision between these hypotheses. Ratings of extended family members and self-ratings from a home–school perspective (as Donald gets older) could help to clarify this picture.

References

Achenbach, T. M. (1966). The classification of children's psychiatric symptoms: A factor-analytic study. *Psychological Monographs, 80*(Whole No. 615).

Achenbach, T. M. (1978). The Child Behavior Profile: I. Boys age 6–11. *Journal of Consulting and Clinical Psychology, 46*, 478–488.

Achenbach, T. M., & Edelbrock, C. S. (1978). The classification of child psychopathology: A review and analysis of empirical efforts. *Psychological Bulletin, 85*, 1275–1301.

Achenbach, T. M., & Edelbrock, C. S. (1979). The Child Behavior Profile: II. Boys aged 6–12 and girls aged 6–11 and 12–16. *Journal of Consulting and Clinical Psychology, 47*, 223–233.

Achenbach, T. M., & Edelbrock, C. S. (1981). Behavioral problems and competencies reported by parents of normal and disturbed children aged 4 through 16. *Monographs of the Society for Research in Child Development, 46*(1, Serial No. 188).

Achenbach, T. M., & Edelbrock, C. S. (1983). *Manual for the Child Behavior Checklist and Revised Child Behavior Profile*. Burlington: Department of Psychiatry, University of Vermont.

Anastasi, A. (1976). *Psychological testing* (4th ed.). New York: Macmillan.

Arnold, L. E., Barneby, N. S., & Smeltzer, D. J. (1981). First grade norms, factor analysis and cross correlation for Conners, Davids, and Quay-Peterson Behavior Rating Scales. *Journal of Learning Disabilities, 14*, 269–275.

Barkley, R. A. (Ed.). (1981). *Hyperactive children: A handbook for diagnosis and treatment*. New York: Guilford Press.

Brown, L. L., & Hammill, D. D. (1978). *Behavior Rating Profile: Manual*. Austin, TX: Pro-Ed.

Brown, R., & Wynne, M. (1982). Correlates of teacher ratings, sustained attention, and impulsivity in hyperactive and normal boys. *Journal of Clinical Child Psychology, 11*, 262–267.

Buss, A., & Plomin, R. (1975). *A temperamental theory of personality development*. New York: Wiley.

Campbell, D. T., & Fiske, D. W. (1959). Convergent and discriminant validation by the multitrait-multimethod matrix. *Psychological Bulletin, 56*, 18–105.

Campbell, S. B., & Steinert, Y. (1978). Comparison of rating scales of child psychopathology in clinic and nonclinic samples. *Journal of Consulting and Child Psychology, 46*, 358–359.

Conners, C. K. (1969). A teacher rating scale for use in drug studies with children. *American Journal of Psychiatry, 126*, 884–888.

Conners, C. K. (1970). Symptom patterns in hyperkinetic, neurotic, and normal children. *Child Development, 41*, 667–682.

Conners, C. K. (1973). Rating scales for use in drug studies with children. *Psychopharmacology Bulletin* (Special Issue: Pharmacotherapy with Children), 24–84.

Conners, C. K. (1982). Parent and teacher rating forms for the assessment of hyperkinesis in children. In P. A. Keller & L. G. Ritt (Eds.), *Innovations in clinical practice: A source book* (Vol. 1). Sarasota, FL: Professional Research Exchange, Inc.

Conners, C. K., & Blouin, A. G. (1980). *Hyperkinetic syndrome and psychopathology in children*. Paper presented at the American Psychological Association, Montreal, Canada.

Conners, C. K., Taylor, E., Meo, G., Kurtz, M. A., & Fournier, M. (1972). Magnesium Pemoline and Dextroamphetamine: A controlled study in children with minimal brain dysfunction. *Psychopharmacologia, 26*, 321–336.

Cooper, W. H. (1981). Ubiquitous halo. *Psychological Bulletin, 90*, 218–244.

Curry, J. F., & Thompson, R.J. (1979). The utility of behavior checklist ratings in differentiating developmentally disabled from psychiatrically referred children. *Journal of Pediatric Psychology, 4*, 345–352.

Curry, J. F., & Thompson, R. J. (1982). Patterns of behavioral disturbance in developmentally disbled children: A replicated cluster analysis. *Journal of Pediatric Psychology, 7*, 61–73.

Cytryn, L., Gilbert, A., & Eisenberg, L. (1960). The effectiveness of tranquilizing drugs plus supportive psychotherapy in treating behavior disorders of children: A double blind study of eighty outpatients. *American Journal of Orthopsychiatry, 30*, 113–129.

Davids, A. (1971). An objective instrument for assessing hyperkinesia in children. *Journal of Learning Disabilities, 4*, 499–501.

DeFilippis, N. A. (1979). Normative and validity data for the Missouri Children's Behavior Checklist. *Journal of Clinical Psychology, 35*, 605–610.

Eaton, W. O. (1983). Measuring activity level with actometers: Reliability, validity and arm length. *Child Development, 54*, 720–726.

Eaves, R. C. (1975). Teacher race, student race and the behavior problem checklist. *Journal of Abnormal Child Psychology, 3*. 1–10.

Edelbrock, C. (1983). Problems and issues in using rating scales to assess child personality and psychopathology. *School Psychology Review, 12*, 293–299.

Edelbrock, C., & Achenbach, T. M. (in press). The teacher version of the Child Behavior Profile: I. Boys aged 6–11. *Journal of Consulting and Clinical Psychology*.

Edelbrock, C., Costello, A. J., & Kessler, M. D. (in press). Empirical corroboration of the attention deficit disorder. *Journal of the American Academy of Child Psychiatry*.

Edelbrock, C., & Reed, M. L. (1983). *Validation of the teacher version of the Child Behavior Profile against observational ratings of classroom behavior*. Manuscript submitted for review.

Epstein, S. (1979a). Explorations in personality today and tomorrow: A tribute to Henry Murray. *American Psychologist, 34*, 649–653.

Epstein, S. (1979b). The stability of behavior: I. On predicting most of the people much of the time. *Journal of Personality and Social Psychology, 37*, 1097–1126.

Epstein, S. (1980). The stability of behavior: II. Implications for psychological research. *American Psychologist, 35*, 790–806.

Epstein, S. (1983). The stability of confusion: A reply to Mischel and Penke. *Psychological Review, 90*, 179–184.

Firestone, P., Kelly, M. J., & Fike, S. (1980). Are fathers necessary in parent training groups? *Journal of Clinical Child Psychology, 9*, 44–47.

Fuller, G. B., & Goh, D. S. (1983). Current practices in the assessment of personality and behavior by school psychologists. *School Psychology Review, 12*, 240–243.

Gajar, A. H., & Hale, R. L. (1982). Factor analysis of the Quay-Peterson Behavior Problem Checklist across racially different exceptional children. *Journal of Psychology, 112*, 287–293.

Ghiselli, E. E., Campbell, J. P., & Zedeck, S. (1981). *Measurement theory for the behavioral sciences*. San Francisco, CA: Freeman.

Gittelman-Klein, R., Klein, D. F., Abikoff, H., Katz, S., Gloisten, A. C., & Kates, W. (1976). Relative efficacy of methylphenidate and behavior modification in hyperkinetic children: An interim report. *Journal of Abnormal Child Psychology, 4*, 361–379.

Glow, R. A. (1979). Cross-validity and normative data on the Conners Parent and Teacher Rating Scales. In K. D. Gadow & J. Loney (Eds.), *The psychological aspects of drug treatment for hyperactivity*. Boulder, CO: Westview Press.

Glow, R. A., Glow, P. H., & Rump, E. E. (1982). The stability of child behavior disorders: A one year test-retest study of Adelaide versions of Conners Teacher and Parent Rating Scales. *Journal of Abnormal Child Psychology, 10*, 33–60.

Goyette, C. H., Conners, C. K., & Ulrich, R. F. (1978). Normative data on revised Conners Parent and Teacher Rating Scales. *Journal of Abnormal Child Psychology, 6*, 221–236.

Hollingshead, A. B. (1957). *Two-factor index of social position*. Unpublished manuscript, Department of Sociology, Yale University, New Haven, CT.

Hollingshead, A. B. (1975). *Four-factor index of social status*. Unpublished manuscript, Department of Sociology, Yale University, New Haven, CT.

Jacob, T., Grounds, L., & Haley, R. (1982). Correspondence between parents' reports on the Behavior Problem Checklist. *Journal of Abnormal Child Psychology, 10*, 593–608.

Jacobsen, R. H., Lahey, B. B., & Strauss, C. C. (1983). Correlates of depressed mood in normal children. *Journal of Abnormal Child Psychology, 11*, 29–40.

Kelly, C. K., & King, G. D. (1980). Normative data on the Missouri Children's Picture Series and the Missouri Children's Behavior Checklist with southern black children. *Journal of Abnormal Child Psychology, 8*, 421–433.

Kendall, P. C., & Brophy, C. (1981). Activity and attentional correlates of teacher ratings of hyperactivity. *Journal of Pediatric Psychology, 6*, 451–458.

King, C., & Young, R. (1982). Attentional deficits with and without hyperactivity: Teacher and peer perceptions. *Journal of Abnormal Child Psychology, 10*, 483–495.

Kivlahan, D. R., Siegel, L. J., & Ullman, D. G. (1982). Relationship among measures of activity in children. *Journal of Pediatric Psychology, 7*, 331–334.

Kupietz, S., Bialer, I., & Winsberg, B. (1972). A behavior rating scale for assessing improvement in behaviorally deviant children: A preliminary investigation. *American Journal of Psychiatry, 128*, 1432–1436.

Lahey, B. B., Green, K. D., & Forehand, R. (1980). On the independentce of ratings of hyperactivity, conduct problems, and attention deficits in children: A multiple regression analysis. *Journal of Consulting and Clinical Psychology, 48*, 566–574.

Lindholm, B. W., & Touliatos, J. (1981a). Development of children's behavioral problems. *Journal of Genetic Psychology, 139*, 47–53.

Lindholm, B. W., & Touliatos, J. (1981b). Mothers' and fathers' perceptions of their children's psychological adjustment. *Journal of Genetic Psychology, 139*, 245–255.

Lindholm, B. W., & Touliatos, J. (1982). Checklist agreement among observers of children. *Psychology in the Schools, 19*, 548–551.

Lueger, R. J. (1980). Person and situation factors influencing transgression in behavior-problem adolescents. *Journal of Abnormal Psychology, 89*(3), 453–458.

Mack, J. L. (1969). Behavior ratings of recidivist and nonrecidivist delinquent males. *Psychological Reports, 25*, 260.

Martin, R. P. (1984). *The Temperament Assessment Battery—Interim Manual*. Athens, GA: Developmental Metrics.

Mash, E. J., & Johnston, C. (1983). Parental Perceptions of child behavior problems, parenting self-esteem, and mother-reported stress in younger and older hyperactive and normal children. *Journal of Consulting and Clinical Psychology, 51*, 86–99.

McCarthy, D. A. (1972). *A manual for the McCarthy Scales of Children's Abilities*. New York: Psychological Corporation.

McMahon, R. C., Kunce, J. R., & Salomak, M. (1979). Diagnostic implications of parental ratings of children. *Journal of Clinical Psychology, 35*, 759–762.

Miller, L. C. (1972). School Behavior Checklist: An inventory of deviant behaviors in children. *Journal of Consulting and Clinical Psychology, 38*, 134–144.

Miller, L. C., Hampe, E., Barrett, E., & Noble, H. (1971). Children's deviant behavior within the general population. *Journal of Consulting and Clinical Psychology, 37*, 16–22.

O'Conner, M., Foch, T., Sherry, T., & Plomin, R. (1980). A twin study of specific behavioral problems of socialization as viewed by parents. *Journal of Abnormal Psychology, 8*, 189–199.

Pfeffer, J., & Martin, R. P. (1983). Comparisons of mothers' and fathers' temperament ratings of referred and non-referred preschool children. *Journal of Clinical Psychology, 39*, 1013–1020.

Porter, B., & O'Leary, K. D. (1980). Marital discord and childhood behavior problems. *Journal of Abnormal Child Psychology, 8*, 287–295.

Quay, H. C. (1983). A dimensional approach to behavior disorder: The revised Behavior Problem Checklist. *School Psychology Review, 12*, 244–249.

Quay, H. C., & Parsons, C. B. (1972). *The differential behavioral classification of the juvenile offender* (2nd ed.). Washington, DC: U.S. Bureau of Prisons.

Quay, H. C., & Peterson, D. R. (1967). *Manual for the Behavior Problem Checklist*. Champaign: Children's Research Center, University of Illinois.

Quay, H. C., & Peterson, D. R. (1975). *Manual for the Behavior Problem Checklist*. Privately printed.

Quay, H. C., & Peterson, D. R. (1979). *Manual for the Behavior Problem Checklist*. Privately printed.

Quay, H. C., & Peterson, D. R. (1983). *Interim manual for the Revised Behavior Problem Checklist*. Coral Gables, FL: University of Miami.

Rapoport, J., Abramson, A., Alexander, D., & Lott, I. (1971). Playroom observations of hyperactive children on medication. *Journal of the American Academy of Child Psychiatry, 10*, 524–534.

Reed, M. L., & Edelbrock, C. (1983). Reliability and validity of the Direct Observation Form of the Child Behavior Checklist. *Journal of Abnormal Child Psychology, 11*, 521–530.

Saal, F. E., Downey, R. G., & Lahey, M. A. (1980). Rating the ratings: Assessing the psychometric quality of rating data. *Psychological Bulletin, 88*, 413–428.

Sandberg, S. T., Wieselberg, M., & Shaffer, D. (1980). Hyperkinetic and conduct problem children in a primary school population: Some epidemiological considerations. *Journal of Child Psychology, Psychiatry, and Applied Disciplines, 21*, 293–311.

Sandoval, J. (1981). Format effects in two teacher rating scales of hyperactivity. *Journal of Abnormal Child Psychiatry, 9*, 203–218.

Sines, J. O., Pauker, J. D., Sines, L. K., & Owen, D. R. (1969). Identification of clinically relevant dimensions of children's behavior. *Journal of Consulting and Clinical Psychology, 33*, 728–734.

Sprague, R. L., Christensen, D. F., & Werry, J. S. (1974). Experimental psychology and stimulant drugs. In C. K. Conners (Ed.), *Clinical use of stimulant drugs in children*. The Hague: Excerpta Medica.

Sprague, R. L., & Sleater, E. K. (1973). Effects of psychopharmacological agents on learning disorders. *Pediatric Clinics of North America, 20*, 719–735.

Stott, D. (1970). *Bristol Social Adjustment Guides: Manual*. San Diego, CA: Educational and Industrial Testing Service.

Thompson, R. J., & Curry, J. F. (1983). A construct validity study of the Missouri Children's Behavior checklist with developmentally disabled children. *Journal of Clinical Psychology, 39*, 691–695.

Thompson, R. J., Curry, J. F., Sturner, R. A., Green, J. A., & Funk, L. G. (1982). Missouri Children's Behavior Checklist ratings of preschool children as a function of risk status for developmental and learning problems. *Journal of Pediatric Psychology, 7*, 307–316.

Thompson, R. J., Curry, J. F., & Yancy, W. S. (1979). The utility of parents' behavior checklist ratings with developmentally disabled children. *Journal of Pediatric Psychology, 4*, 19–28.

Thompson, R. J., & McAdoo, W. G. (1973). A comparison of mothers' and fathers' behavior checklist ratings of outpatient boys and girls. *Journal of Community Psychology, 1*, 387–389.

Touliatos, J., & Lindholm, B. W. (1980). Teachers' perceptions of behavior problems in children from intact, single-parent, and step-parent families. *Psychology in the School, 17*, 264–269.

Touliatos, J., & Lindholm, B. W. (1981). Congruence of parents' and teachers' ratings of children's behavior problems. *Journal of Abnormal Child Psychology, 9*, 347–354.

Trites, R. L., Blouin, A. G., & LaPrade, K. (1979). Factor analysis of the Conners Teacher Rating Scale based on a normative sample. *Journal of Consulting and Clinical Psychology, 80*, 615–623.

Trites, R. L., Dugas, E., Lynch, G., & Ferguson, H. B. (1979). Prevalence of hyperactivity. *Journal of Pediatric Psychology, 4*, 179–188.

U.S. Department of Health, Education and Welfare. (1976). *ECDEU assessment manual for psychopharmacology*. Washington, DC: Author.

von Isser, A., Quay, H. C., & Love, C. T. (1980). Interrelationships among three measures of deviant behavior. *Exceptional Children, 46*, 272–276.

Weissman, M. M., Orvaschel, H., & Padian, N. (1980). Children's symptom and social functioning self-report scales. Comparison of mothers' and children's reports. *Journal of Nervous and Mental Disease, 168*, 736–740.

Werry, J. S., & Sprague, R. L. (1974). Methylphenidate in children—Effects of dosage. *Australia and New Zealand Journal of Psychiatry, 8*, 9–19.

Werry, J. S., Sprague, R. L., & Cohen, M. N. (1975). Conners' Teacher Rating Scale for use in drug studies with children—An empirical study. *Journal of Abnormal Child Psychology, 3*, 217–229.

Behavioral Observation Approaches to Personality Assessment

Harold R. Keller

The use of behavioral observation approaches in the assessment of children and adolescents' personality development is derived from different conceptual frameworks, including behavioral, ethological, ecological, and phenomenological frameworks. This chapter will focus primarily upon observational approaches as conceptualized within a behavioral model. Initially, a behavioral construct system is presented, along with a set of influences that have important implications for the development and use of observational approaches. While assessment can have many purposes, including screening/identification, classification/placement, psychological/educational planning, child/adolescent evaluation, and program evaluation (Salvia & Ysseldyke, 1978; Ysseldyke, 1979), the concern here is primarily with assessment for purposes of developing interventions. As such, the theoretical bases will be discussed as they relate to a conceptualization of change within a particular model. Alternative conceptual models to the use of observation will be discussed briefly. Second, behavioral observation will be discussed within the context of behavioral assessment. Third, specific observational approaches will be described in terms of measures, methods, aids, and psychometric issues. Fourth, a summary of how observational approaches have been used in personality assessment will be presented. This will include a discussion of definitional issues and of target variables (i.e., age, problem domains, and setting). Finally, a case study will be presented in which assessment relied extensively upon the use of behavioral observation. Throughout, knowledge gaps and research needs will be emphasized, as well as the need for continual interaction among practitioners and researchers to more effectively use behavioral observation approaches in the service of our clients.

Theoretical Bases of Behavioral Observation

A common set of theoretical constructs underlies the interrelated areas of behavioral observation and assessment, behavioral consultation, and behavior therapy. Although the names of Skinner and Watson and the constructs of learn-

Harold R. Keller. Department of Psychology and School of Education, Syracuse University, Syracuse, New York.

ing theory are frequently associated with behavioral change approaches, such associations are too narrow. Major conceptual approaches to behavior change include Eysenck's (1982) neobehavioristic (S-R) theory, applied behavior analysis (Baer, 1982), cognitive-behavior therapy (Meichenbaum & Cameron, 1982), and social learning theory (Rosenthal, 1982). Social learning theory and behavior influence research provide perhaps the broadest context for a theory of behavior change and will be emphasized here. Proponents of behavioral approaches argued early for a broader reliance on social learning theory, rather than merely on learning theory (Patterson, 1969; Ullmann & Krasner, 1969). Social learning refers to a rapidly growing body of knowledge dealing with behavioral changes occurring as a function of contingencies that characterize social interaction. Many of the mechanisms that bring about these changes are based upon principles derived from social psychology, in addition to learning theory, and include such processes as persuasion, conformity, modeling, and interpersonal attraction. Bandura (1969, 1977) has made important attempts to integrate this diverse body of knowledge.

A Behavioral Construct System

The basic characteristics and assumptions of a behavioral construct system which can guide behavioral change approaches have been delineated by numerous writers (e.g., Agras, Kazdin, & Wilson, 1979; Haynes, 1978; Krasner, 1971, 1982; G. T. Wilson & Franks, 1982; G. T. Wilson & O'Leary, 1980). Behavioral change strategies are based first upon the assumption that typical and atypical behaviors are learned and maintained in similar manners. Atypical behavior is learned by an individual as a way to cope with the stress and difficulties of living in a changing and increasingly complex physical and social environment; it is not symptomatic of some kind of underlying disease process. Because the learning and maintenance of problem behavior as well as normal behavior occur through social learning processes, it is assumed next that the problem behaviors can be changed (treated) directly through the application of social learning principles (rather than indirectly by first altering intrapsychic phenomena).

A third assumption relates to situational specificity. It is assumed that individuals' personalities and behaviors are best described and understood by determining what they think, feel, and do in particular life situations. More specifically, problem behaviors require an assessment of the individual, the setting, and the interaction between the person and the setting—including other people in the setting. Given this interactional perspective and the assumption that behavioral problems do not reflect intrapsychic or physiological trauma, behavioral change theory rejects psychodynamic and personality trait labels (e.g., dominant, extraverted, ego defended) to describe people and their behavior. These labels would only suggest that an individual's problems originate within or are exclusively caused by the individual. Mischel (1968, 1969, 1973, 1979) has supported this behavioral position through demonstrations that measures from intraindividual models have little cross-measure consistency. Briefly, individual scores on two measures that assess the same trait rarely correlate significantly as intraindividual models would predict. Instead, Mischel has found that situational effects are more important determinants of performance on personality and cognitive measures. This emphasizes the need to directly measure persons, settings, and interactions of persons with settings to best understand personality and specific behavior.

This assumption of situational specificity and the resulting concern with person–environmental interactions leads to a variety of complex issues having serious implications for behavioral assessment and change strategies. Bandura (1977, 1978) delineated alternative conceptualizations of the relationship between person and environment. The most simplistic views of behavior involve no person–environmental interaction. Thus, behavior is a function of personality characteristics of the person (intraindividual models): $B = f(P)$, or, behavior is a function of environment: $B = f(E)$. One interactional conceptualization views the person and environment as both determining behavior in some sort of additive manner, that is, $B = f(P, E)$. Another conceptualization of person–environmental interaction is bidirectional in that it acknowledges that people influence the environment while, at the same time, they are influenced *by* the environment. However, behavior is still viewed as a product of their interaction, that is, $B = f(P \leftrightarrow E)$. Bandura labeled the final form of interaction reciprocal determinism, whereby behavior, person, and environment are mutually and reciprocally influential, that is,

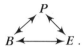

This last conceptualization results in increasingly complex interactional systems to consider for assessment and change.

Based on the assumptions above, the characteristics of the behavioral construct system underlying behavioral change approaches can be delineated. The behavioral construct system relies on the close relationship between assessment (problem identification and problem analyses) and consultation/intervention, and the emphasis on behavioral change as a problem-solving, empirically based process. Considering the former area, behavioral assessment is tailored to the unique characteristics of the referred individual and the targeted environment(s) (see the third assumption above). Behavioral characteristics and determinants are specific to the referred problem or situation; they are observable, quantifiable, and clearly specified such that they may be tested, replicated, or evaluated empirically; and they directly suggest intervention directions with minimal inferential leaps. Thus, behavioral assessment is one part of a larger construct system which focuses primarily on identifying observable person–environment interactions, causalities, and problem resolution directions.

The latter area reinforces the behavioral construct system's emphasis on evaluation as the mechanism demonstrating environmental causalities. Every step within the behavioral construct system should be evaluated: the assessment procedures, the consultation processes, the intervention outcomes. Only then can the practitioner demonstrate that the particular change strategies were indeed responsible for the obtained behavioral changes. The total change process or change strategy, then, becomes a problem-solving process; and this process, in turn, is viewed as evidence of change. Thus, the behavioral construct system is an evolving, self-correcting (cybernetic) system based on the evaluation of empirical data.

The unifying factor in behavioral approaches seems to be their derivation from experimentally established procedures and principles (ad hoc development of techniques rather than post hoc development). G. T. Wilson and O'Leary (1980) point out that behavioral approaches draw upon principles of operant and classical conditioning, but are not restricted to them. These change strategies draw upon principles from other branches of experimental psychology, including social, developmental, and cognitive psychology. The importance of "private events" or cognitive (verbal and imaginal) mediation of behavior also is recognized, as is the role of vicarious and symbolic learning processes (e.g., modeling). Furthermore, they emphasize the importance of the change agent's personal qualities in skillfully and appropriately designing and implementing various behavior change programs.

Krasner (1971, 1982) and Keller (1981) have summarized the historical influences which have crystallized to create the behavioral construct system and the general behavioral–social learning approach to the process of change (see Table 11-1). These historical origins are important to note because they demonstrate the significant breadth of this approach.

To summarize, behavioral observation, as addressed in this chapter, is based upon a theory of change that is derived from a broad-based social learning model which encompasses diverse streams of psychological and social science research and theory. The behavioral construct system underlying the assessment and change strategies include the following assumptions: (*a*) Problem and nonproblem behaviors are acquired and maintained, thus changed, through the action of social learning principles; (*b*) behavior involves complex person–environment interactions; and (*c*) a close relationship exists between assessment and consultation/intervention. The system also includes the characteristics of (*a*) clear specifications of variables and concepts, (*b*) quantification, (*c*) environmental causality, (*d*) recognition of individual differences in behavior and its determinants, leading to idiosyncratic assessment, consultation and intervention, (*e*) emphasis upon public

---

Table 11-1
Streams of Influence on a General Behavioral–Social Learning Approach[a]

1. Experimental psychology and the concept of behaviorism	12. Apparent failure of psychodynamic and psychoanalytic therapies
2. Instrumental conditioning: Thorndike and Skinner	13. Available behavioral, social learning alternatives to disease model of psychopathology
3. Wolpe's work influenced by Pavlov and Hull	14. Potential implementation of Boulder scientist/practitioner model
4. Eysenck as influenced by Hullian concepts	15. Ward milieu and community programs: A. Meyer, H. S. Sullivan
5. Application of learning concepts to problem behaviors: Fuller, M. C. Jones, Mowrer, Guthrie	16. Growth of behavioral assessment as concern in and of itself
6. Dollard and Miller's attempts to translate psychoanalysis into learning terms	17. Attempts at integrating behavioral model and ecological psychology
7. Pavlov-inspired Soviet research	18. Integration of cognitive psychology within the behavioral model
8. Social psychology and sociology	19. Concern with prescriptive matching
9. Utopian conceptualizations emphasizing planning of social environments	20. Research on generalization and transfer
10. Developmental psychology: Bijou, Baer, Gerwirtz, Bandura, Risley, Stevenson	21. Growth of behavioral consultation and application of behavioral approaches to broader community and social concerns through indirect service strategies
11. Research on social influence parameters: hypnosis, placebo effects, demand characteristics, experimenter bias, subject and client expectancy, effects of nonverbal cues in interviews	

[a]From Keller (1981); Krasner (1971, 1982).

events and direct observation of behavior in the natural environment, and (*f*) the cybernetic, or self-correcting, nature of the behavioral construct system and its derived approaches.

Alternative Frameworks for Behavioral Observation

A behavioral construct system is not the only conceptual context within which behavioral observation might be conducted. Other conceptual frameworks include ethological, ecological, and phenomenological approaches. These conceptual frameworks will be described only briefly.

Ethological Framework

Ethological observation (Blurton Jones, 1972; Hutt & Hutt, 1970), originating in research investigating animal behavior, is tied to an evolutionary perspective by examining behavior reflecting a species' adaptation for survival. Adaptation within this model refers to the relationship between a living organism and an environment that demands something of that organism. The relational or interactional aspect of this definition is critical for ethologists. Using this basic notion of adaptation, Charlesworth (1978) has described detailed observational approaches, particularly for understanding how an individual person solves the social, physical, and cognitive problems which confront them in their daily living environments. The individual's problem-solving behaviors are viewed as mediators between the individual and the environment. The child's behavior as well as what precedes and what follows the behavior are observed intensively as they occur spontaneously in the natural environment. Observation occurs in a variety of natural settings, including the home and classroom. Highly specific and descriptive behavioral definitions of adaptation and problem solving are used rather than global categories. Therefore, such observations focus on naturally occurring, adaptive behavior and its interactive function in the settings of concern. The data obtained are both quantitative (frequency counts) and qualitative (descriptive). Leach (1972) has used ethological approaches to examine child–child and mother–child interactions of typical and problem (acute social anxiety) preschoolers. For example, Leach investigated these interactions in terms of 61 specifically defined actions (e.g., approach, bend over, bump, crouch, flap hands), 22 distinct facial expressions (e.g., avert eyes, blush, compress lips, nod head, raise eyebrows), plus numerous other molecular response categories.

Ecological Framework

The ecological model is concerned primarily with the structural, affective, and organizational components of settings. One basic premise of this model is that people adapt and act selectively toward their environment to achieve a harmonious working relationship with it. Specific environments influence individual behavior and have dependable, predictable, and enduring effects on all individuals. For example, children in a sixth-grade reading group generally behave in consistent ways within that group, even though the actual group members change throughout the morning. These consistent ways of behaving (e.g., reading silently, reading aloud when asked by teacher, answering questions about the material) are different from the ways the children act in other segments of the environment (like the playground). A lack of adaptive fit between an individual's behavior and a particular environmental setting is cause for concern. Because this model assumes that behavior and settings are mutually interdependent, an intervention that better fits one child's needs might also cause other children to behave more appropriately in that setting.

The ecological model leads psychologists to examine an individual's naturally occurring behavior, the environment immediately surrounding that behavior, and the ways the individual and the immediate environment are linked. Hilton-smith and Keller (1983) suggest that assessment within this model should focus upon three major components: (*a*) setting appearance and contents (design and ambient features, contents); (*b*) setting operation (organization, communication, and ecological patterns); and (*c*) setting opportunities (nurturance and sustenance, cognitive and social/emotional stimulation). They describe general strategies for gathering information about persons within settings for each of these components. Carlson, Scott, and Eklund (1980) present ecological observational approaches for getting at person-setting linkages. Finally, Conoley (1980) described ecological variables to consider in such organizational assessment. Here, practitioners assess a whole organization, its interlocking systems (e.g., a school district and its buildings, support staff, interrelationships among administration and teachers), and how it influences a child's behavior within a given setting.

Despite numerous calls suggesting the assessment of individuals within a setting's context and including relevant person-setting interactions (e.g., McReynolds, 1979; Sundberg, Snowden, & Reynolds, 1978), setting assessment has rarely moved beyond a conceptual level into research and practice. The importance of assessing existing settings, however, cannot be minimized. School psychologists, for example, are actively working in the context of PL 94-142, which includes mandates both for (special) education in the least restrictive environment and for the assessment of adaptive behavior in school and nonschool settings. Clearly, both mandates must involve a thorough understanding of a child's current and potential educational settings. Similar practical concerns must be addressed by clinical and community psychologists and practitioners working to help effectively deinstitutionalize intellectually and behaviorally disordered individuals. Finally, the growth of community psychology and systems approaches to therapy with children and families typically requires a thorough assessment of setting and persons' interactions with settings. As indicated in Table 11-1, there have been recent attempts to integrate ecological and behavioral models (e.g., Rogers-Warren & Warren, 1977; Wahler, House, & Stambaugh, 1976).

Phenomenological Framework

Participant or qualitative observation developed primarily from sociological theory and research (Bogdan & Taylor, 1975; S. Wilson, 1977). Such work is particularly well suited for obtaining information on phenomenological aspects of behavior, that is, on an individual's view of a setting, her or his own behavior, and the personal meaning and affect attributed to that setting, behavior, and setting–behavior interaction. This framework argues against the establishment of a priori delineated observational schedules because they provide restricted data and, thus, a restricted picture and understanding of the individual and setting. Understanding behavior within this model is best accomplished through intensive, direct naturalistic observation combined with interviews and examinations of permanent records. Bogdan (1976) illustrated the utility of this approach using a case study of a deinstitutionalized adult. Bardon, Bennett, Bruchez, and Sanderson (1976) described a participant observation approach (referred to as psychosituational classroom intervention) that, in addition to providing pertinent observational data, serves as a model for the teacher and pupils while enhancing collaborative consultation. Bersoff and Grieger's (1971) psychosituational assessment, which combines behavioral observation with interviewing from a rational-emotive therapy orientation, is another strategy analogous to this approach.

As indicated above, there are diverse and overlapping conceptual orientations that underlie the development and use of observational approaches and tools. One can use direct observation of a client as part of an assessment conducted within any theoretical framework, not just those described above. It is important, though, to recognize the conceptual bases for the particular tools used in an assessment process. Behavioral observation, conducted within the present focus of a behavioral construct system, is typically done within the context of a broad-based behavioral assessment. The next section will place observational approaches within that context.

Behavioral Assessment

Given a referred child or adolescent, the purposes of behavioral assessment are to specify the problems to be solved, validate those problems, identify the variables that might facilitate solutions for these problems, and specify consultation/intervention plans. The underlying assumption to behavioral assessment is that problems (or, more generally, personality and behaviors) involve people interacting with environments, including settings and other people (Keller, 1980a). Behavioral assessment is characterized by the direct measurement (at least as direct as possible) of behaviors in settings of concern to the consulting practitioner, the referred child, and the referral source. This assessment approach facilitates a closer, more direct relationship between assessment and intervention with a minimum, or a least a reduction, of the inferential leaps common between standardized test assessments and intervention. Behavioral assessment also is characterized by assessment in multiple settings (e.g., in the naturalistic environments of the classroom, school halls, cafeteria, playground, home, neighborhood, and/or in such structured settings as role plays, trial teaching, and some types of interviews). Finally, behavioral assessment approaches are not limited to motoric aspects of the individual–environment interaction. These assessments also might focus upon cognitive, phenomenological (feelings, meanings), physiological, and structural or ecological components of the interaction.

Given the multiple settings and multiple levels at which all assessments occur, it follows that behavioral assessment is characterized by multiple strategies, of which observation is just one. Behavioral assessment uses intensive interviews (Morganstern & Tevlin, 1981), behavior checklists and rating scales (Bellack & Hersen, 1977; R. P. Martin, 1983, chap. 10; Walls, Werner, Bacon, & Zane, 1977; C. C. Wilson, 1980), and systematic observation (Alessi, 1980; Haynes, 1978; Keller, 1980b; Nay, 1977). There has been an explosion of research and interest in behavioral assessment, as indicated by the appearance of articles, books, and two journals (*Behavioral Assessment, Journal of Behavioral Assessment*) devoted specifically to the topic (e.g., Barlow, 1981; Ciminero, Calhoun, & Adams, 1977; Cone & Hawkins, 1977; Goldfried, 1976, 1977; Goldfried & Kent, 1972; Goldfried & Linehan, 1977; Haynes, 1978; Haynes & Wilson, 1979; Hersen & Bellack, 1976, 1981; Keefe, Kapel, & Gordon, 1978; Keller, 1980a; Kratochwill, 1982; Mash & Terdal, 1976, 1981).

Some writers (Cone, 1978; Kanfer & Saslow, 1969; Lazarus, 1973) have described general schemes of behavioral assessment which specify a range of dimensions that should be considered in problem identification and analysis and that are necessary for development of appropriate intervention strategies. Lazarus (1973) describes seven interactive modalities that need to be identified and assessed before an adequate program of change can be implemented. These modalities are referred to by the acronym BASIC ID, using the first letter of each term—behavior, affect, sensation, imagery, cognition, interpersonal relationship, and drugs and diet.

Kanfer and Saslow (1969) present perhaps the most comprehensive set of dimensions for consideration within behavioral assessment. Their proposed dimensions include the following: a detailed description of behavioral excesses, deficits and assets; a motivational analysis including a survey of various incentives and aversive conditions; a developmental analysis including a consideration of biological, sociological, and behavioral changes in the person's history that may be pertinent to the present problem; an analysis of self-control; an analysis of social relationships including others' expectations for the client and the potential for involving important others in the intervention process; and an analysis of the social–cultural–physical environment as it might affect the client.

The multiple strategies, settings, and levels for conducting behavioral assessment are perhaps best viewed within the context of Cone's (1978) three-dimensional taxonomy. His framework consists of behavioral contents, methods, and universes of generalization (see Figure 11-1). Behavioral contents refers to motoric acts (publicly observable events), cognitive contents (private events including thought, images, reported feelings), and physiological contents. Methods of assess-

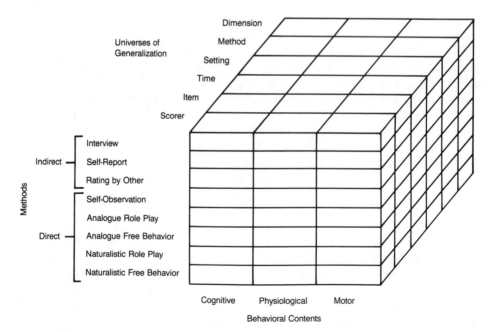

Figure 11-1. Cone's Three-Dimensional Taxonomy of Behavioral Assessment. From Cone (1978).

ment or measurement are ordered along a continuum of directness; that is, methods are ordered on their ability to directly and fully measure any relevant behavior at the time and place of its natural occurrence. Measurement methods include interviews, self-reports, and ratings by others (about past events) at the most indirect end of the continuum, and self, analogue, and naturalistic observation at the most direct end. The third dimension refers to the domains across which we wish to generalize about a given phenomenon. Specific universes of generalization include scorer generalization (interrater reliability), item generalization (referring to how representative a set of responses is to a universe of similar responses), generalization across time, setting generality (to determine the degree of setting specificity or generality of a particular set of behaviors), method generality (referring to the consistency of measuring a given behavior across methods), and dimensions generalization (referring to the comparability of data on two or more different behaviors, which allows us to understand response classes or response clusters).

These behavioral assessment schemes exemplify not only the interactive nature of persons and settings, but also the reality that behavioral observation approaches are only one set of personality assessment strategies, and they are not used in isolation. In using these assessment schemes, one is looking for convergence—across methods, contents, and universes of generalization—in our understanding of a child's problems and, eventually, in our measurement of the efficacy of interventions applied to those problems. Other methods, such as rating scales and interviews, may provide efficient approaches toward identifying problem areas for the subsequent use of detailed observational methods. A description of specific observation approaches will be presented next.

Observational Approaches

Early observation approaches (Wright, 1960) employed open-ended, anecdotal, and narrative recording, where observers were instructed to observe "everything." Such observation generally is found to be less reliable than those approaches that establish a priori observational categories. Observers are necessarily selective and unable to record everything. While the psychometric characteristics of such an approach are problematic, thorough narrative recording has the advantage of providing rich descriptive information that might aid in the development of a specific problem/situation observational system (Bijou, Peterson, & Ault, 1968). Of course, good interviews and/or rating scales might provide the same information for a more specific observational schedule, and in a more efficient manner. As indicated, observational measures with predetermined categories may restrict the scope of an assessment by providing narrower bands to measure; however, they are generally more reliable. Alessi (1980) has described various observational procedures.

Observational Measures

Interval Recording

This measure involves selecting a recording period (e.g., one-half or 1 hour), dividing that period into equal intervals (e.g., 20 seconds observe, 10 seconds record), and recording whether or not a given behavior (or behaviors) occurs within each time interval. This results in a tally of the number of intervals within which the behavior was observed to occur (e.g., John was observed physically aggressing against other children during 12 of the 40 intervals observed). Recording percentages of intervals where the behavior was observed (12/40 = 30%) is then helpful, particularly when recording periods vary in length (resulting in different total numbers of intervals). When reporting the results of interval recording, it is important to note that behavior was engaged in for a specific percentage of intervals observed, not for a percentage of time.

Interval recording is used when a behavior occurs at a moderate but relatively steady rate. This measure is not efficient for events that rarely occur. Interval recording typically does require the use of an external observer. A teacher or staff member would have too many competing demands (e.g., teaching, carrying out interventions) to attend reliably to recording time intervals and behaviors as well.

Time-Sample Recording

This procedure measures the number of times that target behaviors are observed at prespecified sampling points in time (e.g., at the end of every 60-second period, at the end of every 15-minute period, or at randomly selected points of time throughout the day). This procedure also can determine the number of children engaging in particular behavior(s) at prespecified times (by scanning a classroom or developmental unit). For example, Sue was observed studying appropriately at 14 of 20 sampled times (70%); or, observing an entire class, between 60% and 80% of a preschool's children were engaging in cooperative play at the sampled times. Time sampling, like interval recording, requires behavior that occurs at a moderate but steady rate. With relatively long intervals between sampling points, an external observer is not necessary.

The major difference between time sampling and interval recording is that, with time sampling, the individual is observed momentarily and only at the prespecified times, while interval recording requires observation during the entire interval. One advantage of time sampling is that other activities can be engaged in while waiting for the prespecified time (timers or watches with beepers can remind the observer to attend and record at the designated time). The disadvantage is that a much smaller sample of observation time, and thus behavior, is obtained with time sampling. Decreasing the interval between sampling points can address this issue, but this would necessitate an external observer.

Many interval and time-sampling measures allow only the recording of co-occurrences of behaviors (e.g., when the two behaviors, referred child argues with sibling and mother asks referred child to begin studying homework, occur within the same interval or at the same sampled time), without a clear indication of the sequential chain of events occurring (i.e., which behavior preceded the other one at that interval or moment in time). Knowledge of precise behavioral sequences is important in determining events that precipitate or reinforce problem behaviors. Mash, Terdal, and Anderson (1973) have described a response-class matrix for recording sequences of behaviors over time (or reciprocal antecedent–response chains) in parent–child interactions. For example, with their interval recording schedule, we might find that an ambiguously stated parental request is followed by the child's noncompliance, which is followed by a severe parental reprimand, which is followed by a temper tantrum; and a clearly stated parental request is followed by the child's compliance and then at least two intervals of no observable parental response. Sackett (1978a, 1978b) has described other observational approaches that allow sequential analyses of interactions between parents and children and between staff and clients. Such sequential recording procedures allow greater certainty in identifying environmental determinants for the behaviors of participants in social interactions.

Event Recording

This procedure yields a measure of the number of times that a target behavior(s) occurred during an entire observation session. Event recording is preferred for very high- or very low-frequency behaviors (e.g., swearing out loud or physical assaults on staff members), as well as for behaviors that might occur only briefly. In such instances, interval and time-sample recording are less accurate. Event recording is also used for behaviors that result in a permanent product which can be counted (e.g., number of problems solved correctly). The sequential analyses mentioned above with interval and time-sample recording have the disadvantage of circumscribed time intervals. Sequential event recording eliminates this constraint. Multiple events can be recorded in the order in which they occur, and antecedents and consequences can be identified and analyzed.

Duration and Latency Recording

For some behaviors, it may be more important to know how long they occur (duration) or how long it takes (latency) from the end of one behavior (e.g., parental request) to the start of another behavior (e.g., child's compliance or noncompliance) than to know how often (frequency) they occur. In such instances, duration or latency recording, respectively, would be the procedures of choice. For such procedures, it is very important to be able to clearly define the starts and stops of the events or behaviors of interest. Duration and latency recording require timers as observation aids and typically require an external observer.

These observational measures can only be used individually or in combination with other methods of observation, depending on the referral problem and the situations or environments which need to be observed. An individual client or staff member can make self-observations, or the practitioner may need to become an external observer. Finally, professionals may engage in direct naturalistic observation of children, and/or analogue situations such as role plays can be structured for additional observational assessment data.

Methods of Observation

Self-Monitoring

Self-monitoring is a method of observation in which an individual observes and records his or her own behavior. The critical distinction between self-monitoring and self-reports (indirect measures) is that the former involves observation of behavior at the time of its occurrence. It should be noted that self-monitoring can be used as part of a personality or behavioral assessment and/or as a component in a self-control treatment program.

As part of the assessment process, a number of variables have been shown to influence the reliability and validity of self-monitored observation (see R. O. Nelson, 1977a, for a review). Accuracy of self-monitoring data may be influenced by (*a*) training in the use of self-monitoring, (*b*) the use of systematic and formal record forms, (*c*) use of easy to use devices such as wrist counters, (*d*) the timing of self-monitoring (i.e., the closer the recording is to the behavioral occurrence, the more accurate it is likely to be), (*e*) the amount of response competition (either number of responses to be monitored concurrently or the simultaneous occurrence of other behavior during self-monitoring), (*f*) the amount of time and energy required to engage in self-monitoring, (*g*) use of contingent positive reinforcement for accurate recording (particularly important for children), (*h*) the client's awareness of the external assessment of accuracy of self-recording, (*i*) the specific target behaviors selected (e.g., salience, discriminability), and (*j*) client characteristics (e.g., age, ability).

Reactivity (the influence of the observation process on the behaviors being monitored) also can be problematic when self-monitoring is used for assessment purposes. R. O. Nelson (1977b) and Ciminero, Nelson, and Lipinski (1977) reviewed variables influencing the reactivity of self-monitoring, including the following: (*a*) client's motivation to change problematic behavior, (*b*) the valence or value of the behavior to be monitored (with positively valued behaviors likely to increase in frequency and negatively valued behaviors likely to decrease in frequency), (*c*) nature of target behaviors (i.e., their social desirability and whether there are social sanctions for them), (*d*) use of goals, reinforcement, and feedback as part of a self-monitoring system, (*e*) timing of self-monitoring (i.e., before an act or after its occurrence, the former likely to be more reactive), (*f*) the obtrusiveness of the self-monitoring devices, (*g*) number of target behaviors, and (*h*) schedule of self-monitoring. It should be noted that when self-monitoring is engaged in as part of an intervention, reactivity may be desirable; that is, a change in the behavior is a desired outcome with intervention. Self-monitoring has been shown to be an effective change strategy (e.g., Piersel & Kratochwill, 1979) and can enhance the development of self-control (Haynes, 1978; Kazdin, 1974; R. O. Nelson, 1977a; Workman & Hector, 1978).

Despite the need to consider these numerous variables, self-monitoring assessment has a variety of advantages, and, compared to other approaches, it is relatively cost-efficient. This greater efficiency is particularly evident with low-rate behaviors such as seizures or drug ingestion. For private or covert behaviors (such as headaches, daydreams, obsessive thoughts, suicide thoughts, feelings of inadequacy, feelings of helplessness, and covert reinforcing or punishing thoughts), self-monitoring may be the assessment method of choice. Behaviors of extremely high social value also may be most appropriately approached through self-monitoring, since high-value behaviors are often subject to reactivity effects with other assessment strategies (Haynes, 1978). Certainly self-monitoring is less intrusive than other assessment approaches. Self-monitoring can provide additional convergent evidence for the existence of a given problem assessed through other methods.

Analogue Observation

This method involves the creation of structured settings designed to simulate conditions in the natural environment and to provide a controlled situation where behaviors of concern are highly likely to occur (Haynes, 1978; McFall, 1977; McReynolds & DeVoge, 1978; Nay, 1977). The client typically is requested to role play or act as if he or she were in the natural environment, and the results are assumed to represent how the target behaviors typically occur in that environment. Nay (1977) described five types of analogue methods, including paper and pencil, audiotape, videotape, enactment, and role play. Clearly the similarity between stimuli and responses in the analogue setting and problem setting is crucial to the validity of this approach.

Analogue observation provides a number of advantages. For example, variables that contribute to a problem can be controlled more easily (as well as those inconsequential to the problem), allowing systematic analysis of the independent roles of these variables in problem behavior. The problem behaviors also can be broken down into components that can be analyzed separately. Analogue observation can increase observational efficiency, particularly with low-rate behaviors (e.g., response to teasing), and possibly with behaviors likely to be reactive to direct naturalistic observation (such as parent–child disagreements). Further, instructions to role play a set of problematic behaviors may reduce the resistance to exhibiting these behaviors which sometimes occurs when observations occur in a natural environment.

From a negative perspective, analogue observation increases the number of inferences from the assessment setting to the problem setting (e.g., the stimulus–response similarity noted above), and the validity of analogue observation in many problem areas must be determined through further research and other assessments. The importance of these inferences' validity is especially significant in the school setting where, for example, a crucial part of the definition of serious emotional disturbance under PL 94-142 refers to its degree of interference with the individual's ability to profit from instruction. Observation during trial teaching (Smith, 1980, 1983) represents an instance of analogue assessment where the observed behaviors (emotional reactivity and learning performance under specified conditions of instruction) often are quite congruent with the behaviors of concern in the natural classroom environment. Naturally, the practitioner must be quite satisfied with such assessments' validity to avoid unjustified conclusions and recommendations resulting in an inappropriate placement.

Another structured observation approach includes that by Campbell, Schleiter, Weiss, and Perlman (1977) to assess hyperactivity in preschoolers. The situation involves a teacher with a small group of children and three 10-minute time blocks of specified activities—free time at a table with multiple materials available, teacher-structured activity with certain materials, and put-away materials. A coding scheme for behavioral indices of hyperactivity was used. The analogue observation procedure clearly discriminated between independently identified hyperactive children and typical children. Similarly, in Syracuse University's Psychoeducational Clinic, we frequently observe parent–child interactions through a sequence of free play by parent(s) and child, child play while the parent(s) is busy completing information forms at one side of the room, and joint cleanup of play materials. Such a structured sequence can be used to assess behavioral indices of dependence–independence, responsivity to authority demands for compliance, reinforcement–discipline tactics, and potential reinforcing activities within a contingency management system, among other dimensions.

Naturalistic Observation

Jones, Reid, and Patterson (1975) indicate that the three major characteristics of naturalistic observation include the recording of behaviors in their natural settings at the time of occurrence, the use of trained impartial observers, and descriptions of behaviors that require minimal inference by observers-coders. Numerous sources have presented specific observational procedures that might be used, from behavioral (e.g., Bijou *et al.*, 1968, 1969; Goodwin & Coates, 1977; Haynes, 1978;

Jones *et al.*, 1975; Kirschenbaum, Steffen & D'Orta, 1978; O'Leary, Romanczyk, Kass, Dietz, & Santagrossi, 1971; Reed & Edelbrock, 1983; Reid, 1979; Wahler *et al.*, 1976; White, 1975) and nonbehavioral perspectives (e.g., Bell & Low, 1977; Boehm & Weinberg, 1977; Cartwright & Cartwright, 1974; Flanders, 1966, 1970; Hunter, 1977; Lynch, 1977; Medley & Mitzel, 1963; Rosenshine & Furst, 1973; Sackett, 1978a, 1978b; Sitko, Fink, & Gillespie, 1977; Weick, 1968; Wright, 1960). Significantly, while direct observational procedures are used frequently in clinical settings, there is a dearth of available observational instruments (to be critically reviewed later). Numerous reviews of methodological and conceptual issues in naturalistic observation have been written (e.g., Achenbach & Edelbrock, 1984; Alessi, 1980; Baker & Tyne, 1980; Cone & Foster, 1982; Haynes, 1978; Johnson & Bolstad, 1973; Jones *et al.*, 1975; Kazdin, 1981; Keller, 1980b; Kent & Foster, 1977; Kratochwill, 1982; Lipinski & Nelson, 1974; Wildman & Erickson, 1977). Kratochwill (1982) has summarized a number of recommendations derived from the literature on methodological issues in the use of naturalistic observation.

First, observers need to be trained with behavior samples and environmental settings closely approximating the behaviors and settings where assessment will occur. Allen *et al.* (1976) describe procedures for involving and training community volunteers in observational approaches. Second, "booster" training for observers is also needed to maintain observer motivation and accuracy. Third, interobserver agreement should be established among observers during the assessment process. The conditions for determining observer agreement should be maintained in order to ensure consistent levels of agreement. Finally, when using observation to assess treatment progress, observer bias might be reduced by not communicating the specific treatment plan to the observers.

If instruments or coding sheets are unavailable for a particular problem, specific observational codes should be constructed on an a priori basis so that behaviors can be easily coded. (Observational record forms will be discussed in the next section.) Operational definitions should be constructed for each specific behavior to be observed, and the number of codes to be rated at any one time must be kept at a reasonable number (e.g., less than seven). Alessi (1980) and Morris (1976) have presented some helpful pointers for creating behavior definitions. In addition, Rogers-Warren and Warren (1977) suggest the need to be sensitive to incidental behaviors, which differ from the targeted problem behaviors so that unanticipated positive and negative side effects, due to assessment procedures or interventions, may be investigated.

Observations always should be conducted in the most unobtrusive manner possible (see Webb, Campbell, Schwartz, & Sechrest, 1966, for a discussion). Haynes (1978) suggests a variety of strategies for examining obtrusive or reactive observational data (i.e., behavior influenced by the observational process). Measurement of the generality of observational data across diverse settings also should be conducted. Such assessment will ensure an adequate sampling of the behaviors of concern and help determine the extent of the problem and of treatment effects.

As with other assessment approaches, normative data are an important part of observational assessment. Melahn and O'Donnell (1978) described a feasible process for gathering and developing observationally based norms. They developed yearly norms while providing psychological services to 15 Headstart centers. A minimum of 15 minutes per day was spent in normative observation of referred and randomly selected nonreferred children. With such local norms, a referred child can be distinguished from peers in the same setting. When a referred child's behavior is not discrepant from the norms, the referral should be reexamined to determine its appropriateness (i.e., the problem may not exist as a child-centered problem) or its accuracy. Given the latter, a consultant might assist the consultee in a more accurate problem description, possibly resulting in different or additional problems requiring intervention. A comparison of current assessment observations with those normed separately over specific time periods may suggest that an identified problem behavior requires no formal intervention, that it will resolve itself over time. Finally, postintervention observational data can be compared with norms on nonreferred peers to determine the relative success of the intervention program.

An alternative strategy for developing local norms via observation was suggested by R. O. Nelson and Bowles (1975) and Walker and his colleagues (Walker & Hops, 1976; Walker, Mattson, & Buckley, 1971). This alternative involves observing a referred child and randomly selected nonreferred children in the same settings at pre-, during, and postintervention. Again, this approach results in an effective strategy for identifying problems and evaluating change in single children.

The development of local observational norms might allow the practitioner to use observations for screening purposes (e.g., Forness & Esveldt, 1975a, 1975b; Forness, Guthrie, & Hall, 1976; Forness, Guthrie, & Nichira, 1975; C. M. Nelson, 1971; Werry & Quay, 1969). However, much research is needed to determine the utility of observational assessment for screening purposes.

To summarize briefly, observational assessment that includes self-monitoring, analogue, and naturalistic observation has the advantage of being direct and of addressing different behavioral contents (motoric and cognitive). However, such work can be time consuming. Research is needed to determine how most effectively to implement and use observational assessment. There are a number of aids to facilitate observational assessments, and these will be discussed next.

Aids to the Use of Observation

As indicated earlier, target behaviors must be clearly defined when using behavioral observation. Behaviors should be defined so that any two individuals observing the same child at the same time can agree on what did and did not happen. Morris (1976) suggests that each target should be defined so that it passes the IBSO test (or, the Is the Behavior Specific and Objective test). Definitions should deal only with observable events; self-reports of feelings, thoughts, and images are included as observable events (while, admittedly, the feelings, thoughts, and images themselves are not). Alessi (1980) suggests writing behavioral definitions in complete sentences, including active verbs and objects of the verbs. Inferences and verbs "to be" and "to have" should be avoided. For example, "He is independent" is an inference that is not directly observable. "He asks for help immediately following the presentation of directions" and "He remains in close proximity (within 2 feet) to an adult" are both observable. Inferences cannot be observed, but the facts on which inferences are based can be observed. Our task is to gather as many facts pertinent to the assessment questions being addressed, so that we can make sound professional inferences.

Defining behaviors is a skill that requires practice. A suggested learning or training process might have the practitioner (a) select a situation and define a limited set of behaviors, (b) present the definitions to someone else to get feedback about any ambiguities or inconsistencies, (c) observe children in the selected setting with another individual, (d) compare observational records, (e) discuss the sources of disagreement if there are any discrepancies, (f) modify the definitions if necessary, and (g) observe again. When high levels of observational agreement are attained, the definitions are assumed to be clear enough for formal behavioral assessment. Such practice will lead to greater proficiency in defining target behaviors.

Observational Equipment

Morris (1976) has provided a selected list of apparatuses to facilitate observation. Certainly cost factors and the degree of intrusiveness (to the observer and those observed) must be considered when deciding whether to use various observational aids.

Counters (or digital counters) are frequently used to count a wide variety of events and behaviors. Counters can be single or multiple channels. The advantage of multiple channels is that the observer can record the occurrence of more than one behavior on the same equipment. A counter should be reliable (i.e., register a count each time the mechanism is pressed), be error and trouble free, and be easy to operate.

Portable timers or commercially available kitchen timers can be used to record the duration of particular events. Stopwatches can also be used. The length of time that such devices record (typically, from 5 to 60 minutes) is one limitation. Another limitation is their loudness that increases the intrusiveness of the observations. Alternative timers are now commercially available such as the variety of multifunction digital watches, many of which have a stopwatch and/or lap mode. The alarm mode on some watches can also be used to indicate time intervals for interval recording. Timer pocket calculators can also be used. These watches and timer calculators are quieter and less obtrusive, and the digital displays are easier to read. In addition, the calculators (and some watches) can perform various percentage and rate calculations relevant to interval, time sample, and event recording methods.

Other equipment that can aid the observational process includes the use of audiotape recorders, particularly the small cassette ones. Such equipment can be used to record directly events of concern (such as parent–child disagreements and negotiations in the home), or to help human observers by signaling record and observation intervals in interval recording. Use of a Y plug and dual earplugs can dramatically aid interobserver reliability with interval recording formats.

Movie cameras and videotape recorders and cameras can also be used in observational assessment. Such recording equipment certainly has the advantage of providing permanent records that can be examined on numerous occasions (thus enhancing reliability and verticality of observations), and often can be used in the change process itself by providing children and teachers/parents with direct feedback about their styles of interaction. Of course, cost factors and intrusiveness must be considered with such techniques.

Charting equipment is most often used to present the occurrence of a particular behavior, providing the observer and change agent with a graphic description of the progress of a child's program. Such equipment is electrically operated, so that chart paper moves at a fixed speed. Connected to the paper, a pen records a straight line as time progresses. When the pen is electrically activated by a switch held by the observer, a small mark is recorded at a right angle to the line. Such equipment may be single or multichannel event recorders. An expensive device is the Observational System-3, a compact event recorder that records complex sequential data, presents summary data on each behavior, and transmits data to a host computer directly from the field site or from observational records. This device eliminates coding and transcribing steps, which are sources of error in observational data.

Protocol Formats

Because of cost factors and considerations of intrusiveness, many practitioners may not have or use observational equipment. Various alternatives such as prepared observational protocol forms are available to aid the observational process (Alessi, 1980; Simon & Boyer, 1970). Tukey (1977) developed a useful method of tallying behaviors. Dots and lines are used to record behavioral incidents or counts. The first count is represented by a single dot (.), the second by two dots (..), the third by three dots (.:), and the fourth by four dots (: :). The numbers 5–8 are then represented by completing the sides of the box created by the four dots—5 = ⎵:, 6 = ∟:, 7 = ⊔, and 8 = □, with 9 and 10 being ⧄ and ⊠, respectively. Fewer errors in both tabulation and summarization are likely with this system compared to others (e.g., /, //, ///, ////, ~~////~~). Tukey's system also takes less space and can be used with both event and interval recording. Its use and advantage over merely interval recording, particularly for fast rates of behavior, are illustrated in Figure 11-2.

The format of a particular observational protocol will vary depending on the type of problem behavior observed. A school district or agency might develop its own "standard" protocol format that addresses most of the situations that arise. Then, the use of the standard recording protocols allows easy interpretation by other staff, makes the data collected on each child more consistent from one assessment period to another, and makes it easier to train new staff in the recording procedures. Figures 11-3 and 11-4 illustrate two classroom observation record protocols developed by Alessi at Western Michigan University's School Psychology Program. Creativity and practice in the use of various protocol formats for particular problems and situations will enhance the accuracy and usefulness of obser-

BEHAVIORS	Tot.		1	2	3	4	5	6	7	8	9	10	11	12	13	14	15
1. Talk outs by event record	76	R	⊔	⊠	□	⧄	⊔	∟:	⊠		. .	: :	∟:	: .	. .	.	.
	9	C		: :		.		.						. :			
		T															
2.		R															
		T															
		T															
3. Talk outs by interval record	14	R	X	X	X	X	X	X	X	0	X	X	X	X	X	X	X
	4	C	0	X	0	X	0	X	0	0	0	0	0	X	0	0	0
		T															

Figure 11-2. Example of event record within 1-minute intervals. Top part shows event data for talking out behaviors counted within each interval. Bottom part shows same data as scored by interval only method. By comparison one can see that interval scoring is not as sensitive to the dynamics of the high rate of behavior as is the event within interval record. With the event (top) record one can see a sudden decrease in rate of talking out after minute 8. The interval record is insensitive to this change. Likewise, the discrepancy between the two pupils is greater as measured by the actual rate (event) measure and underestimated by the interval (bottom) measure.

Western Michigan University School Psychology Program
CLASSROOM OBSERVATION RECORD PROTOCOL*

Pupil: _Mary_	Comparison: _C.J_	Observer: _School Psychologist (L.C.)_
Age: _6-10_	Age: _6-7_	Reliability: _Social Worker_
Grade: _2nd_		Class Size: _26_
School: _Westwood_		Class Type: _Regular ed._
Teacher: _Mrs. Kaput_		Time Stop: _10:23_
Date: _16/10/78_		Time Start:
		Total Time: _:10_

Reason for observation (What questions do we want to answer?):
To confirm reported discrepancy between Mary's behavior and that of her classroom peers:

Classroom Activity and explicit rules in effect at time of observation:
Activity: Math. — See notes below for details. Rules: 1. Follow teacher's directions: 2. Work quietly; 3. complete work.

Description of Observation Techniques: (interval or time sample and length)
30″ interval for Mary and comparison, 2 minute time sample for class scan check.

Behavior Codes:	Grouping Codes:	Teacher Reaction Codes:
T = On Task	L = large group	AA = attention to all
V = Verbal Off task	S = small group	A+ = positive attention to pupil
M = Motor Off task	O = one-to-one	A- = negative attention to pupil
P = Passive Off task	I = independent Act.	Ao = no attention to pupil
=	F = free-time	An = neutral attention to pupil
=	=	=

	Time	Pupil	Com-parison	Class Scan Check	Anecdotal notes on behavior	Grouping	Teacher Reaction
1.	10:13	P	T		Ma not responding to teacher	L	An
2.		M	T		Standing up — other sitting	L	Ao
3.	10:14	M	T		Te leads Ma back to desk	L	An
4.		M	T	80%	Standing up	L	Ao
5.	10:15	P	T		Sitting staring at others	L	Ao
6.		T	N		Looking at teacher	S	Ao
7.	10:16	T	N	76%	Sitting quietly and listening	S	Ao
8.		T	T		Working at desk	S	AO
9.	10:17	P	T		Looking out window	L	Ao
10.		T	T	83%	Copying math problems	L	Ao
11.	10:18	P	T		Staring at board	L	Ao
12.		M	T		On floor getting pencil	L	Ao
13.	10:19	M	T	80%	On floor getting pencil	L	Ao
14.		M	N		On floor poking other	L	Ao
15.	10:20	P	T		In seat staring	L	Ao
16.		P	T	88%	In seat staring	L	Ao
17.	10:21	T	T		Writing math	S	An
18.		T	T		Writing math	S	Ao
19.	10:22	M	T	80%	Walking in class	S	Ao
20.		T	T		Writing math	S	Ao
Summary:		35% (7/20)	85% (17/20)	81%		L=13; S=7	Ao=17; An=3

Reliability = _83%_

Figure 11-3. Observation protocol based on anecdotal record system. Designed for either interval or time-sample recording. Allows coding for time, behaviors, notes, grouping situation, and teacher reactions.

vational assessment. In addition to protocols described in the literature, there are a limited number of available observational coding systems. The most recognized coding systems, used primarily in research but also in practice, are discussed next.

Observational Schedules

Perhaps the three most recognized general coding systems in use are those developed by Patterson and his colleagues at the Oregon Social Learning Center, by O'Leary and his associates at Stony Brook, and by Wahler and his colleagues at the University of Tennessee. In addition, one other general observational schedule, the Direct Observation Form (DOF) of the Child Behavior Checklist (Reed & Edelbrock, 1983), will be mentioned because of its close ties with Achenbach's (1978; Achenbach & Edelbrock, 1979, 1981) Child Behavior Checklist (CBCL), which has demonstrated utility in the identification of behavioral problems (see Martin, Chapter 10 of this volume, for a review). Each system has its own advan-

Western Michigan University School Psychology Program
CLASSROOM OBSERVATION RECORD PROTOCOL*

Observer: _School Psychologist (K.A.)_
Reliability Observer: _paraprofessional_
Teacher: _Mrs. Graves_
School: _Pine Elementary_
Subject area: _reading — seatwork_
Referred pupil (R): _Chelsea_ Age: _8-6_
Comparison pupil (C): _—_ Age: _8-5_
Class size: _31_ Class Type: _regular_

Date: _28 / 10 / 78_
 day month year

Time Stop: _11:16_
Time Start: _11:09_
Total Time: _:7_

Grouping situation:
(circle one)
L = large group
S = small group
O = one-to-one
(I)= independent act.
F = free time
= _____

Teacher Reaction Codes (T):
AA = attention to all
A+ = positive attention to pupil
A- = negative attention to pupil
Ao = no attention to pupil
An = neutral attention to pupil
= _____

Observation recording method:
(circle one)
(a) Interval: size _30"_.
(b) time sample: size _____.
(c) event count
↦(d) duration for "out of seat"
(e) latency

Explicit classroom rules in effect during observation: _1. work quietly 2. sit at desks 3. raise hand for help._

BEHAVIORS	Tot.		1	2	3	4	5	6	7	8	9	10	11	12	13	14	15
1. Verbal Off Task	8	R	X	O	O	X	X	O	O	X	X	O	O	X	X	O	X
	2	C	O	X	O	O	X	O	O	O	O	O	O	O	O	O	O
		T	Ao	Ao			Ao	An			Ao	Ao			Ao	An		Ao
2. Motor Off Task	4	R	X	O	X	O	O	O	O	O	O	X	X	O	O	O	O
	1	C	O	O	O	O	O	O	O	O	O	O	O	X	O	O	O
		T	Ao		Ao							Ao	An	Ao			
3. Passive Off Task	1	R	O	O	O	O	O	X	O	O	O	O	O	O	O	O	O
	1	C	O	O	O	O	O	O	X	O	O	O	O	O	O	O	O
		T						Ao	An								
4. On Task	3	R	O	X	O	O	O	O	X	O	O	O	O	O	O	X	O
	11	C	X	O	X	X	O	X	O	X	X	X	X	O	X	X	X
		T	Ao	An	An	An		Ao			Ao	Ao	An	Ao		Ao	An	Ao
5. Ask questions	1	R	O	O	O	O	O	O	O	O	O	O	X	O	O	O	O
	3	C	O	O	O	X	O	O	O	O	O	O	X	O	O	X	O
		T				An							An	An		An	
6.		R															
		C															
		T															
7. Out-of-seat (duration)	53"	R	14"	8"	22"	9"											
	6"	C	6"														
		T	A-	A-	An	A-											
8. Raising hand for help.	1	R	O	O	O	O	O	O	O	O	O	O	X	O	O	O	O
	2	C	O	O	O	X	O	O	O	O	O	O	O	O	O	X	O
		T				An							An			An	
9.		R															
		C															
		T															

(left margin, bottom-to-top) Teacher would like to see: less of · · ; none; more of · · ; strengths

Were reliability data collected? (Yes) No   If yes, interobserver % agreement =_83%._
**Specific behavior definitions included on back, as well as comments (strengths, contextual observations, etc.).

Figure 11-4. Observation protocol for use with any five record methods: interval, time sample, event, duration, or latency. Allows record of the behaviors, teacher reactions, and grouping situation. Interval records are marked with "Xs" and "Os," while duration record (7: out-of-seat) includes actual elapsed time out of seat for each successive incident (1–4). Teachers' reactions are coded just below each interval where occurrence of behavior is scored, in the row following (T). Behaviors for the referred pupil are scored in the row of intervals following (R), while those for the comparison pupil are scored in the row of intervals following (C).

tages and disadvantages. Other general and more specific observational schedules will be discussed later.

The Behavioral Coding System (BCS) was developed for both home and school use (Jones *et al.*, 1975; Patterson, 1977; Reid, 1977) and is the most researched instrument of those to be discussed. The BCS uses a time-sampling procedure and has 28 behavioral categories in six response classes (see Table 11-2). The observational schedule permits recording sequences of behavioral interactions between a child and significant others. The BCS is complex, and considerable time and cost is required to train observers for adequate reliabilities. Patterson (1977) provides a brief review of the BCS, and Reid (1977) edited a manual which provides an extensive review of the literature, operational definitions of categories, normative data, training tapes, and procedures for training observers.

Technically, test-retest and interobserver agreement with the BCS have been adequate (Jones *et al.*, 1975; Patterson, 1977; Reid, 1977), though complexity (defined as the number of discriminations required of an observer during a session) was found to be positively correlated with reliability (Taplin & Reid, 1973). Observer bias in the form of observer expectancies was not found to influence the data of well-trained observers (Skindrud, 1972), though it can affect observers' global judgments (Kent, O'Leary, Diament, & Dietz, 1974). Concurrent (Patterson & Reid, 1973) and predictive validity (Jones *et al.*, 1975) have been demonstrated for the BCS. Construct validity has also been demonstrated in that the BCS scores differentiate normal and deviant children (Lobitz & Johnson, 1975) and normal and aggressive boys (Reid & Hendriks, 1973), and BCS scores on deviant behaviors change after treatment (Jones *et al.*, 1975; Patterson, 1977).

O'Leary's observational schedule (O'Leary *et al.*, 1971) was designed specifically for classroom settings. There are nine disruptive child behavior codes plus an on-task code. The system uses interval recording and does not record specific interactional sequences. There are only limited data on reliability and validity, but the O'Leary system is relatively easy to use.

Wahler *et al.* (1976) developed a commercially available system for use in home, school, laboratory, and other settings which therefore allows cross-situational comparisons of data. There are 19 response categories in five general classes of behavior (compliance-opposition, autistic, play, work, and social behaviors) and six stimulus categories that cover both aversive and nonaversive instances of adult instructions and adult and child attention. Wahler's system uses time sampling and, like Patterson's, has the advantage of recording sequential interactions between the child and teachers, parents, and/or peers. Little data exist on the system, but Wahler *et al.* report high interobserver agreement and some validity data.

The Direct Observation Form (DOF) of the Child Behavior Checklist (CBCL) directly parallels the teacher and parent versions of the CBCL in terms of item selection. There are 96 behavior problem items and a measure of on-task behavior on the DOF. Of the 96 items, 86 overlap with the teacher CBCL form and 73 overlap with the parent CBCL form. Clearly, such item congruence allows direct determination of method and source generalizability in a multidimensional assessment.

The DOF was designed to be a simple and efficient observational system, not requiring special equipment, clinically sophisticated observers, or lengthy observer training. With use of a time-sampling approach, a given child is observed for six 10-minute sessions (preferably at different times of the day over

Table 11-2
Six Classes of 28 Behavior Categories in the Behavior Coding System (BCS)

First order	Second order

VERBAL

CM (Command): This category is used when an immediate and clearly stated request or command is made to another person.

CN (Command negative): A command which is very different in "attitude" from a reasonable command or request (CM): (1) immediate compliance is demanded; (2) aversive consequences are threatened if compliance is not immediate; (3) a kind of sarcasm or humiliation directed to the receiver.

CR (Cry): Whenever a person cries, with no exceptions.

HU (Humiliate): Makes fun of, shames, or embarrasses the subject intentionally.

LA (Laugh): A person laughs in a nonhumiliating way.

NE (Negativism): A statement in which the verbal message is neutral, but which is delivered in a tone of voice that conveys an attitude of "don't bug me; don't bother me."

WH (Whine): A person states something in a slurring, nasal, high-pitched falsetto voice.

YE (Yell): The person shouts, yells, or talks loudly.

TA (Talk): This code is used if none of the other verbal codes are applicable.

NONVERBAL

DS (Destructiveness): The person destroys, damages, or attempts to damage any (non-human) object; the damage need not actually occur, but the potential for damage must exist.

HR (High-rate): A repetitive behavior not covered by other categories that if carried on for a long period of time would be aversive or annoying.

IG (Ignore): When person A has directed behavior at person B and person B appears to have recognized that the behavior was directed at him, but does not respond in an active fashion.

(PN) (Physical negative): A subject physically attacks or attempts to attack another person with sufficient intensity to potentially inflict pain.

AT (Attention): When one person listens to or looks at another person and the categories AP or DI are not appropriate.

NO (Normative): A person is behaving in an appropriate fashion and no other code is applicable.

NR (No response): When a person does not respond to another person. Applicable when a behavior does not require a response, or when behavior is directed at another person, but the person to whom the behavior is directed fails to perceive the behavior.

RC (Receive): A person receives a physical object from another person and does not do anything as a result of the contact.

TH (Touch): When the subject touches other people or hands an object to another person.

EITHER VERBAL OR NONVERBAL

AP (Approval): A person gives clear gestural or verbal approval to another individual. Must include some clear indication of positive interest or involvement.

CO (Compliance): A person immediately does what is asked of him.

DI (Disapproval): The person gives verbal or gestural disapproval of another person's behavior or characteristics.

SS (Self-stimulation): Repetitive behaviors that the individual does to himself and cannot be coded by any other codes.

(continued)

Table 11-2 **(Continued)**

First order	Second order
EITHER VERBAL OR NONVERBAL (CONT.)	

DP (Dependency): When person A is requesting assistance in doing a task that he is capable of doing himself, and it is an imposition on the other person to fulfill the request.

NC (Noncompliance): When a person does not do what is requested of him.

PL (Play): A person is playing either alone or with other persons.

TE (Tease): Teasing another person in such a way that the other person is likely to show displeasure and disapproval or when the person being teased is trying to do some other behavior, but is unable to because of the teasing.

WK (Work): A person is working, either alone or with other people: (1) the behavior is necessary for the smooth functioning of the household; (2) the behavior is necessary for a child to perform in order to learn behavior which will help him assume an adult role.

a 2-week period). During the observational period, the observer writes a narrative description of the child's behavior, noting the occurrence, duration, and intensity of any problem behaviors. Following the 10-minute observational period, the DOF is completed, rating each item on a 4-point scale reflecting occurrence and intensity or duration. At the present time, a total behavior problem score is derived by summing across the 96 items.

Reed and Edelbrock (1983) report high interobserver agreement and reliability for both behavior problem and on-task scores. In addition, DOF scores correlated in expected directions with teacher-reported problem behavior, school performance, and adaptive functioning. Further, teacher-referred boys obtained significantly higher behavior problem scores and significantly lower on-task scores than a matched sample of nonreferred boys observed in the same classrooms.

It should be apparent that considerable attention must be directed to the psychometric characteristics of these and other observational assessment approaches. Historically, little attention has been given to psychometric characteristics of observational procedures, perhaps because they have been characterized as informal assessment and because of an implicit assumption that since observation involves direct measurement, it does not need to meet basic assessment criteria (Wildman & Erickson, 1977). If we intend to use observation within psychoeducational planning and decision making, such considerations are necessary (American Psychological Association, 1974).

Psychometric Issues in Behavioral Observation

While direct observational measures allow a reduction in the number of inferences because the problem behavior is directly sampled, concern with reliability and validity must still be addressed. Mental health practitioners should know the definitions of reliability and validity and their importance for measurement. Discussing reliability and validity in terms of various subcategories (e.g., internal consistency, temporal stability, predictive validity) is somewhat cumbersome. Cronbach and his colleagues published a classic text (Cronbach, Gleser, Nanda, & Rajaratnam, 1972) in which they collapsed these various concepts of reliability and validity into a single dimension of generalizability. Cone's (1978) previously cited universes of generalization, within his three-dimensional model of behavioral assessment, is based upon the Cronbach *et al.* generalizability theory. According to Cone, interscorer reliability, for example, is reconceptualized as the extent to which obtained scores are independent of the person doing the scoring. In other words, if independent observers agree with one another, it does not matter which observer's data are used. Similarly, if alternate forms of a test are highly correlated, the scores on one form are generalizable to the correlated alternate forms. The various forms of reliability and validity can be conceptualized in terms of generalizability theory and will be discussed in that context below.

Generalizability over Observers

Checks for interobserver agreement determine the extent to which data about particular behaviors are independent of the observer's personal style or manner of observing. High interobserver agreement indicates that the observational data are not biased by idiosyncracies of individual observers. Agreement between observers, however, does not necessarily imply that either observer is accurate. The need to independently determine accuracy of observational data has been discussed by numerous writers (e.g., Cone & Foster, 1982; Johnson & Bolstad, 1973; Kazdin, 1977a). Briefly, during observer training and periodically throughout observational work, an independently determined accuracy criterion should be established with observers and compared against that objective standard.

Obtaining interobserver agreement is not a simple matter. Numerous variables influence agreement between observers, and there are at least 22 different measures of interobserver agreement (Berk, 1979). Two broad categories of these measures involve calculating observers' percentage of agreements and nonparametric approaches and those providing correlational estimates of coefficients of interobserver reliability. Despite Berk's strong arguments for the superiority of the latter kinds of measures, simple percentage agreement measures characterize the majority of the applied uses of direct observational assessment (Kelley, 1977). Some researchers have empirically compared various measures of interobserver agreement (House, House, & Campbell, 1981; Repp, Deitz, Boles, Deitz, & Repp, 1976).

Haynes (1978) discussed logistical and application issues when calculating reliability estimates. With event (or frequency) recording, the simplest and most common interobserver agreement approach is to divide the number from the observer with the smaller frequency by the number from the observer with the larger. Similarly, with duration recording, the smaller amount of time is divided by the larger amount. Although most common, this "total reliability" approach can lead to artificially inflated percentages of agreement and should not be used. Further, even with a high reliability index, we cannot be certain that the observers are recording the same behavior at any given point in time. Thus, this approach is insensitive to the occurrence of specific events.

With interval recording, the most frequently used method of calculating interobserver agreement is based upon observer agreement and disagreement within each sampling interval (dividing number of agreements by number of agreements plus disagreements). The resulting percentages vary with the rate of behavior and with the formula's inclusion of behavioral occurrences, nonoccurrences, or both. For overall agreement (based upon both occurrences and nonoccurrences), there is a U-shaped relationship between agreement due merely to chance and the frequency of the behavior being observed; that is, using overall agreement will yield relatively high levels of chance agreement for behavior occurring at very low or very high frequencies. Generally, it is suggested that interobserver reliability estimates take into account the probability of chance agreements (e.g., Fleiss, Cohen, & Everitt, 1969; Harris & Lahey, 1978; Haynes, 1978; Yelton, Wildman, & Erickson, 1977).

Among the variables that influence the amount of agreement between observers, the explicitness of the behavioral definitions within the observational system has received little attention (Hawkins & Dobes, 1977). The number of categories in a system (also called code complexity or observer load) influences observer agreement (Mash & McElwee, 1974), though its effect may interact with degree of observer experience (Frame, 1979). Method and materials used in observer training also can influence interobserver agreement. Mash and McElwee (1974) demonstrated that observers trained with audiotapes of unpredictable behavior sequences (rather than predictable sequences) subsequently had higher levels of agreement in the observation of verbal interactions. Kent, Kanowitz, O'Leary, and Cheiken (1977) demonstrated the need to supervise the consistent use of an observational system. Lack of supervision led to inflated interobserver agreement scores.

Merely making interobserver agreement checks can influence interobserver agreement. In a controlled experiment, Taplin and Reid (1973) made continuous agreement checks on three groups of observers, although the directions to the groups differed. One group was told that their observations would not be checked, a second was informed that there would be announced periodic checks, and a third informed that random unannounced agreement checks would be made. The group with announced agreement checks showed the greatest fluctuations in agreement, with the lowest levels of agreement during "unchecked" sessions and the highest correspondence during announced checks. The highest and most consistent agreement scores were obtained by the group that expected random checking. This problem of differential reliabilities can be practically addressed by giving observers in a given setting partially overlapping observational protocols such that at random they are recording the same behaviors for the same child at random times during the observational setting.

A related problem affecting observation reliability is observer drift. This occurs when pairs of observers together shift their definitions of behavior away from those definitions on which they were originally trained (Johnson & Bolstad, 1973). This often happens when observer pairs compare their reliabilities, discuss their definitions of behavioral codes, and arrive at idiosyncratic definitional variations. Reassigning observer pairs on frequent occasions can control this potential problem.

Some of the variables shown to influence interobserver agreement also affect the levels of behavior reported by observers. This creates another possible source of error in observational data. For example, Romanczyk, Kent, Diament, and O'Leary (1973) showed that the rate of behavior and the proportion of behavior categories recorded varied with the presence and absence of agreement checks. Other variables provide additional sources of error. Hay, Nelson, and Hay (1977), using continuous nonparticipant observers, found that both teacher and referred children changed their behaviors when participant observers (teachers) started to record behavior. Observer bias has been investigated by evaluating the effects of different observation instructions on observers' expectancies for change due to treatment effects (Kent *et al.*, 1974). Using O'Leary's classroom observation schedule, they found that none of the specific behavioral categories were influenced by the expectancy manipulation, nor was the composite disruptive behavior category. Observers' general subjective estimates of change, after the observational session, did show a significant bias in the direction of the expectancy manipulations, however. Such a finding suggests that general ratings, not tied to specific behavioral referrants, may be more subject to biasing conditions than direct observation of specific behaviors.

Generalizability over Time

The stability of data over successive administrations of any assessment instrument is as critical for observation as for testing. Instability may be due to inadequacies in the observational procedures or to actual variability in the behaviors being observed. The very nature of observational sampling procedures is likely to lead to some degree of variability. It is important to determine the proportion of observed behavioral variance due to actual behavior variability and the proportion due to error in the observational system. Increased control over situational and historical variables affecting observed behaviors should increase stability. Observing in the same situational context can be helpful here. Analogue observational approaches that reduce variations in environmental stimuli across observational sessions should lead to greater stability, but the relative stability of naturalistic and analogue observation has not been empirically investigated. Correlational internal consistency measures and/or graphic analyses may be used to estimate the stability of those behaviors sampled (Haynes, 1978; Parsonson & Baer, 1978).

Generalizability over Settings

This generalization area is concerned with whether data collected in one observational context are representative of those obtainable in other contexts. Formally, setting refers to any specific stimulus environment. Settings can refer to relatively gross stimulus complexes such as school, home, clinic, and office. They can also refer to more specific stimulus configurations such as total class instruction, small group reading, independent seatwork, or recess. There are few comparisons of identical behaviors across general settings. Wahler (1975) compared the deviant behaviors of boys in home and school settings, but his concern was primarily with interresponse relationships rather than intrabehavior–intersetting relationships. Lobitz and Johnson (1975) compared parent–child interactions in home and clinic settings for referred and nonreferred children. Tasks varied across settings, so it is not clear whether behavioral differences were due to task or setting differences. There does seem to be evidence for considerable setting specificity to behaviors.

The question of setting generalizability is particularly important when using analogue observation as part of the assessment process. Role play analogue assessment of assertiveness and social skills has been examined particularly closely. Research on setting generalizability in this area shows considerable inconsistency. Response variations are related to the specific analogue tasks (Bellack, Hersen, & Lamparski, 1979; Bellack, Hersen, & Turner, 1979; S. Martin, Johnson, Johansson, & Wahl, 1976), the sex of the participants (Eisler, Hersen, Miller, & Blanchard, 1975), the number of responses required (Galassi & Galassi, 1976), the degree of elaboration provided for setting the stage for the role play (Bellack, 1979; Eisler *et al.*, 1975), and whether the individual responds to a live or taped analogue presentation (Taskey & Rich, 1979). Similarly, research with analogue assessment has shown that role play instructions, or demand characteristics, can greatly influence behavior. Behavioral avoidance tests for fear assessments appear particularly susceptible to demand characteristics (Kern, 1984). Kern showed that self-report measures of fear were better predictors of naturalistically observed fear (i.e., approach of the feared object) than obtrusive behavior avoidance tests. In fact, the analogue measures of fear overestimated the efficacy of treatment effects.

Reactivity is a specific setting variable in that the setting (or environmental ecology) changes through the act of observation itself. Reactivity refers to the influence of the observer's presence upon the behaviors of those being observed. The research on reactivity effects has been reviewed recently (e.g., Baum, Forehand, & Zegiob, 1979; Haynes & Horn, 1982; Kent & Foster, 1977), so this work will only be summarized. Reactivity has been studied through one of three basic paradigms: habituation, varying the level of observer conspicuousness, and manipulating the subject's awareness of being observed. While reactivity is not always found in behavioral observation (e.g., Dubey, Kent, O'Leary, Broderick, & O'Leary, 1977; Hagen, Craighead, & Paul, 1975; Johnson & Bolstad, 1975; Kent, O'Leary, Dietz, & Diament, 1979; R. O. Nelson, Kapust, & Dorsey, 1978; Weinrott, Garrett, & Todd, 1978), under some conditions it does occur.

Haynes and Horn (1982) indicated a number of effects due to reactivity. These included increases in behavior rates, decreases in behavior rates, differential effects on behavior rates for different behaviors of the same subject, differential effects on behavior rates for different subjects, increased variability in behavior rates, systematic changes in behavior rates over time, changes in behavior rates consistent with demand conditions in the assessment situation, orientation toward observers, deficits in task performance, and changes in behavior rates by mediators (such as teachers or parents) in the clients' environment. Variables that appear to influence these reactive effects include the obtrusiveness of the observers or the observation process, the novelty of the observation process, client characteristics (age, sex, degree of disturbance, expectations, evaluative anxiety), and target response characteristics (such as the social sensitivity or social valence of the target behavior). Given these variables, a number of practical conclusions are evident. It is apparent that structured analogue observations may increase reactivity relative to naturalistic observation. A classroom where the presence of strangers is common is likely to result in less reactivity than a classroom where outside visitors are rare. Individuals being observed might react differently to the presence of an observer as a function of prior history of being observed (or being tested by the observer). Finally, people who are more or less sensitive to social sanctions or social desirability may react differently to observation. For example, behaviors subject to a high level of social sanction (e.g., masturbation, drug intake) might be highly reactive.

While rates of behavior are often influenced by observation, the validity of the assessment is not necessarily threatened, because the relationships among the behaviors and their controlling events may still remain despite the changed behavior rates. Haynes (1978; Haynes & Horn, 1982) has suggested a number of strategies to minimize reactive effects of observation. These approaches include using product measures (e.g., work output, homework sheets), participant observers, and covert observation; minimizing the intrusiveness of the observers and the observation process, and client–observer interactions and other discriminative properties of observers; using telemetry, video cameras, or tape recorders; instructing those being observed to "act natural" and/or fully disclosing the beneficial purposes of observation; allowing sufficient time for dissipation of reactive slope and variability in observation data; and using a number of observers so that differential effects cancel out. In addition, phenomenological reports from those being observed and from others in the setting may be used to corroborate or question observational data.

The material discussed above on psychometric issues relates to traditional discussions of reliability. The remainder of this section relates to traditional notions of validity.

Generalizability over Behavior

Generalizability over behavior implies that discrete behaviors can be combined into larger classes of behavior and ultimately into general response categories or dimensions. In an informal way, this is how behavior rating scales cluster individual behaviors into broad-band and narrow-band factors (see Martin, Chapter 10 of this volume). Of particular importance here, behavior generalization evaluates the construct validity of behaviors as they relate to general response categories. This potentially addresses the universality of behaviors and categories over time and across different referred populations.

With adequate construct validity, a general response category may be used to identify individuals' behavioral similarities, even though they manifest different specific behaviors which belong to that particular category. The response category may then suggest potentially successful interventions which may have been overlooked had the practitioner focused only on the specific behaviors. Much of the research in this area takes an interindividual approach (e.g., Reed & Edelbrock, 1983) rather than the intraindividual approach, which is the concern of the clinician working with individual clients. Exceptions to this approach include Wahler's (1975) work with deviant children in school and home settings, Bakeman's (1978) research on mother–infant interactions, and Patterson and Moore's (1979) work on parent–child interactions in distressed families.

Generalizability over Methods

Generalizability over methods is concerned with the degree of congruence among the methods of assessment that comprise the entire personality assessment battery. Because personality assessment is a coordinated process of generating hypotheses, testing these hypotheses, and seeking convergence with respect to a referred problem, the assessment battery's various methods should be chosen for their contribution to problem analysis and intervention and for their convergent validity.

Given the time-consuming nature of observational assessment, it is particularly important to evaluate the individual contribution of observational data compared to less time-consuming methods such as interviews, self-reports, or behavior rating scales. Through cross-method comparisons, practitioners can evaluate the consistency and accuracy (convergent validity) and redundancy of observational data compared with other data. Across a number of referred children, these comparisons can provide a sense of behavioral observation's (or any other method's) effectiveness and efficiency in the assessment battery. This information can dictate the practitioner's need for observational assessment for particular cases in the future.

When using cross-method comparisons to assess convergent validity, a particularly important issue involves response equivalence (Cone, 1979). Practitioners must ensure that different assessment methods are focusing on the same operationalization of a particular behavior (e.g., a self-report of school avoidance should be consistent with directly observed school avoidance). If response equivalence does not occur, assessment method and results may be confounded, behavioral differences cannot be clearly accounted for, and convergent validity is difficult to determine. The degree of relationship among behavioral observations and self-reports, other ratings, and self-monitoring vary tremendously. It is generally found that the more specific the ratings (self or other) and the greater the response equivalence (rarely addressed in research thus far), the greater the relationship to observational data (Cone & Foster, 1982).

The previously cited Direct Observation Form (Reed & Edelbrock, 1983) was specifically designed to address this need for method generalizability by paralleling its development with the teacher and parent forms of the Child Behavior Checklists (Achenbach, 1978; Achenbach & Edelbrock, 1979, 1981). Research with the Behavioral Coding System (Jones *et al.*, 1975; Patterson, 1977; Reid, 1977) has shown it to have considerable method generalizability as well.

Utility of Behavioral Observation

Determining the utility of behavioral observation for the assessment of personality and socioemotional problems requires examining the purposes for conducting such assessment and the conceptual models which determine the specific assessment procedures used. As indicated in the introduction to this chapter, behavioral observation is not concerned with the description, identification, or diagnosis of personality traits. Rather, behavioral observation is typically conducted as part of an assessment process which identifies or suggests relevant interventions. Indeed, Reschly (1979), while discussing nonbiased assessment, argues that assessments that do not result in effective interventions should be regarded as useless. The reader is encouraged to reread the section on theoretical bases of behavioral observation. The central point in that discussion is that personality and problem and nonproblem behaviors (including socioemotional problems) are acquired, maintained, and thus changed through involvement in complex person–setting interactions.

In other to discuss the utility of behavioral observation for the assessment of socioemotional problems, some definitional issues will be discussed first. These will be illustrated through a presentation of definitions of emotional disturbance in school-aged children.

Definitional Issues in Emotional Disturbance

When a child is referred for possible school placement in a program for emotionally disturbed children, the first assessment decision relates to whether the child exhibits those behaviors required to classify him or her as emotionally disturbed under state guidelines. Of course, such a classification decision is necessary only in a categorically based special education or funding system, a system prevalent in most states. A needs-based system (Hobbs, 1975) would not have to address this general classification decision.

New York State regulations for the education of children with handicapping conditions can be used to illustrate the definition of emotional disturbance (New York State Education Department, 1981) and the potential for behavioral assessment. The definition of an emotionally disturbed child is as follows:

> A pupil who exhibits one or more of the following characteristics over a long period of time and to a marked degree, which adversely affects educational performance:
> (i) An inability to learn which cannot be explained by intellectual, sensory, or health factors.
> (ii) An inability to build or maintain satisfactory interpersonal relationships with peers and teachers.
> (iii) Inappropriate types of behavior or feelings under normal circumstances.
> (iv) A generally pervasive mood of unhappiness or depression.
> (v) A tendency to develop physical symptoms or fears associated with personal or school problems.
> The term does not include socially maladjusted pupils unless it is determined that they are emotionally disturbed.

The pervasiveness of the problem in terms of duration and intensity is an important and observable part of this definition. Interference with educational performance implies the need to observe the child in an educational setting. Finally, while the exclusionary part of the definition (i) requires other assessment strategies, all other parts (ii–v) are potentially observable—i.e., quality of peer and adult interpersonal relationships, behaviors and reported feelings under various environmental contexts, pervasive moods of unhappiness or depression, and physical symptoms or fears associated with personal or school problems.

Given the requirements of PL 94-142 for education in the least restrictive environmental setting, Tombari (1981) argues that the classification decision for emotional disturbance requires addressing three concerns. First, it must be determined that behavioral, cognitive, or affective problems interfere with the child's learning, development, and interpersonal relationships and those of his peers. Second, the child must be significantly impaired as a result of these problems in comparison to his peers. Third, it must be determined that the kinds of tasks, degrees of classroom structure, and motivational levels that must be provided to help the student are beyond the capacity of the regular classroom program. Related to the last point is the need to assess possible alternative placements and programs in order to determine the most appropriate, least restrictive educational setting (Hiltonsmith & Keller, 1983). None of the above definitions of emotional disturbance and related concerns necessitates the identification of personality traits or the determination of hypothesized underlying dynamics. The classification of emotional disturbance under this and similar definitions can be addressed within the context of the conceptual framework and observational procedures presented in this chapter.

Similarly, for community mental health placements, many of the categories in the third edition of the *Diagnostic and Statistical Manual* (DSM-III) (American Psychiatric Association, 1980) can be addressed at least partially through behavioral assessment, and particularly through observational approaches (Taylor, 1983). While DSM-III still has numerous problems, such as its reliance upon a medical model and its related assumptions concerning the within-individual nature of psychological problems, it does represent an improvement in the generally descriptive nature of the categories of mental disorder. DSM-III attempts to operationalize the criteria for classification of mental disorders, though there is still considerable pseudospecificity with many criteria (Taylor, 1983). Such specification of classification criteria allows the possible use of observational approaches as one important set of assessment strategies with socioemotional problems.

Research with DSM-III through the use of observational approaches should facilitate the further operationalization of classification criteria. Freeman and Ritvo (1982) have described such a process of operationalization for the syndrome of autism by reviewing theirs and others' work based heavily upon direct observation. The Behavior Observation Scale (BOS) for autism (Freeman, Ritvo, Guthrie, Schroth, & Ball, 1978) has been found to be a highly reliable analogue measure (in that it is conducted in a clinic playroom setting) that discriminates among autistic, mentally retarded, and normal children.

Observational approaches to assessment have been used with a broad range of socioemotional problem areas, age ranges, and settings. The next section will summarize this breadth of coverage. Haynes and Wilson (1979) critically evaluate behavioral assessment methods and present comprehensive lists of applications (in terms of age range, problems, and settings) for naturalistic observation, analogue observation, and self-monitoring.

Target Variables

As indicated above, the breadth of coverage through the use of behavioral observation assessment approaches is tremendous. Rather than citing all articles relevant to the various categories of target variables and observational approaches, the categories will be indicated in text and tables. The lists are based upon thorough reviews by Haynes and Wilson (1979) and, in the area of naturalistic observation of conduct disorders, the review of McIntyre and colleagues (1983). The interested reader should refer to these sources for specific references and critical evaluations of the area. In addition, a selective review was made of more recent (since 1979) articles in *Behavioral Assessment* and *Journal of Behavioral Assessment* plus other behavioral therapy journals and issues of the APA *PsycSCAN: LD/MR* and *PsycSCAN: Clinical Psychology*.

Examination of these sources indicates that naturalistic observation is by far the most frequently used general observational method for the assessment of children and youth. Haynes and Wilson (1979) list 137 observational studies with children and youth. McIntyre *et al.* (1983) reviewed 43 additional naturalistic observation studies conducted in home settings with conduct-disorderd children. Haynes and Wilson (1979) cited 54 analogue observation and 12 self-monitoring clinically relevant studies with children and youth.

With regard to settings where the observational assessments took place, self-monitoring occurred in naturalistic environments, while analogue observations generally were conducted in clinic settings. Haynes and Wilson's (1979) review showed that assessment of children and youth via naturalistic observation occurred most frequently in school settings (65), followed by home observations (42 plus the 43 cited by McIntyre *et al.*, 1983) and institutional setting (24), with the fewest done in community settings (6).

It is interesting to note that despite the emphasis upon an interactional model within the behavioral construct system, most of the observational studies cited in Haynes and Wilson (1979) have children or youth as the sole targets of observation. In fact, a full 78% of the naturalistic and analogue observational studies cited have the problematic child/youth as the object of observation. The remaining 22% observed interactional sequences among parents and children or teachers and pupils. All studies of conduct-disordered children in the home, cited by McIntyre *et al.* (1983), were interactional. Collapsing across interactional and noninteractional studies cited by Haynes and Wilson, it is apparent that elementary school-aged children represent the primary focus of observational assessment (72%), followed by preschoolers, infants, and adolescents in descending order (14%, 9%, 5%, respectively). Clearly adolescents have not been the targets of observational assessment to any great extent. At the same time, college students (not counted in the above figures) have been the targets of observational studies, particularly for assessment of fears and phobias, assertiveness, social skills, heterosexual interaction problems, and prosocial behaviors. Table 11-3 presents the numbers of studies in the various categories of observational method, setting, and age range.

The importance of interactional observational data cannot be overemphasized. For example, Cohen and Minde (1983) demonstrated that naturalistic observation differentiated among three groups of hyperactive children (varying with regard to symptom pervasiveness) and a group of normal children, while biological measures and standard psychological tests did not differentiate among the groups. Prior, Leonard, and Wood (1983) demonstrated that observational assessment of mother–child interactions differentiated hyperactive from normal children better than approaches that focused upon just the child. Similarly, Mash and Johnston

Table 11-3
Numbers of Observational Studies: Method, Setting, Age Range[a]

| Setting | Naturalistic Observation | | | | |
	Adult/child interactions	Infants	Preschoolers	Elementary school-aged children	Adolescents
Family	13	6	0	23	0
Institution	1	1	0	17	5
Schools	8	0	15	40	2
Community	2	0	0	4	0
		Analogue observation			
Clinic adult–client Interactions		4	0	12	2
Clinic client		6	12	17	1
		Self-monitoring			
Diverse	0	0	0	12	0

[a]Cited in Haynes and Wilson (1979).

(1982) showed the value of such mother–child interactional observations in differentiating hyperactive and normal children. Dubey, O'Leary, and Kaufman (1983) demonstrated the utility of observational assessment of parent–child interaction for the development and evaluation of treatment procedures focusing upon parent training. Other investigators have illustrated the value of sequential observational data for parent–child interactions with conduct-disordered children (McIntyre *et al.*, 1983), with hyperactive children and interactions with their siblings (Mash & Johnston, 1983), for peer interactions with learning-disabled children (Pearl, Bryan, & Donahue, 1983), for teacher–pupil interactions with behavior-disordered children and youth (Forness, 1983), and for parent–adolescent interactions with disturbed but nonpsychotic adolescents (Asarnow, Lewis, Doane, Goldstein, & Rodnick, 1982).

Socioemotional problems can be experienced by any child or youth, from typical children to mentally retarded, learning-disabled, gender-disturbed, conduct-disordered, and more seriously emotionally disturbed children and youth. Table 11-4 indicates the diversity of child/youth categories that have been the targets of observational assessment approaches. Table 11-5 illustrates the broad range of behavioral categories that have been the target problem areas of observational assessment. The categories indicated represent broad summary labels, each of which has one or more specific operational behavioral responses associated with it. Again, the interested reader should refer to Haynes and Wilson (1979) and McIntyre *et al.* (1983) for specific references in order to obtain information on the behavioral definitions and specific observational schedules.

The diversity of target behaviors in Table 11-5 reflects a desirable individualization of client assessment. At the same time, it presents problems for researchers and clinicians; that is, cross-laboratory/clinician comparisons are difficult, making replication, discrimination, and implementation of observational schedules problematic. There is a clear need for more uniform and concise observational procedures. The observational schedules reported in the literature are highly

Table 11-4
Targets of Observational Assessment: Child/Youth Categories[a]

Naturalistic observation	Analogue observation	Self-monitoring
Adolescent Psychiatric	Autistic	Children with Academic Problems
Autistic	Behavior Problem/ Behavior Disordered	Gender Disturbed
Conduct Problems	Children of Schizophrenics	
Emotionally Handicapped	Distressed Mother–Adolescent Dyads	
Gender Disturbed	Disturbed but nonpsychotic Adolescents	
Hyperactive	Emotionally Handicapped	
Learning Disabled	Gender Disturbed	
Mentally Retarded	Hyperactive	
Predelinquent	Mentally Retarded	
Withdrawn	Withdrawn	

[a]Cited in Haynes and Wilson (1979).

Table 11-5
Targets of Observational Assessment:
General Behavioral Categories[a]

Naturalistic observation	Analogue observation	Self-monitoring
Academic Behaviors/Skills	Aggression	Academic Behaviors/ Skills
Activity Level	Anxiety	Compulsive Rituals
Aggression	Assertiveness	Hallucinations
Anxiety	Compliance/Noncompliance	Obsessive Ruminations
Assertiveness	Conflict Resolution	Sex-Typed Mannerisms
Classroom Environment (Forness, Guthrie, & MacMillan, 1982)	Drug Reactions	Sex-Typed Play
Compliance/Noncompliance	Echolalic Speech	
Conflict	Parent–Child Interactions	
Cross-Gender Behaviors	Parenting Skills	
Disruptive Behaviors	Self-Stimulation	
Eating Behaviors	Sex-Typed Mannerisms	
Enuretic Behaviors	Social Skills	
Fears/Phobias	Tantrums	
Oppositional Behaviors	Temperament (Greenberg & Field, 1982)	
Parent–Child Interactions	Verbal Responsiveness	
Parenting Skills		
Ritualistic Behavior		
Self-Care		
Self-Injurious Behavior		
Social Interactions		
Theft		

[a]Cited in Haynes and Wilson (1979).

sophisticated, with sequential recording techniques (allowing precise description of interactional sequences within and/or among individuals) being used in 60% of those studies reported by McIntyre *et al.* (1983). Further, researchers and clinicians using observational assessment need to address the social validity of the behaviors being observed (Kazdin, 1977b; Wolf, 1978); that is, it is important to demonstrate that the changes measured as a result of intervention are clinically significant. Social validity can be evaluated by asking the clients themselves and/or important others in the client's environment, or by comparing clients with typical individuals in targeted environments.

This need for normative comparison data is particularly pertinent to analogue observational methods. Analogue observation has been used primarily for research purposes rather than as a clinical tool. Where it has been used for treatment evaluation, little normative or discriminative validity data are available concerning the behavioral measures derived from the structured settings. Similarly, while naturalistic observation has been used primarily in treatment evaluation, it has been used less as a preintervention assessment strategy. To enhance its usefulness as part of preintervention assessment, more discriminant validity studies are needed where observational data are shown to discriminate among clinical and typical populations. More research like Cohen and Minde's (1983) previously cited work is needed to show the ability of observational approaches to differentiate socioemotional problems relative to other assessment strategies. In addition, we need to determine how best to pragmatically integrate observational procedures and data within the comprehensive assessment of clients.

Case Study

The following case study is taken from Tombari (1981) and illustrates a behavioral assessment of a child referred for possible emotional disturbance. As implied throughout this chapter, the observations described in the case study are merely part of a comprehensive behavioral assessment.

BEHAVIORAL ASSESSMENT

Name: Terry Stones
D.O.B.: 2/1/68
Dates of assessment: 10/5–10/19

Problem Identification

Terry was referred by his classroom teacher, Mrs. Cash, because of extensive acting-out behavior in class. In the 30-minute interview with her, she specified acting-out behavior as getting out of his seat at least 30–40 times a day, hitting, touching other students, calling out, using abusive language, and refusing to follow directions. She also stated that Terry has no friends. The other students dislike him because he is constantly bothering them and getting them into trouble.

Mrs. Cash stated that she has several other children who break classroom rules, but none to the extent that Terry does. She reported that Terry has exhibited these behaviors since the first week of school and that his cumulative folder details a similar history since second grade.

Terry's reading and math skills are more than 2 years below grade level. According to Mrs. Cash, he appears totally unable to converse in any pleasant manner with adults or peers. Based on my interview with Mrs. Cash, the following problems were identified:

1. Behavioral excesses: fighting, out of seat, cursing, general disruptiveness.
2. Behavioral deficits: no skills in making friends or communicating with adults.
3. Academic deficits: below grade level in reading and math.

Behavioral Observations

Mrs. Cash and I observed and recorded Terry's classroom behavior for 1 week. Mrs. Cash kept a frequency count of disruptive behavior for 5 days. Terry averaged 50 disruptive acts a day. I observed Terry for six randomly chosen intervals of 10-minutes' duration over a period of 2 days. My observations validated those of Mrs. Cash. Using a 20-second interval recording pace, Terry was observed to engage in disruptive behavior in 25% of the intervals. In addition, I recorded disruptive acts by other classmates. The total amount of disruption from others amounted to only 5% of recorded intervals.

Other school personnel were asked to observe and record any instances of the following behaviors: conversing with adults, cooperative play with other students, initiating social interactions with peers or adults. They observed for 1 week in the cafeteria, play areas, and during recess. Terry was never observed conversing with adults, playing cooperatively with other students for more than 10% of the time, or initiating any social interactions.

Interview with Terry (30 minutes)

This interview took place in the counselor's office. I explained to Terry who I was, why I was interviewing him, and that I had observed him in class. Terry was aware that he was "in trouble," but he believed that he was being picked on by his teacher. He was tired of being given "baby readers to read and kindergarten math." When I explained that his reading and math skills were not up to sixth-grade level, he replied that other kids made fun of him because he was doing what the little kids do. He said he just can't learn to do reading and math well. He reported that he can't wait to get out of the "stupid school" and get to junior high where things were nicer. At junior high, he said, you travel to different classes and don't sit bored with the same "old bitch" all day.

He believed that the principal, Mr. Bran, picked only on the black kids. He also indicated that his parents are fed up with the constant harassment by the school in the form of notes sent home and phone calls. When I told him that a lot of what I observed in class was started by him and I saw no one picking on him, he retorted, "Well, then, you need new glasses."

I asked if he felt there was any way the situation could be improved. He said, "Yes! When I get out of this damn school." When I explained to Terry that he had 8 months of school left and that the situation can't remain as it is, he indicated that "it's up to them [teachers and principal] to make it better." He expressed little sense of control over the school situation.

From this interview, the following possible problems can be identified:

1. Irrational thoughts that he is picked on because of his race, that teachers have it in for him.
2. Self-defeating, self-verbalizations: that is, can't do reading and math, can't control the situation.
3. Affective responses: "Others are laughing at me and that's awful"; concerns over what others think of him.

Assessment of Environment–Behavior Interaction

Terry's behavior varies throughout the school day, apparently depending on such variables as difficulty of tasks assigned, reinforcers in the environment, classroom structure in terms of specificity of rules and consequences for breaking them, and amount of adult attention. From observations and teacher reports, it appears that Terry's behavior is worse in settings where adult attention to behavior is sporadic and tasks are inappropriate for his ability level. Mrs. Cash has 31 students in her class and has difficulty attending to Terry when he is behaving well and ignoring many of his attention-getting behaviors. Likewise, Terry's peers are a constant source of reinforcement for inappropriate behavior. The only consequences the school uses for bad behavior are "time-out" in the principal's office and a letter home or parent conference. None of these work with Terry because he wants to get out of class and his parents are at odds with the school.

PE class is another story. Terry enjoys the activities, receives much praise and encouragement from the teacher, and the class has explicit rules and routines which Terry respects. The consequences for misbehavior also are explicit: removal from the gym.

The remedial reading teacher reports that Terry is no problem in her classes which run for 30 minutes. Terry works in a group of six, in a reader at his level. His teacher also has set up a token reinforcement program to which Terry responds very well. She is quick to praise him for appropriate behavior and knows which behaviors to ignore and which to punish by loss of tokens. Terry has averaged over 90% of his tokens for the past 4 weeks.

Results of Trial Effort to Improve Terry's Behavior in Mrs. Cash's Room

Despite some reluctance, Mrs. Cash agreed to the use of a good behavior checklist for 7 school days to see if Terry's behavior would improve over what we observed at baseline. Four simple rules were specified, and Terry received a check mark every 15 minutes for the absence of any rule violations. Mrs. Cash also was to make an effort to give him more social praise. A total of 80% of all possible checks allowed Terry extra gym time every day. Terry received 80% the first day, 75% the second, 50% the third and fourth, and then refused to keep the checklist any more. His inappropriate behavior returned to the level it was at baseline.

Failure may be attributed to a number of factors: Terry's academic tasks still were too difficult for him; peer attention for inappropriate behavior continued; Mrs. Cash was too busy with other students to regularly give Terry social praise; Terry's belief that Mrs. Cash doesn't like him remained unchanged. The program could be improved, but it would require more time and attention than Mrs. Cash could give.

Intellectual Skills Assessment

During both IQ and achievement testing, Terry behaved in a manner similar to that described by his remedial reading teacher: He attended to directions and tasks even though some were difficult, and he expressed pleasure at doing well. On the Brigance Skills Inventory, he worked to his frustration point but expressed such comments as, "I can't do well on these." These comments were particularly evident on math problems. Terry clearly demonstrated that he can control his behavior in situations requiring sustained attention to sometimes tedious tasks, given close adult supervision, liberal social praise, and attention for appropriate behavior.

Terry's IQ on the WISC-R was well within the average range, indicating ability to succeed at academic tasks.

Results of assessment using the Brigance indicated skill levels in reading at late second grade and in math at early third grade. A more detailed breakdown of the specific skills that Terry has and has not mastered can be ascertained from the attached record forms.

Summary of Problem Areas in Need of Change

Behavior: Terry must learn to
1. Stay in seat and complete work,
2. Speak out at appropriate times,
3. Initiate and engage in conversation with adults,
4. Initiate and engage in appropriate social interactions with peers,
5. Ask for help when he cannot do work, and
6. Improve in reading and math skills.

Affect
1. Improve attitude toward school, and
2. Express anger in socially appropriate ways.

Thoughts
1. Decrease irrational thoughts (e.g., "Teachers don't like me. The principal picks on me because I am black. Everybody picks on me."),
2. Decrease self-defeating beliefs (e.g., "I can't learn to read well."),
3. Increase positive self-statements related to academic skills, and
4. Develop more realistic beliefs about why he is failing in school and why he is being disciplined.

Interpersonal Relationships
   1. Increase friendships, and
   2. Play games cooperatively.

Recommendations

Terry's school-related problems are significant enough to impede his learning and the learning of others in his classroom. His behavior is markedly worse than that of others in his classroom. This is particularly evident in large-group situations where adult attention is sparse. The learning tasks that Terry can succeed at, the level of adult attention required to keep him on task and learning, and the immediacy of reinforcement and punishment needed are beyond the resources of a regular classroom setting. He also requires cognitive therapy to change certain thoughts and beliefs that interfere with his adjustment to school rules and school learning. For the above reasons the following recommendations are offered:

   1. Terry should be placed in a special education program under the classification of emotionally disturbed, pending parent approval.
   2. The objectives of such a program should include those listed under "Summary of Problem Areas in Need of Change."
   3. The details of this program should be worked out in a joint meeting with teachers, parents, school psychologist, and special education staff.
   4. The program should include sufficient mainstreaming to allow the evaluation of progress toward program objectives using data-gathering techniques described in this report.
   5. At the meeting described in (3), strategies to help Terry to meet objectives and methods to evaluate progress will be mutually discussed and decided upon.[1]

This case illustrates many of the points presented in the chapter. The first teacher interview was used to define the referral problem and to specify the behaviors to be observed initially. Both participant observation by the teacher and external observation were conducted to validate the interview data concerning the problem. Additionally, this initial observation provided comparative (in-setting normative) data on the child and peers. Observation took place in multiple settings indicating those environmental contexts where the child's problematic behaviors were most and least likely to be manifested. Observations were conducted in an unsuccessful trial effort to maintain appropriate behavior in a mainstreamed setting (a strategy crucial to classification). Finally, an explicit recommendation was made to use observational approaches during intervention. Observation was therefore helpful during the preintervention assessment for problem identification, aided in classification and selection of intervention focuses and strategies, and served as one evaluation component of intervention efficacy.

Summary

This chapter has examined the use of behavioral observation approaches in the assessment of children's and adolescents' personality development within the context of a behavioral construct system, though such approaches can be used

---

[1]As a general rule, specific details of a program should be worked out jointly with those responsible for its execution. This helps to dispel the all-too-prevalent notion that school psychologists are unrealistic and dogmatic about their recommendations and insensitive to the demands of classroom teachers.

within any theoretical construct system. The central assumption of a behavioral construct system is that personality and problem and nonproblem behaviors (including socioemotional problems) are acquired and maintained and thus changed through involvement in complex person–setting interactions. Assessment within this context includes the use of multiple methods (of which observation represents one important approach) to measure diverse behavioral contents (motoric, cognitive, affective, and physiological) under diverse conditions.

A variety of observational measures were presented, including interval recording, time-sample recording, event recording, and duration and latency recording. Each of these measures has advantages and disadvantages with respect to various problems and methods of observation. Observation may be conducted via self-monitoring, analogue observation (in settings structured to simulate natural conditions), and naturalistic observation. Various aids to the use of observation were presented; four highly recognized general observational coding systems were evaluated.

As with any assessment tool for decision making, psychometric issues are very important. Such issues were critically discussed within the context of generalizability theory. Specifically, generalizability over observers, time, settings, behaviors, and methods were addressed. The problem of reactivity in behavioral observation was also discussed.

Behavioral observation has been used with a diversity of child and adolescent populations in a variety of environmental settings. A broad range of problems have been assessed via behavioral observation. This diversity in the utility of observational approaches was presented. Finally, a case study illustrating the use of observation within the context of comprehensive behavioral assessment of a child referred for possible emotional disturbance was presented.

References

Achenbach, T. M. (1978). The Child Behavior Profile: I. Boys aged 6–11. *Journal of Consulting and Clinical Psychology, 46,* 478–488.

Achenbach, T. M., & Edelbrock, C. S. (1979). The Child Behavior Profile: II. Boys aged 6–12 and girls aged 6–11 and 12–16. *Journal of Consulting and Clinical Psychology, 47,* 223–233.

Achenbach, T. M., & Edelbrock, C. S. (1981). Behavioral problems and competencies reported by parents of normal and disturbed children aged four through sixteen. *Monographs of the Society for Research in Child Development, 46,* (1, Serial No. 188).

Achenbach, T. M., & Edelbrock, C. S. (1984). Psychopathology of childhood. *Annual Review of Psychology, 35,* 227–256.

Agras, W. S., Kazdin, A. E., & Wilson, G. T. (1979). *Behavior therapy: Toward an applied clinical science.* San Francisco: W. H. Freeman.

Alessi, G. J. (1980). Behavioral observation for the school psychologist: Responsive-discrepancy model. *School Psychology Review, 9,* 31–45.

Allen, G. J., Chinsky, J. M., Larcen, S. W., Lochman, J. E., & Selinger, H. V. (1976). *Community psychology and the schools: A behaviorally oriented multilevel preventive approach.* New York: John Wiley.

American Psychiatric Association. (1980). *Diagnostic and statistical manual of mental disorders* (3rd ed.). Washington, DC: Author.

American Psychological Association, American Educational Research Association, National Council on Measurement in Education. (1974). *Standards for educational and psychological tests.* Washington, DC: Author.

Asarnow, J. R., Lewis, J. M., Doane, J. A., Goldstein, M. J., & Rodnick, E. H. (1982). Family interaction and the course of adolescent psychopathology: An analysis of adolescent and parent effects. *Journal of Abnormal Child Psychology, 10,* 427–442.

Baer, D. M. (1982). Applied behavior analysis. In G. T. Wilson & C. M. Franks (Eds.), *Contemporary behavior therapy: Conceptual and empirical foundations* (pp. 277–309). New York: Guilford Press.

Bakeman, R. (1978). Untangling streams of behavior: Sequential analyses of observational data. In G. P. Sackett (Ed.), *Observing behavior: Vol. 2. Data collection and analysis methods* (pp. 63–78). Baltimore, MD: University Park Press.

Baker, E. H., & Tyne, T. F. (1980). The use of observational procedures in school psychological services. *School Psychology Monograph, 4*, 25–44.

Bandura, A. (1969). *Principles of behavior modification*. New York: Holt, Rinehart, & Winston.

Bandura, A. (1977). *Social learning theory*. Englewood Cliffs, NJ: Prentice-Hall.

Bandura, A. (1978). The self system in reciprocal determinism. *American Psychologist, 33*, 344–358.

Bardon, J. I., Bennett, V. C., Bruchez, P. K., & Sanderson, R. A. (1976). Psychosituational classroom intervention: Rationale and description. *Journal of School Psychology, 14*, 97–104.

Barlow, D. H. (Ed.). (1981). *Behavioral assessment of adult disorders*. New York: Guilford Press.

Baum, C. G., Forehand, R., & Zegiob, L. E. (1979). A review of observer reactivity in adult-child interactions. *Journal of Behavioral Assessment, 1*, 167–178.

Bell, D. R., & Low, R. M. (1977). *Observing and recording children's behavior*. Richland, WA: Performance Associates.

Bellack, A. S. (1979). Behavioral assessment of social skills. In A. S. Bellack & M. Hersen (Eds.), *Research and practice in social skills training* (pp. 75–106). New York: Plenum Press.

Bellack, A. S., & Hersen, M. (1977). Self-report inventories in behavioral assessment. In J. D. Cone & R. P. Hawkins (Eds.), *Behavioral assessment: New directions in clinical psychology* (pp. 52–76). New York: Brunner/Mazel.

Bellack, A. S., Hersen, M., & Lamparski, D. (1979). Role-play tests for assessing social skills: Are they valid? Are they useful? *Journal of Consulting and Clinical Psychology, 47*, 335–342.

Bellack, A. S., Hersen, M., & Turner, S. M. (1979). Relationship of role playing and knowledge of appropriate behavior to assertion in the natural environment. *Journal of Consulting and Clinical Psychology, 47*, 670–678.

Berk, R. (1979). Generalizability of behavior observations: A clarification of interobserver agreement and interobserver reliability. *American Journal of Mental Deficiency, 83*, 460–472.

Bersoff, D. M., & Grieger, R. M. (1971). Psychosituational assessment. *American Journal of Orthopsychiatry, 41*, 483–493.

Bijou, S. W., Peterson, R. F., & Ault, M. H. (1968). A method to integrate descriptive and experimental field studies at the level of data and empirical concepts. *Journal of Applied Behavior Analysis, 1*, 175–181.

Bijou, S. W., Peterson, R. P., Harris, F. T., Allen, K. E., & Johnston, M. S. (1969). Methodology for experimental studies of young children in natural settings. *Psychological Record, 19*, 177–210.

Blurton Jones, N. (Ed.). (1972). *Ethological studies of child behavior*. London: Cambridge University Press.

Boehm, A. E., & Weinberg, R. A. (1977). *The classroom observer: A guide for developing classroom skills*. New York: Teachers College.

Bogdan, R. (1976). The judged, not the judges: An insider's view of mental retardation. *American Psychologist, 31*, 47–52.

Bogdan, R., & Taylor, S. J. (1975). *Introduction to qualitative research methods*. New York: Wiley.

Campbell, S. B., Schleiter, M., Weiss, G., & Perlman, T. (1977). A two-year following of hyperactive preschoolers. *American Journal of Orthopsychiatry, 47*, 149–162.

Carlson, C. I., Scott, M., & Eklund, S. J. (1980). Ecological theory and method for behavioral assessment. *School Psychology Review, 9*, 75–82.

Cartwright, C. A., & Cartwright, G. P. (1974). *Developing observation skills*. New York: McGraw-Hill.

Charlesworth, W. R. (1978). Ethology: Its relevance for observational studies of human adaptation. In G. P. Sackett (Ed.), *Observing behavior: Vol. I. Theory and applications in mental retardation* (pp. 7–32). Baltimore, MD: University Park.

Ciminero, A. R., Calhoun, K. S., & Adams, H. E. (Eds.). (1977). *Handbook of behavioral assessment*. New York: Wiley.

Ciminero, A. R., Nelson, R. O., & Lipinski, D. P. (1977). Self-monitoring procedures. In A. R. Ciminero, K. S. Calhoun, & H. E. Adams (Eds.), *Handbook of behavioral assessment* (pp. 195–232). New York: Wiley.

Cohen, N. J., & Minde, K. (1983). The "hyperactive syndrome" in kindergarten children: Comparison of children with pervasive and situational symptoms. *Journal of Child Psychology and Psychiatry and Allied Disciplines, 24*, 443–455.

Cone, J. D. (1978). The behavioral assessment grid (BAG): A conceptual framework and a taxonomy. *Behavior Therapy, 9*, 882–888.

Cone, J. D. (1979). Confounded comparisons in triple response mode assessment research. *Behavioral Assessment, 1*, 85–95.

Cone, J. D., & Foster, S. L. (1982). Direct observation in clinical psychology. In P. C. Kendall & J. N. Butcher (Eds.), *Handbook of research methods in clinical psychology*. New York: Wiley.

Cone, J. D., & Hawkins, R. P. (Eds.). (1977). *Behavioral assessment: New directions in clinical psychology* (pp. 311–354). New York: Brunner/Mazel.

Conoley, J. C. (1980). Organizational assessment. *School Psychology Review, 9*, 83–89.

Cronbach, L. J., Gleser, G. C., Nanda, H., & Rajaratnam, N. (1972). *The dependability of behavioral measures*. New York: Wiley.

Dubey, D. R., Kent, R. N., O'Leary, S. G., Broderick, J. E., & O'Leary, K. D. (1977). Reactions of children and teachers to classroom observers: A series of controlled investigations. *Behavior Therapy, 8*, 887–897.

Dubey, D. R., O'Leary, S. G., & Kaufman, K. F. (1983). Training parents of hyperactive children in child management: A comparative outcome study. *Journal of Abnormal Child Psychology, 11*, 229–246.

Eisler, R. M., Hersen, M., Miller, P. M., & Blanchard, E. B. (1975). Situational determinants of assertive behaviors. *Journal of Consulting and Clinical Psychology, 43*, 330–340.

Eysenck, J. H. (1982). Neobehavioristic (S-R) theory. In G. T. Wilson & C. M. Franks (Eds.), *Contemporary behavior therapy: Conceptual and empirical foundations* (pp. 205–276). New York: Guilford Press.

Flanders, N. A. (1966). *Interaction analysis in the classroom: A manual for observers* (rev. ed.). Ann Arbor: University of Michigan.

Flanders, N. A. (1970). *Analyzing teacher behavior*. Reading, MA: Addison-Wesley.

Fleiss, J. L., Cohen, J., & Everitt, B. S. (1969). Large sample standard errors of Kappa and weighted Kappa. *Psychological Bulletin, 72*, 323–327.

Forness, S. R. (1983). Diagnostic schooling for children or adolescents with behavioral disorders. *Behavioral Disorders, 8*, 176–180.

Forness, S. R., & Esveldt, K. C. (1975a). Classroom observation of learning and behavioral problem children. *Journal of Learning Disabilities, 8*, 383–385.

Forness, S. R., & Esveldt, K. C. (1975b). Prediction of high-risk kindergarten children through classroom observation. *Journal of Special Education, 9*, 375–387.

Forness, S. R., Guthrie, D., & Hall, R. J. (1976). Follow-up of high risk children identified in kindergarten through direct classroom observation. *Psychology in the Schools, 13*, 45–49.

Forness, S. R., Guthrie, D., & MacMillan, D. L. (1982). Classroom environments as they relate to mentally retarded children's observable behavior. *American Journal of Mental Deficiency, 87*, 259–265.

Forness, S. R., Guthrie, D., & Nichara, K. (1975). Clusters of observable behavior in high-risk kindergarten children. *Psychology in the Schools, 12*, 263–269.

Frame, R. (1979). Interobserver agreement as a function of the number of behaviors recorded simultaneously. *Psychological Record, 29*, 287–296.

Freeman, B. J., & Ritvo, E. R. (1982). The syndrome of autism: A critical review of diagnostic systems, follow-up studies, and the theoretical background of the behavioral observation scale. *Advances in Child Behavioral Analysis and Therapy, 2*, 1–39.

Freeman, B. J., Ritvo, E. R., Guthrie, D., Schroth, P., & Ball, J. (1978). The Behavior Observation Scale for Autism. *Journal of the American Academy of Child Psychiatry, 17*, 576–588.

Galassi, M. D., & Galassi, J. P. (1976). The effects of role-playing variations on the assessment of assertive behavior. *Behavior Therapy, 7*, 343–347.

Goldfried, M. R. (1976). Behavioral assessment. In I. B. Weiner (Ed.), *Clinical methods in psychology* (pp. 281–330). New York: Wiley.

Goldfried, M. R. (1977). Behavioral assessment in perspective. In J. D. Cone & R. P. Hawkins (Eds.), *Behavioral assessment: New directions in clinical psychology* (pp. 3–22). New York: Brunner/Mazel.

Goldfried, M. R., & Kent, R. N. (1972). Traditional versus behavioral assessment: A comparison of methodological and theoretical assumptions. *Psychological Bulletin, 77*, 409–420.

Goldfried, M. R., & Linehan, M. M. (1977). Basic issues in behavioral assessment. In A. R. Ciminero, K. S. Calhoun, & H. E. Adams (Eds). *Handbook of behavioral assessment* (pp. 15–46). New York: Wiley.

Goodwin, D. L., & Coates, T. J. (1977). The teacher-pupil interaction scale: An empirical method for analyzing the interactive effects of teacher and pupil behavior. *Journal of School Psychology, 15*, 51–59.

Greenberg, R., & Field, T. (1982). Temperament ratings of handicapped infants during classroom, mother, and teacher interactions. *Journal of Pediatric Psychology, 7*, 387–405.

Hagen, R. L., Craighead, W. E., & Paul, G. L. (1975). Staff reactivity to evaluative behavioral observations. *Behavior Therapy, 6*, 201–205.

Harris, F. C., & Lahey, B. B. (1978). A method for combining occurrence and nonoccurrence interobserver agreement scores. *Journal of Applied Behavior Analysis, 11*, 523–527.

Hawkins, R. P., & Dobes, R. W. (1977). Behavioral definitions in applied behavior analysis: Explicit or implicit. In B. C. Etzel, J. M. LeBlanc, & D. M. Baer (Eds.), *New developments in behavioral research: Theory, methods and application. In honor of Sydney W. Bijou* (pp. 167–188). Hillsdale, NJ: Erlbaum.

Hay, L. R., Nelson, R. O., & Hay, W. M. (1977). The use of teachers as behavioral observers. *Journal of Applied Behavior Analysis, 10*, 345–349.

Haynes, S. N. (1978). *Principles of behavioral assessment*. New York: Gardner Press.

Haynes, S. N., & Horn, W. F. (1982). Reactivity in behavioral observation: A review. *Behavioral Assessment, 4*, 369–385.

Haynes, S. N., & Wilson, C. C. (1979). *Behavioral assessment: Recent advances in methods, concepts, and applications*. San Francisco, CA: Jossey-Bass.

Hersen, M., & Bellack, A. S. (Eds.). (1976). *Behavioral assessment: A practical handbook*. Oxford: Pergamon Press.

Hersen, M., & Bellack, A. S. (Eds.). (1981). *Behavioral assessment: A practical handbook* (2nd ed.). Oxford: Pergamon Press.

Hiltonsmith, R. W., & Keller, H. R. (1983). What happened to the setting in person-setting assessment? *Professional Psychology: Research and Practice, 14*, 419–434.

Hobbs, N. (1975). *The futures of children*. San Francisco, CA: Jossey-Bass.

House, A. E., House, B. J., & Campbell, N. (1981). Measures of interobserver agreement: Calculation formulas and distribution effects. *Journal of Behavioral Assessment, 3*, 37–57.

Hunter, C. P. (1977). Classroom observation instruments and teacher inservice by school psychologists. *School Psychology Monograph, 3*, 45–88.

Hutt, S. J., & Hutt, C. (1970). *Direct observation and measurement of behavior*. Springfield, IL: Charles C. Thomas.

Johnson, S. M., & Bolstad, O. D. (1973). Methodological issues in naturalistic observations: Some problems and solutions for field research. In L. A. Hamerlynck, L. C. Handy, & E. J. Mash (Eds.), *Behavior change: Methodology, concepts, and practice* (pp. 7–68). Champaign, IL: Research Press.

Johnson, S. M., & Bolstad, O. D. (1975). Reactivity to home observation: A comparison of audio recorded behavior with observers present or absent. *Journal of Applied Behavior Analysis, 8*, 181–187.

Jones, R. R., Reid, J. B., & Patterson, G. R. (1975). Naturalistic observation in clinical assessment. In P. McReynolds (Ed.), *Advances in psychological assessment* (Vol. 3, pp. 42–95). San Francisco, CA: Jossey-Bass.

Kanfer, F. H., & Saslow, G. (1969). Behavioral diagnosis. In C. M. Franks (Ed.), *Behavior-therapy: Appraisal and status*. New York: McGraw-Hill.

Kazdin, A. E. (1974). Self-monitoring and behavior change. In M. J. Mahoney & C. E. Thorenson (Eds.), *Self-control: Power to the person* (pp. 218–246). Moneterey, CA: Brooks/Cole.

Kazdin, A. E. (1977a). Artifact, bias, and complexity of assessment: The ABC's of reliability. *Journal of Applied Behavior Analysis, 10*, 141–150.

Kazdin, A. E. (1977b). Assessing the clinical or applied importance of behavior change through social validation. *Behavior Modification, 1*, 427–451.

Kazdin, A. E. (1981). Behavioral observation. In M. Hersen & A. S. Bellack (Eds.), *Behavior assessment: A practical handbook* (2nd ed., pp. 101–124). Oxford: Pergamon Press.

Keefe, F. J., Kapel, S. A., & Gordon, S. B. (1978). *A practical guide to behavioral assessment*. New York: Springer.

Keller, H. R. (Ed.). (1980a). Behavioral assessment. *School Psychology Review, 9*.

Keller, H. R. (1980b). Issues in the use of observational assessment. *School Psychology Review, 9*, 21–30.

Keller, H. R. (1981). Behavioral consultation. In J. C. Conoley (Ed.), *Consultation in schools: Theory, research, procedures* (pp. 59–100). New York: Academic Press.

Kelley, M. B. (1977). A review of the observational data-collection and reliability procedures reported in the *Journal of Applied Behavior Analysis. Journal of Applied Behavior Analysis, 10*, 97–101.

Kent, R. N., & Foster, S. L. (1977). Direct observational procedures: Methodological issues in applied settings. In A. Ciminero, K. S. Calhoun, & H. E. Adams (Eds.), *Handbook of behavioral assessment* (pp. 279–328). New York: Wiley.

Kent, R. N., Kanowitz, J., O'Leary, K. D., & Cheiken, M. (1977). Observer reliability as a function of circumstances of assessment. *Journal of Applied Behavior Analysis, 10*, 317–324.

Kent, R. N., O'Leary, K. D., Diament, C., & Dietz, A. (1974). Expectation biases in observational evaluation of therapeutic change. *Journal of Consulting and Clinical Psychology, 42*, 774–780.

Kent, R. N., O'Leary, K. D., Dietz, A., & Diament, C. (1979). Comparison of observational recordings in vivo, via mirror, and via television. *Journal of Applied Behavior Analysis, 12*, 517–522.

Kern, J. M. (1984). Relationships between obtrusive laboratory and unobtrusive naturalistic behavioral fear assessments: Treated and untreated subjects. *Behavioral Assessment, 6*, 45–60.

Kirschenbaum, D. S., Steffen, J. J., & D'Orta, C. (1978). An easily mastered social competence classroom behavioral observation system. *Behavioral Analysis and Modification, 2*, 314–322.

Krasner, L. (1971). Behavior therapy. *Annual Review of Psychology, 22*, 482–532.

Krasner, L. (1982). Behavior therapy: On roots, contexts, and growth. In G. T. Wilson & C. M. Franks (Eds.), *Contemporary behavior therapy: Conceptual and empirical foundations* (pp. 11–64). New York: Guilford Press.

Kratochwill, T. R. (1982). Advances in behavioral assessment. In C. R. Reynolds & T. B. Gutkin (Eds.), *The handbook of school psychology* (pp. 314–350). New York: Wiley.

Lazarus, A. A. (1973). Multimodal behavior therapy: Treating the "Basic ID." *Journal of Nervous and Mental Disease, 156*, 404–411.

Leach, G. M. (1972). A comparison of the social behaviour of some normal and problem children. In N. Blurton Jones (Ed.), *Ethological studies of child behaviour* (pp. 249–284). London: Cambridge University Press.

Lipinski, D., & Nelson, R. O. (1974). Problems in the use of naturalistic observation as a means of behavioral assessment. *Behavior Therapy, 5*, 341–351.

Lobitz, G. K., & Johnson, S. M. (1975). Normal versus deviant children: A multimethod comparison. *Journal of Abnormal Child Psychology, 3*, 353–374.

Lynch, W. W. (1977). Guidelines to the use of classroom observation instruments by school psychologists. *School Psychology Monograph, 3*, 1–22.

Martin, R. P. (Ed.). (1983). Personality assessment: The rating scale approach. *School Psychology Review, 12*, 226–299.

Martin, S., Johnson, S. M., Johansson, S., & Wahl, G. (1976). The comparability of behavioral data in laboratory and natural settings. In E. J. Mash, L. A. Hamerlynck, & L. C. Handy (Eds.), *Behavior modification and families* (pp. 189–203). New York: Brunner/Mazel.

Mash, E. J., & Johnston, C. (1982). A comparison of mother-child interactions of younger and older hyperactive and normal children. *Child Development, 53*, 1371–1381.

Mash, E. J., & Johnston, C. (1983). Sibling interactions of hyperactive and normal children and their relationships to reports of maternal stress and self-esteem. *Journal of Clinical Child Psychology, 12*, 91–99.

Mash, E. J., & McElwee, J. D. (1974). Situational effects on observer accuracy: Behavioral predictability, prior experience, complexity of coding categories. *Child Development, 45*, 367–377.

Mash, E. J., & Terdal, L. G. (Eds.). (1976). *Behavior therapy assessment: Diagnosis, design, and evaluation*. New York: Springer.

Mash, E. J., & Terdal, L. G. (Eds.). (1981). *Behavioral assessment of childhood disorders*. New York: Guilford Press.

Mash, E. J., Terdal, L., & Anderson, K. (1973). The response-class matrix: A procedure for recording parent-child interactions. *Journal of Consulting and Clinical Psychology, 40*, 163–164.

McFall, R. M. (1977). Analogue methods in behavioral assessment: Issues and prospects. In J. D. Cone & R. P. Hawkins (Eds.), *Behavioral assessment: New directions in clinical psychology* (pp. 152–177). New York: Brunner/Mazel.

McIntyre, T. J., Bornstein, P. .H., Isaacs, C. D., Woody, D. J., Bornstein, M. T., Clucas, T. J., & Long, G. (1983). Naturalistic observation of conduct-disordered children: An archival analysis. *Behavior Therapy, 14*, 375–385.

McReynolds, P. (1979). The case for interactional assessment. *Behavioral Assessment, 1*, 237–247.

McReynolds, P., & DeVoge, S. (1978). Use of improvisational techniques in assessment. In P. McReynolds (Ed.), *Advances in psychological assessment* (Vol. 4). San Francisco, CA: Jossey-Bass.

Medley, D. M., & Mitzel, H. E. (1963). Measuring classroom behavior by systematic observation. In N. Gage (Ed.), *Handbook of research on teaching* (pp. 247–328). Chicago, IL: Rand McNally.

Meichenbaum, D., & Cameron, R. (1982). Cognitive-behavior therapy. In G. T. Wilson & C. M. Franks (Eds.), *Contemporary behavior therapy: Conceptual and empirical foundations* (pp. 310–338). New York: Guilford Press.

Melahn, C. L., & O'Donnell, C. R. (1978). Norm-based behavioral consulting. *Behavior Modification, 2*, 309–338.

Mischel, W. (1968). *Personality assessment.* New York: Wiley.

Mischel, W. (1969). Continuity and change in personality. *American Psychologist, 24,* 1012–1018.

Mischel, W. (1973). Toward a cognitive social learning reconceptualization of personality. *Psychological Review, 80,* 252–283.

Mischel, W. (1979). On the interface of cognition and personality: Beyond the person-situation debate. *American Psychologist, 34,* 740–754.

Morganstern, K. P., & Tevlin, H. E. (1981). Behavioral interviewing. In M. Hersen & A. S. Bellack (Eds.), *Behavioral assessment: A practical handbook* (2nd ed.). Oxford: Pergamon Press.

Morris, R. J. (1976). *Behavior modification with children: A systematic guide.* Cambridge, MA: Winthrop.

Nay, W. R. (1977). Analogue measures. In A. R. Ciminero, K. S. Calhoun, & H. E. Adams (Eds.), *Handbook of behavioral assessment* (pp. 233–278). New York: Wiley.

Nelson, C. M. (1971). Techniques for screening conduct disturbed children. *Exceptional Children, 37,* 501–507.

Nelson, R. O. (1977a). Assessment and therapeutic functions of self-monitoring. In M. Hersen, R. Eisler, & P. M. Miller (Eds.), *Progress in behavior modification* (Vol. 5, pp. 264–309). New York: Academic Press.

Nelson, R. O. (1977b). Methodological issues in assessment via self-monitoring. In J. D. Cone & R. P. Hawkins (Eds.), *Behavioral assessment: New directions in clinical psychology* (pp. 217–240). New York: Brunner/Mazel.

Nelson, R. O., & Bowles, P. E. (1975). The best of two worlds—observation with norms. *Journal of School Psychology, 13,* 3–9.

Nelson, R. O., Kapust, J. A., & Dorsey, B. L. (1978). Minimal reactivity of overt classroom observations on student and teacher behaviors. *Behavioral Therapy, 9,* 659–702.

New York State Education Department (1981 April). New Part 200 of the Regulations of the Commissioner of Education Effective July 1, 1982. Albany, NY: Author.

O'Leary, K. D., Romanczyk, R. G., Kass, R. E., Dietz, A., & Santagrossi, D. (1971). *Procedures for classroom observations of teachers and children.* Unpublished manuscript, State University of New York at Stony Brook.

Parsonson, B. S., & Baer, D. M. (1978). The analysis and presentation of graphic data. In T. R. Kratochwill (Ed.), *Single subject research: Strategies for evaluating change* (pp. 101–166). New York: Academic Press.

Patterson, G. R. (1969). Behavioral techniques based upon social learning: An additional base for developing behavior modification technologies. In C. M. Franks (Ed.), *Behavior therapy: Appraisal and status* (pp. 341–374). New York: McGraw-Hill.

Patterson, G. R. (1977). Naturalistic observation in clinical assessment. *Journal of Abnormal Child Psychology, 5,* 309–322.

Patterson, G. R., & Moore, D. (1979). Interactive patterns as units of behavior. In M. E. Lamb, S. J. Suomi, & G. R. Stephenson (Eds.), *Social interaction analysis* (pp. 77–96). Madison: University of Wisconsin Press.

Patterson, G. R., & Reid, J. B. (1973). Intervention for families of aggressive boys: A replication study. *Behavior Research and Therapy, 11,* 383–394.

Pearl, R., Bryan, T., & Donahue, M. (1983). Social behaviors of learning disabled children: A review. *Topics in Learning & Learning Disabilities, 3,* 1–14.

Piersel, W. C., & Kratochwill, T. R. (1979). Self-observation and behavior change: Applications to academic and adjustment problems through behavioral consultation. *Journal of School Psychology, 17,* 151–161.

Prior, M., Leonard, A., & Wood, G. (1983). A comparison study of preschool children diagnosed as hyperactive. *Journal of Pediatric Psychology, 8,* 191–203.

Reed, M. L., & Edelbrock, C. (1983). Reliability and validity of the direct observation form of the child behavior checklist. *Journal of Abnormal Child Psychology, 11,* 522–530.

Reid, J. B. (Ed.). (1977). *A social learning approach to family interaction: Vol. 2. A manual for coding family interactions.* Eugene, OR: Castalia.

Reid, J. B. (1979). *Observation in home settings: A social learning approach to family intervention* (Vol. 2). Champaign, IL: Research Press.

Reid, J. B., & Hendriks, A. F. C. J. (1973). A preliminary analysis of the effectiveness of direct home intervention for treatment of pre-delinquent boys who steal. In L. A. Hamerlynck, L. C. Handy, & E. J. Mash (Eds.), *Behavior change: Methodology concepts and practice* (pp. 209–219). Champaign, IL: Research Press.

Repp, A. C., Deitz, D. E., Boles, S. M., Deitz, S. M., & Repp, C. G. (1976). Differences among common methods for calculating interobserver agreement. *Journal of Applied Behavior Analysis, 9*, 109–113.

Reschly, D. (1979). Nonbiased assessment. In G. D. Phye & D. J. Reschly (Eds.), *School psychology: Perspectives and issues* (pp. 215–256). New York: Academic Press.

Rogers-Warren, A., & Warren, S. F. (Eds.). (1977). *Ecological perspectives in behavior analysis.* Baltimore, MD: University Park Press.

Romanczyk, R. G., Kent, R. N., Diament, C., & O'Leary, K. D. (1973). Measuring the reliability of observational data: A reactive process. *Journal of Applied Behavior Analysis, 6*, 175–186.

Rosenshine, B., & Furst, N. (1973). The use of direct observation to study teaching. In R. Travers (Ed.), *Second handbook of research on teaching* (pp. 122–183). Chicago, IL: Rand McNally.

Rosenthal, T. L. (1982). Social learning theory. In G. T. Wilson & C. M. Franks (Eds.), *Contemporary behavior therapy: Conceptual and empirical findings* (pp. 339–366). New York: Guilford Press.

Sackett, G. P. (Ed.). (1978a). *Observing behavior: Vol. I. Theory and applications in mental retardation.* Baltimore, MD: University Park Press.

Sackett, G. P. (Ed.). (1978b). *Observing behavior: Vol. II. Data collection and analysis methods.* Baltimore, MD: University Park Press.

Salvia, J., & Ysseldyke, J. E. (1978). *Assessment in special and remedial education.* Boston, MA: Houghton-Mifflin.

Simon, A., & Boyer, E. G. (Eds.). (1970). *Mirrors of behavior: An anthology of observation instruments continued* (Supplement, Vol. A and B). Philadelphia, PA: Research for Better Schools.

Sitko, M. C., Fink, A. H., & Gillespie, P. H. (1977). Utilizing systematic observation for decision-making in school psychology. *School Psychology Monographs, 3*, 23–44.

Skindrud, K. D. (1972). *An evaluation of observer bias in experimental-field studies of social interaction.* Unpublished doctoral dissertation, University of Oregon, Portland.

Smith, C. R. (1980). Assessment alternatives: Non-standardized procedures. *School Psychology Review, 9*, 46–57.

Smith, C. R. (1983). *Learning disabilities: The interaction of learner, task, and setting.* Boston, MA: Little, Brown.

Sundberg, N. D., Snowden, L. R., & Reynolds, W. M. (1978). Toward assessment of personal competence and incompetence in life situations. *Annual Review of Psychology, 29*, 179–221.

Taplin, P. S., & Reid, J. B. (1973). Effects of instructional set and experimenter influence on observer reliability. *Child Development, 44*, 547–554.

Taskey, J. J., & Rich, A. R. (1979). *Effects of demand characteristics and format variations in role-playing assessment.* Paper presented at the meeting of the American Psychological Association, New York.

Taylor, C. B. (1983). DSM-III and behavioral assessment. *Behavioral Assessment, 5*, 5–14.

Tombari, M. L. (1981). Nonbiased assessment of emotionally disturbed students. In T. Oakland (Ed.), *Nonbiased assessment* (pp. 123–140). Minneapolis: University of Minnesota.

Tukey, J. W. (1977). *Exploratory data analysis.* Reading, MA: Addison-Wesley.

Ullmann, L. P., & Krasner, L. (1969). *A psychological approach to abnormal behavior.* Englewood Cliffs, NJ: Prentice-Hall.

Wahler, R. G. (1975). Some structural aspects of deviant child behavior. *Journal of Applied Behavior Analysis, 8*, 27–42.

Wahler, R. G., House, A. E., & Stambaugh, E. E. (1976). *Ecological assessment of child problem behavior: A clinical package for home, school, and institutional settings.* Oxford: Pergamon Press.

Walker, H. M., & Hops, H. (1976). Use of normative peer data as a standard for evaluating classroom treatment effects. *Journal of Applied Behavior Analysis, 9*, 159–168.

Walker, H. M., Mattson, R. H., & Buckley, N. K. (1971). The functional analysis of behavior within an experimental class setting. In W. Becker (Ed.), *An empirical basis for change in education.* Chicago, IL: Science Research Associates.

Walls, R. T., Werner, T. J., Bacon, A., & Zane, T. (1977). Behavior checklists. In J. D. Cone & R. P. Hawkins (Eds.), *Behavioral assessments: New directions in clinical psychology* (pp. 77–146). New York: Brunner/Mazel.

Webb, E. J., Campbell, D. T., Schwartz, R. D., & Sechrest, C. (1966). *Unobtrusive measures: Nonreactive research in the social sciences.* Chicago, IL: Rand McNally.

Weick, K. E. (1968). Systematic observational methods. In G. Lindzey & E. Aronson (Eds.), *The handbook of social psychology* (2nd Ed., Vol. 2, pp. 357–451). Reading, MA: Addison-Wesley.

Weinrott, M. R., Garrett, B., & Todd, N. (1978). The influence of observer presence on classroom behavior. *Behavior Therapy, 9,* 900–911.

Werry, J. S., & Quay, H. C. (1969). Observing classroom behavior of elementary school children. *Exceptional Children, 35,* 461–467.

White, M. S. (1975). Natural rates of teacher approval and disapproval in the classroom. *Journal of Applied Behavior Analysis, 8,* 367–372.

Wildman, B. G., & Erickson, M. T. (1977). Methodological problems in behavioral observation. In J. D. Cone & R. P. Hawkins (Eds.), *Behavioral assessment: New directions in clinical psychology* (pp. 255–274). New York: Brunner/Mazel.

Wilson, C. C. (1980). Behavioral assessment: Questionnaires. *School Psychology Review, 9,* 58–66.

Wilson, G. T., & Franks, C. M. (Eds.). (1982). *Contemporary behavior therapy: Conceptual and empirical foundations.* New York: Guilford Press.

Wilson, G. T., & O'Leary, K. D. (1980). *Principles of behavior therapy.* Englewood Cliffs, NJ: Prentice-Hall.

Wilson, S. (1977). The use of ethnographic techniques in educational research. *Review of Educational Research, 47,* 245–265.

Wolf, M. M. (1978). Social validity: The case for subjective measurement of how applied behavior analysis is finding its heart. *Journal of Applied Behavior Analysis, 11,* 203–214.

Workman, E. A., & Hector, M. A. (1978). Behavioral self-control in classroom settings: A review of the literature. *Journal of School Psychology, 16,* 227–236.

Wright, H. F. (1960). Observational child study. In P. Mussen (Ed.), *Handbook of research methods in child development* (pp. 71–138). New York: Wiley.

Yelton, A. R., Wildman, B. G., & Erickson, M. T. (1977). A probability-based formula for calculating interobserver agreement. *Journal of Applied Behavior Analysis, 10,* 127–132.

Ysseldyke, J. E. (1979). Issues in psychoeducational assessment. In G. D. Phye & D. J. Reschly (Eds.), *School psychology: Perspectives and issues* (pp. 87–122). New York: Academic Press.

12
Family Assessment Approaches and Procedures

Marla R. Brassard

Traditional methods of personality assessment with children and adolescents have utilized a child-focused perspective that largely ignores family, school, peer, community, and societal influences on behavior (Green & Fine, 1980; Plas, 1981). This focus on the individual has not been the exclusive perspective of school or child mental health practitioners. Indeed, the history of scientific thinking, from the Greeks and Egyptians on, has been dominated by analyses of individuals and their characters or temperaments (Gottman, 1982). Personality theory and research in this century has certainly been influenced by this line of thinking. Thus, personality, defined as "those enduring properties of individuals that tend to separate them from other individuals" (Pervin, 1975, p. 3), has been studied primarily by those interested in reliably measuring the noted "enduring properties" (Hogan, DeSoto, & Solano, 1977; Mischel, 1968, 1977). The interactive or ecological factors determining and influencing personality development have been obliquely referred to (i.e., the mother–child relationship), but largely ignored.

In the past two or three decades, however, there has been a dramatic theoretical shift away from the study of individuals toward an emphasis on the context in which individuals develop the stable characteristics comprising "personality." While a number of major theoretical perspectives and events influenced this shift, one of the most significant was the general systems theory (Hoffman, 1981; von Bertalanffy, 1968).

Ludwig von Bertalanffy is credited with the creation and promotion of general systems theory when, as a European biologist during the 1920s, he became interested in some obvious gaps in the research and theory of biology. He felt that the mechanistic or random view of evolution and biology just did not fit the phenomena he observed. Life to him appeared to be, if anything, highly organized—not random and chaotic in its general manifestations. Von Bertalanffy began to advocate, with vehement resistance, an organismic conception of biology (and later of other sciences and mathematics) which considered organisms as wholes

Marla R. Brassard. Department of Educational Psychology, University of Georgia, Athens, Georgia.

or systems. He proposed that biology's major objective should be the discovery of principles of organization at various levels. When game theory, information theory, and cybernetics appeared after World War II and were related to systems theory, a cross-discipline shift occurred resulting in a more organismic view of individuals and an emphasis on understanding animate and inanimate behavior in context (Bateson, 1979; von Bertalanffy, 1968).

General systems theory has had an impact on the mental health field to a large extent through the work of Gregory Bateson and his 10-year research project on communication at Palo Alto, California (Bateson, Jackson, Haley, & Weakland, 1956; Hoffman, 1981). Influenced by the theories of Bateson and his group, family therapists in the late 1950s and early 1960s began to study the influences of family communications on symptomatic behavior and schizophrenia, in particular. Serendipitously, they began seeing families for treatment (Haley, 1959), although Ackerman in New York, a true revolutionary, had been doing this since the late 1930s (N.W. Ackerman, 1937; N.W. Ackerman & Sobel, 1950; Gottman, 1982).

Based on these developments and the research produced by family and marital therapists, it was generally concluded within the field that information from personality measures with the individual explained very little about the quality of family or marital groups. Further, these measures contributed little insight into the origins of individuals' maladaptive behaviors. As the most useful and necessary information is assumed to be interpersonal or interactive in nature (see Gottman, 1979, for a review), the clear result, with some empirical support, indicated that individual pathology can be understood and influenced only within the context where it occurs and has meaning. While the focus of this research was on the family, Petrie and Piersel (1982) pointed out that this model, in the case of children and adolescents, applies equally well to schools as a system.

In addition to family systems therapy, other forces have influenced this system-oriented trend: For example, ethology has stimulated developmental psychologists to look at developing infants' species-specific interactions with social environments (Ainsworth & Bell, 1970; Parkes & Stevenson-Hinde, 1982), and ecology has guided many disciplines to examine individual behavior and adaption within environmental contexts. Conceptually, the ecological approach (Belsky, 1980; Bronfenbrenner, 1977, 1979; Hobbs, 1966, 1975; Rhodes, 1967) has had a large influence on the fields of developmental psychology, child abuse, and increasingly, school psychology (e.g., Anderson, 1983; Knoff, 1983). This approach is discussed in some depth in Chapter 13 of this volume. The dramatic increase in the divorce rate and the prevalence of new family structures have also focused community and professional attention on larger cultural and parental determinants of child and adolescent behavior (Guidubaldi, 1980; Guidubaldi, Cleminshaw, Perry, & McLoughlin, 1983; Hetherington, Cox, & Cox, 1979; Kurdek, 1983). Together, these intellectual and cultural forces have strongly challenged the "medical model" view of symptomatic individuals as ill or victims of specific disease elements.

From an applied perspective, there are many child psychologists and mental health practitioners who complete personality assessments (Prout, 1983). Exactly what they are assessing is sometimes difficult to define. Perhaps Koppitz (1982) provided one of the better definitions of personality when she defined it as "feelings, conflicts, motives, and attitudes" (p. 273). She further stated that personality assessment with school-aged children serves four important functions:

(*a*) determining behavioral and learning styles; (*b*) discovering pupils' motives, attitudes, and modes of adjustment to school and the curriculum; (*c*) assessing self-concept and ability to relate to others; and (*d*) evaluating whether undue anxiety, serious emotional disturbance, or thought disorders are present and require further evaluation or intervention. Although Koppitz's definition is directed toward young children in school settings and takes a child—rather than a family or systems—focus, it is relevant to this chapter because it illustrates the value and importance of family assessment as part of a comprehensive approach to personality assessment. This chapter will emphasize that family assessment not only offers some of the more relevant answers to questions involving the four functions noted above, but also provides its own unique information and perspective as well.

Conceptualizing Family Assessment

Children and adolescents often are referred for personality assessment by concerned or exasperated adults who want some explanation for their inappropriate behavior, feelings, or attitudes at home, at school, or in the community (Evans & Nelson, 1977). Appropriate or expected behavior is determined by the adults in charge of a particular setting and thus, a large measure of subjective or relative judgment may be involved in a decision to refer a child (Lobitz & Johnson, 1975). For example, mothers' referrals of children have been shown to be affected by depression (Forehand, Wells, McMahon, Griest, & Rodgers, 1982; Griest, Wells, & Forehand, 1979), teachers' referrals by the type of problem exhibited by a child (Lorion, Cowen, & Caldwell, 1974), and juvenile court referrals by social class (Gordon, 1967). Thus, the act of getting referred is actually a systems event and should be acknowledged as part of the embedded relationship between the referred child and the environment that the practitioner is trying to assess. The referral source, the setting constraints, the capabilities of the referred child to function within those constraints, and the presence or absence of family and/or ecological stresses and supports should all be considered part of a personality assessment in order to respond most responsibly to referral questions and concerns.

In most cases, the family's positive or negative perspective and involvement in the referred child's behavior is an important aspect of the personality assessment. Presenting problems may reflect many types of family involvement: (*a*) marital difficulties and unresolved parental issues with their families of origin; (*b*) parental incompetence such as mild deficiencies in management skills, or deficiencies that arise from alcoholism or severely impaired physical or mental health; (*c*) environmental stress on the family or its community such as an economic depression or the presence of a toxic waste dump; (*d*) characteristics of a presenting child that have resulted in family stress such as in the case of an autistic or Down's syndrome child; or (*e*) tension or a lack of cooperation between home and other settings, such as the school, that affects the healthy development of the family, referred child, and significant others (Bronfenbrenner, 1979). Practitioners should be alert to the role of such family or ecological stressors in the presenting problem, indeed, throughout the personality assessment process.

All school or community mental health agency referrals may include a family-related difficulty at the heart of the problem. However, certain presenting problems are much more likely to involve family issues than others. In general, family assessments can be divided into two broad categories according to their purpose:

(*a*) assessments where the probable source of the presenting problem lies within the family (e.g., covert marital discord), and (*b*) assessments where the family may need support for a problem that is not directly within their control or responsibility (e.g., mental retardation). These categories are by no means mutually exclusive.

The first category above includes those presenting problems that have been clinically and empirically associated with maladaptive family functioning. Thus, when a child or adolescent is referred for one of these problems, the practitioner should be alerted to the probable role of the family and complete a full family interview and a formal family assessment. Obviously, this rule does not hold in all cases. For example, the author has encountered a case of school refusal, usually associated with an overly close relationship between a child and a parent, where the child was actually attempting to avoid a sexually abusive school janitor.

The psychological problems falling into this first category include anorexia nervosa (Minuchin, Rosman, & Baker, 1978), conduct problems and juvenile delinquency (Achenbach, 1982; Atkeson & Forehand, 1981; Hetherington & Martin, 1979), depression and suicidal gestures (Goodman & Guze, 1979; Jacobs, 1971; Lavigne & Burns, 1981; McConville, 1983), school phobia or refusal (Lavigne & Burns, 1981), running away (Thomas, 1982), substance abuse (Barnes, 1977; Brook, Lukoff, & Whiteman, 1978), child abuse (Belsky, 1980, 1984; Egeland, Sroufe, & Erickson, 1983; Parke & Collmer, 1975), and psychosomatic illness such as asthma (Melamed & Johnson, 1981; Minuchin *et al.*, 1975, 1978). Attention-deficit disorder with hyperactivity may also fall in this category (Barkley, 1981; Cantwell, 1972, 1978).

The second category includes presenting problems that may require school or clinic support for family efforts, but not necessarily "therapeutic" family intervention. Prominent among these are the developmental disabilities such as mental retardation, cerebral palsy, autism, neurological disorders, as well as cases of attention-deficit disorder, severe learning disabilities, and chronic illnesses such as juvenile diabetes and congenital heart disease. Obviously, family problems (i.e., exemplified in the first category) can occur along with the stresses of having an ill or handicapped child in a family, stresses that strain even the highest functioning family (see Lavigne & Burns, 1981, chaps. 13 and 14 for a review of the literature). For example, it is not uncommon for siblings of handicapped children to have more behavioral problems or psychosomatic symptoms, and marital relationships are frequently strained as the mother becomes overly involved with the handicapped or ill child while the father turns to his work.

Depending on the type of problem and the level of parental functioning, many families benefit from a variety of support services. In the case of autism, close home–school cooperation, parental support groups, and training in behavior modification techniques for parents and siblings have proved desirable and useful by the involved families and the professionals involved in producing comprehensive treatment programs for these individuals (Jenson & Young, in press; Lovaas, 1978). Similarly, families with other types of handicapped or ill members have benefited from crisis counseling, short-term family counseling, long-term planning, the identification of formal and informal community support services, training in behavior modification techniques, and other forms of cooperative and pragmatic help from involved schools or agencies (Barkley, 1981; Forehand *et al.*, 1979; Murphy, Pueschel, & Schneider, 1973; Yates & Lederer, 1961).

The referred handicapped or ill child or adolescent is frequently ignored when it comes to personality assessment. This is unfortunate given the relatively high level of anxiety, low self-esteem, and serious emotional disturbance in this population (Lavigne & Burns, 1981). In addition, these individuals are also at greater risk for child abuse (Gil, 1968, 1970). Thus, a careful personality and family assessment is just as important with families falling in this second category, although the focus and depth of the assessment will vary and the interventions are likely to be very different.

The remainder of the chapter will describe and illustrate an approach that can be used in school, child-oriented clinics, or family treatment settings; specific limitations are discussed in the section following this one. The approaches described are not exhaustive. They are limited to interview, self-report, and rating measures that can be administrated and scored by the mental health practitioner as part of an intake or developmental/social history in an office setting. Thus, structured observation methods which can provide valuable interactional information are not included in this section (see Keller, Chapter 11 of this volume). While observation methods have long been touted by behavioral psychologists as the assessment method of choice, there is little evidence that they are more valid than self-report or rating scale measures (Mash & Terdal, 1981). In fact, self-report or rating measures are actually preferable when assessing low-frequency events, and they are unquestionably more convenient (Huston & Robins, 1982). Also omitted are relevant parent and self-rating measures (e.g., the Personality Inventory for Children) which tap parental perceptions of children's behavior (see Lachar, Chapter 9 of this volume). Finally, the approach described is appropriately used as but one component of a comprehensive assessment in a psychoeducational setting; it could, however, serve as the sole approach in a family treatment setting.

The Stages of the Family Assessment Process

Family assessment as presented here consists of four stages: (a) preparing for the interview, (b) clarifying the presenting problem and its components, (c) gathering descriptive and dynamic information about the family, and (d) deciding on an intervention and the degree of family involvement in it. The basic guidelines of family assessment are (a) to obtain a clear description of the need for and purpose of the assessment; (b) to begin the assessment with the least threatening and intrusive measures, moving toward questions requiring more personal information and depth; and (c) to assess until some resolution is reached as to the nature of the problem, its functional relationship with other variables, and the context in which it occurs.

Preparing for the Interview

In a school setting, where the referral source is most often a teacher or administrator, the psychologist or mental health practitioner usually has access to a potentially vast amount of past and present information about a child, even before completing a family interview. This information includes, for example, academic history and achievement information; a description and, ideally, an actual observation of the child's current classroom (or other setting-specific) performance; a description of the problem of concern to the referral source; and an intimate awareness of the ecology of the school and its demands and expectations.

Given this information, tentative hypotheses may be developed that can focus the family interview and make it more productive. Not infrequently, the practitioner may already know the child and may have met the parents or other siblings, a major advantage when entering an assessment interview.

Practitioners working in an agency or hospital setting typically are more limited in the information available to them about a family prior to the interview. This does depend to a large extent, however, on how and by whom the family is referred. When the referral is school-facilitated, more information may be shared with the agency as records are released from the school's files (with parent permission) and telephone contacts between the school and agency occur. Otherwise, some general information about the referral may be taken over the phone. This information can help to determine who should come into the initial interview session, what the general referral concerns are, and what possible intake and assessment directions may be useful.

Clarifying the Presenting Problem

The presenting problem is the raison d'être, at least ostensibly, for the family assessment. Thus, given the need to gear assessments and interventions to referral questions, it is appropriate to focus the opening stages of the family interview on problem clarification. "Why are you here?" addressed to one or both of the parents is a good opening question when the referral comes from the parents or when the parents have been referred by one agency to another (e.g., from juvenile court to a clinic). When the family has been invited in by a referral source (such as a school), a description of the perceived problem by the referral source is helpful in focusing the group on the initial agenda for the meeting. Here, "How do you see the problem?" addressed first to one parent, then the other, to any older siblings, to the individual being referred, and finally to any other siblings is a good beginning. This question elicits the family's perspective on the problem, and the questioning done in a hierarchical order reinforces the leadership of the parents and avoids placing the referred child in the "hot seat" (Karpel & Strauss, 1983, p. 118).

There are a number of ways to elicit information about the referred problem, depending on the theoretical perspective of the practitioner. Karpel and Strauss (1983), taking a systems and family treatment orientation, focus on the onset, severity, and previous family responses to the problem. They suggest asking when the problem started, what was going on at the time, and what does the family think precipitated the problem's onset. Severity questions are addressed by asking what impact the problem has had on the family (e.g., nightly marital arguments over the recent addition of the husband's adolescent son, by a first marriage, into the household) and how the problem has developed and changed since its onset (i.e., was there a variable pattern of impact or has the problem led to consistently negative changes?). Questions related to family coping address what the family has done (have they actively confronted the problem or avoided it?), what has been attempted, and how has it worked. Family responses to these questions may reflect the family's decision-making ability, motivation for treatment, and crisis intervention skills, all important observations which will help the practitioner to develop appropriate interventions. Karpel and Strauss (1983) recommend spending only about the first 15 minutes of the initial interview on the presenting problem to leave sufficient time for a more global family assessment.

Mash and Terdal (1981) approach the referred problem from a behavioral perspective that is similar to the family system approach presented above, but more specifically tied to clarifying the patterns of social reward and punishment that are maintaining the objectionable behavior. They suggest directing the interview toward answering the following questions: (*a*) Is there a problem (i.e., is the child's behavior nonnormative)? (*b*) What is the child or adolescent doing or not doing that is bringing him or her in conflict with the environment? and (*c*) What variables potentially control these behaviors? Once a tentative diagnosis has been formulated, the questioning takes an even more specific, concrete direction with a focus on information that is directly related to potential treatment strategies. As the authors state succinctly:

> This gathering of information includes further specification and measurement of potential controlling variables (e.g., patterns of social reward and punishment), determination of the child's own resources for change (e.g., behavioral assets, and/or self-controlling behaviors), assessment of potential social and physical environmental resources that can be utilized in carrying out treatment, assessment of the motivation for treatment for both the child and significant others, indication of potential reinforcers, specification of realistic and specific treatment objectives, and recommendation of the types of treatment that are most likely to be effective. (p. 15)

A comparison of these two approaches reveals that the systems practitioner spends relatively little time on the presenting problem, focusing most of the session on assessing the family as a whole. With the behavioral psychologist, however, the presenting problem *is* the focus of the interview.

Karpel and Strauss (1983) suggest asking a final question to close this section of the family assessment. The question is, "Let me ask all of you again, in recent months, have there been any other changes for people in the family as a whole or any other problem areas besides the situations you've mentioned so far?" (p. 131). This question very successfully elicits information that the family has avoided or information they may not have thought was relevant.

Gathering Descriptive and Dynamic Information

This phase involves gathering information on the family's context (historical, social, and familial environment), structure and dynamics (e.g., role assignments, power structure, alliances, values, style of interaction, pattern of communication), and level of adaptation or health (coping strategies and experiences, satisfaction, and mental health of family members) (see Table 12-1). To some extent, this division of assessment techniques and measures into specific categories is arbitrary and reflects what the author considers most important. However, the choices are consistent with the literature.

The importance of the historical, social, and familial context has been particularly stressed by Bowen (1978), who developed the genogram, and by Carter and McGoldrick (1980a) in their book on the family life cycle. Hill (1964, 1970; Hill & Rogers, 1964), Duvall (1977), Haley (1973), and Minuchin (1974) have all noted the importance of the developmental stages of the family and its members and the interaction of those stages with the social circumstances of the time and the place in which the family exists.

The importance of structure in assessing and treating toward family health has been most associated with Minuchin (1974), under the rubric of structural

Table 12-1
Domains of Family Functioning and the Measures That Assess Them[a]

	Domains		
Measures	*Context: Historic and present*	*Structure and dynamics*	*Level of adaptation/health*
Ecomap	X	(X)	(X)
Description of Neighborhood/Day	X	(X)	
Genogram	X	(X)	(X)
Family Life Cycle	X	(X)	
FILE	X		
FACES II		X	
FES		X	
Marital Inventory		X	(X)
Parent–Adolescent Communication		X	(X)
Parent Perceptions Inventory		X	(X)
RATC		X	(X)
Family Satisfaction			X
Quality of Life			X
F-COPES			X

[a]An X connotes the primary domain assessed by the measure, and an (X) that the measure may provide supplementary information in regard to a domain.

family therapy, but it has not been ignored by other researchers or clinicians (see Hoffman, 1981). Family dynamics refers to those aspects of families that have been called more broadly the typology of families (Olson *et al.*, 1983; Olson & Portner, 1983) or the family environment (Moos & Moos, 1981, 1983).

Finally, the level of adaption or mental health of the family has been the impetus for much scale development by the University of Minnesota group (Olson *et al.*, 1983), and the responsibility to be aware of individual member's functioning has been stressed by others (e.g., Karpel & Strauss, 1983).

Intervention Decision Making and Treatment Planning

Good intervention decision making and treatment planning result from carefully focused assessments that are sensitive to the presented and identified referral problems and the contingencies supporting them. A clearly conceptualized case initially involves an identification of the primary problems (as noted above), their severity, and their remediability. After this, interventions that logically follow the various assessments can be identified along with possible intervention agents (e.g., a preferred psychologist, marriage counselor, or support group). Finally, the receptivity of the family to the suggested intervention program should be evaluated such that the presentation of recommendations will increase the likelihood of implementation.

The severity of a presenting problem often affects a family's and a referral source's (e.g., school or agency) motivation to seek treatment. This, in turn, affects the resources available to treat the problem and the number of ecological levels it is necessary to involve to make the intervention work. For example, an intervention may involve the child alone, parent alone, family, family and school, or youth, family, school, and community together, as in the case of a teenage sex offender participating in a community-based treatment program. The assessment of problem severity and family or agency motivation is individualistic and situation-specific in nature; that is, a very severe problem could either motivate a family toward quick, decisive action or paralyze them into helplessness and hopelessness. Regardless, this dimension must be considered prior to the intervention process.

The severity of a referral problem and the motivation of a family and referral source toward treatment reflect a problem's remediability. The remediability of a referred problem significantly influences decision making because practitioners, families, and agencies must decide whether or not an intervention program is advisable, defensible, or warranted, given the potential for successful change. In the author's opinion, the most resources should be allocated to cases that are amenable to remediation. Too often, chronically dysfunctional families consume enormous resources with little demonstrable change in terms of treatment outcome.

When intervention is necessary and advisable, the practitioner next generates a list of treatment recommendations prioritized by their importance for child and family health. (This list may be limited by available school, agency, or community resources.) Concurrently, the practitioner needs to consider who will implement the intervention(s). Sometimes, this choice is obvious (e.g., using the very skilled middle school resource room teacher), but frequently, especially when family and/or individual child treatment require complex mental health treatments, a referral to an external professional is necessary.

When deciding whether to keep a case for treatment beyond a family assessment or to make an external referral, practitioners should examine their own or their staff's training, their rapport with the family, the appropriateness of the case for their particular setting or institution (school or agency), and the case load within the institution. If the practitioner does not have the requisite training, he or she should not handle the case. Exceptions to this general rule would include those situations where there are no other professional resources (e.g., in rural settings) and where the practitioner, upon consultation (if possible) with other appropriately trained professionals, is fairly certain that the family would not be harmed by the treatment. When practitioners do proceed with an external referral, they are responsible for having thorough and up-to-date knowledge of referral resources and these resources' skills, fees, specialities, and general success records with particular types of cases.

The final consideration in treatment planning involves communicating recommendations to families so that they will be likely to implement them. A well-presented recommendation constitutes a major intervention in and of itself, and it can require considerable therapeutic skill. Although a thorough discussion of this process requires a separate chapter at a minimum, a few general statements can be made. Successful recommendations tend to specifically address the problems that family members have expressed concern over; they are clear and in terms that the family can comprehend; they offer explicit payoffs or rewards to family members for changing (see Alexander & Parsons, 1982); and they reorganize or relabel problems, making them acceptable to the family yet advisable to change (Hoffman, 1981; Papp, 1977; see Knoff, Chapter 15 of this volume).

Family Assessment Techniques and Measures

The third stage of the family assessment process, gathering descriptive and dynamic information, was briefly described above along with three components: information on context, on structure and dynamics, and on levels of adaptation or health. In this section, these three components will be presented in greater detail along with specific, respective techniques and measures which facilitate family assessment.

Assessing Context: The Family in Space and Time

The family's development over time, its developmental stage when referring a specific problem to a practitioner, and the context in which the family and the problem are embedded relate directly to problem analysis and treatment planning. The techniques and measures described in this section are the ecomap, and descriptions of the home, the neighborhood, and the typical daily routine of family members to assess the current environment; the genogram and family life cycle to assess family history, patterns, and current developmental stage; and the Family Inventory of Life Events (FILE and A-FILE, the adolescent version) to assess the number and kinds of stressful events that have occurred over the past year.

The Ecomap

The ecomap is increasingly popular in the field of social work (Hartman, 1979; Holman, 1983) as a tool for family assessment. This method was first developed by Hartman to help public welfare workers assess individual family needs, and its rationale emanates from a growing body of literature documenting the relationship between social support systems and the mental health of adults (Henderson, Byrne, & Duncan-Jones, 1982; Henderson, Duncan-Jones, Byrne, & Scott, 1980) and the inverse relationship between extrafamilial contacts and child maltreatment (Salzinger, Kaplan, & Artemyeff, 1983; Wahler, 1980). Practically, the ecomap visually portrays or maps a family's ecological system showing the interactions of each member with outside resources such as churches, extended family, schools, health care, friends, work, and so forth. By also portraying the nature and flow (uni- or bidirectional) of the relationships between the family or its members and these outside resources, the ecomap identifies stresses and supports within the family system as well as areas where individual or family needs are unmet and where untried resources might be available.

Holman (1983) suggests involving as many family members as possible in the ecomap's development because this provides the practitioner and the family with a comprehensive understanding of the family's perceptions of its ecological system. Holman recommends sitting down with the family or several members grouped around the ecomap protocol (or a large sheet of white cardboard) with the usual environmental resources drawn in (see Figure 12-1). Initial nonthreatening and nonintrusive questions can then be asked such as "Do you have much family?" and "Do you work at a job?" with more specific questions gradually appearing such as "Have you worked there for a while?" and "How do you get along with the family?" Because the ecomap is a visually and intrinsically interesting picture of a family's social environment, family members tend to feel comfortable

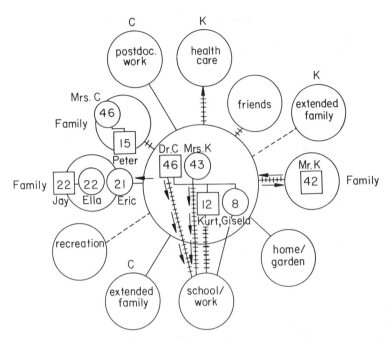

Figure 12-1. Ecomap of the Koehler/Cottingwood Family. The nature of interactions or connections is depicted by different lines which indicate a strong (———), tenuous (–––), or stressful (+ + +) connection. Arrows depict the flow of resources or energy. Adapted from Hartman (1979) and Holman (1983).

providing the information requested and additional information that might not typically be volunteered (Hartman, 1979). In fact, this technique is particularly recommended for nonverbal or easily threatened families who are reluctant to divulge information.

When drawing the ecomap, the nuclear family first can be drawn into the center circle in the fashion of genograms with squares for males, circles for females, and generational connections between (see the following section for a description). Then, the family as a whole or individual members can be connected with important extrafamilial systems. Different types of lines are used to illustrate the type of relationships involved (e.g., unidirectional, high intensity, tenuous, conflicted). For example, if one of the children was a behavior problem in school, the connecting line could be a solid cross-hatched line with arrows pointing from the school to the child to indicate the amount and direction of energy expended by the school in dealing with this problem. After these system connections are portrayed, empty black circles can be used to individualize the ecomap for the family. For example, a talented 10-year-old ice skater with Olympic aspirations might have strong ties with a private coach who plays an influential role in dictating family routines, vacations, and financial expenditures.

Having created an ecomap, a practitioner should possess a great deal of information on the family's social environments, its significant sources of stress, and available used and unused sources of social support. A good measure for an initial interview, the ecomap generates much information in a short amount of time. This makes it especially useful when more time-consuming, standardized measures of social support, family stress, or family social environment cannot be administered or are not important to the overall assessment. Finally, the ecomap's self-reported information can be verified by independent sources or by comparisons to other family-completed measures if its results or validity are in doubt.

To summarize, the ecomap, when given along with other family measures, serves to specify and individualize the strains, conflicts, and available resources within a family system and to generate as comprehensive a family picture as possible within a time-limited interview. Given these characteristics, the ecomap is rivaled only by the genogram.

Description of Home/Neighborhood and Typical Day

As part of the family assessment, it is often useful to ask the family to describe their home and neighborhood and to obtain a detailed description of each family member's typical weekday and weekend. This information is also nonthreatening, yet it provides the practitioner with salient environmental constraints and patterns that are useful when planning interventions. With respect to the home description, it is useful to obtain the number and types of rooms, who sleeps where, number of bathrooms and where they are located, and where the family usually spends time together (Karpel & Strauss, 1983). Neighborhood characteristics might include its socioeconomic level, the number of nearby children within the same ages as family members, religious or ethnic influences, accessibility of recreational facilities, and safety and environmental quality (e.g., noise level, beauty). Finally, information regarding each member's typical weekday and weekend routine might involve morning rising habits and sequences; how meals are handled, who attends them, and where different individuals sit; the comings and goings of members during the day and arrivals home; how evenings and weekends are spent; or what family conversations and general interactions are like (e.g., silent, inquisitional, catch as catch can).

The Genogram

Based on the concept of a genological family tree or family pedigree, the genogram is a visual description of a family over at least three generations (see Figure 12-2 for an example). The genogram provides a great deal of information quickly by identifying all the family members, their biological and emotional relationships to one another, and their proximities. Family patterns and the emotional responses to critical events can all be elicited in a nonthreatening manner through the genogram process, encouraging the family to see itself as a unit (Holman, 1983). Bowen (1978) is credited with the introduction of the genogram into clinical practice, and its popularity is attested to its frequent use in illustrating case studies in family therapy books (e.g., Alexander & Parsons, 1982; Carter & McGoldrick, 1980a; Papp, 1977).

In the author's experience, families seem to enjoy the genogram technique. However, as the information requested tends to be quite personal, it is best completed after the ecomap technique or after some trust has developed between the practitioner and the family. A brief introduction such as "This is an exercise that might help me see who is in the family and help all of us understand more about the problem" is usually sufficient to get the family involved. Then, with the family gathered in a circle around a table, the practitioner can ask individual family members specific, necessary questions. A large, white, cardboard sheet of paper

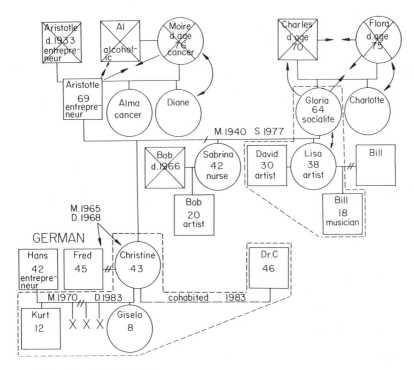

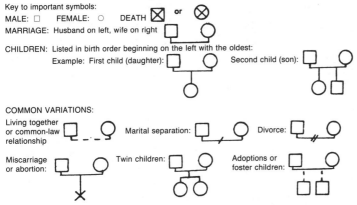

Figure 12-2. Mrs. Koehler's Genogram.

A genogram is a map that provides a graphic picture of family structure and emotional process over time. IT was developed by Murray Bowen, M.D., as part of his family systems theory, and it has become a standard form among clinicians for describing families. Our version of the genogram is used in case examples throughout this book. Bowen uses other symbols to denote other details. Also, to provide more space for dates and notations about each family member, he uses a different way of connecting the spouses rather than the line between the spouses, □   ○, used by the authors in this book. The following is a key to some important points in the genogram.

A complete genogram should include:

    1. Names and ages of all family members.
    2. Exact dates of birth, marriage, separation, divorce, death, and other significant life events.
    3. Notations with dates, about occupation, places of residence, illness, and changes in life course, on the genogram itself.
    4. Information on three or more generations.

Key to important symbols:

MALE: □   FEMALE: ○   DEATH ⊠ **or** ⊗

MARRIAGE: Husband on left, wife on right

CHILDREN: Listed in birth order beginning on the left with the oldest:

    Example: First child (daughter):   Second child (son):

COMMON VARIATIONS:

Living together or common-law relationship   Marital separation: Divorce:

Miscarriage or abortion: Twin children: Adoptions or foster children:

Figure 12-2a. Key to the Use of the Genogram. Note: (Copyright, Murray Bowen, M.D., 1980. Reprinted with permission of M. Bowen, M.D., Georgetown University Hospital, Washington, D.C. 20007.)

is used to integrate the elicited information into the genogram while providing plenty of room to draw and an area that the entire family can see.

At a minimum, the following information should be obtained for the genogram: (*a*) family members' given names, first and middle; (*b*) dates of birth, death, marriage, divorce, separations, major illnesses; (*c*) places of birth and series of residences; (*d*) occupations; (*e*) family members' health and occurrences of mental illness, mental retardation, postpartum depressions, involvement with the legal system, suicides, learning disabilities, and hereditary degenerative diseases or common causes of death; (*f*) identifications such as social class, and ethnic and religious affiliation; and (*g*) two-word descriptions that may give some idea of family myths and individual member's role assignments. For information regarding the last item, Karpel and Strauss (1983) suggest asking, "What word or two, what pictures come to mind when you think about this person?" (p. 56).

As with the ecomap, the practitioner can comment on patterns observed (e.g., a history of pregnancy-induced marriages across generations in the mother's family; high levels of achievement among adult members and resulting expectations for the younger generation). Other observations, such as nonnormative or unusual events (e.g., a life-threatening health scare in a relatively young parent), severed relationships among family members, or the impact of historical events on family experiences (e.g., the role of World War II and the GI Bill on the family moving from lower to middle-class status), are identified given their relevance to a historical or evolving family identity and to the current family/child difficulties.

The genogram helps family members to take a step back and look at themselves as a current functioning yet historically influenced entity or unit. Biological and cultural roots and the almost deterministic influence of past family experiences on current family functioning are particularly highlighted by this technique. Indeed, the genogram frequently reminds family members of the significance of some critical events, particularly embarrassing or painful events (e.g., a parent or grandparent's mental illness or a mother's out-of-wedlock teenage pregnancy) on their lives and interactions. While important to discuss, the practitioner must nonetheless be sensitive to a parent's possible discomfort when these events may be shared in front of children. This information and discussion may be better addressed in an individual session or when only the parents (or spouses) are present.

The information provided by the genogram is so useful that the author recommends administering it routinely as part of all parent interviews, social history batteries, and family assessments. The genogram covers the major family bases systematically and efficiently, quickly orienting the practitioner to the complex and multifaceted world of any human family.

The Family Life Cycle

Many authors deserve credit for the conceptual framework that has become known as the family life cycle (Duvall, 1977; Haley, 1973; Hill, 1970). The family life cycle is based on the notion that the family proceeds through time as a developmental unit, as opposed to a collection of individuals with independent developmental progressions. For example, while each family member and generation has its own tasks to accomplish and master, this still affects the successful achievement of different tasks by other family members and generations (Carter & McGoldrick, 1980b). Thus, a young adult's unsuccessful attempts to leave home and establish an independent life prevents his parents from renegotiating the marital system as a dyad and developing adult-to-adult relationships with their grown children.

Carter and McGoldrick (1980b) define the family as "the entire family emotional system of at least three generations" (p. 9). Thus, the nuclear family is only one subsystem of a larger network that "is reacting to both past and present relationships within the larger three-generational system" (p. 9). Within this model, family stress or anxiety evolves from two sources. The "vertical" flow of anxiety comes from generationally transmitted patterns of relating and functioning that are usually passed on through intergenerational coalitions. Included within this source of stress are "all the family attitudes, taboos, expectations, labels, and loaded issues with which we grow up" (p. 9). The "horizontal" flow includes the stresses that the family encounters as it moves through developmental and historical time. This includes normative (the first child entering adolescence) and nonnormative (war death of a young husband, birth of a handicapped child) events that occur. Carter and McGoldrick contend that all families will become dysfunctional if enough stress (i.e., external and developmental stressors) is placed on the horizontal axis. Then, even a small amount of vertical stress will result in disruption beyond that already caused by the pressures along the horizontal axis.

Carter and McGoldrick (1980b) believe that families manifest disruptive symptoms when vertical and horizontal stressors converge to produce dysfunction. The following incident illustrates how this can happen:

> Mandy is the unplanned child of elderly parents who have already raised three older children. A very religious and hardworking couple, the parents economically struggled through the Depression and had little time to attend to the emotional and social needs of their offspring. Because of her parents' guilt over their perceived poor caretaking of the older siblings, Mandy, born during World War II, received all of their adoration and attention. Now an adolescent, Mandy is beginning to find their adoration oppressive. The couple is terrified of being alone together: They have not spent much time sharing their lives, nor have they slept in the same room since early in their marriage. Mandy is dating an attractive boy over her parents objections, creating the first real distance in their parent–child relationship.
>
> Uninstructed in sexual matters, Mandy is overwhelmed when she becomes pregnant—not only because of the implications of the pregnancy, but because she violated a family myth that all family members are righteous. Afraid to tell her parents, she binds her stomach until the seventh month of her pregnancy when her mother confronts her by asking if she is married. A hasty marriage is arranged by the mortified family. Mandy drops out of high school and bears a mentally retarded and deformed daughter. A month later, her father has a near-fatal heart attack which the family blames on Mandy.

Using this model, the practitioner must assess general life stress, normative developmental stress, and the extent to which these stresses connect with inherited themes and labels. The vertical stressors in this short case example are the parents' guilt over the neglect of their older children, the distant marital relationship of the parents that is triangulated with the children and their busy jobs, the taboo around sexual issues, and the myth of family righteousness. The horizontal stressors are Mandy's developmental need to separate from her family of origin, the resulting renegotiation of her parents' marital dyad, and the accumulated stress of 30 years of working two jobs and smoking three packs of cigarettes per day on the father's health.

Carter and McGoldrick (1980b) present a 6-stage outline of the family life cycle that requires a specific emotional process for a family's transition from one stage to the next (see Table 12-2). The outline also details second-order changes in family status that are necessary for developmental progress. As these stages are modeled on late twentieth-century middle-class Americans, it is important to note that individuals of other cultures and socioeconomic classes may differ tremendously in the breakdown of their stages and transitional tasks. Finally, a model for proceeding developmentally through divorce, postdivorce, and remarriage—a fairly common life cycle derailment—is also presented by the authors.

The family life cycle is a powerful therapeutic paradigm which child-oriented practitioners, who often think developmentally, can easily integrate into their personal theoretical frameworks. A conscious awareness in an interview of the family's status relative to vertical and horizontal stresses often directs the assessment in therapeutically relevant directions and toward treatment recommendations.

The FILE

The Family Inventory of Life Events and Changes (FILE; McCubbin & Patterson, 1983), one of a number of self-report inventories developed by the family social science group at the University of Minnesota, assesses normative and nonnormative family stresses. Completed simply by having family members check off whether a particular life event or strain has occurred over the past year, the FILE, nevertheless, does *not* assess individuals. Unlike the Social Readjustment Rating Scale by Holmes and Raye (1967), the FILE is a family inventory where an event or change experienced by one family member is assumed to affect, and thus is recorded for, all members. The measure's 71 items are completed separately by both members of a couple, while adolescents in the family use the A-FILE (Adolescent-FILE), a life stress measure which is similar but shorter in length. McCubbin and Patterson (1983) assume that families, at any point in time, are dealing concurrently with numerous stresses and strains. Noting that the FILE measures the combined effects of these stresses, these authors refer to it as "an index of a family's vulnerability to crisis" (McCubbin & Patterson, 1983, p. 280).

The FILE was normed on a national, stratified, cross-sectional sample of intact couples representing all stages of the family life cycle (independent husband sample: $N = 1,330$; independent wife sample: $N = 1,410$). Overall, this normative sample tended to be more midwestern in region, more Lutheran in religious orientation, and more inclusive of first marriages than the nation as a whole. Factor analytic studies then grouped the FILE's 71 items into nine subscales: conflict between family members, marital conflict, pregnancy and childbearing strains, finance and business strains, work–family transitions and strains, illness and family care strains, family losses such as the breakup of a relationship or loss of health, family transitions in or out of the nuclear family, and family legal strains. From here, five possible FILE scores are possible, depending on the needs of the researcher or practitioner: the Family Readjustment score, Family Life Events score, Family–Couple Life Events score, Family–Couple Discrepancy score, and a score called the Family Pileup for which normative data are available.

The FILE (particularly its Family Pileup score) is adequately reliable for research purposes, but its $r = .81$ (using Cronbach's alpha) seems a little low for individual diagnosis. However, the authors note that the FILE's internal consistency is reduced by including infrequently occurring life events, such as the death of a child, which are conceptually necessary yet psychometrically weakening.

Table 12-2
The Stages of the Family Life Cycle[a]

Family life cycle stage	Emotional process of transition: Key principles	Second order changes in family status required to proceed developmentally
1. Between Families: The Unattached Young Adult	Accepting parent off-spring separation	a. Differentiation of self in relation to family of origin b. Development of intimate peer relation-ships c. Establishment of self in work
2. The Joining of Families Through Marriage: The Newly Married Couple	Commitment to new system	a. Formation of marital system b. Realignment of relationships with extend-ed families and friends to include spouse
3. The Family With Young Children	Accepting new members into the system	a. Adjusting marital system to make space for child(ren) b. Taking on parenting roles c. Realignment of relationships with extend-ed family to include parenting and grand-parenting roles
4. The Family With Adolescents	Increasing flexibility of family boundaries to include children's independence	a. Shifting of parent-child relationships to permit adolescent to move in and out of system b. Refocus on mid-life marital and career is-sues c. Beginning shift toward concerns for older generation
5. Launching Children and Moving On	Accepting a multitude of exits from and en-tries into the family system	a. Renegotiation of marital system as a dyad b. Development of adult to adult relation-ships between grown children and their parents c. Realignment of relationships to include in-laws and grandchildren d. Dealing with disabilities and death of parents (grand parents)
6. The Family in Later Life	Accepting the shifting of generational roles	a. Maintaining own and/or couple function-ing and interests in face of physiological decline; exploration of new familial and social role options b. Support for a more central role for middle generation c. Making room in the system for the wis-dom and experience of the elderly; sup-porting the older generation without over-functioning for them d. Dealing with loss of spouse, siblings and other peers and preparation for own death. Life review and integration.

[a]From Carter and McGoldrick (1980a, p. 17). Copyright 1980 by Gardner Press, Inc. Reprinted by permis-sion.

Similarly, while three of the nine subscales (Intrafamily Strains, Finance and Business Strains, and Family Legal Strains) have adequate reliability, the remaining six do not (*r*s range from .16 to .56). Again, this is largely due to the infrequency of some important stressful events. Test-retest reliabilities stand up well over a 4- to 5-week period with an *r* of .80 for the total scale and *r*s of .64 to .84 for the subscales. The FILE's validity, derived from factor analyses of two independent samples, revealed virtually identical factor structures, a predicted inverse relationship between positive family functioning on the Family Environment scale and Family Pileup, and a similar relationship between family stress and changes in the health status of children with cystic fibrosis (McCubbin & Patterson, 1983).

Interpretation with the FILE is not difficult, but needs to be sensitively addressed with the family. Instead of alarming families about their high level of stress, McCubbin and Patterson (1983) suggest focusing in on the following:

> (1) the family's vulnerability to future stressful life events or strains; (2) the family's use of important psychological, interpersonal, and tangible resources and strengths that may be exhausted in the near future; (3) specific stressors and specific strains that may need their attention; (4) the family's coping skills and abilities in meeting these demands (that is, what they are going to do to help themselves); (5) the family's feelings about their circumstances and difficulties; and (6) the family's problem-solving ability to resolve or eliminate some of the more manageable demands. (pp. 288–289)

Families may find this approach very useful, especially when incorporated into a full family assessment or used in conjunction with other techniques such as the ecomap that supplies more comprehensive information.

Assessing Structure and Dynamics

Assessing a family's structure and dynamics involves the clinical observations and information gleaned from the initial family interview and the data collected from the many research/clinical inventories that have been developed to tap family values, communication patterns, cohesiveness, adaptability, discipline, and other stylistic features of the family. Two of the most widely used family measures are reviewed in this section: the Family Environment Scale (FES) and the Family Adaptability and Cohesion Evaluation Scale (FACES II). The FES is the most widely researched family instrument currently in the literature, and FACES II is supported by the strongest theoretical base of any family measure. Parent–child communication and interaction inventories from both the parent and the child's perspectives and a projective measure of children's perceptions of family interactions round out this area of family assessment.

By this stage of the interview and assessment process, the family should be feeling comfortable enough, if all is going well, to share more personal information. If this is not the case, the material in this section can be obtained in short meetings with individual members (see Karpel & Strauss, 1983, for a discussion of this point) or in meetings after inventories like those discussed below have been administered and scored. Some important areas to explore at this time include (*a*) family rules, (*b*) family alliances and coalitions, and (*c*) how family disagreements are addressed.

Queries relating to rules might investigate how household chores are divided among family members, what happens if rules are broken, how discipline is handled and by whom, whether punishments fit the crime and the age of the offender, if parents and children agree in their perceptions, and the family's overall comfort with its approach to rules and discipline.

Karpel and Strauss (1983) recommend a series of questions to address family alliances, starting with: "I'd like to get a better idea of who spends a good deal of time with whom in the family; whom is each of you most likely to talk to if something is on your mind?" (p. 142). Alternative questions in this area include "Who sticks up for whom?" and "Who worries about whom in the family?" Obviously, not all of these questions need to be asked, but when asked, the practitioner should avoid questions that sound like "Who's on your side and who's on the other side when there are family disagreements?" Responses to these questions can be depicted on the genogram if the family feels comfortable with this process. Ultimately, this may help to elucidate family boundaries, subgroups, power structures, and, through this, some of the critical difficulties within the family.

Finally, for questions about family disagreements, Karpel and Strauss (1983) recommend introducing the topic with the following question: "Every family has certain areas of disagreement, areas they frequently disagree about, but these areas differ from one family to another. I wonder if you could fill us in on the kinds of disagreements your family tends to have most often?" (p. 144). Knowing the major players in family arguments often highlights family coalitions. The sequence of fights and their consequences to members also suggest the needs and payoffs that members receive for these interactions (see Alexander & Parsons, 1982, for an excellent presentation of a functional analysis of family dynamics). Detailed and verbatim descriptions best pinpoint the controlling variables and consequences during these types of interactions.

In addition to these specific areas, the practitioner also can identify and evaluate the adult models within the nuclear and extended family who are available to children in the family being assessed. Who is admired and who is not? What would the parents like the children to become? Do the children accept or reject the available models? What types of nonfamily members (e.g., Mary Lou Retton, Billy Graham) does the family admire? This information can be gleaned from the genogram, from comments made in the interview, and from specific questions if necessary.

The Family Adaptability and Cohesion Evaluation Scale

FACES II, a 30-item, self-report measure, reflects the Circumplex Model of Marital and Family Therapy (Olson, Russell, & Sprenkle, 1979; Olson, Sprenkle, & Russell, 1979), which was developed to "integrate the seemingly diverse theoretical and therapeutic concepts used to describe families" (Olson *et al.*, 1983, p. 16). The Circumplex Model focuses on three dimensions considered central to family dynamics: cohesion, adaptability, and communication. The authors provide impressive support for the centrality of these dimensions (see Olson *et al.*, 1983, for a review of the literature).

Family cohesion is defined as "the emotional bonding that family members have toward one another" (Olson *et al.*, 1983, p. 48). In the Circumplex Model, this ranges from disengaged (very low) to enmeshed (very high). Separated (low to moderate) and connected (moderate to high) represent central levels of this spectrum which most healthy families fall into, depending on their developmental stage. Sixteen of the FACES II items measure cohesion, with two items addressing each of eight concepts related to this dimension. These concepts are emotional bonding, family boundaries, time, space, coalitions, friends, decision making, and interests and recreation. An example of an item measuring family boundaries on the cohesion subscale is "Family members feel closer to people outside the family than to other family members."

Family adaptability is defined as the "ability of a marital or family system to change its power structure, role relationships, and relationship rules in response to situations or developmental stress" (Olson *et al.*, 1983, p. 48). In the model, the levels of adaptability range from rigid (very low) to chaotic (very high), with structured (low to moderate) and flexible (moderate to high) as central levels. Fourteen items measure adaptability, with two to three items assessing each of six component areas: negotiation style, role relationships, family power (assertiveness, control, discipline), and relationship rules. An example of an item measuring relationship rules on the adaptability subscale is "It's hard to know what the rules are in our family."

Family communication is the third dimension of the Circumplex Model; it is defined as a facilitating dimension that is critical toward change on the other two dimensions. It is not measured by a subscale of FACES II, but with two separate instruments: the Parent–Adolescent Communication scale and the marital communication subscale from the ENRICH marital inventory (see below).

Based on their scores in FACES II's adaptability and cohesion dimensions, an individual family is placed into 1 of 16 marital or family system types. The primary scoring categories are extreme, midrange, and balanced, referring to distance of the family or couple's mean score from the center of the Circumplex Model. Couples that obtain a central rating on both scales are categorized as balanced; there are four such types. An extreme rating on one scale and central rating on the other constitutes a midrange categorization; there are eight such types. Extreme categorizations result when families receive extreme scores on both scales; there are four extreme types.

FACES II was derived from the 111-item FACES. Reduced to 50 items on the basis of reliability data and factor analysis, the final version consists of 30 items. However, most of the reliability and validity information was gathered on the 50-item version of the scale. FACES II norms were based on the same large, national, cross-sectional study mentioned earlier when describing the FILE (Olson *et al.*, 1983); 2,082 parents and 416 adolescents constituted the sample. As gender differences were nonsignificant, these two subsamples were collapsed for additional analyses.

The FACES II norms revealed large differences in family members' ratings. Correlations between spouses on the cohesion subscale was .46, and the *r* for the adaptability subscale was .32. Parent–child correlations were even lower. On the cohesion subscale, the *r* was .46 for fathers and adolescents and .39 for mothers and adolescents. On the adaptability scale, the *r* was .31 for fathers and adolescents and .21 for mothers and adolescents. The authors use these findings to emphasize the importance of obtaining ratings from as many family members as possible to obtain a complete and reliable picture of the family systems.

Cronbach's alpha was used to assess the internal consistency of FACES II, resulting in an *r* of .87 for cohesion, .78 for adaptability, and .90 for the total scale using a large cross-sectional sample of 2,498 family members. Test-retest reliability over an unspecified period of time was .83 for cohesion, .80 for adaptability, and .84 for the total scale.

Construct validity for the instrument is supported by (*a*) the moderate to low correlations (.31–.55) of FACES II with other family and marital measures, and (*b*) findings in a national survey of over 1,140 couples and families from 31 states roughly distributed over seven developmental stages in the life span, which supported the Circumplex Model. This survey's results generally supported the hypothesis that balanced family types tend to function more competently across the family life cycle, although this varied by developmental stage. In addition, a number of family variables (e.g., resources, stress levels, coping strategies) were used to predict two family types, balanced and extreme, with 100% accuracy. This was not the case, however, for midrange families where prediction was poor. A possible reason for the poor prediction with midrange families lies in the FACES II normative sample. Biased toward healthy family functioning, the norms do not include a true clinical sample. Thus, the cutting scores appear to place healthy families in the midrange and even extreme range. One independent study that examined a clinical population found that families at high risk for adolescent abuse fell into the extreme range. They were chaotically enmeshed, while those at low risk were flexibly connected and in the balanced range (Garbarino, Sebes, & Schellenbach, 1984).

The FACES II manual makes this scale easy to administer, score, and interpret (Olson *et al.*, 1982). There is a family form and a couples form for partners with no or grown children. Individuals make two separate ratings along different 5-point Likert scales for each of the 30 statements: How true is this statement of your family now, and how would you like your family to be, given the implications of this statement. Interpretation involves using cutting scores to place the family into the Circumplex Model, and then plotting their perceived and ideal scores for further analysis.

Olson and Portner (1983) suggest a number of clinical uses for the FACES II: as a tool assisting in diagnosis, a vehicle allowing family members to share their perceptions and levels of satisfaction with family interactions (by comparing perceived and ideal scores), and an instrument suggesting treatment goals which are individualized to the family's structure, dynamics, and current developmental stage. This last use, resulting in comparisons with the national, normative data, is particularly important to practitioners working with children and adolescents because adaptive family styles differ greatly for families with children across different age levels (Olson *et al.*, 1983).

FACES II provides useful information revealing a family's unique perspective of its own family dynamics and structure. It can identify and analyze the genesis and source of family conflicts that may be creating or maintaining a referred child or adolescent's functioning. Finally, the instrument's therapeutic orientation often directly suggests treatment issues and directions. This may be a strength or a weakness; it would be a weakness if the assessing practitioner unintentionally moves into therapeutic intervention with the FACES II when assessment is the only objective.

The Family Environment Scale

The Family Environment Scale (FES; Moos & Moos, 1981) is one of the first inventories developed to assess family characteristics. It is a 90-item, 10-subscale, self-report inventory that assesses individuals' perceptions of the social and environmental characteristics of their families. There are three parallel forms of the FES, but only the Real Form (Form R) is normed on a large, somewhat representative sample of normal and distressed families. Form R assesses individuals' perceptions of their own families or families of origin. Form E (the Expectation Form) measures the individuals' anticipated family environments and is used, for example, in premarital counseling. Form I (the Ideal Form) taps the goals and value orientations of family members, that is, what they would like the family to be like.

The FES is one of nine social climate scales designed in the early 1970s which assess a variety of social environments such as educational, psychiatric, and work settings (Moos & Insel, 1974). Moos and Moos (1983) developed these scales to measure three domains shared across all nine settings: the quality of interpersonal relationships, environmental emphasis on personal growth goals, and the degree of structure and openness to change. The quality of interpersonal relationships is assessed by the FES's cohesion, expressiveness, and conflict subscales. An example of an item from the expressiveness subscale is "We say anything we want to around home." The personal growth domain is tapped by five subscales: independence, achievement orientation, intellectual–cultural orientation, active–recreational orientation, and moral–religious orientation. An example of an item from the active–recreational orientation is "Watching TV is more important than reading in our family." Finally, the system maintenance and change domains are measured by two subscales: organization, which addresses the clarity and structure of family responsibilities, and control, which assesses the use of rules and set procedures in directing family life. "We can do whatever we want to in our family" is an example of an item from the control subscale.

Scale norms were developed for Form R using a sample of 1,125 normal and 500 distressed families. While "normal" was left undefined, this group included 294 families drawn randomly from census tract data in the San Francisco area, and other families from "all areas of the country" (Moos & Moos, 1981, p. 4), which included single parent, minority, and multigenerational families of all age groups and all family developmental stages (e.g., retired, families with adolescents). Since the random subsample means and standard deviations resembled those of the rest of the normal families, the authors concluded that the normative data were representative of the range of normal families.

The distressed families were drawn from groups of psychiatric patients, alcohol users, probation and parole department clients, psychiatrically oriented family clinic clients, and families with problem children or adolescents. As predicted, this group scored significantlty lower on cohesion, expressiveness, independence, intellectual, and recreational orientations, and significantly higher on the subscales of conflict and control than their normal sample counterparts. There were no significant differences on the organization and moral–religious emphasis subscales. Even when socioeconomic and family background variables were controlled, the differences on the seven subscales remained. Each subscale's standard scores in the manual are based on the normal family data. Comparisons with the distressed families can be obtained by deriving standard scores from the subscale means and standard deviations in the manual. For the Ideal Form, preliminary norms are available based on 281 normal and distressed families. There are no norms yet available for the Expectations Form.

The reliability data for the Form R subscales are adequate for research purposes, but a little low for individual family diagnosis; Cronbach's alpha correlations range from .61 to .78 (median = .72). Test–retest data assessed at 2 months ($N = 47$), 4 months ($N = 35$), and 12 months ($N = 241$) indicate that test results are quite stable, with rs at the 2-month level ranging from .68 to .86 and at the 12-month level from .52 to .89. The instrument's sensitivity to family change is demonstrated by six published studies cited in the manual where families in various intervention programs changed several FES subscale scores in a positive direction, while control families evidenced no change. However, not all of these subscale changes reached statistical significance. Finally, the use of all 10 subscales appears to be justified, as the scale intercorrelations, ranging from .00 to .44 for adults, are low.

Many researchers have employed the FES despite its relatively short history (75 studies are reported in the 1981 manual and over 100 research projects have used the measure), underlining the demand for well-constructed family instruments. The FES has been used to describe variations of normal family types (e.g., Mexican–American families), to determine characteristics of families with a member in crisis (e.g., depressed or delinquent member), to predict and assess treatment outcomes, to relate FES subscales to other aspects of family life (e.g., adult career patterns and occupational and child-rearing attitudes), to examine the relationship between families of origin and nuclear family climates, and for cross-cultural research on family environments (see Moss & Moss, 1981, for specific citations). Altogether, the evidence supports both the construct and predictive validity of the FES.

The FES authors examined gender and generational differences in the normative sample's perceptions of the family environment (Moos & Moos, 1981). Overall, they found few gender differences. Wives perceived family climate as slightly more positive on the intellectual and recreational orientation, the organization, and the moral–religious emphasis subscales than did husbands. Boys perceived slightly greater achievement orientations in their family climates than did girls. Parent–child differences, though small, were not apparent. When parental ratings were compared with adolescents' ratings, less favorable views on the part of the children were evident. They reported less cohesion, expressiveness, independence, and intellectual and religious orientation, and greater conflict and emphasis on achievement. The authors attribute this to the general finding that those in power rate their environment more positively.

The FES Form R is very easy to administer and score. A neatly printed 5½″ × 8½″ reusable booklet is used with a half-page scoring sheet. Subjects are simply asked to mark each item true if the item accurately describes their family or false if it is inaccurate. A template is provided, making scoring an easy task. As each column on the response sheet constitutes a subscale, the scorer needs only to count the x's that appear in the circles on the template to tabulate the score for each subscale. Individual raw scores or family averages on each subscale are converted to standard scores using a table in the manual, and these scores are then plotted on a profile roughly similar to that used by the PIC. For family assessment, it is usually most useful to plot the profiles of each family member old enough to take the FES. Forms I and E are reworded versions of Form R; they are administered and scored similar to the description above.

In addition to individual subscale scores, a family incongruence score can be obtained to measure family members' disagreements concerning the family environment (the reading level may be too difficult for children under 12). This interesting and important family characteristic results when the absolute differences between each pair of family members on each of the 10 subscales is calculated and summed over all 10 subscales. The mean of these summed scores yields a measure of incongruence. A table in the manual can then be used to convert the family mean to a standard score, with the normal family sample of 1,125 families as the reference group.

Specific to personality assessment, the FES is quite useful, as it provides an insider's view of the family context in which a child or adolescent is developing (Olson & Portner, 1983). By highlighting this context, the instrument can help to identify factors that have shaped and maintained deviant behavior as well as personality strengths; it also can identify family resources that might be useful to shape an intervention program or to determine a prognosis for the current situation. By administering the FES to both parents and adolescents, reasons for satisfactions or dissatisfactions about the family environment may be illuminated. The Ideal Form can be used to identify family members' goals and values, while discrepancies between the Real and Ideal Forms may target possible areas for family or individual therapy. Similarly, the Expectation Form can provide guidance when assessing children or families for foster care or child custody placements. Expectations of family life often represent unexamined assumptions that are relevant later to decisions or potential adjustments to proposed changes.

Marital Inventories

A number of studies have shown that the quality of marital relationships and marital harmony is positively related to the emotional health of children and adolescents (Westley & Epstein, 1969), and that extreme disharmony, such as that which results in a divorce, is detrimental to the functioning of children (Guidubaldi *et al.*, 1983; Hetherington *et al.*, 1979), depending on the age (Wallerstein & Kelly, 1980) and sex (Guidubaldi *et al.*, 1983) of the individual. In addition, a number of family therapists have asserted, on the basis of their clinical experience, that covert marital discord frequently is evident in the emotional or behavioral symptoms of children or adolescents (N. Ackerman, 1980; Alexander & Parsons, 1982; Hoffman, 1981). Thus, there are critical reasons to assess the quality of the marital relationship as part of a family assessment.

While many school psychologists (Brassard & Anderson, 1983), and probably much of the public, do not consider marital intervention as a legitimate school role, it is often very appropriate in a clinic or community agency setting. Unfortunately, however, the extensive literature in this area cannot be suitably covered here. Two books edited by Filsinger (1983) and Filsinger and Lewis (1981) are recommended for further reading on this topic: *Marriage and Family Assessment* and *Assessing Marriage: New Behavioral Approaches*, respectively. The ENRICH marital inventory, developed by the Minnesota group, is described in a chapter in the Filsinger book, as well as in the Olson *et al.* Family Inventories (1982) and their book describing the results of their national survey of intact families (Olson *et al.*, 1983).

The Parent–Adolescent Communication Scale

As presented above, communication is the third dimension of Olson, Sprenkle, and Russell's (1979) Circumplex Model. It is defined by the authors as the facilitating dimension that is critical toward change on the other two dimensions of the model, cohesion and adaptability. The authors hypothesized that "effective communication facilitates movement to, and maintenance of, systems at the desired (Balanced) level on the two major dimensions of the model. Further, ineffective communication minimizes and may prevent movement toward balanced levels of adaptability and cohesion" (Olson *et al.*, 1982, p. 33). Within the Circumplex Model, this third dimension is measured intergenerationally by the Parent–Adolescent Communication scale and maritally by the communication scale of ENRICH. No scale has been developed by the Minnesota group for children under the age of about 12.

In Family Inventories, Olson *et al.* (1982) present a condensed but thorough review of the literature supporting their hypotheses with respect to communication. The majority of studies cited involve the use of self-report measures administered to spouses; few of the studies examined differences in perceptions among family members. The Parent–Adolescent Communication scale, while employing a self-report format, goes beyond these past measures, because it compares the separate perceptions of each parent directly to the adolescent's perceptions of each respective parent.

The Parent–Adolescent Communication scale is a 20-item scale composed of two subscales containing 10 items each. The Open Family Communication subscale measures the "more positive aspects of parent–adolescent communication," with a focus on the "freedom or free flowing exchange of information, both factual and emotional as well as on the sense of lack of constraint and degree of understanding and satisfaction experienced in their interactions" (Olson *et al.*, 1982, p. 37). The Problems in Family Communication subscale "focuses on the negative aspects of communication, hesitancy to share, negative styles of interaction, and selectivity and caution in what is shared" (p. 37). For each of the items, adolescents are asked to respond to a 5-point Likert scale with choices ranging from "strongly disagree" to "strongly agree." For each item, they first rate their relationship with their mother and then their relationship with their father. "I openly show affection to my mother/father" is an example of an item from the Open Family Communication subscale. The parent form differs only in that "child" is inserted instead of "mother/father."

Items from the subscales are intermixed. The Open Family Communication items are positively worded, while the Problem in Family Communication items are negatively phrased. As the total score is a sum score, the point values from the negatively worded items are reversed to score the protocol. Percentile norms are provided for fathers, mothers, adolescents' ratings of their mothers, and adolescents' ratings of their fathers. Separate norms are provided because data in the national sample indicated that parents' perceptions of parent–child communication were much more positive than the adolescent sample's perceptions. This was particularly true for mothers, who perceived greater openness in communication than did fathers. Adolescents also perceived greater openness when communicating with their mothers, but they expressed consistent difficulty when trying to communicate with *both* parents. Overall, the authors reported that adolescent responses toward each parent were similar enough to warrant a combined set of norms.

Cronbach's alpha was used to assess the internal consistency of the Parent–Adolescent Communication scale. The findings from a total sample of parents and adolescents ($N = 1,841$) pulled from a larger national sample revealed r values which were quite satisfactory for research purposes, although a little low for diagnostic use: .87 for the Open Family Communication subscale, .78 for the Problems in Family Communication subscale, and .88 for the total scale.

Construct validity is based on early work which led to this scale's final development. Items initially were generated from a list of variables which previous studies had identified as relevant to parent–adolescent communication. From this pool, 35 items were selected and written at readability levels suitable for at least a 12-year-old. The first form of the instrument was piloted on 433 high school and college young people, all primarily in the 16- to 20-year-old age range. Factor analysis identified three factors with eigen values above 1.0 when two methods were used: the two mentioned above and a third factor called Selective Family Communication. As this latter factor involved negative aspects of communication and collapsed into the second factor (Problems in Family Communication) when the analysis was restricted to two factors, only the first two factors were retained as subscales after a second pilot study using 20 items. Data from the national survey replicated these results from the second pilot study.

The uses and implications of this scale in clinical work are fairly obvious, as communication difficulties do affect family balance and can be relatively easy to remediate. If communication problems are causing family or parent–child distress, a thorough analysis of the problem may lead to appropriate intervention. Quality of communication also theoretically affects the amount of change that is possible on the cohesion and adaptability dimensions of the Circumplex Model. Thus, this scale can be useful, particularly in conjunction with FACES II, in pinpointing other correlates of the difficulty and in assessing the potential for comprehensive positive change.

The Parent Perception Inventory (PPI)

The Parent Perception Inventory (Hazzard & Christensen, no date; Hazzard, Christensen, & Margolin, 1983) is an 18-item measure of children's perceptions of positive and negative parental behaviors. Evidently appropriate for elementary school-aged children (the authors have used it with children ages 5–13), the child rates each parent separately on the same items. Items are presented in a written/oral manner and are rated in a pictorial/written fashion (i.e., variably filled beakers correspond to the "never," "a little," "sometimes," "pretty much," and "a lot" ratings for each item). Half of the items reflect positive behaviors (positive reinforcement, comfort, talk time, involvement in decision making, time together, positive evaluation, allowing independence, assistance, and nonverbal affection), while the other half involve negative behaviors, although a number of them may well be appropriate parenting behaviors, depending on the circumstances (privilege removal, criticism, commands, physical punishment, yelling, threatening, time-out, nagging, and ignoring).

The PPI instructions ask the examiner to read each item's specific examples repeatedly until understood by the child. (This should be necessary only with very young or intellectually slow children.) An item assessing parental comfort reads "How often does your Mom (Dad) talk to you when you feel bad and help you to feel better, help you with your problems, comfort you?" The PPI yields four subscales entitled Mother Positive (9 items), Father Positive (9 items), Mother Negative (9 items), and Father Negative (9 items), with total scores ranging from 0 to 36. Items are scored 0 for "never" to 4 for "a lot."

PPI reliability and validity is based on a study of 75 children (ages 5–13) who participated in a university research project that examined differences in distressed and nondistressed families (Hazzard *et al.*, 1983). Positive and negative items were all significantly correlated with the appropriate scale. Cronbach's alpha for each of the four subscales were as follows: .84 for Mother Positive, .78 for Mother Negative, .88 for Father Positive, and .80 for Father Negative. For older children alone (ages 10–13), the alphas ranged from .74 to .89, and from .81 to .87 for younger children (ages 5–9). Convergent validity was assessed by computing correlations between the PPI subscales, a measure of children's self-concept, and a parental measure of conduct disorders. The results were in the predicted directions with high positive behavior correlated with high self-esteem and high negative behavior correlated with high scores on the conduct disorder measure. In addition, negative PPI scores were positively related to the conduct disorder measure.

To examine discriminant validity, the PPI subscales were correlated with two measures not expected to be related to them, an achievement and an intellectual deficiency measure. Findings were as predicted in six of the eight correlations. There were no age effects and only two gender effects: Boys rated their parents more positively than girls and both sexes perceived their mothers as performing more negative behaviors than their fathers.

Overall, children in distressed families viewed their parents' behavior more negatively than the nondistressed group, with lower scores on the positive items and higher scores on the negative items. These differences, however, only reached significance for ratings of mothers. Interestingly, children from nondistressed families perceived their parents as acting in similar ways significantly more often than children from distressed families. The authors interpreted this as support for the family systems theory notion that family distress is caused by a couple's lack of unity in their parental role and the formation of parent–child coalitions (Hazzard et al., 1983).

As one of the relatively few scales to look at the parent–child relationship from the young child's perspective, the PPI is clinically useful not only for the information that it provides, but also for its role in helping the younger child feel included in the assessment process. In this author's experience, children beam with pleasure when asked for their opinion of their parent's behavior, particularly when older members of the family are at work completing their own instruments. Finally, as the validity study shows, the PPI can identify family distress and parent–child difficulties. Designed to evaluate family therapy outcomes, particularly behaviorally oriented outcomes, the PPI targets children's perceptions of parent behaviors in need of change and their perceptions of parent change after an intervention program (Hazzard et al., 1983; Margolin & Fernandez, 1983).

The Roberts Apperception Test for Children (RATC)

The RATC is a new projective instrument that has generated some immediate interest (Margolin & Fernandez, 1983; Roberts, McArthur, Roid, Zachary, & Reynolds, 1983). Developed to assess children's (ages 6–15) perceptions of frequently occurring interpersonal situations (McArthur & Roberts, 1982), the RATC differs from similar apperception tests in that it portrays children in family-oriented situations. Themes of sibling rivalry; parental discipline, affection, conflict, and support; and conflict with peers are featured. This makes this technique particularly useful for mental health practitioners who typically work with individual children as the identified clients; that is, the RATC may alert them to the need for family as opposed to individual child treatment. THE RATC has already been described by Obrzut and Boliek-Uphoff; the reader is referred to Chapter 6 of this volume for a detailed discussion.

Assessing Levels of Adaptation and Health

Assessment results that reveal a family's level of adaptation to their environment, their strengths as a family unit, their styles of coping and ability to cope with life experiences, and the mental health of individual family members relate directly to intervention planning and prognosis. Like the assessment of other areas of family functioning, the interview process, observations during the interview, and self-report measures are the primary means of evaluating these family characteristics.

The central questions when assessing a family's levels of adaptation and health are "How has the family attempted to handle the particular referred problem or crisis?" and "What have been their approaches to past family crises?" Karpel and Strauss (1983) suggest addressing these areas by asking for the following information:

> It will help us in dealing with the present problem to learn something about any previous problem the family has experienced, or that any members of the family have gone through themselves. Any past situation that has been especially upsetting to the family or put stress on it would be of interest to us, as would any previous problems that required professional help. (p. 146)

Chronic illnesses, divorce, psychiatric hospitalizations, a grandparent's move into the home, the birth of a handicapped or unwanted child, or a teenage pregnancy are all relevant past problems that reveal a great deal about individual family members, family themes, and coping strategies at specific stages in a family's historical development (Carter & McGoldrick, 1980b; Karpel & Strauss, 1983).

Once uncovered, past problems can be compared and contrasted to current problems (e.g., this is the third adolescent in the family to have trouble with illegal drug use and promiscuity) to explore for the current crisis that could be "an acute exacerbation of a chronic family difficulty" (Karpel & Strauss, 1983, p. 147). These comparisons may reveal long-standing family organization, decision making, and structure and judgment processes. For example, in one family where the 13-year-old boy, the youngest of four, was the identified problem child, the father's recent and serious bout with cancer was revealed only to the oldest daughter, a college student. This communication gap left the boy highly anxious and distrustful of his parents, a significant issue behind his presenting problems. These past problems may also identify individuals who are particularly vulnerable and who may need to be treated with care (e.g., a father who has been hospitalized for manic-depressive illness which appears to run in his family). Any intervention program must consider the implications and effects of any past problems so that unnecessary additional stress is avoided.

If a family has received treatment before or has survived a significant crisis, it is often useful to ask what they've learned from the experience. An inability to answer may indicate an impaired ability to learn from experience or to respond to treatment (for whatever reasons). Well-considered, insightful responses to crises indicate a favorable prognosis, a family's resources to resolve problems and issues, and a family's motivation for treatment or assistance.

Finally, it is extremely important for the practitioner to note any signs of distress or impairment in a family member throughout the assessment process. Depression, tangential or loose thinking, intense anxiety, paranoid-sounding expressions, or any other signs of acute distress in a family member should be evaluated in an individual meeting with the person, followed by a meeting with the parents or spouse, in the case of an adult.

In addition to the interview, there are three instruments, all developed by the University of Minnesota group, that relate to family adaptation and health. The ecomap, described earlier, also provides information of direct relevance to this aspect of the family.

The Family Satisfaction Inventory

This inventory, designed by Olson and Wilson (1982, in Olson et al., 1982) for the Circumplex Model, is the only measure of family satisfaction in existence, according to its authors. Each inventory item assesses 1 of the 14 concepts (8 for cohesion and 6 for adaptability) on FACES II. Individuals taking the test simply rate their level of satisfaction with the specified aspect of family life. For example, satisfaction with emotional bonding is tapped with the item "How satisfied are you with how close you feel to the rest of the family?" The scale is scored simply by tallying an unweighted total score for the 14 items. Interpretation is aided by the use of percentile norms, with means and standard deviations from the national survey.

The Family Satisfaction Inventory's original 28 items were reduced to 14 using a factor analysis of the responses of 438 university students. Items selected had high communality, variance, and factor loadings on the first factor, with 9 of the final 14 items loading at greater than .40 on the first rotated factor. The final instrument, which was normed on the large national sample described above, has only one factor with every item loading on it at .50 or greater on the first principal component. Cronbach's alpha for the total scale was .92, .84 for the adaptability subscale, and .85 for the cohesion subscale. Test-retest data over a 5-week period ($N = 106$) indicated rs of .75 for the total scale, and .76 and .67 for the cohesion and adaptability subscales, respectively.

Construct validity for this inventory is based on a significant positive correlation between family and life satisfaction (.68 for individuals and .67 for couple means) in the national survey of intact families (Olson et al., 1983). The correlation between family satisfaction and marital satisfaction was also high, .70 for couple means. In addition, family satisfaction was significantly, though "moderately" (a specific correlation was not reported) correlated with nearness to the center of the Circumplex Model using both individual and couple data. This means that the more balanced the family type, the higher the family satisfaction. The most impressive correlations here involve the degree to which family satisfaction is related to adaptability and cohesion (for couple means the rs are between $-.33$ and $-.40$); that is, satisfied families were those experiencing little stress.

Because this scale is so related to FACES II, the two measures complement one another and should be used together. Identified areas of dissatisfaction or differences in perceived satisfaction between spouses or parents and adolescentss can trigger discussion or negotiation in the interview or later treatment sessions.

The Quality of Life Inventory

Also developed by the Minnesota group (Olson and Barnes, in Olson et al., 1982), the Quality of Life Inventory uses a subjective, as opposed to an objective, statistical approach. Instead of assessing actual social and economic indicators, parents are asked to rate their degrees of satisfaction with 12 domains of life satisfaction (40 items) and adolescents to rate 11 domains of satisfaction (25 items). The domains assessed are marriage and family life, friends, extended family, health, home, education, time, religion, employment, mass media, financial well-being, and neighborhood and community. The adolescent scale does not have an employment item and assesses family life as opposed to marriage and family life. The inventory's items also differ in their wordings, which are slanted toward the concerns of the respective age groups.

Construct validity is based on a factor analysis (varimax rotation) of the total scale. Twelve factors were delineated which generally supported the initial conceptual structure of the scale. Cronbach's alpha for the national sample data was .92 for adults ($N = 1,950$) and .86 for the adolescents ($N = 399$). The instrument is scored using a total scale unweighted sum score and interpreted using percentile norms for husbands, wives, and male and female adolescents.

Throughout most of the life cycle, using the cross-sectional data, wives' life satisfaction scores were lower than husbands', although both were less satisfied with their quality of life than with their family or marital satisfaction. Satisfaction for both groups was higher during the "launching children" and "retirement" stages than at the "family with young children" stages. Finally, both parents' life satisfactions declined when the oldest child entered adolescence.

The Quality of Life measure complements the ecomap, FILE, and A-FILE, helping the family and practitioner to identify areas where support (satisfaction) and stress (dissatisfaction) subjectively impact family members. Families (and individuals) vary in their need for support and the levels of stress they find optimal. Using a number of measures gives a more comprehensive picture of the ecology of family life.

The Family Coping Strategies Inventory (F-COPES)

This inventory, also by the Minnesota group, was "created to identify effective problem-solving approaches and behaviors used by families in response to problems or difficulties. It was initially designed to integrate family resources and the meaning perception factors identified in family stress theory into coping strategies" (Olson *et al.*, 1982, p. 101). The authors refer to family resources as the use of social support networks and problem-solving strategies. Perception meaning factors are considered to be the meaning a family attaches to a stressful event to explain or make sense out of it, and how the family uses the event to later help them rearrange their social environment.

On the basis of their research and the findings of others, the authors contend that family coping strategies are developed and modified over time. They have identified five components of coping that successful families manage simultaneously, producing a balance in the family system:

> (1) maintaining satisfactory internal condition for communication and family organization, (2) promoting member independence and self-esteem, (3) maintenance of family bonds of coherence and unity, (4) maintenance and development of social supports in transactions with the community, and (5) maintenance of some efforts to control the impact of the stressor and the amount of change in the family unit. (Olson *et al.*, 1982, p. 102)

The initial inventory (used by both parents and adolescents) was developed to assess two dimensions of family coping, internal and external family strategies. A review of the literature identified 49 coping strategies. A factor analysis with a varimax rotation on a sample of 119 college students reduced the item pool to 30 items, with eight factors of eigen values greater than one. A replication of this initial construct validity study, using the 30-item instrument, was conducted on the national sample by dividing it in half for purposes of cross-validation. Findings from both studies resulted in five factors and a 29-item instrument. The five factors are Acquiring Social Support, Reframing, Seeking Spiritual Support, Mobilizing Family to Acquire and Accept Help, and Passive Appraisal.

Cronbach's alphas, calculated for both halves of the total sample, were .86 and .87. Subscale alphas ranged from .62 (Passive Appraisal) to .84 (Acquiring Social Support). While not high enough for use in individual or family diagnosis, the alphas are sufficient for use in research, screening, and to supplement other information gleaned during a family assessment.

Individuals taking the F-COPES rate their level of agreement with its 29 items on a 5-point Likert scale. "When we face problems or difficulties in our family, we respond by attending church services" is an example of an item that taps the Seeking Spiritual Support factor as a means of coping. A sum score is obtained for each subscale, as well as a total score which measures the number and degree of coping strategies that individuals perceive their families using. Percentile norms for husband, wife, and male and female adolescents are provided for subscales and total scores, as well as means and standard deviations for each group.

F-COPES is clinically useful when coordinated with the FILE, A-FILE, the family life cycle, and the ecomap. When family stress is a component of a referred problem or an additional pressure in a difficult situation, an appraisal of family coping strategies may well identify unused strategies that could facilitate a resolution or decrease in stress. In this regard, practitioners should note that coping strategies often vary by sex and developmental stage, type of family, and quality of family functioning. Practitioners interested in using F-COPES are encouraged to read the Olson *et al.* (1983) book, *Families: What Makes Them Work*. Even a professional working on a more superficial level with parents may find this scale useful. According to cross-sectional data, families with young children and families where the oldest child is an adolescent (including single parent families, divorced, and reintegrated families) are the two most stressed and least satisfied types of families in the life cycle. Thus, many parents seen by professionals may benefit from a discussion or assessment of their current stress levels and coping skills.

Critique and Discussion of Family Assessment Approaches

Utility in Finding Atypical Children

Obviously, family assessment is not a preferred means for identifying atypical or exceptional children and adolescents. It is a relatively time-consuming approach to understanding and developing interventions for already identified individuals. At the elementary school-age level, this is usually done through teacher or parent referrals to the school psychologist (guidance counselor, social worker) or to a clinic. Occasionally, districts will utilize screening procedures such as the very effective *A Process for the Assessment of Effective Student Functioning* (Lambert, Hartsough, & Bower, 1979). With adolescents, administrator and self-referrals are most common in the schools; at clinics, parent-, other agency-, or school-facilitated referrals serve in problem identification. Once the family is involved in the assessment, other children or adolescents in the family who are at risk for developing psychological difficulties may be identified.

Use with Adolescents versus Children

Family assessment is as useful for families with elementary school children as it is with adolescents. Adolescents, however, are easier to assess in many ways. Their greater verbal skills, the greater availability of self-report measures, their increased status within the family, their expertise in serving as a force for change within the family, their ability to ally with the practitioner, and their superior observation skills make them a relatively good identified client with which to work. On the other hand, separation, sexual, and boundary issues are explosive adolescent conflicts confronting families. The major structural transition that a family experiences when the first child leaves the family unit is probably the most traumatic of those changes in the family life cycle stages (N. Ackerman, 1980). The emotionality displayed by teenagers and parents and the unpredictability of adolescents in general require much flexibility, empathy, and a certain toughness on the part of the practitioner.

In the case of children, any type of personality assessment is more prone to error given the wider range of normal variability, the rapidity of developmental change, their limited verbal skills, and their relatively powerless position in the family. Thus, practitioners must evaluate the validity and reliability of data assessing children's cognitive and emotional structures. Psychologically immature, children may have great difficulty in coping with the complexities of a formal family assessment, that is, understanding its purposes and their role in it. They are less able to speak for themselves and thus may need to be assessed less directly through projective techniques or adult ratings of their behavior. The major advantage of dealing with younger children is that they frequently present milder difficulties or less entrenched maladaptive patterns, and thus they are more amenable to remediation.

Educational versus Clinical Settings

Mental health practitioners working in educational settings are restricted in their work with families by the goals of the institutions that they work for. As adjuncts to teaching professionals, they are charged with diagnosing and developing remedial plans for students who are not learning at rates commensurate with their tested abilities or who are behaving in socially inappropriate ways. As such, these practitioners represent the institution or public's interest in children, although they may also act as child advocates. The family is the practitioner's third concern in terms of loyalty or client status; the family and the parents are almost necessarily viewed as allies (or hinderances) helping the student to perform at expected or optimal levels at school. Parents are seen by practitioners or other school personnel to obtain information and to determine the family's role in a child's problem. Unlike many clinics where practitioners decide to treat a family through marriage counseling because the marital relationship is triggering many of the child's or youth's problems, the school is not in a position to do this. The school practitioner may reach the same conclusion, but would have to refer the family elsewhere.

These restrictions of client, role, and resources affect the ways that schools conduct family assessments; these restrictions point out difficulties that practitioners (and school psychologists, in particular) should be aware of when planning assessments. First, there is the issue of training. Many school psychologists have little experience or training in working with families (Brassard & Anderson, 1983). Taking a developmental and family history from a mother and giving feedback on the results of a psychoeducational evaluation may be the extent of school psychologists' past involvement with families. Many of the techniques presented in this chapter would work well in a school setting even without special training. The ecomap, a less detailed genogram, the family life cycle, and the measures for children and adolescents (A-FILE, Parent–Adolescent Communication, Roberts Apperception Inventory, and the Parent Perception Inventory) would all complement most school psychologists' repertoires of assessment techniques. Other measures' use could depend not only on a greater background in family assessment and family therapy approaches, but also on a service-delivery orientation that allows for greater involvement with families.

This leads directly into the second point that needs to be considered, namely, how one differentiates family evaluation from family treatment. Rapport and trust facilitate a good assessment atmosphere, but a therapeutic set is also created by this atmosphere. The assessment process usually involves receiving a great deal of intimate and personal information. These points raise several ethical questions. Under Principle 5 of the APA Ethical Principles of Psychologists (American Psychological Association, 1981), one is obligated to avoid undue invasion of privacy. A formal family assessment may go well beyond identifying family conflicts that influence a student's school performance. If serious problems become apparent within the assessment, the school psychologist is not usually in a position to offer treatment, only to make an outside referral. The family is then in the predicament of having entered a quasi-therapeutic relationship, aroused many powerful feelings during the assessment process, and exposed some personal aspects of their lives—only to be offered a referral. As some choose not to follow through with outside referrals to mental health services (Conti, 1975; Zins & Hopkins, 1981), the psychologist may have helped the family focus on sources of anguish while raising hopes for changes that may not soon be resolved.

On the other hand, the more knowledge school psychologists have about a family, the better they are able to suggest appropriate referral resources and to motivate the family to follow through. And, there are other advantages when a school practitioner knows a family well and has established a therapeutic relationship with it. For example, some problem children pose difficulties throughout their school career; thus, frequent parent–practitioner interactions over many years are not uncommon whether focused on that particular child or on other problem children from the same family. A strong practitioner–family bond in these cases may produce a powerful positive impact on the student's social and educational progress, thus fully justifying a formal family assessment.

In a clinic or hospital setting, training and service delivery orientations still affect how and why families are assessed. However, family or marital treatment is much more likely to be the focus of these assessments. Families go to these settings acknowledging, in many cases, that there is a difficulty which needs to be addressed. Unlike the schools, these settings have a built-in set for sharing intimate information. Yet, problems can arise when the service delivery model demands a quick turnaround time on cases, even when they are not therapeutically resolved.

Utility with Various Types of Exceptional Children or Adolescents

As mentioned above, some clinical or school referrals may have a family difficulty at the heart of the problem. Certain types of presenting problems, however, have been associated clinically and empirically with maladaptive family functioning. If the practitioner, through a careful assessment and examination of the presenting problem and its controlling variables and consequences, has determined that the primary locus of the problem does not reside in other environmental settings or interactions between settings, then it may well be that only a family-oriented treatment program will produce the desired results. An important consideration in these cases is the family's motivation for treatment and the overall prognosis. It is very easy in both clinic and school settings to spend an enormous amount of clinical time on a few families who make little or no progress over the course of many years.

Almost all families with significantly handicapped children or adolescents can benefit from a close, supportive relationship with the school. This gives these parents and youngsters in the family (handicapped or not) someone to call or see when stress at home, school, or with the peer group becomes dysfunctional and difficult to bear.

A Family Assessment Case Study

Background and Reason for Referral

Mrs. Koehler called the school psychologist asking for an appointment at the suggestion of her son's sixth-grade homeroom teacher. She was concerned about 12-year-old Kurt's dramatic drop in school performance (from a B + to a C – average) and his behavior at home and when visiting his father. She explained briefly that she, a social worker at another school in the district, and the superintendent of the psychologist's district had been living together for the past 2 years. Her children from another marriage, Kurt and Gisela, age 8, lived with them while their father lived alone on a nearby estate. The divorce, recently finalized, had been typically unpleasant, but the children had seemed to adapt to the new situation and they liked Dr. Cottingwood, her lover. Recently, Kurt's behavior had gotten much worse and his poor grades had caused some bad arguments with his father. In addition, Mrs. Koehler had been diagnosed as having a fatal disease, had undergone surgery, and then had been sent home being told that her cells had fooled the excellent pathologists treating her. She assumed that the problems with her son were related to the stress the family had undergone, and she requested some help.

Because of the apparent role of the family in Kurt's reported difficulties, Mrs. Koehler was invited to come in for an appointment with Dr. Cottingwood and the two children. Prior to the family interview, Kurt's school records were examined, his teachers interviewed briefly, and he was unobtrusively observed in the lunchroom and the classroom.

The records indicated that Kurt had historically done well in school and had been involved in band and in school plays where he had had a number of lead roles and writing and directing positions. He was liked by his teachers, although they commented that he worked to draw attention to himself; "self-dramatizing" was the word one teacher used. His work, once conscientious and oriented toward obtaining teacher approval, had recently become sloppy and assignments were frequently late. Kurt usually associated with a stable circle of three other boys. Recently, however, he was spending more time alone, often because of quarrels with one or more of his friends.

Interview and Assessment

Session 1

The Koehler/Cottingwood family appeared for the first of their four afterschool appointments dressed for work or school. Mrs. Koehler wore a well-cut tailored dress with tasteful, expensive gold and diamond jewelry. She had the look of a lady of the manor—handsome, voluptuous, and gracious. The superintendent was more casually dressed in a corduroy jacket, tie, slacks, and loafers. Outdoorsy, athletic, and down-to-earth, his style presented a contrast to Mrs. Koehler. The children, particularly Kurt, resembled their mother in coloring, voluptuous features, and poise. The children seemed to like Dr. Cottingwood; they frequently touched him and initiated eye contact and verbal moves to engage his attention. He responded warmly to them.

The adults sat next to each other with a child on each side, Gisela next to her mother. After the psychologist briefly explained what had initiated the meeting, she asked the adults how they saw the problem. Dr. C. began by saying that he felt that Kurt was feeling the stress of the divorce, was torn apart by feelings of loyalty to his Dad and his growing feelings for Dr. C., and had been extremely worried that his mother was going to die. Mrs. K. agreed, but felt that conflicts between she and Dr. C. were also being felt by Kurt. She referred to the adjustment in life styles that the adults had made: She had moved from wealth and high social status to a middle-class existence, while Dr. C., financially strained by alimony, child support, and college tuition payments for one son, had increased his affluence by moving in with her. Gisela commented next that the divorce was the problem, but declined to elaborate with a shy smile. Kurt began by agreeing with Dr. C., and then he talked about the pressures he'd been under. He then burst into tears, sobbed loudly for a moment, and then walked quickly from the room crying that he just couldn't talk about it in front of a stranger.

After discussing the situation with the adults, the psychologist followed Kurt to the outer office, leaving the rest of the family to fill out several nonthreatening survey instruments. Kurt was standing with his back to the psychologist, facing a corner of the room, holding a tissue to his eyes. The psychologist commented on the pressure he seemed to be feeling to which he responded, "Sometimes I feel no one has gone through what I've gone through. I wish I could just vanish!"

"Are you referring to the divorce and your Mom's health scare?" the psychologist asked. Nodding yes, Kurt sobbed, "I don't want to be like my Dad. He's cheating us financially. He wants me to be perfect. He wants me to go to private school and then to Harvard. I'm *not* that smart! He got me a tutor for the summer 'cause my grades in advanced math were C's!" Crying again, he paused and then whispered, "He doesn't understand me."

Kurt calmed and began talking about the many things that were pressuring him: difficulty communicating with his father, resentment over his sister getting along better than he with their father, the few demands made on Gisela by his father, her much nicer bedroom in the mansion, and his role in maintaining the relationship between his parents. "I feel like I'm just seeing him to be nice so he'll give us money and things." Kurt tearfully nodded yes when the psychologist asked him if he felt like he was using his father at times. He expressed his desire to get away from all the worries about his mother's health, the divorce, school, and friends—to pretend these things weren't happening. "I just can't cope. Even sitting beside Mom's bed in the hospital, I was doing homework." Another problem was his sister who was spending less and less time with him and more time with a particularly close friend. Kurt felt shut out. Finally, his closest friend had called up three times to cancel plans saying that he was going with another friend or had to do something on his paper route.

After 30 minutes of discussing these issues, Kurt had regained his composure and was willing to return to a full family session. With Kurt's permission, the psychologist briefly summarized Kurt's concerns before resuming the family session.

Context: The Family in Space and Time

Following the initial discussion of the problem as perceived by each family member, the interview moved to a more general assessment phase. This began with the completion of the family's ecomap, with the psychologist and family all sitting around a table. Most notable in the ecomap was the strong and somewhat stressful relationship most of the family members had with the local school district; only Gisela's relationship here was unstressful (see Figure 12-1). Mrs. Koehler's relationship with her doctors, each adult's interactions with their former spouse, and Kurt's relationships with his friends and his father were other areas of stress for the family. In addition, Kurt and Gisela, once very close, were fighting more now that Gisela was spending increasing amounts of time with girlfriends.

Areas of particular enjoyment for the whole family, and Mrs. K. in particular, centered around decorating the new home and garden. Dr. C. expressed satisfaction with his new postdoctoral program. Social support was provided by Dr. C.'s large, extended family; Mrs. Koehler's family served more as a stressor in that her mother and sisters traditionally looked to her for emotional support. Friends were largely unavailable as both adults' divorces had taken away most of their social circle and close friends; both felt somewhat bitter about this. Favorite hobbies such as high country camping for Dr. C. and antiques for Mrs. K. had been neglected in the press of the current life situation.

Overall, both adults and Kurt were experiencing difficulties in primary relationships, in work/school situations; further, they were feeling isolated and did not have the time or energy to engage in those activities which they found pleasurable. Getting along with her father and her peers at school, Gisela appeared relatively unstressed. She was doing well academically and in gymnastics, horseback riding, and her music lessons.

The adults were struck by their isolation and lack of social support and by the stress apparent in *every* aspect of Kurt's life. This generated some discussion that led directly into gathering further information on their life-style and living environment.

The family described their new home and neighborhood in the mountains around a popular intermountain region ski village. Located in an affluent neighborhood, their new colonial house and barn gave their several acres a country feeling. A few children of the "right" ages lived nearby. A formal garden had been designed by Mrs. K. in the spring with the actual work carried out by Dr. C. and Kurt. The spacious house "dripped" with valuable antiques that Mrs. K. had been able to salvage from her former mansion home and her "vindictive and selfish" former spouse. Done in a mid-nineteenth-century decor, the home was lovingly decorated and maintained. The family room-kitchen was the area in which the family congregated. It was cozy, attractive, and very lived in. The family had three pets, two dogs and a cat, all with pedigree papers. The adults slept together in the large master suite and each child had his or her own bedroom and bath.

In terms of the typical routine, on weekdays Dr. C. woke first and then roused Kurt as they both needed to be at school at 7:30. Mrs. K. and Gisela joined them for breakfast at 7:00 and then readied themselves to be at school by 8:00. Kurt arrived home by bus at 2:45, and Gisela arrived home with her mother 3 days of the week at 4:15 following her gymnastics practice. On the other 2 days, she arrived at home at 3:30 by bus. A teenaged girl worked in the house from 2:00 to 4:30 every weekday afternoon, cleaning and caring for the children. Both children played at home or at an approved neighbor's house until dinner at 5:30. Dr. C arrived home between 4:30 and 5:00.

Dinner was somewhat formal, with everyone attending and sitting with the adults at the head of the table. Family members' daily activities were discussed along with projects for the house, vacation plans, and relatives. After dinner, homework, chores, and the practice of musical instruments occupied the children until 8:00 when they were allowed to watch television or read before bed at 9:00 and 9:30, respectively. The adults gardened, painted parts of the house or did other chores, and argued with former spouses over the phone until the children went to bed. Weekends were spent working on the house or grounds, visiting relatives, watching the children engage in sports, or attending school district functions. On every other weekend that the children spent with their father (he had a reason for not taking them approximately every third time), the adults would dine out or attend an art show or concert.

The family expressed an interest in continuing the evaluation and an appointment was scheduled for the next week. Family members were sent home with a number of survey instruments to fill out alone for the next session. Mrs. K. suggested that the psychologist meet with her former husband to get his input on the family situation and Kurt's difficulties.

The psychologist agreed to this if Mr. Koehler was willing. They arranged for Mrs. Koehler to telephone later in the week after talking with Mr. Koehler.

Session 2

For the second session, the family returned with their completed test protocols; Dr. C. admitted to having filled out the lot of them just prior to the meeting. The protocols were collected, and the family was again asked to gather around the table and a large sheet of white cardboard paper.

Given the complexity of each family, a genogram was completed first for the Koehler family (see Figure 12-2) and then for the Cottingwood family (see Figure 12-3). Mrs. K.'s family consisted of a series of strong, dominant women marrying foreign-born entrepreneurs. A tendency toward artistic talent, and histories of cancer and headaches were also present. Mrs. K. came from a monied family that placed a high value on nice things. Her upbringing was very traditional in that her father did not believe in higher education for women. While her mother disagreed (she herself came from a family of well-educated women), Mrs. K. still felt pushed to put herself through college on a scholarship. Her role in the family was to fix things or "mother" her mother and sisters. She often took on her dictatorial father, a role her mother grew weary of over the years. Thus, Mrs. K. seemed to adopt overfunctioning (e.g., doing more than she needed or was expected to do, taking on others' responsibilities in addition to her own) as a means of coping with unmet emotional needs. Lately, she had been providing both emotional and some financial support to her mother who was recovering from a serious and, for a long time undiagnosed, dysfunction of the thyroid gland.

Dr. C.'s family contrasted sharply with that of Mrs. K.'s along a number of dimensions (see Figure 12-3). From a small rural town in the mountains of the intermountain region, Dr. C. grew up in a large religious family as the oldest and only male of five children. Dr. C.'s parents were gentle, pious people who raised him in an environment that valued independence, hard work, survival skills and crafts useful in the wilderness and rural areas, as well as the managerial skills that his father used in his work. With many kin from both

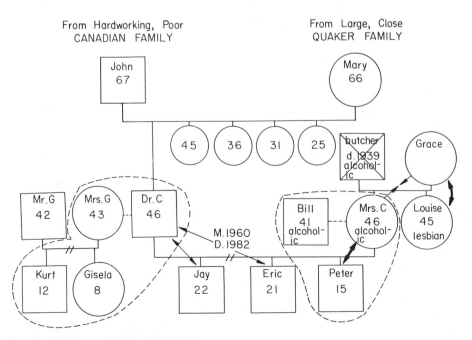

Figure 12-3. Dr. Cottingwood's Genogram.

sides of the family nearby, Dr. C. developed early a strong, positive sense of his roots, knowing most of his neighbors and kin from birth. Along the way, he collected a library of folk sayings appropriate for the various situations confronting him as a superintendent of schools, and an air of authority from supervising four younger sisters. Needless to say, both his staff and the community liked his folksiness and his no-nonsense, take-charge style of administration.

Dr. C. married a woman he had met at their state college after graduation. Mrs. C. was the daughter of an alcoholic butcher and a mother who worked in a shoe factory. Five years after their marriage and the birth of two sons, Mrs. C. developed a serious drinking problem. Already dependent, she became increasingly childlike and dysfunctional. A third child, Peter, was born 6 years after the second child. Fetal alcohol syndrome was later suspected as the source of this son's endocrinological, neurological, and learning problems and his obesity and effeminacy. Dr. C. rejected this child, Peter, who, from birth on, seemed pathologically close to his mother. Over the years Peter had passive-aggressively and aggressively demanded his father's attention in various ways (e.g., school failure, behavior problems, temper tantrums), and he caused much conflict when he moved into the Koehler/ Cottingwood household for 1 year and 4 months. The conflict appeared to have resulted from the change from a more permissive, child-centered rearing style where Peter functioned in a parental role with his mother to an orderly parent-run household style.

Dr. C. did many things to inadvertently support his wife's drinking habit. He relieved her of all home responsibilities, picked her up and put her to bed when she fell into a stupor, and protected the kids from many visible signs of her disease. Dr. C. would have stayed with the marriage had Mrs. C. not initiated an acting-out stage that resembled an adolescent rebellion. As this involved an affair with Dr. C.'s closest friend, he finally moved to discontinue the relationship.

In his distress, Dr. C. sought some formal supportive counseling from a local family counselor. She helped him realize the extent to which he was maintaining his wife's dysfunctional behavior and motivated him initially to push for couple counseling and an alcoholism treatment program. After a year's worth of intermittent treatment and several attempts to reunite with his wife, Dr. C. began informally discussing his troubled family situation with the district's social worker, Mrs. K. Further discussions brought Dr. C. to the point of realizing that he no longer loved Mrs. C. and was becoming increasingly interested in Mrs. K.

At this point in the session, the psychologist introduced the notion of the family life cycle, a concept with which Mrs. K. was familiar. Specifically, the postdivorce and family reintegration issues were presented. Each family member was asked for their overall appraisal on these developmental family issues. Carter and McGoldrick (1980b) identified two developmental stages confronted by the postdivorce custodial family: (*a*) making flexible visitation arrangements with the ex-spouse and his extended family, and (*b*) rebuilding the divorced spouse's social network. Mrs. K. felt she and Mr. K. were still working on their co-parenting relationship. At times, things would proceed smoothly, particularly in regard to Gisela. However, Kurt's fights with his father or his discomfort in being with him would sometimes lead to phone calls to his mother and requests to be taken home. This would precipitate an argument between his parents, and often between him and one or both of his parents. At this point, Kurt commented, "It seems like when Mom is getting along with Dad, I'm not; and when I'm getting along with him, she isn't."

Dr. C. had virtually given up trying to co-parent with Mrs. C. He felt that she sabotaged most of his efforts to get Peter's life back on track. Mrs. K. volunteered that Peter was so difficult to manage and caused so much disruption in their home that she had become unwilling to risk the family's emotional well-being by having him live with them again.

The rebuilding of their social networks had begun sporadically for both adults. Fortunately, the children maintained most of their friendships because there was no change in school district. Mr. Koehler's mother and grandmother had stopped communicating with Mrs. Koehler and with the children. They did not answer letters and no longer sent gifts at Christmas and birthdays. However, since Mr. Koehler had had a long-standing rift with his mother that had improved with Mrs. K's encouragement, it was unclear what had motivated this complete break.

The remarried family formation, also developed by Carter and McGoldrick (1980b), applied to some extent to the Koehler/Cottingwood family, although remarriage had not occurred. When this was presented, Dr. C. interrupted, asking that this discussion be held without the children present. With Kurt protesting mildly, the children were sent to play in the gym. Dr. C. then broached what he considered a major source of conflict—Mrs. K.'s unwillingness to marry him. Facing a third marriage, Mrs. K. used financial concerns as the primary reason for her hesitation. She felt that she had lost financially through both marriages, and she was concerned that it would happen again. Her hesitation, however, had not prevented her from purchasing a house with Dr. C., with her money constituting the bulk of the down payment.

Dr. C. felt embarrassed living with a woman in his position as a community leader. This also went against his religious values and his personal style of making commitments and sticking with them. He admitted to getting very angry over the situation. He felt uncomfortable expressing his anger; he did not want to badger Mrs. K. on the issue, and he was unwilling to issue an ultimatum or to leave. Dr. C. also felt that Mrs. K. was still overly involved with her former husband, and that she was still mourning aspects of their relationship. Thus, from what he said (and Mrs. K. voiced little disagreement), Mrs. K. had not "emotionally divorced" Mr. K. completely and the family was unable to move toward resolving the first developmental issue of the remarried family—recommitment to marriage and forming a new family. A discussion of this point took up the rest of the session.

Another appointment was scheduled to give the family feedback on their responses to the survey instruments. This appointment was arranged to follow the psychologist's interview with Mr. K.

Session 3

Mr. K. presented himself as a well-groomed sophisticated looking man in his early 40s. Tall, thin, and fair, he spoke with a slight German accent. He began the interview by politely telling the psychologist that he doubted that she could be much help to him since she had never gone through a divorce. He had agreed to the interview, however, because he wanted to improve his relationship with his son and wanted his son's grades to improve.

Mr. K. continued by stating frankly that many of his feelings about the divorce were unresolved and that one needn't push too hard to hit upon very raw material. The psychologist reassured him that rehashing the divorce was not her purpose. Mr. K. admitted to being "very jealous" of Dr. C.'s current father role to his children. He had bought the beautiful estate that he now lived alone in as a family home to be passed down through the generations; the divorce had crushed that dream. His marriage had been a permanent commitment and he had been generally happy in it. Mrs. K. had been a wonderful homemaker who also offered shrewd advice about business deals; she had supported his judgments and gave him confidence in himself when he first started out in business.

Mr. K. now felt that Mrs. K. had never really loved him. Instead, she had coolly recognized his social background and future earning power, and she couldn't resist the temptation to snare him. He felt she could never trust him because he was a gambler by nature (a necessary characteristic given his business), and because she saw him as a Nazi (his father had run his German factory during the war and generally supported the German cause). In addition, he felt she was a hypochondriac. When he found out that the doctors thought she had cancer, he had laughed. It was one more exotic illness without a biological base. Thus, Mr. K. felt the risks of his business, which grew greater as he became more successful, his lack of sympathy for his wife's chronic health problems, and his frequent travel caused her to become more insecure about their relationship and her control over him. Ultimately, she accused him of having affairs on his international trips. And, as her insecurity increased, she became open to the overtures of Dr. C. who was supportive, believed her health stories, and provided a good, stable father role for the children. For these reasons, and not for love of either man, did she leave Mr. K. for Dr. C.

As for the children, Mr. K. was happy with his relationship with Gisela, but felt frustrated and baffled in his dealings with Kurt. He felt that his son was too pampered by his mother and that his interests weren't developing in a manly direction. For example, Kurt preferred music, acting, and drawing to sports. And he complained bitterly if he had to do work around the grounds or wash cars when staying with his father.

Mr. K. lay much of the blame for his poor relationship with his son on his former spouse. Mrs. K. often hostilely attacked him in front of the children for cheating *them* out of *their* share of the material goods acquired during their marriage. He would remind her of their settlement and the fact that anything that he still possessed was in his home and available to the children on their visits; the children had not lost anything. Mr. K. felt that Mrs. K. played the martyr role to the hilt, just as she had when her first marriage had ended.

Mr. K.'s ecomap pictured a socially isolated man whose life revolved around his work. A couple living with their two children on the estate constituted "family" for him when he was at home. (The woman was the best friend that Mrs. K. lost in the divorce.) Most primary relationships were strained. (Mrs. K. commented later that this was because of his pattern of setting himself up for rejection by hurting and betraying those close to him in his own interest.) Mr. K. was cut off from his mother, sister, and brother-in-law because of long-standing money squabbles. He said that he had not attempted to repair the relationship because of his suspicion, in recent years, that his mother was having an affair with his sister's husband. The Koehler/Cottingwood tie was conflictual, and he infrequently contacted an illegitimate infant son, Terrence, and the boy's mother.

This child was conceived shortly after the divorce and was kept secret from Mrs. K. and the children until the divorce was finalized. The children had noticed the pregnancy prior to the divorce; in fact, Mrs. K. had questioned Mr. K. about it, but he denied it. The topic appeared to be a source of embarrassment to Mr. K. The mother was a socially prominent young woman who, on becoming pregnant, had decided to keep the child against Mr. K.'s wishes. After rejecting the two outright, Mr. K. had been persuaded by Mrs. K. to acknowlege, visit, and provide some support for the child. Mrs. K. made a point of introducing Kurt and Gisela to their half-brother. (When asked about this later, Mrs. K. said that she did this for Kurt and Gisela's sake; she wanted to intervene in Mr. K.'s pattern of cutting himself off from kin before he cut them off.)

Mr. K.'s sources of support at this time were a nonstressful work situation, some good friends in Germany who were seen infrequently, a good relationship with his father and his father's mistress, his house and grounds, and a rare book business that he owned. The relationship with his father was recent (within the last 6 years); they had spent much of Mr. K.'s adulthood cut off from one another.

The genogram portrayed an interesting German background and history. Mr. K. was born to a bricklayer and the daughter of a watchmaker who became wealthy factory owners. They lived in a small town whose inhabitants mostly worked in the factory. Mr. K. had no peers other than his older sister, Lina. While his father had had extramarital affairs for many years, his mother grew tired of it 15 years into the marriage and withheld sexual relations as punishment. Years later when the factory was in some financial trouble, Mr. K.'s father put his assets into his wife's name. Shortly thereafter, she filed for divorce. Mr. K.'s mother moved in with her daughter who was married to a much older and very wealthy man, also a factory owner. This marriage was quite strained, and eventually sister Lina had an affair and was caught with her lover in a car accident. As a result, her husband sent her out of the country for a number of years while her mother remained and ran her son-in-law's large household. Mr. K. reported that his mother was a very powerful person; he found it necessary to sever their relationship in order to move out on his own. This break occurred around the time he first met Mrs. K. (Mrs. K. said the break was due to Mr. K. borrowing $60,000 from his mother and refusing to repay it, claiming it was his father's money and not his mother's.) His mother was very critical and originally unaccepting of her daughter-in-law.

Reviewing and summarizing Mr. K.'s ecomap and genogram, there were themes involving sexual and financial acting out, harsh separations rather than a working through of separation or other issues, attachments to strong older women (mother, sister, Mrs. K.), a notion of marriage as an institution that carries on regardless of the couple's feelings toward one another, and values toward financial success and manorial living.

Session 4

The fourth session, the third session overall with the Koehler/Cottingwood family, was arranged to discuss some of the assessment results with the family. This was done by first describing each measure, what it evaluates, and what the family's responses might mean. As Kurt refused to complete any of the survey instruments, only the adults' and Gisela's responses were presented.

The Family Inventory of Life Events (FILE) is presented here first, since it is the last of the five measures to assess context. The total Family Pileup score for Dr. C. and Mrs. K. placed them in the extremely high stress range. Their combined score of 41 (31 out of 72 items were checked by one or both) placed them over three standard deviations above the mean of the national sample ($M = 8.8$, $SD = 5.9$). This indicates an increased vulnerability to crisis. Major stressors fell in the Finances and Business category (9 of 12 items checked) where enormous expenses for medical care, tuition, and the new home and car were exacerbated by delays in child-care payments from Mr. K. and some declining family investments. Marital Status strains noted included the unresolved issues mentioned above. Intrafamily Strains, Work/Family Transitions each had 3–4 stressors checked. The Illness category contained only one item, but that was the diagnosis of Mrs. K.'s major illness. Loss of close friends and Dr. C.'s return to school completed the list of stressors.

Other Assessment Results

Structure and Dynamics

This component of the family assessment was initially addressed by investigating some key areas of family functioning: rules, alliances, and conflicts or disagreements. Interview questions and test results indicated a reasonable and effectively maintained structure of family rules. For example, each child had age-appropriate chores. If chores were not completed or if rules were broken, both parents responded with fairly similar reactions (according to self-reports and Gisela's ratings on the Parent Perception Inventory). Punishments consisted of time-out in one's bedroom for short periods of time and removal of privileges. While Mrs. K. would sometimes nag or remind her children to do their chores, both parents were capable of affectionate and supportive responses.

Coalitions were not a major factor within the household. Generation boundaries were maintained which is a generally positive sign of healthy family functioning. External boundaries were a problem in that Mr. K. and Mrs. K. were often overly close, yet at other times, Mrs. K. would become overly involved in Kurt's relationship with his father. Similarly, in the Cottingwood family, Mrs. C. had formed a fused relationship with Peter which was often aligned against Dr. C. and, to a lesser extent, the two older sons.

Areas of disagreement fell into two major categories. The first general category involved the unresolved emotional divorce between Mr. K. and Mrs. K. This caused conflict between Mrs. K. and Dr. C., Mrs. K. and Mr. K., and between Mr. K. and Kurt. It prevented Kurt from maintaining a stable, positive relationship with his father, because he felt pulled in to help his mother maintain a balancing act between her old and new relationships. It prevented Dr. C. and Mrs. K. from establishing a boundary around themselves as a family so they could begin to resolve the issues involved in that process. Other areas of disagreement mentioned by the family could be incorporated into this general area; Kurt's behavior which caused problems for all three adults, Mr. K. and Kurt's difficulties with one another, Mrs. K.'s interventions in the relationship between Kurt and his Dad and her financial squabbles with Mr. K. as a means of maintaining that relationship, and Kurt's resentment of Gisela's increasing time with friends. He appeared to seek Gisela out as a berth in the storm. Uninvolved in parental machinations, she was moving ahead developmentally while Kurt was stuck given his family role.

Also related was Kurt's very normal conflict over his growing attachment to Dr. C. and diminishing attachment to his father. Mr. K. and Kurt had not been close prior to the divorce. Dr. C.'s warmth, continuous and reliable presence, and responsiveness were new and very welcome to Kurt, as well as to Gisela. Kurt felt pressured by his mother to maintain a good relationship with his father (he interpreted this as an imperative to ensure continuous financial support by keeping Dad happy with him) and, consequently, felt terribly guilty for not caring enough about his Dad and for using him.

The second general area of conflict was Dr. C.'s manner in handling certain situations involving his children. Mrs. K. felt that he was too financially generous, allowing them to impose on him by asking for favors that affected the Koehler/Cottingwood household unreasonably. For instance, Dr. C. agreed to pay for an expensive music camp when the money had to come either from a loan or from Mrs. K.'s savings. Mrs. K. felt that Dr. C. should turn his children down rather than allowing them to believe that he could and would provide for their every need. This pattern may have developed during Dr. C.'s first marriage where, concerned about his wife's impairment, he would provide for his children regardless of the personal cost or the reasonableness of the requests.

The Family Adaptability and Cohesion Scales (FACES II) indicated that both adults' responses placed the family in the midrange. Mrs. K. saw the family as connected-chaotic, and Dr. C. as separated-chaotic. Both felt that the current family structure and family dynamics were close to ideal. The extreme level of adaptiveness indicated by the chaotic range appeared to be related to the uncertainty in the couple's relationship, the number of major crises that the family had weathered, and the flexibility needed when a family in the "young children stage" merges to some extent with a family in the "launching children stage." Mrs. K.'s placement of the family in the connected-chaotic range coincided with the range considered most adaptive for families with young children.

On the Family Environment Scale (FES), the couple again strongly agreed on the family's climate. Both saw the family as high in cohesion, expressiveness, and organization, and low in moral–religious orientation. Dr. C. viewed the family as higher on intellectual–cultural orientation, achievement orientation, and control than Mrs. K., who rated these areas as average in emphasis. Mrs. K. rated the family as low on independence and dependent while Dr. C. rated these areas as average. Overall, the family was perceived as relationship and achievement oriented, with a high degree of organization and an average amount of conflict.

ENRICH, the marital inventory developed by the Minnesota group (Olson *et al.*, 1982), was used to assess the couple's relationship. Both rated their sexual relationship, overall marital satisfaction, the egalitarian nature of their relationship, and their lack of religious involvement as highly positive. The Children and Marriage subtest was generally positive for both, although some conflict in the relationship was attributed to the children.

On the remaining six ENRICH subtests, Dr. C. noted many concerns (4 to 7 out of 10 possible items were checked as being problematic), while Mrs. K. noted few problems (0 to 3 out of 10 items were checked as problematic). Finances and Personality Issues were the areas with the most specific complaints. Financially, Dr. C. was worried about financial priorities, the amount of money saved, credit card use, couple responsibility for handling finances, and debt level. Mrs. K. was concerned about credit card use, debts, and decisions about saving. The Personality Issues subtest elicited many complaints from Dr. C. He saw Mrs. K. as too critical and negative in her outlook, unhappy and withdrawn at times, possessing a temper, stubborn, moody, and too domineering. Mrs. K. reported Dr. C. as somewhat moody.

The Family and Friends subtest revealed Dr. C.'s desire for more time with family and friends, his concern about not liking his partner's friends (and vice versa), and his belief that his partner was too influenced by family, and that certain relatives were creating tension in their relationship. Mrs. K., on the other hand, was contented with the status quo.

Similarly, the Communication subtest elicited only one concern from Mrs. K.: that Dr. C. did not share his feelings as often as she would like. Dr. C., however, noted four problems: He sometimes felt uneasy expressing negative feelings to his partner, thinking she would get angry; his partner made comments which put him down; he often didn't tell his partner what he was thinking, although he thought she should know; and he had trouble expressing his true feelings.

The Conflict Resolution subtest fit the same pattern. Dr. C. reported that he often gave up too quickly to end an argument, that he couldn't always tell his partner what was bothering him, that arguments don't get resolved, that he doesn't always openly share his feelings in a disagreement, and that after an argument he ended up feeling that the argument was his fault. Mrs. K. reported some serious arguments over unimportant issues, unresolved conflicts, and being unhappy with the degree to which she felt her partner understood her. She reported no difficulty expressing her true feelings openly.

In the Leisure area, both adults indicated that their partner did not have enough time or energy for recreation with them. Dr. C. felt that they did not enjoy some of the same leisure activities, he didn't like the way holidays were spent, and he felt that there was not enough balance between leisure time spent together and separately.

On the general questions concluding the ENRICH inventory, both agreed that leadership was shared, that they didn't spend enough time having fun, that they often depended on their partner, and that rules were clear and flexible. Some lack of congruence was evident as Mrs. K. reported that disagreements were settled after some discussion, with both sharing final problem decisions; Dr. C. reported much discussion, but no clear decisions. Mrs. K. reported feeling close to her partner while Dr. C. felt very close.

The Parent–Adolescent scale was given to Kurt's parents to assess their perceptions of the quality of communication between each of them and Kurt. As the Circumplex Model posits that quality of communication influences the potential for change within a family, this is an important variable to assess. Kurt, at age 12, fell on the borderline between an elementary school age and adolescence, so the instrument was used.

Mrs. K.'s ratings placed her at the 43rd percentile for mothers' ratings of their communication with teenage children. On the first factor of Open Family Communication, responses were rated as being very open. On the second, Problems in Family Communication, a number of problems were noted. These involved having trouble believing everything said by her child, being afraid to make requests to her child, having the child insult her when angry, and having a child who sometimes verbalized things better left unsaid. Interestingly, Mr. K. noted many of the same problems on the second factor; he reported the last three problems described above and having to be careful about what he said to his child. In addition, Mr. K. negatively rated two responses on the Open Family Communication factor, that his child was not a good listener and that he didn't get honest answers to some of his questions. His ratings placed him at the 18–22nd percentile for fathers' rating their communication with teenage children.

Overall, the parents presented a consistent perceived communication pattern with Kurt. Both appeared to be a little afraid of Kurt's emotionality and his responses when upset. Kurt's honesty with them was also of some concern. It was unfortunate that Kurt's responses to the same items were not available.

Level of Adaptation and Health

This component of family functioning was obtained (a) from general observations, (b) from specific questions on the family's coping mechanisms with past trials, and (c) from family responses to several survey instruments measuring adaptive functioning and health.

Other than the recent crises of divorce and health, the Koehler family as a whole had not suffered any major crises. The adults, however, had had individual crises in their pasts. Mr. Koehler had a major confrontation with the law during the 1960s, resulting in a major battle with his father who lost confidence in his competence to inherit the family business. At that time and with his mother's support, he left Germany for the United States. Shortly thereafter, he met Mrs. K. and relations with his mother became strained. Relying on a strong woman thus seemed to be his major means of coping with crisis. The divorce, coupled with his severed relationship with his mother, forced him to develop and rely on his own resources. Periodically he would call on Mrs. K. to provide some emotional support, a role that she occasionally accepted.

Both Mrs. K. and Dr. C. tended to overfunction when in a crisis. They would make lists of work that needed to be done and then occupy themselves so there was no time to dwell on the problem. They modified this approach somewhat during the recent crisis over Mrs. K.'s health, when they openly vented their feelings to one another in the middle of the night—a time when they knew the children could not hear them. At daylight, they returned to the focus on work and practical issues. Until the moment of surgery, Mrs. K. was on the phone to her substitute social worker in the district and covering fine points of her will with her lawyer. None of the adults had received prior mental health treatment aside from the family counselor Dr. C. saw prior to his divorce.

The Quality of Life measure was designed to identify areas of support and stress. Mrs. K. scored over two standard deviations below the mean, somewhere below the 12th percentile. Her mean response was 2.4 ("somewhat dissatisfied"), with responses ranging from 1 ("extremely dissatisfied") to 3 ("generally satisfied"). Areas of relative support were marriage and family, house, job, and neighborhood. Areas of relative stress were friends, health, time, financial well-being, extended family, amount of education, and job security.

Dr. C.'s responses placed him at the 26–31st percentile on this measure. His mean response was 3.1 ("generally satisfied"), with responses ranging from 2 ("somewhat dissatisfied") to 5 ("extremely satisfied"). Areas of relative support were employment, community, extended family, nuclear family, neighborhood, money for necessities, religion, home, new educational endeavors, own health, and friends. Areas of relative stress were partner's health, his children, time, money for luxuries, and saving. In general, information from this measure was consistent with the ecomap, FILE, and interview information.

F-COPES is a measure of family coping strategies. Of the five coping strategies, four were used by Dr. C. and Mrs. K. Reframing was the most used by the couple (94th and 91st percentiles, respectively). Acquiring Social Support was used frequently by Mrs. K. (95th percentile) and less by Dr. C. (53rd percentile). Passive Appraisal (28th percentile for Dr. C. and 57th for Mrs. K.) and Mobilizing the Family to Seek and Accept Help from community (57th percentile for Dr. C. and 44th for Mrs. K.) were also utilized. Neither partner resorted to Spiritual Support. On the total scale, Dr. C. fell at the 39th percentile, while Mrs. K. fell at the 55th.

Overall, Mrs. K. was much more active in exploiting coping resources than was Dr. C. He was particularly less likely to reach out to friends, perhaps because of his feelings of isolation when he lost his best friend and/or due to the perceived awkwardness caused by his relationship in the community. Both wanted and needed more friends. Therapy, joint or individual, might also provide some support; they were both open to the use of professionals as a means of coping.

The Family Strengths instrument, developed by the Minnesota group but not discussed earlier in this chapter, was the last given to the couple. Consisting of 12 items, it taps two factors: Family Pride, which identifies loyalty, pride, trust, and respect within the family toward the family as a whole; and Accord, which taps a family's self-perception of competence. On the total scale, Dr. C. fell at the 67th percentile with high family pride and moderate accord; he noted particular concerns about recurring problems and conflict. Mrs. K. fell at the 39th percentile, also with high family pride, but with fairly low accord. She noted difficulties in accomplishing things, recurring problems, and a tendency to worry about things and to be critical of one another.

Family Responses to Feedback

Session 4 Continued

The results of the assessment stimulated much discussion among the family. Generally, the discussion highlighted Kurt's role bridged between his parents. While Kurt had learned to thrive on the attention this role gave him, the pressures had gotten too great. He clearly wanted and needed relief.

Dr. C. agreed with the psychologist's interpretation of the assessment findings, but was concerned about the impact on Mrs. K. Mrs. K. did not deny the interpretation, but initially seemed unsure of how to respond to the information. She acknowledged her mild depression and agreed that it related to her impaired sense of physical integrity as a result of her surgery and to her loss of social status and wealth. She was unsure of its relationship to any unresolved mourning over her broken marriage. Late adolescent experiences that impaired her ability to trust men were explored after the children were asked to leave at their mother's request.

Mrs. K. was surprised by the extent to which Dr. C. was unhappy about aspects of their relationship. Personality issues and their handling of finances and conflicts were of particular interest to her. Although Mrs. K. had been taking the attitude that she was not going to marry and Dr. C. could do what he wanted to about it, it was clear that she was very concerned about his level of satisfaction with the situation. An exploration of the feelings of both partners in relation to areas of concern identified by ENRICH consumed the remainder of the session. A final session with the couple was scheduled. They were asked to think, over the course of the next week, of ways in which conflict generated by unfinished business over the Koehler divorce might be resolved. Strategies for rebuilding a social circle, increasing social support for the relationship, increasing amounts of time spent having fun together and separately, and reducing life stress were also identified for discussion at the final session with the couple.

Because the family had given their permission for the psychologist to write up their case for inclusion in a book chapter, they were given a copy of the write-up to review prior to the final session. They were asked to read the report for clinical accuracy, as well as for their comfort with the degree to which the psychologist disguised the family to protect its privacy.

The Fifth and Final Session

The couple returned alone for the final session. Mrs. K. was concerned about the psychologist's conclusion in the report that many of the family's difficulties stemmed from the unresolved "emotional divorce" between the Koehlers. While she admitted that she and Mr. Koehler were still emotionally involved with one another, she felt that she had done everything she could to strengthen Kurt's relationship with his father. She denied that she, Kurt, and Mr. Koehler were involved in a triangle that was immobilizing Kurt developmentally. In addition, both Mrs. Koehler and Dr. Cottingwood noted some minor inaccuracies in the facts reported. (These have been amended into the final version of this case study as presented above.)

The psychologist and Dr. C. helped Mrs. K. explore her interpretation of family dynamics before Dr. C. presented his view. He agreed with the psychologist that two triangles were operating that were destructive to family relationships, i.e., the Kurt, Mr. K., and Mrs. K. threesome and the Mr. K., Mrs. K., and Dr. C. triangle. He felt that not only did Kurt have problems when his mother drew too close to his father, but so did he. Additional comments that Kurt had made, presented in this report, were mentioned by Dr. C. in support of his position.

After much discussion of the three adult relationships, the couple moved to describing changes they had made in response to the information from ENRICH, the marital inventory. Much of their focus on the report at home had centered on Dr. C.'s hesitance in sharing his feelings and Mrs. K.'s unsettled feelings as a result of being informed about his views. They felt that they had grown much closer through hashing over the validity of the report as it related to couple interactions.

The session then shifted to a focus on the issue of marriage. The couple decided not to force things given the amount of stress they had undergone in the last year. However, they planned to set a rough timeline by which to make a decision. In the interim, they planned to look into legal ways that Mrs. K. might protect her antiques and personal property if a divorce occurred after they married. Mrs. K. had talked to Mr. K. and they had reached an agreement that she would not argue with him in front of the children or harangue him about the divorce settlement if he would get his child support payments in on schedule. They had also decided, with Kurt's originally tentative consent, that Kurt would go to Europe with his father on a 3-week trip early in the summer.

In regard to increasing social support and reducing stress, a number of ideas were generated within the session. To increase the amount of fun time the couple had together, they decided to set aside an adults-only-cocktail-hour-and-unwinding-session at home. The children would be asked to play elsewhere during that period. Dr. C. also planned to take a 7-day camping trip with one of his sons and Kurt early in the summer, while Mrs. K. went on a museum and shopping trip with Gisela and her mother in a nearby city.

The remaining issues of financial conflict, Dr. C.'s reluctance to share his feelings, Dr. C.'s relationship with his children, and the rebuilding of their social circle were discussd thoroughly with no firm plans formulated. The couple did not feel, and the psychologist agreed, that they needed ongoing marriage or family counseling. The adults ended the session with an agreement that they and/or Kurt would feel free to return if further difficulties arose. They would use the information from the assessment and their own family and individual strengths to attempt to resolve their problems before seeking further assistance.

Postscript

Mrs. K. and Dr. C. dropped by the psychologist's office after school one and a half months after the fifth session. They were in a good mood, holding hands and joking. They announced that they were planning to set a wedding date soon. Since the last meeting, Mrs. K. had sharply curtailed her interactions with Mr. K., and Kurt was getting along better with his father, teachers, and peers. Dr. C. was playing racketball regularly with several men, which was helping him deal with increased pressure at work, and the couple had instituted a monthly overnight getaway for the two of them. Mrs. K. was still having health problems of a minor but irritating nature, and she needed her own fun activity comparable to racketball to help her unwind. She was looking into various activities she could do with a girlfriend.

They wanted the psychologist to know that the assessment experience had been *very* helpful for them. They particularly liked having a written report, even though they realized that it was not part of the standard procedure. Having the report to go back to, as opposed to their memories of what had been said in the family sessions, allowed them to return to it and the issues it addressed repeatedly and more fruitfully. Mrs. K. also said that she liked being able to challenge the therapist on some misconceptions that Mrs. K. would have been unaware of without the knowledge of what the psychologist thought. Mrs. K. wondered in her own work how often she and her clients left a session with very different perceptions of what had occurred. Without a report, or regular contact, there was no opportunity to discuss and interact with assessment information and resultant treatment recommendations.

Summary

Family assessment is of definite value and importance to the comprehensive assessment of child and adolescent personality; this chapter has presented its unique contribution and perspective to the assessment process. Within the family assessment approach, an ecological and systems perspective was endorsed emphasizing that child and adolescent behavior is systemically embedded in the context where it occurs, has meaning, and is interactive. When integrated into the stages of family life, this assessment process involves (*a*) gathering information on the referred child's relevant history, current behavior, and academic functioning in the school (and other settings); (b) a formal interview with the entire family, if possible, for clarification of the presenting problem and examination of its functional relationship to school and family factors; (c) gathering descriptive and dynamic information on the family's historical and current environment, structure and dynamics, and levels of adaptation and health; and (d) integrating all significant individual and family variables and characteristics so that decision making in regard to treatment planning and intervention can proceed.

Family assessment was divided into two general and overlapping categories according to their purpose: (a) assessment where the probable source of the presenting problem lies within the family (e.g., covert marital discord), and (b) assessment where the family may need support for a problem that is not directly within their control or responsibility (e.g., childhood autism). The tailoring of the approach and procedures according to assessment purpose was discussed.

Specific procedures and measures were described that could be used in school or child-oriented clinic and family treatment settings. The approaches were limited to interview, self-report, and rating instruments that could be administered and scored by mental health practitioners in office settings. The approach described is appropriately used as but one component of a comprehensive assessment in a psychoeducational setting, but it could serve as the only method in a family treatment setting.

A detailed case study illustrated the use of the family assessment approach and its specific evaluation measures with a family where the identified problem individual was a child with mild learning and behavioral difficulties which related to a parental divorce and family reintegration. The method presented in the case study is much more extensive than would likely be done in either a school, clinic, or family treatment setting. However, the rich detail obtained through the use of multiple interviews and measures was thought to best illustrate the potential of the approach and the specific information obtained with each instrument.

References

Achenbach, T. (1982). *Developmental psychopathology* (2nd ed.). New York: Wiley.

Ackerman, N. (1980). The family with adolescents. In E. A. Carter & M. McGoldrick (Eds.), *The family life cycle: A framework for family therapy* (pp. 147–169). New York: Gardner Press.

Ackerman, N. W. (1937). The family as a special and emotional unit. *Bulletin of the Kansas Mental Hygiene Society, 12,* 1–8.

Ackerman, N. W., & Sobel, R. (1950). Family diagnosis: An approach to the study of the pre-school child. *American Journal of Orthopsychiatry, 20,* 744–752.

Ainsworth, M. D. S., & Bell, S. M. (1970). Attachment, exploration, and separation: Illustrated by the behavior of one-year-olds in a strange situation. *Child Development, 41,* 49–67.

Alexander, J., & Parsons, B. V. (1982). *Functional family therapy.* Monteray, CA: Brooks/Cole.

American Psychological Association. (1981). *Ethical principles of psychologists* (rev. ed.). Washington, DC: Author.

Anderson, C. (1983). An ecological developmental model for a family orientation in school psychology. *Journal of School Psychology, 21,* 179–189.

Atkeson, B. M., & Forehand, R. (1981). Conduct disorders. In E. J. Mash & L. G. Terdal (Eds.), *Behavioral assessment of childhood disorders* (pp. 185–219). New York: Guilford Press.

Barkley, R. A. (1981). Hyperactivity. In E. J. Mash & L. G. Terdal (Eds.), *Behavioral assessment of childhood disorders* (pp. 127–184). New York: Guilford Press.

Barnes, G. (1977). The development of adolescent drinking behavior: An evaluative review of the impact of the socialization process within the family. *Adolescence, 12,* 571–591.

Bateson, G. (1979). *Mind and nature*. New York: E. P. Dutton.

Bateson, G., Jackson, D. D., Haley, J., & Weakland, J. (1956). Toward a theory of schizophrenia. *Behavioral Science, 1*, 251–264.

Belsky, J. (1980). Child maltreatment: An ecological integration. *American Psychologist, 35*, 320–335.

Belsky, J. (1984). The determinants of parenting: A process model. *Child Development, 55*, 83–96.

Bowen, M. (1978). *Family therapy in clinical practice*. New York: Jason Aronson.

Brassard, M. R., & Anderson, C. W. (1983). *A family orientation for school psychology: The results of a national survey*. Unpublished manuscript available from Marla Brassard, Department of Educational Psychology, 325 Aderhold Hall, University of Georgia, Athens.

Bronfenbrenner, U. (1977). Toward an experimental ecology of human development. *American Psychologist, 32*, 513–531.

Bronfenbrenner, U. (1979). *The ecology of human development: Experiments by nature and design*. Cambridge, MA: Harvard University Press.

Brook, J., Lukoff, I., & Whiteman, M. (1978). Family socialization and adolescent personality and their association with adolescent use of marijuana. *Journal of Genetic Psychology, 133*, 261–271.

Cantwell, D. P. (1972). Psychiatric illness in the families of hyperactive children. *Archives of General Psychiatry, 27*, 414–427.

Cantwell, D. P. (1978). Hyperactivity and antisocal behavior. *Journal of the American Academy of Child Psychiatry, 1*, 252–262.

Carter, E. A., & McGoldrick, M. (1980a). *The family life cycle: A framework for family therapy*. New York: Gardner Press.

Carter, E. A., & McGoldrick, M. (1980b). The family life cycle and family therapy: An overview. In E. A. Carter & M. McGoldrick, (Eds.), *The family life cycle: A framework for family therapy* (pp. 3–20). New York: Gardner Press.

Conti, A. P. (1975). Variables related to contacting/not contacting counseling services recommended by school psychologists. *Journal of School Psychology, 13*, 41–50.

Duvall, E. (1977). *Marriage and family development* (5th ed.). Philadelphia, PA: Lippincott.

Egeland, B., Sroufe, L. A., & Erickson, M. (1983). The developmental consequences of different patterns of maltreatment. *Child Abuse and Neglect: The International Journal, 7*, 459–469.

Evans, I. M., & Nelson, R. O. (1977). Assessment of child behavior problems. In A. R. Ciminero, K. S. Calhoun, & H. E. Adams (Eds.), *Handbook of behavioral assessment* (pp. 603–681). New York: Wiley.

Filsinger, E. E. (Ed.). (1983). *Marriage and family assessment*. Beverly Hills, CA: Sage Publications.

Filsinger, E. E., & Lewis, R. A. (Eds.). (1981). *Assessing marriage: New behavioral approaches*. Beverly Hills: Sage Publications.

Forehand, R., Sturgis, E., McMahon, R. J., Aguar, D., Green, K., Wells, K. C., & Breiner, J. (1979). Parent behavorial training to modify child noncompliance: Treatment generalization across time and from home to school. *Behavior Modification, 3*, 3–25.

Forehand, R., Wells, K. C., McMahon, R. J., & Griest, D., & Rodgers, T. (1982). Maternal perception of maladjustment in clinic referred children: An extension of earlier research. *Journal of Behavioral Assessment, 4*, 145–151.

Garbarino, J., Sebes, J., & Schellenbach, C. (1984). Families at risk for destructive parent-child relations in adolescence. *Child Development, 55*, 174–183.

Gil, D. G. (1968). Incidence of child abuse and demographic characteristics of persons involved. In R. E. Helfer & C. H. Kempe (Eds.), *The battered child* (pp. 19–40). Chicago, IL: University of Chicago Press.

Gil, D. G. (1970). *Violence against children: Physical child abuse in the United States*. Cambridge, MA: Harvard University Press.

Goodman, D. W., & Guze, S. B. (1979). *Psychiatric diagnois*. London & New York: Oxford University Press.

Gordon, R. A. (1967). Issues in the ecological study of delinquency. *American Sociological Review, 32*, 927–944.

Gottman, J. M. (1979). *Marital interaction: Experimental investigations*. New York: Academic Press.

Gottman, J. M. (1982). Temporal form: Toward a new language for describing relationships. *Journal of Marriage and the Family, 44*, 943–962.

Green, K., & Fine, M. J. (1980). Family therapy: A case for training school psychologists. *Psychology in the Schools, 17*, 241–248.

Griest, D., Wells, K. C., & Forehand, R. (1979). An examination of predictors of maternal perceptions of maladjustment in clinic referred children. *Journal of Abnormal Psychology, 88*, 277–281.

Guidubaldi, J. (1980). The status report extended: Further elaborations on the American family. *School Psychology Review, 9*, 374–379.

Guidubaldi, J., Cleminshaw, H. K., Perry, J. D., & McLoughlin, C. S. (1983). The impact of parental divorce on children: Report of the nationwide NASP study. *School Psychology Review, 12*, 300–323.

Haley, J. (1959). The family of the schizophrenic: A model system. *Journal of Nervous and Mental Disease, 129*, 357–374.

Haley, J. (1973). *Uncommon therapy: The psychiatric techniques of Milton H. Erickson.* New York: Norton.

Hartman, A. (1979). *Finding families: An ecological approach to family assessment in adoption.* Beverly Hills, CA: Sage Publications.

Hazzard, A., & Christensen, A. (no date). *Parent Perception Inventory.* Available from Andrew Christensen, Department of Psychology, University of California, Los Angeles, CA.

Hazzard, A., Christensen, A., & Margolin, G. (1983). Children's perception of parental behaviors. *Journal of Abnormal Child Psychology, 11*, 49–60.

Henderson, A. S., Byrne, D. G., & Duncan-Jones, P. (1982). *Neurosis and the social environment.* New York: Academic Press.

Henderson, S., Duncan-Jones, P., Byrne, D. G., & Scott, R. (1980). Measuring social relationships: The interview schedule for social interaction. *Psychological Medicine, 10*, 723–734.

Hetherington, E. M., Cox, M., & Cox, R. (1979). Play and social interaction in children following divorce. *Journal of Social Issues, 35*, 26–49.

Hetherington, E. M., & Martin, B. (1979). Family interaction. In H. C. Quay & J. S. Werry (Eds.), *Psychopathological disorders of childhood* (2nd ed., pp. 247–302). New York: Wiley.

Hill, R. (1964). Methodological problems with the developmental approach to family study. *Family Process, 3*, 5–22.

Hill, R. (1970). *Family development in three generations.* Cambridge, MA: Schenkman.

Hill, R., & Rogers, R. (1964). The developmental approach. In H. T. Christensen (Ed.), *Handbook of marriage and the family.* Chicago, IL: Rand McNally.

Hobbs, N. (1966). Helping disturbed children: Psychological and ecological strategies. *American Psychologist, 21*, 1101–1115.

Hobbs, N. (1975). *The futures of children.* San Francisco, CA: Jossey-Bass.

Hoffman, L. (1981). *Foundations of family therapy.* New York: Basic Books.

Hogan, R., DeSoto, C. B., & Solano, C. (1977). Traits, tests, and personality research. *American Psychologist, 32*, 255–264.

Holman, A. M. (1983). *Family assessment: Tools for understanding and intervention.* Beverly Hills, CA: Sage Publications.

Holmes, T. H., & Raye, R. (1967). The social readjustment rating scale. *Journal of Psychosomatic Research, 11*, 213–218.

Huston, T. L., & Robins, E. (1982). Conceptual and methodological issues in studying close relationships. *Journal of Marriage and the Family, 44*, 901–925.

Jacobs, J. (1971). *Adolescent suicide.* New York: Wiley-Interscience.

Jenson, W. R., & Young, R. K. (in press). Childhood autism: Developmental considerations and behavioral treatment through core management programs by staff, family, and peers. in R. McMahon & R. DeV. Peters (Eds.), *Childhood disorders: Behavioral-developmental approaches.* New York: Brunner/Mazel.

Karpel, M. A., & Strauss, E. S. (1983). *Family evaluation.* New York: Gardner Press.

Knoff, H. M. (1983). Personality assessment in the schools: Issues and procedures for school psychologists. *School Psychology Review, 12*, 391–398.

Koppitz, E. (1982). Personality assessment in the schools. In C. R. Reynolds & T. B. Gutkin (Eds.), *Handbook of school psychology* (pp. 273–295). New York: Wiley.

Kurdek, L. A. (Ed.). (1983). *Children and divorce.* San Francisco, CA: Jossey-Bass.

Lambert, N. M., Hartsough, C. S., & Bower, E. M. (1979). *Process for the assessment of effective student functioning: Administration and use manual.* Monteray, CA: Publisher's Test Service, CBT/McGraw-Hill.

Lavigne, J. V., & Burns, W. J. (1981). *Pediatric psychology: An introduction for pediatricians and psychologists.* New York: Grune & Stratton.

Lobitz, G. K., & Johnson, S. M. (1975). Normal versus deviant children: A multimethod comparison. *Journal of Abnormal Child Psychology, 3*, 353–374.

Lorion, R. P., Cowen, E. L., & Caldwell, R. A. (1974). Problem types of children referred to a school-based mental health program. *Journal of Consulting and Clinical Psychology, 42*, 491–496.

Lovaas, O. I. (1978). Parents and therapists. In M. Rutter & E. Schoplear (Eds.), *Autism: A reappraisal of concepts and treatments* (pp. 369–378). New York: Plenum Press.

Margolin, G., & Fernandez, V. (1983). Other marriage and family questionnaires. In E. E. Filsinger (Ed.), *Marriage and family assessment: A sourcebook for family therapy* (pp. 317–338). Beverly Hills, CA: Sage Publications.

Mash, E. J., & Terdal, L. G. (1981). Behavioral assessment of childhood disturbance. In E. J. Mash & L. G. Terdal (Eds), *Behavioral assessment of childhood disorders* (pp. 3–76). New York: Guilford Press.

McArthur, D. S., & Roberts, G. E. (1982). *Roberts Apperception Test for Children Manual*. Los Angeles, CA: Western Psychological Services.

McConville, B. (1983). Depression and suicide in children and adolescents. In P. D. Steinhauer & Q. Rae-Grant (Eds.), *Psychological problems of the child in the family* (2nd ed., pp. 277–292). New York: Basic Books.

McCubbin, H. I., & Patterson, J. M. (1983). Stress: The family inventory of life events and changes. In. E. E. Filsinger (Ed.), *Marriage and family assessment: A sourcebook for family therapy* (pp. 275–315). Beverly Hills, CA: Sage Publications.

Melamed, B. G., & Johnson, S. B. (1981). Chronic illness: Asthma and juvenile diabetes. In E. J. Mash & L. G. Terdal (Eds.), *Behavioral assessment of childhood disorders* (pp. 529–572). New York: Guilford Press.

Minuchin, S. (1974). *Families and family therapy*. Cambridge, MA: Harvard University Press.

Minuchin, S., Baker, L., Rosman, B., Liebman, R., Milman, L., & Todd, T. (1975). A conceptual model of psychosomatic illness in children. *Archives of General Psychiatry, 32*, 1031–1038.

Minuchin, S., Rosman, B. L. & Baker, L. (1978). *Psychosomatic families: Anorexia nervosa in context*. Cambridge, MA: Harvard University Press.

Mischel, W. (1968). *Personality and assessment*. New York: Wiley.

Mischel, W. (1977). On the future of personality measurement. *American Psychologist, 32*, 246–254.

Moos, R. H., & Insel, P. M. (Eds.). (1974). *Issues is social ecology*. Palo Alto, CA: National Press Books.

Moos, R. H., & Moos, B. S. (1981). *Family Environment Scale Manual*. Palo Alto, CA: Consulting Psychologists Press.

Moos, R. H., & Moos, B. S. (1983). Clinical applications of the Family Environment Scale. In E. E. Filsinger (Ed.), *Marriage and family assessment: A sourcebook for family therapy* (pp. 253–273). Beverly Hills, CA: Sage Publications.

Murphy, A., Pueschel, S., & Schneider, J. (1973). Group work with parents of children with Down's Syndrome. *Social Casework, 54*, 114–117.

Olson, D. H., McCubbin, H. I., Barnes, H., Larsen, A., Muxen, M., & Wilson, M. (1982, June). *Family Inventories*. Can be obtained by writing to Dr. David Olson, Family Social Science, 290 McNeal Avenue, University of Minnesota, St. Paul, MN 55108.

Olson, D. H., McCubbin, H. I., Barnes, H., Larsen, A., Muxen, M., & Wilson, M. (1983). *Families: What makes them work*. Beverly Hills, CA: Sage Publications.

Olson, D. H., & Portner, J. (1983). Family adaptability and cohesion and evaluation scales. In E. E. Filsinger (Ed.), *Marriage and family assessment: A sourcebook for family therapy* (pp. 299–315). Beverly Hills, CA: Sage Publications.

Olson, D. H., Russell, C. S., & Sprenkle, D. H. (1979). Circumplex model of marital and family systems II: Empirical studies and clinical intervention. In J. Vincent (Ed.), *Advances in family intervention, assessment and theory*. Greenwich, CT: JAI.

Olson, D. H., Sprenkle, D. H., & Russell, C. S. (1979). Circumplex model of marital and family systems: I. Cohesion and adaptability dimensions, family types, and clinical application. *Family Process, 18*, 3–28.

Papp, P. (Ed.). (1977). *Family therapy: Full length case studies*. New York: Gardner Press.

Parke, R. D., & Collmer, C. W. (1975). Child abuse: An interdisciplinary analysis. In E. M. Hetherington (Ed.), *Review of child development research* (Vol. 5, pp. 509–590). Chicago, IL: University of Chicago Press.

Parkes, C. M., & Stevenson-Hinde, J. (Eds.). (1982). *The place of attachment in human behavior*. New York: Basic Books.

Pervin, L. (Ed.). (1975). *Personality: Theory, assessment and research* (2nd ed.). New York: Basic Books.

Petrie, P., & Piersel, W. C. (1982). Family therapy. In C. R. Reynolds & T. B. Gutkin (Eds.), *The handbook of school psychology* (pp. 580–590). New York: Wiley.

Plas, J. M. (1981). The psychologist in the school community: A liaison role. *School Psychology Review, 10*, 72–81.

Prout, H. T. (1983). School psychologists and social emotional assessment techniques: Patterns in training and use. *School Psychology Review, 12*, 377–383.

Rhodes, W. C. (1967). The disturbing child: A problem of ecological management. *Exceptional Children, 33*, 637–642.

Roberts, G., McArthur, D., Roid, G., Zachary, R. A., & Reynolds, C. (1983). Development of a new apperception test for children (Summary). *Proceedings of the Convention of the National Association of School Psychologists*, 11–12.

Salzinger, S., Kaplan, S., & Artemyeff, C. (1983). Mothers' personal social networks and child maltreatment. *Journal of Abnormal Psychology, 92*, 68–76.

Thomas, A. (1982, October). Runaways. In J. Grimes (proj. coord.). *Psychological approaches to problems of children and adolescents* (pp. 157–177). Iowa Dept. of Public Instruction.

von Bertalanffy, L. (1968). *General systems theory*. New York: George Braziller.

Wahler, R. G. (1980). The insular mother: Her problems in parent-child treatment. *Journal of Applied Behavior Analysis*, 13, 207–219.

Wallerstein, J. S., & Kelly, J. B. (1980). *Surviving the breakup: How children and parents cope with divorce*. New York: Basic Books.

Westley, W. A., & Epstein, N. B. (1969). *Silent minority: Families of emotionally healthy college students*. San Francisco, CA: Jossey-Bass.

Yates, M., & Lederer, R. (1961). Small short term group meetings with parents of children with mongolism. *American Journal of Mental Deficiency, 65*, 467–472.

Zins, J. E., & Hopkins, R. A. (1981). Referral out: Increasing the number of kept appointments. *School Psychology Review, 10*, 107–111.

13

Ecological Assessment Procedures

James Garbarino
Shagufa Kapadia

This chapter has been written with two primary goals in mind. First, the rationale and implications of ecological assessment are presented as one necessary component of the comprehensive assessment of child and adolescent personality. Second, the mechanics of some actual ecological assessment procedures are considered and analyzed. A definition and understanding of the ecological assessment of personality is first necessary, however, as a prelude to meeting these goals.

Introduction: What Is an Ecological Assessment of Personality?

The expression "ecological assessment of personality" has two allied meanings. The first involves an evaluation of the character of human collectives, that is, the personality of a natural or artificially collected group. Historians, historically oriented sociologists, and social and community psychologists have been preeminent in developing this approach. Indeed, the study of "national character" has organized and focused much of this work. For example, David Potter's *People of Plenty* (1954) is a most successful treatise on the crucial role of affluence in forming the distinctively American character. Others in this tradition include Webb's *The Great Frontier* (1952), Slater's *The Pursuit of Loneliness* (1970), Riesman's *The Lonely Crowd* (1950), and Marcuse's *One-Dimensional Man* (1964). All have something to say about collective personality. They are joined by social psychologists such as Lewin (1951; see also Lewin, Lippitt, & White, 1939), who sought to assess the character of small groups, using terms like "democratic," "laissez-faire," and "authoritarian."

The second meaning of "ecological assessment of personality" refers to the evaluation of one's personality and/or behavior which results from the interplay

James Garbarino. Erikson Institute for Advanced Study in Child Development, Chicago, Illinois.
Shagufa Kapadia. Department of Individual and Family Studies, College of Human Development, The Pennsylvania State University, University Park, Pennsylvania.

of individual organism and environmental systems. This approach is more in keeping with conventional individually oriented personality studies and seeks to understand personality as the joint product of a developing individual and a developing environment. While this assessment may lead to a concern with national character, it places greater emphasis on the active contribution of individual human variation (such as temperamental differences) in producing individual character. This second definition leads to a concern with more sociobiological and psychohistorical orientations. Exemplifying this tradition are Freud's *Civilization and Its Discontents* (1930), Horney's *The Neurotic Personality of Our Time* (1937), Naroll's *The Moral Order* (1983), and Wilson's *Sociobiology: The New Synthesis* (1975).

The concern in this chapter is the assessment of environmental systems which interact with individual characteristics on a community and institutional rather than a national or societal level. As other chapters in this book deal extensively with assessing individual psychology and Chapter 12 deals with family assessments, this ecological discussion will focus on environmental systems beyond the family—school, neighborhood, and peer groups in the community. It thus concentrates on identifying the analogue to theories of individual personality. Previously, the interplay between environmental systems and individual characteristics has been analyzed on the basis of psychodynamic, behavioral, and cognitive-mediation approaches.

Psychodynamic approaches to individual personality emphasize the existence of powerful forces working behind the behavioral scenes in motivated ways; that is, they view behavior as the manifestation of a set of primal forces seeking expression and goal-directed fulfillment. Id, superego, and ego all have agendas, according to psychoanalysts; behavior is but the instrumentality realizing those goals. Some analysts believe that environments beyond the individual and family systems are similarly driven. These individuals detect the indirect expression of such forces in the often subtle and operationally unpredictable interplay among extrafamily systems. Forrester (1971) refers to this in commenting upon the often counterintuitive nature of solutions to system problems. Hardin and Baden (1977) refer to the first law of ecology that "you can never do only one thing" (meaning that unintended and unanticipated consequences are all but inevitable when intervening in systems because systems are driven by internal forces and react to the behavior of other systems on that basis).

Those using a behavioral approach to address the individual-by-environment interplay use environmental assessment to catalogue the balancing and sequencing of reinforcement contingencies. They see no motivating forces at work beyond those operationalized by the reinforcement contingencies themselves. Moos (1976), for example, refers to the principle of progressive conformity—the idea that over time individuals increase their congruence with their environment because of what that environment reinforces. Or, in Winston Churchill's words, "We shape our surroundings and then our surroundings shape us."

From the cognitive-mediation perspective, individuals "create" the environment, and thus it is the phenomenology of "person in the world" that counts most heavily in assessing the ecology of personality. Drawing upon Lewin (1935) and MacLeod (1947), Bronfenbrenner's *Ecology of Human Development* (1979) best exemplifies this tradition. Bronfenbrenner believes that the essence of assessing development lies in analyzing the phenomenology of social experience: "The developmental status of the individual is reflected in the substantive variety and structural complexity of the . . . activities which he initiates and maintains in the absence of instigation or direction by others" (1979, p. 55).

An ecological systems approach emphasizes the complex interdependence of biological, psychological, and social forces in generating personality and the need to address all these forces in conducting personality assessments. Perhaps the distinctive character of this tradition will become clear in counterpoint to an examination of its cousins, ecological psychology and sociological ecology.

Ecological Psychology: The Psychology of Context

Devereux (1977) succinctly states the basic premise of the psychological ecologists: If you want to study the socialization of children, you must study the actual conditions to which they are exposed in whatever part of the real world they are growing up in. Or, as Barker and Wright (1955/1971) put it,

> Psychology has been predominately an experimental science . . . Experimental procedures have revealed something about the laws of behavior, but they have not disclosed, nor can they disclose, how the variables of these laws are distributed in different cultures and conditions of life. . . . Psychologists know little more than laymen about the frequency and degree of occurrence of their basic phenomena in the lives of men—of deprivation, of hostility, of freedom, of friendliness, of social pressure, of rewards and punishments. . . . Because we lack such records, we can only speculate on many important questions like these:
>
> What changes have occurred over the generations in the way children are reared and in the way they behave? How does life differ for children in large and small families? . . . How, in psychological terms, does life differ for rural, town, and urban families? (pp. 1–2)

From Barker and Wright's perspective, any psychological progress in the study of socialization had to begin with greater attention to the actual environmental conditions that impinge upon growing children and shape their developing personalities. This implied the study of socialization in its natural contexts. In making this assertion, however, the ecological psychologists were aligning themselves with a broader ecological perspective which transcended psychology.

Any ecological discussion of human development must consider the contexts or settings in which development occurs. Like the biologist who must study an animal in context by learning about the animal's habitat, sources of food, predators, and social practices, the complete study of people involves examining how people live and grow in the social wild. The term "environment" here includes everything outside the organism. The developing child's setting includes family, friends, neighborhood, and school, as well as less immediate forces such as laws, social attitudes, and institutions that directly or indirectly affect the child (Garbarino et al., 1982). The environment is not an undifferentiated medium in which people are immersed; it clearly involves a variety of active or dynamic processes which selectively spur, guide, and restrain behavior. Thus, these dynamic processes must be studied within the environment.

What is more, the social environment is motivated: It actively penetrates the psychological world of children and modifies their behavior. That is, behavioral opportunities and constraints come from the environment or setting as a social system. Once entered, the setting elicits and reinforces a distinct package of behaviors, a package that constitutes an analogue to personality. To an extent that depends upon the totality of the setting and the duration of involvement, the child ultimately comes to incorporate and manifest the personality of the milieu (Gump, 1975).

Relating Setting to Personality

Some work has been done to translate the basic assumptions, principles, and hypotheses discussed above into approaches for personality assessment. Of particular interest are efforts to assess the predominant character of environmental settings. Such assessments may provide information analogous to the results of individual, person-oriented assessments while also providing insight into the dynamic relationship between the setting and the individual.

Devereux (1977) aptly suggests that an understanding of a setting's functioning as an ecological system (or ecosystem) is based on one's knowledge about its structure and the dynamic processes involved in its operation. Here the task of a psychological ecologist is twofold. Initially, the ecologist must extend descriptions of the psychologically relevant characteristics of local settings to include and analyze the ways that these behavioral settings are actually used by children. Barker and Schoggen (1973) operationalize this analysis through a classification system which was developed to describe the various dimensions of the two intensively studied towns (Midwest and Yoredale). Barker and Schoggen identified four components to their comprehensive analysis of settings. Each refers to an important aspect of setting: source of authority, locus of autonomy, expectations for attendance, and relation to child well-being.

1. Authority is a classification according to the source of authority controlling the town's behavior settings. This includes churches, government agencies, private enterprises, schools, and voluntary associations. Each mixes one or more source of authority—spiritual, legal, contractual, historical, or consensual. A church has spiritual authority as its primary basis and some authority on the basis of its traditions of service to members and the community, but it has no legal authority. Government agencies, in contrast, have no spiritual authority but much legal and contractual authority.

2. Autonomy is a classification according to whether the locus of authority lies within the town or outside of it. There are three categories: high, medium, or low local autonomy. The existence of state laws for government agencies, cardinals for Catholic churches, corporate headquarters for local factories, and national councils for clubs all illustrate how local autonomy can be low.

3. Attendance is a classification of behavior settings based on whether attendance by children or adolescents is required, encouraged, neutral, discouraged, or prohibited. School is at one end of this continuum, while adult-only theaters are at the other.

4. Child or adolescent beneficence is a classification of behavior settings based on whether they are intended to benefit children or adolescents directly or indirectly, whether they are neutral in this respect, or whether they provide opportunities for children or adolescents to benefit others. A school is direct, while a factory hiring the child's parents is indirect.

Each of these setting characteristics has an approximate analogue in the personality of individuals. We might appropriately liken the authority dimension to the various maturational patterns associated with authoritarianism, N achievement, N affiliation, and the like; the autonomy dimension to internal/external locus of control; the attendance dimension to compulsive approach versus phobic avoidance; and the child/adolescent beneficence dimension to the kind of self versus other orientation identified by Carol Gilligan (1982) in her analysis of male and female personality development.

The ecologist's second task is to determine the proportion of a child's whole life-space that is spent in settings with specific characteristics, for example, in school classes, in church, or at home. Life-space refers to the Lewinian (1931, 1935, 1951) idea that "the environment of greatest relevance for the scientific understanding of behavior and development is reality not as it exists in the so-called objective world but as it appears in the mind of the person" (Bronfenbrenner, 1979, p. 23). This is the "psychological field" in which meaningful behavior takes place. Ideally, the creation of setting-specific or local "norms" will discriminate how these patterns of usage differ for children of different ages, genders, and social classes. Such information enables the psychological ecologist to make some inferences or to generate hypotheses about possibly different socialization outcomes. In general, the psychological ecologist assumes that the total habitat is more than simply an additive summation of its parts. Rather, it is a meaningful whole, and this is likely to affect a habitat's influence as a socialization setting for its children. Thus, for example, the psychological effects of a "permissive" family setting existing in conjunction with an authoritarian school or church may be quite different from the same family setting reinforced by an equally permissive school or church. Devereux's (1977) perspective, then, argues for an appreciation for the interactive or synergistic effects of settings that "exist" phenomenologically as life-spaces for human action.

The assessment technique proposed by the ecological psychologists to evaluate the second task is the "specimen record"—a detailed account of the moment-by-moment movement of a target individual into and out of specific settings (see Appendix C for an example). This specimen record then becomes the raw material for a classification scheme. The special language of that classification scheme has proved daunting to many investigators (see Barker & Schoggen, 1973, for its elements). It includes a plethora of concepts such as "centiurb," "action pattern," "behavior mechanisms," "operatives," "environmental force units," "program," and "synomorphic." The basic idea of conducting an ecological assessment on the basis of specimen records remains appealing, however, and we will return to it later. The big issue is whether it is possible to use the technology apart from the prohibitive jargon (Devereux, 1977).

Perhaps the most striking application of the principles and techniques of ecological psychology came in Barker and Gump's (1964) classic study of midwestern high schools (Devereux, 1977). Using school size as an intervening variable, the total habitat of a high school was found to vary significantly up through a ceiling size where additional effects were negligible (Garbarino, 1980c; Garbarino & Asp, 1981). Barker and Gump's study revealed that although the small high schools had fewer settings (units of the school system: types of classes, athletic contests, clubs, extracurricular activities) than the larger high schools (those with a grade 9–12 enrollment of 500 or more), the ratio of students to settings was nonetheless lower.

Additional evidence suggested that these schools evidenced different characters or personalities as a function of size (Garbarino, 1980c). For example, the big schools were characterized by more passive and elitist functions, the smaller schools by active involvement and incentives for participation; that is, big school activities most often cast youth in the role of "observer," "audience," or "follower"; only the most competent elites had active leadership roles. Small schools presented settings that resulted in more experience in active leadership roles for more youth and a greater subjective sense of involvement and responsibilities. In short, small schools presented a different life-space than did big schools for most youth. This is because the big schools were "overmanned" (more people available than required to operate the behavioral settings) while the small schools were "undermanned" (less people than required). According to Barker and Gump, when a particular setting is undermanned, there is more pressure per member to fill responsible roles because more people must be active to competently complete the task. Thus, in the smaller schools, on the average, more students would be pressured to get involved in a broader range of different settings and in more responsible or pivotal roles in them. Indeed, in the small schools of their study, the median number of extracurricular activities of graduating seniors was 10.5, while the comparable figure for the larger school was only 3.4. From this ecological psychology perspective, this environmental pressure or demand should affect individual students' general personality and behavioral styles and development. The personality of students should come to reflect the personality of their school.

Ecological psychology's second major application has been to small towns and, later, to urban neighborhoods (Devereux, 1977; Gump & Adelberg, 1978). Barker and Wright (1955/1971) theorized extensively about how a small undermanned town such as Midwest might compensate to provide the necessary socialization experiences for its children. They hypothesized that the town with a small total population relative to its total number of settings will expect its people to participate more broadly and intensely in these settings. The formative population groups, including the town's children and teenagers, will be encouraged to participate and accept responsible roles in order to keep the system functioning. This would result in more mixed-age settings where children and teenagers would work with or for adults and have increased opportunities to observe and learn about adults in roles beyond the typical parent, teacher, and youth leader roles. Results obtained tended to confirm these hypotheses in contrasting small and big towns and self-contained versus diffuse urban neighborhoods, respectively (Gump & Adelberg, 1978).

Bronfenbrenner (1979), expanding the primarily objective character of Barker and Wright's ecological psychology, discusses the "phenomenology of human ecology." What is more, he answers Devereux's (1977) criticism that ecological psychology is cut off from the "primary forces" shaping community life, that is, socioeconomic, demographic, political, and cultural change forces. Bronfenbrenner attempts to assess and understand what a particular ecological context means to the persons in it *and* how the primary forces reach down into the life-space of children. Different behavior settings have different impacts on infants, children, adolescents, and adults, in part because they "construct" it differently; that is, every individual's life-space differs. As we shall see, this phenomenological orientation has important applications for techniques of ecological assessment. But first, the "objective" physical and social environments that provide the raw material for one's life-space must be addressed.

Objective Conditions: Environmental Psychology

Wohlwill and van Vliet (1984) state that in spite of the general tendency for psychologists to disregard the physical environment as a factor, behavior is functionally related to characteristics and attributes of the physical environment. He distinguishes among three forms of this relationship. First, behavior necessarily occurs in some particular environmental context. The environment structures, organizes, and defines the range of behaviors permissible in it and often encourages or restricts particular aspects or patterns of individual behavior. For example, an environment devoid of printed material provides no occasion for reading and may lead to diminished self-esteem if the individual encounters settings in which success depends upon literacy. Second, certain qualities of the environment, such as under- or overstimulation and crowding or isolation, may elicit generalized behavior or reactions which affect broader systems of response within the individual. For example, a dangerous environment may discourage exploratory behavior and promote parental restrictiveness. Third, specific attributes of an environment may combine with individual characteristics in powerful ways. For example, a person confined to a wheelchair may be "liberated" by a barrier-free school or "enslaved" by one that has no ramp access or elevators, with a corresponding enhancement of diminution of self-esteem.

Once again, we are drawn to some approximate analogue in the domain of individual personality. Biologically oriented students of individual personality direct our attention to the neurological substrates of emotion and thought. Similarly, students of temperament tell us that general reaction styles color personality traits. Finally, the psychoanalytic and behaviorist views are united in asserting that specific fears can inhibit development.

Basing his approach upon Murray's (1938) conceptualization of the dual process of "personal needs" and "environmental press," Moos (1975) has suggested an empirical approach to assessing "social climate." This conception begins with the axiom that every institution has a personality, a set of characteristic goals, motivations, and styles of operation. The basic idea behind the Moos technique is that the consensus of participants in an environment constitutes a measure of that environment's social climate (Moos, 1975). How does one assess social climate? What does one ask? One asks people to respond to a series of descriptive and evaluative statements about the environment in which they participate. What are the themes? They are three in number: Relationship, Personal Development/Personal Growth, and System Maintenance/System Change. The respondent's true/false responses to the Real Program, the Ideal Program, and the Expected Program tell the story.

Relationship focuses on the quality and character of personal relationships in an environment in terms of support, help, spontaneity, free and open expression, and involvement. Of course, these dimensions are operationalized somewhat differently for different settings (e.g., family vs. prison vs. university). Personal Development refers to the individual mission of the setting. For example, autonomy is important for correctional facilities and hospitals, while academic achievement is a big issue for schools and families (Moos, 1975). System Maintenance/System Change is a similar issue across types of settings: order, clarity of expectations, maintaining control, and responsiveness to change. The nine variations of the Social Climate Scale reflect commonalities and variabilities across settings on these three primary concerns (i.e., Relationship, Development, and System).

Research conducted by Moos and others documents that the social climate of settings and the interaction between setting and individual account for a major proportion of the variance in behaviors linked to personality, for example, from "aggressivenes" to "talkativeness" (Moos, 1975). Research employing the Social Climate Scale has demonstrated its usefulness in uncovering differences in correctional institutions, juvenile delinquency intervention programs, schools, hospitals, families, and other settings. The Scale provides an important technology for conducting a comprehensive personality assessment by operationalizing the environment term in the classic theorem that states that behavior is a function of person and environment.

The Developmental Nature of Ecological Psychology

As has been said, from the perspective of ecological psychology, "behavior settings are coercive of behavior. People who enter a setting are pressed to help enact its program (while at the same time using the setting for their own purposes)" (Gump & Adelberg, 1978, p. 174). The presence, strength, and dynamic balance among environmental forces differ across contrasting settings. "Environmental press" (Murray, 1938) refers to the combined influence of forces working in an environment to shape the behavior and development of individuals in that setting; it is the force that alters personality to conform to setting through modeling, reinforcing, and extinguishing the specific behaviors, thoughts, and feelings that comprise personality. Environmental press arises when environmental circumstances surround and confront an individual, generate a psychosocial momentum, and guide that individual in a particular direction. Indeed, when the setting is "total," personality changes can be quite dramatic (Goffman, 1961). Apart from the environment's contribution to these individual–environment transactions, the individual possesses and contributes specific personal resources and a developmental status to the situation. Thus, the complement of environmental forces does not exclusively determine all outcomes for an organism; the individual organism is (or can be) a significant influence as well in its own right.

Individual personality, therefore, can play a major role in mediating the impact of environmental conditions. For example, research on the personality of neglectful mothers (the "Apathy/Futility Syndrome") indicates that they are less likely to perceive and act positively within their neighborhood as a social environment. Such individuals evidence a chronic, vicious cycle in which their own self-isolating attitudes and behaviors interact with the distancing rsponses of neighbors (to produce ever-increasing and profound social isolation) (Polansky, Chalmers, Buttenwieser, & Williams, 1981).

Different people may react differently to the same environment, and the same environment may interact differently with the same person at different times. For example, the same busy street that is a life-threatening and fear-instigating challenge to a 4-year-old child may be a developmentally appropriate challenge that enhances the self-esteem of a 9-year-old child. For the personality development of a teenager, it may be irrelevant because it is only a mild inconvenience. The same street may go unnoticed by a 30-year-old single adult, but become an obsession for the parent of a young child. Finally, this street may be an impenetrable barrier that destroys the self-esteem of a feeble elder. In a similar vein, consider the personality effects of a dangerous neighborhood on two 8-year-olds, one of whom is without adult supervision and protection after school (i.e., a latchkey child), the second of whom comes home to a parent. Preliminary research indicates that problems of fear, impaired school performance, and social isolation are more likely to result when the latchkey experience takes place in a threatening rather than a safe neighborhood environment (Galambos & Garbarino, 1983; Garbarino, 1980b). The relevance of neighborhood safety as an influence on child personality is apparently mediated by parental caregiving and supervision (Long & Long, 1983).

Assessing the personality risk involved in the latchkey phenomenon thus requires an ecological perspective. The same can be said for other social issues affecting personality, such as day care and adolescent sexuality. This leads us to consider the sociological side of environmental assessment.

Sociological Ecology: The Sociology of Context

In contrast to ecological psychology, sociological ecology focuses on developing social entities beyond the interpersonal settings that are Barker and Moos's main focuses. Hawley (*Human Ecology*, 1950) defines human ecology as the study of territorially based systems. This designation refers to a concern with the processes and the form of human adjustment to environment, or more broadly, the prevailing adjustment techniques that maintain a population in its habitat. According to the human ecology perspective, the focus for understanding adjustment is not on individuals acting independently, but on individuals acting collectively to create and maintain cooperative procedures for the division of labor. Adjustment, then, is a collective achievement; the unit of observation is not the individual or even the interpersonal dyad, but the aggregate. Hawley (1950) emphasizes that human ecology deals with one of the central problems of sociology, that is, the development and organization of the community.

The basic hypothesis of human ecology is that as a population develops an organization, it increases its chances of survival in its environment (Hawley, 1950). Organization refers to the entire system of interdependencies among the members of a population which enables them to sustain the community as a unit. Different parts of such a system, such as families, clubs, shops, and factories, cannot be self-sustaining; they can only survive within a network of supporting relationships. This differentiates human ecology from ecological psychology in which the behavioral settings are treated as functionally independent units (cf. Devereux, 1977).

Defining and operationalizing the boundaries of social units has been a persistent problem for sociological human ecology. Also at issue has been the conception of individual human beings as actors within those units. As much as ecological psychology warrants criticism for treating individuals and communities as error variance or black boxes in its calculations, so sociological ecology is justifiably accused of ignoring individuals and social entities as active elements in community evolution. Both approaches lack a developmental focus at the individual level and have social blind spots as well (for one it is the community, for the other it is the behavioral settings).

To establish a comprehensive ecological perspective on human development, we need to expand and integrate ecological psychology and sociological ecology. As Devereux (1977) aptly observes, ecological psychology examines the inner life of human settings without adequately attending to how the community's primary economy produces, maintains, and terminates those settings. Traditional human ecology, on the other hand, focuses precisely on that community role without really attending to how the settings themselves function. Each complements the other. But neither alone nor both together really incorporates the developing and phenomenologically oriented individual organism as an active agent in the human ecology. For example, the newborn shapes the feeding behavior of its mother but, largely confined to a crib or a lap, has limited means of communicating its needs and wants. Its development reflects its own biological agenda, the social psychology for its immediate setting, and the broader economic, demographic, and political forces at work shaping its neighborhood and community. The infant's personality reflects its temperament, the structure and content of parent–child relations, the economic resources available to its parents, the degree to which its birth is normative with respect to parental age and marital status, and the family's access to interpersonal support through its social network.

The 10-year-old, on the other hand, presents different challenges and calls into play new settings. He or she influences many adults and children located in many different settings and has many ways of communicating. His or her development is clearly under the influence of multiple settings within the larger community. No one factor or explanation can adequately convey the course of personality development. The adolescent's world is still larger and more diverse, as is the ability to influence it. The adolescent actively chooses or influences immediate settings in many respects and comes into ever greater contact with the evolving community. The individual and the environment negotiate their relationships over time through a process of reciprocity—neither is constant and each depends on the other.

An Ecological Integration

Once we break out of the circumscribed boundaries of ecological psychology and sociological ecology, we are faced with the enormous challenge of a comprehensive ecological integration. Bronfenbrenner (1979) has provided a useful ecological perspective on human development that integrates ecological psychology and sociological ecology, adding an individual development perspective. He recognizes the importance of individual behavior and development by including the individual as an active biopsychological system in his or her own right. Bronfenbrenner sees the individual's experience "as a set of nested structures, each outside the next, like a set of Russian dolls" (p. 22). Beyond the individual's biopsychological representation are four levels of social systems, which may contain unique sources of developmental risk and opportunity (Garbarino *et al.*, 1982). The placement of these systems in the individual's life-space or phenomenological field constitutes a process of social mapping—with the map projected outward from a specific target individual. Each person's map is somewhat different, as we shall see.

Microsystem
The level most immediate to the developing individual is the microsystem, the actual setting in which the individual experiences and creates day-to-day reality. One of the most important aspects of the microsystem is the existence of relationships that go beyond simple dyads. Microsystems include settings such as

the home, school, and workplace and approximate the behavior setting of ecological psychology (but go beyond that to incorporate the Lewinian phenomenology of life-space). The large body of research on family influences on personality is (to some extent) research on the microsystem.

Mesosystem

The interrelations among major settings containing the developing person constitute the mesosystem. Mesosystems represent the interactions between ecosystem levels and subsystems. They link microsystems such as family and school, peer group and church, and camp and workplace. Thus, they contain the potential for linking different individuals, groups, and cultures. The stronger and more diverse the links between settings, the more powerful the influence of the mesosystem on the individual's development. For example, research on outcomes of residential institutions serving youth shows that postrelease success depends mainly upon how well the institution is linked to enduring social support systems outside (Whittaker, 1979, 1983).

Exosystem

Exosystems are situations where the individual is not directly involved, but which nonetheless have a bearing on the individual's development. They include the major settings in which institutional decisions are made (e.g., local government and corporate headquarters) and settings in which key figures in the individual's life (but not the individual him- or herself) are directly active, thus indirectly influencing the individual (e.g., the parent's workplace in the case of the child). Mapping exosystems illustrates the phenomenological foundation of Bronfenbrenner's ecological approach. One individual's exosystem can be a microsystem for someone else. For example, the workplace is an exosystem for the child, but a microsystem for the parent. Research by Kohn (1977) documents that parental work (and social class) affects child-rearing style; for example, more autonomous work leads to greater value on autonomy.

Macrosystem

The meso- and exosystems are set within the broad ideological and institutional patterns of a particular culture or subculture. This is the macrosystem, a "blueprint" for the ecology of human development. As such, it reflects shared assumptions about "how things should be done" and "human nature." In designating a macrosystem, we are recognizing a coherent set of values and principles suffusing the institutional life of a society, for example, Communist, Capitalist, Democratic, Fascist, Judeo-Christian, Islamic. Research on moral development, for example, shows that national political climate is linked to the content and progress of moral development in childhood and adolescence (Garbarino & Bronfenbrenner, 1976).

This returns us to where we started, namely, "national character." Having come this far, we can begin again with specific issues in ecological assessment. These specific assessment approaches directed at the ecology of children and youth provide guidance for personality assessment and include assessments of childbirth, neighborhood, and social networks.

Case 1: Childbirth: "Family Centeredness" of Hospital Environments

Childbirth is a social event, that is, "an experience in which the roles and status of the participants have a significant effect on their behavior and on the outcomes of the event" (Garbarino, 1980a, p. 6). The character of the birth experience is thus an ecological variable which depends upon the degree of the new mother and father's active participation and the extent to which their "birth process roles" reinforce their later roles as parents. Indeed, a family-centered approach to childbirth can provide an occasion to improve the relationship within families, thus creating potent prosocial support systems.

When we speak of family-centered childbirth, we refer to the creation of an institutional social climate that increases maternal control and awareness, that improves maternal evaluation of the childbirth experience, that increases paternal participation, and that enhances early parent–child attachment (Benn, 1984; Benn & Garbarino, 1982; Garbarino, 1980a). Childbirth is a social act (Newton, 1979) and is not simply a matter of individual temperament, training, physical status, or personality. Sosa, Kennell, Klaus, Robertson, and Urrutia (1980), for example, report empirical documentation for the proposition that the presence of an emotionally responsive companion improves the experience of childbirth and enhances the quality of maternal–infant interaction. Presence of the husband, in particular, in the case of difficult births (e.g., Caesarean sections) is linked to a better prognosis (Benn, 1984).

This appears to apply particularly to economically and socially impoverished families, wherein " . . . we can expect that family-centered childbirth can lead to more normal relationships between the parent and the social environment by spinning off social skills, involvements, and motivation. It can *directly* improve family functioning, and thus *indirectly* enhance child development" (Garbarino, 1980, p. 6). Family-centered childbirth has been linked to preventing child abuse, for example (Garbarino, 1980a).

In a broader context, Danziger (1979a) documents the importance of asymmetry between the layperson (patient) and expert (physician and nurse) as a feature of the social climate in which the childbirth process takes place. She delineates two major variables that contribute to this asymmetry: (*a*) the setting of the interaction, and (*b*) the role repertoire of the individuals. First, the locale and social organization of the encounter is important. For example, one would expect different interactions based on whether the patient visits the physician or the doctor makes house calls—one source of difference being an unfamiliar versus a familiar setting. Second, the pattern of deference versus control exhibited during the encounter may or may not be related to what either party does in other situations. For example, the most submissive patient may be the most noncompliant when out of the doctor's office. Danziger (1979b) also emphasizes the communication with hospital staff as a mediating influence upon the childbearing experience and thereby the initial parenting experience, Block and Block (1975) reported that the more oriented hospital staff were toward family-centered childbirth (in the form of Lamaze training), the less pain women experienced and the better they were able to control pain. The social climate *does* make a significant difference.

Appendix A presents a simple assessment form for determining the degree of family-centeredness in a hospital's obstetrical/pediatric policies and practices

(Garbarino, 1980a). It can serve as a starting point (perhaps in combination with a Moos Social Climate Scale) in assessing the relevance of the setting to personality issues.

Case 2: Childhood: Support and Stress in the Neighborhood

Weiss (1980) maintains that the neighborhood is one of the most proximate and potentially coercive external forces to help shape families as developmental systems. The neighborhood is the place in which parents and children interact with each other and with others independently of the children. Children are participants in the neighborhood too, and are often given the freedom to socialize without the presence of the parents. The quality of the support, encouragement, and feedback given by the neighborhood to the family has an effect upon the child's development (Garbarino *et al.*, 1982). For example, Garbarino and his colleagues (Garbarino & Crouter, 1978; Garbarino & Sherman, 1980) found that the social and economic characters of the neighborhood are linked to the incidence of child maltreatment. High-risk neighborhoods were characterized by negative patterns of interaction *between* families that parallel the patterns *within* families (Burgess & Conger, 1977).

Weiss (1980), discussing a study of different neighborhoods, presents two examples which serve to illustrate the multidimensional power of neighborhoods defined in physical, social, and interactional terms. The cases represent two unmixed extremes, a benevolent versus a malevolent neighborhood influence on childbearing. The two sets of neighborhood perceptions are from white single mothers living on welfare income in a housing project. The following are brief examples from the two cases.

Mrs. Smith is 36 years old and has four children. She says that her neighborhood in the Tallman-South area of Syracuse "could be improved." She is white and feels there is a great deal of racial hostility in her area. She has lived in the neighborhood for 7 months, but does not know any of her neighbors.

Mrs. South, 38 years old with one child, presents a completely different view. She lives in the Eastwood North area of the city and says that "I've got one of the best courts of them all . . . *all* my neighbors are fantastic. . . . We all get along and it's give and take. . . ." Mrs. South feels very secure in her area because "People watch out for everyone" (pp. 64–65).

The two descriptions indicate how different neighborhood ecologies can be, and in turn, suggest what powerful effects they can have on parents and children alike.

Weiss (1980) suggests that there are three dimensions of a neighborhood which are especially important to the parents of small children: (*a*) physical characteristics (e.g., the presence of a park and the upkeep of yards), (*b*) social characteristics (e.g., race, age, and income of neighbors), and (*c*) perceptions of the ways in which the interactions of people in the area affect parenting and child activities. Neighborhood ecologies are not passive; rather, they are actively coercive in the ways they shape the activities of everyday life (Gump, 1975). Appendix B presents an approach designed to assess the neighborhood and community as sources of stress and support for parents. It thus approaches the exosystems and microsystems impinging on the developing child's life. Note that for each domain of life the approach starts with open-ended questions, and it concludes with a scaled evaluation (including a rating by the interviewer). This reflects the phenomenological orientation to life-space. In using this instrument, the open-ended quantitative data are used both to illustrate the analysis of the scaled evaluative ratings and as the basis for content analysis. This approach may be contrasted with the ecological psychologist's specimen records which are narrative in form and reflect an attempt by the observer to be "objective" rather than phenomenological.

Specimen Records

Barker and Wright (1955/1971) made extensive use of specimen records in their classic experiment in Midwest. As they put it, "The specimen record is a detailed, sequential narrative of a long segment of a child's behavior and situation as seen by skilled observers. It describes in concrete detail the stream of the child's behavior and psychological habitat" (p. 15). The social environment of the child, as recorded in specimen records, displays readily recognizable properties of directedness with regard to the child (Barker & Schoggen, 1973).

The scope of specimen records is indeed very wide. Specimen records give a multivariate picture of the molar and molecular characteristics of behaviors and situations. Preserving the continuity of behavior, they enable a study of interrelationships between simultaneous and successive conditions by gathering and reporting behavioral phenomena at the time of their occurrence. One central, distinctive aspect of the specimen records is their theoretically neutral character. Thus, they can serve as useful tools in objectively assessing the psychological aspects of a setting—and perhaps thereby providing a complement to phenomenological reports such as those presented in Appendix B. Appendix C presents a specimen record approach to ecological assessment. Presenting the Barker-style ecological analysis of these raw data is beyond the scope of this chapter (see Barker & Schoggen, 1973).

Using specimen records to document two different communities, Midwest and Yoredale, Barker and Schoggen (1973) determined that the habitat differences between the two towns are associated with certain behavioral differences in their human components. The authors demonstrated how a series of differences in various aspects of the two settings produced different behavioral outcomes. One was described as a "melting pot system" because it encouraged widespread exchange and homogenization of experiences. The other was characterized an "enlightened colonial system" because it involved more rigid distinctions and barriers to entering settings due to the control of high-status gatekeepers. Devereux (1977) attributes these differences to the undermanned (i.e., low ratio of people to settings) nature of Midwest in contrast to Yoredale. This led to the greater situational demands for participation by Midwest's children (e.g., for adults to be spectators at school and community performances), which were 10 times more common in Midwest than in Yoredale. This parallels the big school/small school analysis and is one of the most significant and common findings from ecological psychology with a bearing on personality.

Barker and Schoggen (1973) concluded that the behavioral consequences occurred because the habitat differences evoke psychological differences. People and their behavior are essential elements of the program and maintenance systems of the settings that constitute the towns' habitats. The inhabitants of Midwest and Yoredale inevitably reflected the differences that existed in the habitats which included them as interdependent components. Whatever the substance of the analysis, the specimen record provides the empirical foundation.

Family Social Network

Family social networks and neighborhoods serve as sources of interpersonal influence, as sources of direct or indirect material and emotional assistance, and as reference groups or status arenas (Unger & Powell, 1980). A family social network consists of family members' relations with relatives, friends, neighbors, co-workers, and other acquaintances who interact with a family member in regard to an emotional or material issue. The common characteristic of different members of a network is their relationship to the family.

Cochran and Brassard (1979) suggest that personal social networks influence parents by providing access to emotional and material assistance, by providing childrearing controls, and by serving as sources of role models. They further theorize that social networks have a direct influence on the child by providing cognitive and social stimulation, role models, and opportunities for engaging in significant social relations. Appendix D presents a social network assessment instrument (Garbarino & Sherman, 1980). Once again, it is possible to classify and analyze social network data in several ways. For example, we can compute measures of density (who knows whom within the network), size (how many people are part of the network), diversity (how many different types of relationships are contained within the network), and activity (what do network members do with and for each other) (Mitchell & Trickett, 1980).

Case 3: Adolescence: Peers and Social Network

In adolescence, the key ecological assessments involve the character of peer networks of youth that exist in institutions such as schools. Of course, peer groups have long been a major topic in adolescence. Most of this work has involved efforts to determine the relative influence of peers versus adults (usually parents), using only adolescents and/or their parents as respondents. Condry and Siman (1974), however, actually solicited data from peers which assessed actual congruence and discrepancy (as opposed to perceived congruence and discrepancy). This constitutes a potentially major but as yet underdeveloped assessment strategy. It could be expanded to assess social networks as well if those named as part of the adolescent's social network actually were also assessed on their views and responses to the adolescent.

Another line of adolescent-related ecological assessment concerns the demographic characteristics of residential environments for youth. Mapping an adolescent's social environment provides a useful vehicle for assessing elements of social cognition, the status of adolescent relationships, and the direction of development (Garbarino et al., 1985). Others have assessed the social networks of children and youth directly as a way of assessing the ecology of youth (Garbarino & Crouter, 1978). Appendix E presents this approach developed by Blyth, Garbarino, Thiel, and Crouter (1977).

Conclusion

Ecological assessments of personality can become important adjuncts to individual and family assessments. As yet, however, their potential for augmenting and complementing individual-level assessments is only partially developed. Research to date has demonstrated that our understanding of personality is only partial if we do not incorporate an ecological perspective on individual functioning. As ecological assessment approaches are refined, they will be able to provide data on the person in the world that is essential for a complete evaluation of personality. As a review of Appendices A–E shows, these assessments reveal a mix of quantitative (and potentially quantifiable) information plus qualitative information. When worked together, these simultaneous outputs can provide a picture of the person in the world that may be tailored to the special needs of a particular clinical or research problem.

Appendix A: Hospital Assessment to Determine Family-Centeredness of Obstetrical/Pediatric Policy and Practice[a,b]

A. PRENATALLY

1. Does the hospital sponsor prenatal classes?

0	2	3	4
none	irregularly, at request of expectant parent		scheduled on a regular basis for expectant parents

2. Does the hospital systematically assess whether or not expectant parents are "at risk" for child maltreatment and make this a basis for providing services?

0	2	3	4
not at all	informally		on a regular, formalized basis

3. Does the hospital sponsor classes in prepared childbirth (e.g., Lamaze) and encourage participation in such a program by fathers?

0	2	3	4
not at all	optional classes offered		sponsors classes and urges further participation

4. Are arrangements for delivery and hospital stay negotiated and planned to make prospective parents aware of arrangements that can facilitate early contact?

0	2	3	4
not at all	opportunities available upon special request— patient-initiated		routine briefing of expectant parents of opportunities

[a]From Garbarino (1979).

[b]Scoring: This hospital assessment measure has not been subjected to psychometric analysis. As developed, it was used to assess eight hospitals within a single metropolitan area. A simple scoring system is used to provide a basis for institutional comparisons and to provide a baseline for documenting changes in institutional policy and practice.

Scale A: Prenatally: Items 1–4; Total score ranges from 0 to 16.

Scale B: Delivery and the First 12 Hours: Items 1–7; Total score ranges from 0 to 28.

Scale C: First 5 Days: Items 1–7; Total score ranges from 0 to 28.

B. DELIVERY AND THE FIRST 12 HOURS

1. Does the hospital support the presence of prepared fathers in the delivery room through cooperative hospital staff action?

0	2	3	4
not at all	accepts father participation		encourage father participation

2. Does the hospital support effective participation by mothers in the delivery room through staff assistance in labor and delivery?

0	2	3	4
not at all	staff tolerates active participation		staff has special interest in encouraging maternal participation

3. Does the hospital support and encourage mothers who wish to minimize the use of drugs during labor and delivery?

0	2	3	4
not at all	staff tolerates maternal efforts to limit drug use		staff actively encourages minimal drug use

4. What in-service training is provided for staff working in the delivery and labor rooms? Who provides this training and what are its goals?

0	2	3	4
none	optional sporadic in-service		regular required training, high priority

5. What is the standard length of separation of parents and child after delivery?

0	2	3	4
several hours	1 hour		none

6. What is the typical duration of contact between infant and parents immediately after delivery, i.e., in the first hour?

0	2	3	4
none	quick look		sustained contact of 45 minutes or more

7. How soon after delivery do nursing mothers begin nursing?

0	2	3	4
within 24 hours	within 5 hours		within first hour

C. FIRST 5 DAYS

1. What provisions are made for "rooming-in?" (How is rooming-in defined? What support and assistance is given? What arrangements are made for women who change their minds?)

0	2	3	4
none	limited options, early boarding decision		full support for mother's choice

2. What are the visitation policies for fathers and children?

0	2	3	4
limited fathers only	fathers anytime, children limited		unlimited

3. What kind of feeding schedule is encouraged?

0	2	3	4
rigidly scheduled	scheduled; some flexibility		on demand

4. What instruction and support are given to mothers for breastfeeding? What provision is made for women who have difficulty breastfeeding or who changed their minds? (What proportion breast-feed?)

0	2	3	4
little breastfeeding; discouraged	depends upon nurse and mother		breastfeeding encouraged and supported

5. What provisions are made for routinely assessing the adequacy of parent–infant relationships, e.g., expressions of negative affect concerning the child and desire for separation?

0	2	3	4
none	sporadic; informally done		regular, high priority

6. What support and assistance are provided to families with medically high-risk infants?

0	2	3	4
none	arranged on ad hoc basis		high level; regular program

7. What instruction is given in the care of the newborn? Who is involved, e.g., fathers? What provision is made for contact after hospital discharge?

0	2	3	4
none	routine skills		major effort involving family, with postdischarge follow-up

Appendix B: Neighborhood and Community Assessment[1]

1. NEIGHBORHOOD

First I'd like to find out some things about the neighborhood and to hear what you think of it.

1.01 How long have you and your family been living here?
       ____years ____months

1.02 Does the neighborhood have a name? What is it?

1.03 Could you describe the boundaries of this neighborhood? Are there specific streets where it ends?

1.04 What is it like to bring up a child in this neighborhood?
PROBE:
  (a) Are there other children in the neighborhood? Are they the same ages? Do they play together?
  (b) Are there places for children to play?
  (c) Is this a safe neighborhood? If not, why not?
  (d) What are the people like around here?
  (e) Is your house (apartment) a good place for your family to live in?

1.05 Moving in
  (a) Why did you choose this neighborhood to move into?
  (b) How easy/hard was it to get used to the neighborhood?

[1]From Garbarino, J., & Sherman, D. (1980). High-risk neighborhoods and high-risk families: The human ecology of child maltreatment. *Child Development, 51*, 188–198.

(c) Using a scale – 4 to + 4 (from very difficult to very easy), how would you rate the neighborhood?

1.06 What kinds of help do you give to or get from your neighbors? How often?
(PROBE: Can you give an example?)

1.07 Are there any neighborhood problems? What kinds? What is usually done?

1.08 Has the neighborhood changed since you've lived here? In what ways?

1.09 How long do you think you will stay in this neighborhood? Why?
(PROBE: Are there things about this neighborhood that would make it difficult to leave?) Specify.
(PROBE: Are there things about this neighborhood that sometimes make you want to leave?) Specify.

1.10 OVERALL RATING
Taking everything into account, how would you rate this neighborhood as a place for parents with children to live and raise their family? Present card (score – 4 to + 4).

       Interviewer's Rating   *Respondent's Rating*

Comments:

2. CHURCH

2.01 Now let's talk a bit about your family and church. Do you attend or does anyone in your family attend church? How regularly?

    ☐ More than weekly   ☐ Year or less frequently
    ☐ Several times a month   ☐ Never
    ☐ Several times a year

2.02 What is your religious preference?

2.03 Has this changed much since _____ was born? How?

2.04 Are there any ways in which the church helps you in terms of bringing up _____?

2.05 Have you made any friends through your contact with the church?

3. CHILD CARE ARRANGEMENTS

3.01 Now let's talk about some of the things involved in caring for your child. Who has the main job of taking care of _____ during their waking hours? For example, mealtime, bedtime, playtime, etc.? What % of the care do you, your husband/wife, or another person do?

	Respondent	*Spouse*	*Other*
Feeding	_____	_____	_____
Bedtime	_____	_____	_____
Playing	_____	_____	_____

3.02 How much time are you able to spend with _____?

    Circle: too much   about right   too little

    IF TOO LITTLE: What would you like to be able to do with _____ that you aren't doing?

3.03 Does anyone else besides you—and your husband/wife—care for _____ here at home? (For example, a relative, neighbor, babysitter, or friend?) How much time do you leave the child with her/him or others?
(PROBE: How many hours per week with each person?)

3.04 Does anyone else take care of _____ outside the home? How much time?

3.05 How difficult or easy is it to find someone to take care of _____? Can you usually find the right kind of person?

3.06 Who would care for _____ if you were home sick on a school day?

3.07 What happens when _____ comes home from school? Who else is there then?

3.08 OVERALL RATING

In general, how would you rate the kind of care _____ is getting when you yourself are not around? Present card (-4 to $+4$).

Interviewer's Rating   *Respondent's Rating*

Comments:

4. EMPLOYMENT, SCHOOLING, VOLUNTEER WORK

4.01 In addition to being a parent, are you also employed, going to school, or doing anything else that takes a lot of your time? Specify.

Circle: YES   NO

If YES: What?

4.02 How much time does that involve? Record part-time, full-time hours.

From ____ to ____ ____ days a week

Overtime: ____

4.03 Is your husband presently employed, going to school, etc.?

Circle: YES   NO

If YES: What does he do?

4.04 What are his hours like?

From ____ to ____ ____ days a week

Overtime: ____

4.05 How do your work situations work out in terms of _____?

4.06 OVERALL RATING

Taking everything into account, how would you rate the work situation in terms of bringing up a young child?

Interviewer's Rating   *Respondent's Rating*

Comments:

5. RECREATION

Now lets talk a little bit about the spare time you, your husband/wife and children have.

5.01 How much time do you feel you have to do things you would like to do?

Circle: Too much   About right   Too little   None

5.02 What kinds of things do you do for recreation?

(PROBE: Sports, social activities?)

5.03 What kinds of things do you do together with your family?

5.04 How much of this time is spent with your family? (PROBE: What %?)

Alone _____   Children _____

Spouse _____   Children and Spouse _____

5.05 OVERALL RATING

Taking everything into account, how would you rate your chances to enjoy recreation?

Interviewer's Rating   *Respondent's Rating*

Comments:

6. FINANCES

6.01 How is the money situation working out in terms of being a parent of a young child?

6.02 OVERALL RATING

In general, how would you rate the money situation?

Interviewer's Rating   *Respondent's Rating*

Comments:

7. *HEALTH*

7.01 Since _____ was born, has she/he had any serious health problems, been hospitalized?

(INTERVIEWER: A serious health problem is one that has prevented the child from carrying out a normal daily schedule for at least a week.)

    Illness   Age of Child when Ill   Duration   How Often

    1.
    2.
    3.

7.02 Who took care of him/her then? And how did that work out?

(PROBE: When she/he was at home?)

    1.
    2.
    3.

7.03 Has anyone else in the family including yourself had a serious health problem, or been hospitalized since _____ was born?

    Name   Age When Ill   Illness   Duration   How Often

    1.
    2.
    3.

7.04 What happened in terms of _____? Who took care of him them?

7.05 OVERALL RATING

In general, how much of a problem has health been in your family (-4 to $+4$)?

    Interviewer's Rating   Respondent's Rating

Comments:

8. *FAMILY ORGANIZATIONS, PROGRAMS, SERVICES*

8.01 Now I'd like to ask you about some of the services, programs, and organizations in the community. Could you check off the ones on this list that you know something about and those you have used since _____ was born?

(Interviewer: Present list of services. See next page. Have respondents check columns for familiarity, use, and evaluation of the organization.)

8.02 Are any of these services that you feel you could use but aren't using?

Why? (PROBE: Unfamiliar, transportation, unsure of eligibility, spouse disapproves, no one to go with)

8.03 Are there any other services or organizations you know about or have used? Repeat questions.

FAMILY ORGANIZATIONS

Knows Something About	How Often Used	Would Recommend Yes	No	No.	Name
				1	BIG BROTHERS/BIG SISTERS OF THE MIDLAND
				2	SALVATION ARMY BOOTH MEMORIAL RESIDENCE AND HOSPITAL
				3	CATHOLIC SOCIAL SERVICE
				4	CHILD SAVING INSTITUTE
				5	FAMILY SERVICE OF OMAHA-COUNCIL BLUFFS
				6	JEWISH FAMILY SERVICE
				7	LEGAL AID SOCIETY OF OMAHA-COUNCIL BLUFFS
				8	LUTHERAN FAMILY AND SOCIAL SERVICE
				9	UNITED CATHOLIC SOCIAL SERVICE OF THE ARCHDIOCESE OF OMAHA

Knows Something About	How Often Used	Would Recommend		No.	Name
		Yes	No		
				10	BOYS CLUB OF OMAHA
				11	BOY SCOUTS OF AMERICA, MID-AMERICA COUNCIL
				12	OMAHA COUNCIL OF CAMP FIRE GIRLS
				13	CHRIST CHILD SOCIETY
				14	THE OMAHA GIRLS CLUB
				15	GIRL SCOUTS, GREAT PLAINS COUNCIL
				16	JEWISH COMMUNITY CENTER
				17	SOCIAL SETTLEMENT ASSOCIATION OF OMAHA
				18	UNITED METHODIST COMMUNITY CENTER
				19	WOODSON CENTER
				20	OMAHA-COUNCIL BLUFFS Y.M.C.A.
				21	Y.M.C.A.
				22	GREATER OMAHA ASSOCIATION FOR RETARDED CITIZENS
				23	DR. LEE R. MARTIN THERAPY CENTER
				24	MEALS ON WHEELS
				25	POTTAWATTAMIE MENTAL HEALTH CENTER
				26	VISITING NURSE ASSOCIATION OF OMAHA
				27	AMERICAN RED CROSS DOUGLAS/SARPY COUNTY CHAPTER
				28	INFORMATION AND REFERRAL SERVICE OF UNITED WAY OF THE MIDLANDS
				29	SALVATION ARMY
				30	URBAN LEAGUE OF NEBRASKA
				31	VOLUNTEER BUREAU OF UNITED WAY OF THE MIDLANDS
				32	OMAHA AREA COUNCIL ON ALCOHOLISM
				33	INDIAN-CHICANO HEALTH CLINIC
				34	ALCOHOLISM INFORMATION CENTER
				35	AID TO DEPENDENT CHILDREN
				36	B'NAI B'RITH
				37	CHURCH OR SYNAGOGUE ORGANIZATION
				38	COMMUNITY BABY SITTING PROGRAM
				39	COOP-IN-BABY SITTING CENTER
				40	DAY-CARE AND CHILD DEVELOPMENT COUNCIL
				41	DAY-CARE PROGRAM (If used, name)
				42	DENTAL CLINIC
				43	DEPARTMENT OF SOCIAL SERVICES
				44	FOOD STAMPS
				45	FAMILY AND CHILDREN'S SERVICES
				46	INFORMATION AND REFERRAL SERVICE
				47	LA LECHE LEAGUE
				48	PUBLIC LIBRARY PROGRAMS
				49	MENTAL HEALTH ASSOCIATION
				50	MENTAL HEALTH CLINIC
				51	PRE-SCHOOL PROGRAM (If used, name)
				52	SINGLE PARENTS ORGANIZATION
				53	WOMEN'S COMMUNITY BUILDING
				54	Y.M.C.A.

9. *RAISING THE CHILDREN*

9.01 Now let's talk about _____ for a while. Are there things about _____ that make him easy or difficult to bring up?

(PROBE: Behavior, personality-similarity to self or spouse, health)

(a) Behavior at School   (c) Personality

(b) Behavior at Home   (d) Health

                      (e) Other

9.02 How does _____ compare in this way with their brothers and sisters?

9.03 OVERALL RATING

In general, how would you rate _____ in terms of how easy or difficult it is to bring him/her up?

Present card (−4 to +4).

        Interviewer's Rating   *Respondent's Rating*

Comments:

10. *TELEVISION*

10.01 Do you have a television?

10.02 In what ways has TV made it easier or more difficult to bring up _____?

(PROBE: Is it entertaining, educational, harmful, or poor quality?)

10.03 In general, how would you rate television from the point of view of a parent?

Present card (−4 to +4).

        Interviewer's Rating   *Respondent's Rating*

Comments:

11. *PARENTING INFORMATION*

11.01 We're interested in knowing about how people learn to be parents. How did you learn to be a parent? (PROBE: Where do you turn for advice—family, neighbors, TV or books, professionals?)

	Yes	*No*	*Who/Which Ones*
Family	——	——	_____
Neighbors	——	——	_____
TV or Books	——	——	_____
Professional Agencies	——	——	_____

11.02 Which of the above sources has been the most important to you? Rank the above in importance.

	Rank
Family	——
Neighbors	——
TV or Books	——
Professional Agencies	——

11.03 Are there any particular people who are helpful to you as a parent? In what way? (What about friends, relatives, neighbors, professionals, people at work?)

11.04 Are there any people who cause problems for you personally or for your family? In what way?

(PROBE: Are there any who you think may be making some problems for _____?)

11.05 How about other children? Do your own or other people's children make problems for you?

11.06 From your point of view as a parent of a child, how does the school situation look?

(PROBE: Is school a help or a problem to you?)

11.07 How involved are you and your spouse with the schools?

(PROBE: Are you a member of PTA? Do you volunteer time?)

11.08 How much contact do you have with _____ teachers?

Circle: 1. Once a week   5. Several times a year
           2. Twice a month   6. Once a year
           3. Monthly   7. Never or very rarely
           4. Every couple of months

11.09 OVERALL RATING

In general, how satisfied are you with the kind of help you get as a parent? Present card (-4 to $+4$).

	Family	Friends	Neighbors	Professionals (doctors, ministers, social workers, books and TV)
Interviewer's Rating:	____	____	____	____
Respondent's Rating:	____	____	____	____

Comments:

12. *FUTURE*

Now I'd like to ask you some questions about the future.

12.01 Do you plan to have any more children?

Circle: YES   NO

12.02 What are the main reasons for your decision?

12.03 If you had it to do over again, would you have (x number of) children? Why?

13. *SELF AS A PARENT*

13.01 We're getting to the end of the first part of the interview now. Could I ask you—Is there anything about you, yourself, which makes it easier or harder to bring up _____ the way you want to?

(PROBE: personality traits, abilities?)

13.02 In general, how satisfied are you with yourself as a parent? Present card (-4 to $+4$).

Appendix C: Specimen Record[2]

SETTING: Playing Field, Town

SUBJECT: Maers Holman   AGE: 9 yrs. 6 mos.   SEX: Female   Class III

DAY AND DATE: Saturday, July 6, 1957   TIME: 3:59–4:11 p.m.

OBSERVER: Louise Barker

DESCRIPTION OF SUBJECT: Maers Holman is a physically energetic, slight girl. She has straight black bobbed hair and hazel eyes. The fact that she is not a member of group 1A would indicate that she is one of the slower children academically. She is the youngest in her family.

DESCRIPTION OF SETTING: The Playing Field belongs to the community. It is cared for by the Playing Field Committee. The school uses the field for football and cricket. At the top end of the field there are benches and apparatus. The field is completely walled and is also used as pasture. There is a low revolving platform with radial bars to hold on to that the children called a "teapot." There is a big seesaw, there are three baby swings like chairs, and three regular swings. There is an apparatus like a gymnasium horse, except larger, which will rock backward and forward, that a number of children can sit on at once and rock. There is a higher revolving platform that a child would have to be 7 or so to be able even to get up on, with bars to hold on to. This undulated as well, so the children called it "ocean waves." There is also a climbing apparatus which is two parallel bars with two crossbars; they must be 10 feet from the ground. That, too, is arranged so that small children can't easily get up on it because they couldn't reach the bar from standing on the ladder. As I came up to the playing field I met Suzette Thornoon and Hesford Broadly, who were just leaving. Up on the playing field were Helen Kingsley, Maers Holman, and Shirley Woodbine. With Helen Kingsley was a baby, a boy

[2]From Barker, Wright, Barker, and Schoggen (1961, pp. 259–260).

about 18 months old, Benjamin Deldon. She had a stroller for him and Hesper Holden had a little boy named Michael Autin; he was 2 also, with a stroller. With Helen were her cousins, Patricia and Clifford Hacket, and quite on their own were Stephanie Evans, and Grindel Evans. They are the youngest sister and brother of Oran Evans. The Evans and Hacket families are neighbors. As I got up there Hesper handed Michael a bottle with orange juice in it. Michael took it with pleasure.

	Age (yr., mo.)	Class
Hesper Holden	3–6	111
Helen Kingsley	10–1	111
Maers Holman	9–6	111
Shirley Woodbine	8–11	11
Stephanie Evans	5–6	111
Grindel Evans	3–0	111

Tipping Seesaw

3:59 Maers and Shirley walked up the seesaw till it tipped, going down with a bang.

They walked back, tipping it again.

Helen Kingsley and Hesper called in a very school-teacherist way, "You'll break it, don't do that, Shirley."

Noting Girls Leave

4:00 Helen and Hesper with the two babies and Patricia and Clifford Hacket left. They said it was time for tea.

Maers noticed them leave.

Playing on "Teapot"

Maers and Shirley ran to the teapot.

Maers ran along beside it as she started it rotating.

She climbed on.

Shirley scrambled on.

Stephanie ran after them and managed to get on after they had started getting it to go round. Grindel ran up and said urgently, "I want to get on, I want to get on with you." Stephanie said firmly to him, "You can't come on now."

Maers jumped off the teapot as it was still running.

Tipping Seesaw

She ran away to run up on the seesaw to tip it.

She ran up the seesaw till it tipped.

She ran down with great energy.

She repeated this three times.

Playing on "Teapot"

She ran back to the teapot.

Stephanie was trying to make it go by running around.

Maers jumped on the teapot. She climbed up onto the iron bars that are for the children to hold on to.

Balancing in Center

She stood in the very center, balanced on the iron bars as the teapot revolved. She seemed to be enjoying herself very much.

This was a feat. She jumped down.

Swinging

She ran to the little swings.

There she just for a moment swung on one of the little swings.

Playing on Ocean Wave

She ran over to the ocean wave.

Rocking the "Horse"

She left it and went to the rocking horse.

4:05 Maers climbed onto the rocking horse.

She worked vigorously at getting it to rock back and forth.

Shirley got on behind her.

Maers continued to make the horse rock back and forth.

Maers jumped off the rocking horse.

Playing on Horse	She went over to the ocean wave.
	This offered more scope because there are bars coming down to hold up the platform which goes around, and these offered a place to climb on.
	4:06 Both girls started climbing around on the bars.
	Maers hung by her hands and pulled up her knees.
	Shirley remarked approvingly, "Oh, lovely."
Looking At Ladybug	In the meantime Stephanie and Grindel had found a ladybird beetle and Stephanie had brought it over to show me.
	Maers jumped off the ocean wave and, followed closely by Shirley, ran over to the bench where I was sitting.
Commenting to Stephanie	Maers said to Stephanie, "Oh, have you found my ladybug," as she looked at it with great interest and appreciation.
	Stephanie said, "She's funny." I said, "What's funny about her?" She said, "When I see her she laughs."
	Shirley ran to the teapot and climbed on.
	She announced firmly, "No one can come on this time."
Playing on "Teapot"	Maers ran over.
Responding to Jean	She said, "Except me," and jumped on.
	Maers then succeeded in climbing to a standing position on the cross pieces.
	Shirley tried to do the same.
	She didn't quite make it and she said, "I wasn't properly up then," and then she tried again and failed.
Responding to Shirley's Warning	Shirley said something of a warning nature to Maers.
	Maers answered, "No fear."
	4:08 Although the bars are low on this apparatus, Maers managed to hang by them and turn herself thru her arms, that is "skin the cat," as we say.
Depreciating Own Feat	Shirley said admiringly, "I'll try it."
	Maers said, depreciating it, "Oh, it's simple."
	Maers jumped off the teapot while it went around.
Playing with Shirley on Seesaw	She and Shirley ran over to the seesaw.
Singing "Allouette"	They started a song they had been singing in school, "Allouette."
	They sang it as they played on the seesaw.
	They both walked the length of the seesaw, tipping it.
	They both walked back and tipped it again.
	Then they walked to the center and stood holding hands in the middle.
	Shirley, moving a little bit, tipped it one way.
	Maers, moving the other way, tipped it the other way.
	They almost seemed to be doing a little dance step together as they moved up and down on the seesaw, tipping it first one way and then the other as they sang.
Commenting re: Heat	Shirley, who was wearing a skirt and knit upper, said, "I wish I could take my pullover off."
	Maers said, "I wish I could take my dress off."
	I was warm sitting still.
	4:10 Maers and Shirley jumped off the seesaw and ran to where I was sitting.

Stephanie and Grindel were standing near me. Maers looked at the ladybug, which Stephanie was letting walk around her arm and shoulder, with some interest.

She said, "It's really mine, because I found it."

4:11 I stopped the observation at this point because the children started to talk to me. They gave me the names of the different apparatuses at this time and Maers said she loved to come up here and play. She said that she liked best of all the climbing apparatus and that Clifford Matthew had taught her how to use it. She wanted to show me what Clifford taught her. So she and Shirley ran down to the climbing apparatus. Maers climbed up quickly and swung herself from bar to bar till she got to the center, then she pulled herself up and hung by her knees. Shirley said she was going to try it, though she had never done it before. She did it successfully and was very pleased. Then they said they would show me how they raced. They started to come up, one at each end at the same time and raced by hanging and moving along till they got to the center, to see which one got there first. They seemed to do it really very well. I said it was time for my tea and I thought I'd better go along then and they decided it was time for their tea, too, so the four of us started out across the field, but the two little Evans decided to stay up longer. It seemed kind of lonesome for a 5-year-old and a 3-year-old up in this walled field, but the other girls said they had come up by themselves and they would be all right, so we left them.

Appendix D: Social Networks Interview—Family[3]

(INTERVIEWER: If you haven't already established the composition of the household, do so now. Record on the first page.)

We've now finished the first section of the interview. We would like to get more of an idea about the important people in your family's life, who are not living in your home. Let's begin by making a list of the people outside your immediate family who you know best or who know you best.

(PROBE: Is there anyone else [of any age] you know well, or who knows you very well?)

(INTERVIEWER: Couples who are seen together, and not visited as separate people, should be counted as one person.)

1a. NAMES OF THE PEOPLE YOU KNOW BEST

	Name	Relationship	Others Known (Interviewer: Identify by No.)
___	1. _____	_____	_____
___	2. _____	_____	_____
___	3. _____	_____	_____
___	4. _____	_____	_____
___	5. _____	_____	_____
___	6. _____	_____	_____
___	7. _____	_____	_____
___	8. _____	_____	_____
___	9. _____	_____	_____
___	10. _____	_____	_____
___	11. _____	_____	_____

[3]From Garbarino, J., & Sherman, D. (1980). High-risk neighborhoods and high-risk families: The human ecology of child maltreatment. *Child Development, 51*, 188–198.

	Name	*Relationship*	*Others Known (Interviewer: Identify by No.)*
____ 12.	_____	_____	_____
____ 13.	_____	_____	_____
____ 14.	_____	_____	_____
____ 15.	_____	_____	_____
____ 16.	_____	_____	_____
____ 17.	_____	_____	_____
____ 18.	_____	_____	_____
____ 19.	_____	_____	_____
____ 20.	_____	_____	_____
____ 21.	_____	_____	_____
____ 22.	_____	_____	_____

I would like to know a little more about the things you do with the people who are especially important to you. Let us start by picking the 10 people who are most important to you. (Place an X in front of the appropriate names.). What is the relationship of _____ to you? Does _____ know any of the other people on your list?

1b. NETWORK CONTACTS

Person Known	How often do you see or talk with _____?	What do you usually do together?
1. _____	_____	_____
2. _____	_____	_____
3. _____	_____	_____
4. _____	_____	_____
5. _____	_____	_____
6. _____	_____	_____
7. _____	_____	_____
8. _____	_____	_____
9. _____	_____	_____
10. _____	_____	_____

2. Have you belonged to any clubs, groups, or organizations since _____ was born? (PROBE: such as bowling league, church group, social club, etc.?)

What kind of things do you do with that group, and how much time do you spend with them?

	Group Name	*Activities*	*Dates of Membership*	*Frequency of Meetings*	*Leadership*
1.	_____	_____	_____	_____	_____
2.	_____	_____	_____	_____	_____
3.	_____	_____	_____	_____	_____
4.	_____	_____	_____	_____	_____
5.	_____	_____	_____	_____	_____
6.	_____	_____	_____	_____	_____
7.	_____	_____	_____	_____	_____
8.	_____	_____	_____	_____	_____

3. Besides yourself, who are the people who know your children best? How much time do they spend with the children?

INVOLVEMENT WITH CHILDREN

	Name	*Relationship to the child*	*How often do they see the child*	*How long have they known child*	*Activities*
1.	____	_____	_____	_____	_____
2.	____	_____	_____	_____	_____
3.	____	_____	_____	_____	_____
4.	____	_____	_____	_____	_____

	Name	Relationship to the child	How often do they see the child	How long have they known child	Activities
5.	____	_____	_____	_____	_____
6.	____	_____	_____	_____	_____
7.	____	_____	_____	_____	_____
8.	____	_____	_____	_____	_____
9.	____	_____	_____	_____	_____
10.	____	_____	_____	_____	_____

4. Now I would like to ask you about concerns that you may have had. Tell me if this has happened. . . .

	Last month	Last year	Never
(a) Felt so depressed that it ruined your day.	____	____	____
(b) Child not doing well or having behavior problems at school.	____	____	____
(c) Child seems out of control at home.	____	____	____
(d) Child doesn't eat or sleep well.	____	____	____
(e) Got so tense at work that you "blew up."	____	____	____
(f) Wanted to change jobs.	____	____	____
(g) Wanted to move out of the neighborhood because of problems.	____	____	____
(h) Wanted to change the division of duties with your husband/wife.	____	____	____
(i) Had a disagreement with your husband/wife.	____	____	____
(j) Other (specify) _____			

(INTERVIEWER: If at least one concern is indicated continue. If none, go to Question 8.)

5. Whom did you talk to about these concerns? (Check all that apply.)

1. Co-worker	____	6. Counselor	____
2. Friend	____	7. Teacher	____
3. Relative	____	8. Doctor	____
4. Spouse	____	9. Neighbor	____
5. Clergy	____	10. Police	____

6. Which of these things happened when you talked with Person #____?

	#1	#2	#3	#4	#5	#6	#7	#8	#9	#10
(a) They just listened to me.	—	—	—	—	—	—	—	—	—	—
(b) They asked me questions.	—	—	—	—	—	—	—	—	—	—
(c) They told me who else to see.	—	—	—	—	—	—	—	—	—	—
(d) They told me to see someone else.	—	—	—	—	—	—	—	—	—	—
(e) They showed me a new way to look at things.	—	—	—	—	—	—	—	—	—	—
(f) They took some action about the matter.	—	—	—	—	—	—	—	—	—	—

7. How satisfied were you with the help from _____?
Were you:

	#1	#2	#3	#4	#5	#6	#7	#8	#9	#10
Very satisfied	—	—	—	—	—	—	—	—	—	—
Somewhat satisfied	—	—	—	—	—	—	—	—	—	—
Neither satisfied nor dissatisfied	—	—	—	—	—	—	—	—	—	—
Somewhat dissatisfied	—	—	—	—	—	—	—	—	—	—
Very dissatisfied	—	—	—	—	—	—	—	—	—	—

8. Interviewer: Have the respondent fill out the following page.

9. Did you talk with any of the following people when these things happened? (Check all that apply.)

1. Co-worker	____	6. Counselor	____
2. Friend	____	7. Teacher	____
3. Relative	____	8. Doctor	____
4. Spouse	____	9. Neighbor	____
5. Clergy	____	10. Police	____

10. Which of these things happened when you talked with Person #____?

	#1	#2	#3	#4	#5	#6	#7	#8	#9	#10
(a) They just listened to me.	—	—	—	—	—	—	—	—	—	—
(b) They asked me questions.	—	—	—	—	—	—	—	—	—	—
(c) They told me who else to see.	—	—	—	—	—	—	—	—	—	—
(d) They told me to see someone else.	—	—	—	—	—	—	—	—	—	—
(e) They showed me a new way to look at things.	—	—	—	—	—	—	—	—	—	—
(f) They took some action about the matter.	—	—	—	—	—	—	—	—	—	—

11. How satisfied were you with the help from _____?
Were you:

	#1	#2	#3	#4	#5	#6	#7	#8	#9	#10
Very satisfied	—	—	—	—	—	—	—	—	—	—
Somewhat satisfied	—	—	—	—	—	—	—	—	—	—
Neither satisfied nor dissatisfied	—	—	—	—	—	—	—	—	—	—
Somewhat dissatisfied	—	—	—	—	—	—	—	—	—	—
Very dissatisfied	—	—	—	—	—	—	—	—	—	—

11. HISTORY OF RESIDENCE

We would also like to get an accurate picture of where you have lived in the past ten years. Let's start with your present address and move back in time.

	Address	*Reason for Change*	*Satisfaction Rating* (1 to 5)
1978	_____	_____	_____
1977	_____	_____	_____
1976	_____	_____	_____
1975	_____	_____	_____
1974	_____	_____	_____
1973	_____	_____	_____
1972	_____	_____	_____
1971	_____	_____	_____
1970	_____	_____	_____
1969	_____	_____	_____
1968	_____	_____	_____

*RATINGS:

Very Satisfied = 5	Somewhat Dissatisfied = 2
Somewhat Satisfied = 4	Very Dissatisfied = 1
Neither Satisfied nor Dissatisfied = 3	

Appendix E: Social Networks of Youth[4]

Now I would like you to help me make a list of some of the people in your life.

1. First of all, who are the people you consider your *friends*?

[4]From Blyth, Garbarino, Thiel, and Croutes (1977).

PROBE: Are there any other people who are your friends?

FOR ALL FRIENDS LISTED ASK
   A. How old is this person?
   B. What grade is this person in?
   C. What school does this person go to? _____ (name)
   D. Is this person a male or a female?   MALE   FEMALE
   E. Is this person black or white?   BLACK   WHITE
   F. Where does this person live?   (1) IN THE NEIGHBORHOOD
       (2) IN OR AROUND OMAHA   (3) OUTSIDE OMAHA
   G. Where do you usually see this person?   (1) AT SCHOOL
                                                (2) OUTSIDE SCHOOL (at clubs or on teams)
                                                (3) AROUND THE NEIGHBORHOOD
   H. Is _____ the kind of person your parents would like you to be friends with?
           YES   NO
   I. Do your parents know this person?   YES   NO
   J. Is this person friends with _____?   (INTERVIEWER: GO THROUGH ALL OTHER
       NAMES ON THE LIST.)
   K. Who are your five closest friends?   (INTERVIEWER: NUMBER THEM IN THE
       ORDER THEY ARE MENTIONED.)

FRIENDS

Name	A. Age	B. Grade	C. School	D. Sex	E. Race	F. Where does this person live?	G. Where do you see this person?	H. Is _____ kind of person parents would like you to be friends with?	I. Do your parents know this person?	J. Is this person friends with _____?	K. Top 5 friends
1.											
2.											
3.											
4.											
5.											
6.											
7.											
8.											
9.											
10.											

IF KID MENTIONS MORE THAN 10 FRIENDS CHECK HERE ( ) AND PROCEED WITH INTERVIEW

2. Aside from the friends you've just mentioned, are there any other people that you feel *you know well*? These could be kids, adults, members of your family or other relatives.

   PROBE: Who else do you know well?

For all persons listed ask:
   A. Who is this person?
   B. Is this person a male or a female?   MALE   FEMALE
   C. About how old is this person?
       If necessary ask: Is this person . . .
           1 –a little kid
           2 –someone your age
           3 –a teenager
           4 –an adult, or
           5 –an elderly person?

PEOPLE R KNOWS WELL

Name	A. Relationship	B. Sex M F	C. Age

3. Are there any other people that you see a lot or *spend a lot of time with*? These could be parents, brothers or sisters, teachers or anyone else.

   PROBE: Is there anyone else you can think of?

   For all listed ask:
   A. Who is this person?
   B. Is this person a male or a female?   MALE   FEMALE
   C. About how old is this person?
      If necessary ask: Is this person . . .
         1 –a little kid
         2 –someone your age
         3 –a teenager
         4 –an adult, or
         5 –an elderly person?

PEOPLE R SPENDS TIME WITH

Name	A. Relationship	B. Sex M F	C. Age

4. Now I'd like to find out if there are any people who *know you* well that we haven't talked about.

   PROBE: Who else do you feel really knows you well?

   For all people listed ask:
   A. Who is this person?

B. Is this person a male or a female?   MALE   FEMALE
C. About how old is this person?
   For probing if necessary: Is this person . . .
   1 –a little kid
   2 –someone your age
   3 –a teenager
   4 –an adult, or
   5 –an elderly person?

PEOPLE WHO KNOW R WELL

Name	A. Relationship	B. Sex M F	C. Age

5. Now, of all these people we've talked about who would you say are the 10 PEOPLE THAT REAL-LY KNOW YOU BEST?

INTERVIEWER: ONLY IF NECESSARY—GO BACK AND READ ENTIRE LIST OF NAMES
               ''WHO KNOW R WELL'' AND WORK BACK TO HIS FRIENDS.

FOR 10 LISTED ASK:
   A. Where does this person live?
      1 –in the neighborhood
      2 –in or around Omaha
      3 –outside Omaha
   B. How many years have you known this person?   _____years
   C. Do you see this person . . .
      1 –almost every day
      2 –two or three times a week
      3 –once a week
      4 –every two or three weeks, or
      5 –less than once a month
   D. Sometimes you see people in different places. At what kinds of places do you see this
      person?
      1 –at your home
      2 –at his or her home
      3 –at school
      4 –at a club or sports activity
      5 –someplace else, where? _____
   E. Does this person know _____? INTERVIEWER: GO THROUGH ALL THE NAMES
      ON THIS LIST ONLY
   F. How much would you want to be like this person? (SHOW CARD)

FOR TOP 10 ONLY

Name	A. Where does this person live?			B. How many years have you known this person?	C. How often do you see this person?					D. Where do you see this person?					E. Does this person know ___?	F. How much would you like to be like this person? (show card)
	in the neighborhood	in or around Omaha	outside Omaha		almost every day	2-3 times a week	once a week	every 2-3 weeks	less than once mo.	at your home	at his/her home	at school	at a club or sports activity	someplace else, where?		
1.																
2.																
3.																
4.																
5.																
6.																
7.																
8.																
9.																
10.																

References

Barker, R. G., & Gump, P. (1964). *Big school, small school*. Stanford, CA: Stanford University Press.

Barker, R. G., & Schoggen, P. (1973). *Qualities of community life*. San Francisco, CA: Jossey-Bass.

Barker, R. G., & Wright, H. (1971). *Midwest and its children*. Hamden, CT: Archon Books. (Reprinted from Harper & Row, 1955)

Benn, J. (1984). *Determinants of childbirth experience*. Unpublished doctoral dissertation. Pennsylvania State University, University Park.

Benn, J., & Garbarino, J. (1982). The ecology of childbearing and child rearing. In J. Garbarino and Associates (Eds.), *Children and families in the social environment*. Chicago, IL: Aldine.

Block, C., & Block, R. (1975). The effect of support of the husband and obstetrician on pain perception and control in childbirth. *Birth and the Family Journal, 2*, 43–47.

Blyth, D., Garbarino, J., Thiel, K., & Crouter, A. (1977). *Transition to adolescence study: Sixth grader's interview*. Boys Town, NE: Center for the Study of Youth Development.

Bronfenbrenner, U. (1979). *The ecology of human development: Experiments by nature and design*. Cambridge, MA: Harvard University Press.

Burgess, R., & Conger, R. (1977). Family interaction patterns related to child abuse and neglect. *Child Abuse and Neglect, 1*, 269–278.

Cochran, M., & Brassard, J. (1979). Social networks and child development. *Child Development, 50*, 601–616.

Condry, J., & Siman, M. (1974). Characteristics of peer- and adult-oriented children. *Journal of Marriage and the Family, 36*, 543–554.

Danziger, S. (1979a). The medical context of childbearing: A study of social control and doctor-patient interaction. *Social Science and Medicine, 2*, 159–172.

Danziger, S. (1979b). On doctor watching. *Urban Life, 7*(4), 22–29.

Devereux, E. (1977, August). *A critique of ecological psychology*. Paper presented at the Conference on Research Perspectives in the Ecology of Human Development, Cornell University, Ithaca, NY.

Forrester, J. (1971). Counterintuitive behavior of social systems. *Technological Review, 73*, 3–30.

Freud, S. (1930). *Civilization and its discontents*. London: Hogarth Press.

Galambos, N., & Garbarino, J. (1983). Identifying the missing links in the study of latchkey children. *Children Today, 12*(4), 2–4.

Garbarino, J. (1980a). Changing hospital childbirth practices: A developmental perspective on prevention of child maltreatment. *American Journal of Orthopsychiatry, 50*, 588–597.

Garbarino, J. (1980b). Latchkey children. *Vital Issues, 30* (November), 1–4.

Garbarino, J. (1980c). Some thoughts on school size and its effects on adolescent development. *Journal of Youth and Adolescence, 9*, 19–31.

Garbarino, J., & Asp, E. (1981). *Successful schools and competent students*. Lexington, MA: Lexington.

Garbarino, J., *et al.* (1982). *Children and families in the social environment*. Hawthorne, NY: Aldine.

Garbarino, J., *et al.* (1985). *Adolescent development: An ecological perspective*. Columbus, OH: Charles E. Merrill.

Garbarino, J., & Bronfenbrenner, U. (1976). The socialization of moral judgment and behavior in cross-cultural perspective. In T. Lockona (Ed.), *Moral development and behavior* (pp. 70–83). New York: Holt, Rinehart, & Winston.

Garbarino, J., & Crouter, A. (1978). Defining the community context of parent-child relations: The correlates of child maltreatment. *Child Development, 49*, 604–616.

Garbarino, J., & Sherman, D. (1980). High-risk neighborhoods and high-risk families: The human ecology of child maltreatment. *Child Development, 51*, 188–198.

Gilligan, C. (1982). *In a different voice: Psychological theory and women's development*. Cambridge, MA: Harvard University Press.

Goffman, E. (1961). *Asylums*. New York: Doubleday.

Gump, P. (1975). Ecological psychology and children. in E. M. Hetherington (Ed.), *Review of child development research* (pp. 75–126). Chicago, IL: University of Chicago Press.

Gump, P., & Adelberg, B. (1978). Urbanism from the perspective of ecological psychologists. *Environment and Behavior, 10*, 171–191.

Hardin, G., & Baden, J. (1977). *Managing the commons*. San Francisco, CA: Freeman.

Hawley, A. (1950). *Human ecology: A theory of community structure*. New York: Ronald Press.

Horney, K. (1937). *The neurotic personality of our time*. New York: Norton.

Kohn, M. L. (1977). *Class and conformity: A study in values* (2nd ed.). Chicago, IL: University of Chicago Press.

Lewin, K. (1935). *A dynamic theory of personality*. New York: McGraw-Hill.

Lewin, K. (1951). *Field theory in social science, selected theoretical papers*. New York: Harper.

Lewin, K., Lippitt, R., & White, R. K. (1939). Patterns of aggressive behavior in experimentally-created "social climates." *Journal of Social Psychology, 10*, 271–299.

Long, L., & Long, T. (1983). *Latchkey children and their parents*. New York: Arbor House.

MacLeod, R. (1947). The phenomenological approach to social psychology. *Psychological Review, 54*, 193–210.

Marcuse, H. (1964). *One-dimensional man*. Boston, MA: Beacon Press.

Mitchell, R., & Trickett, E. (1980). Task force report: Social support networks as mediators of social support. *Community Mental Health Journal, 16*, 27–44.

Moos, R. (1975). *Evaluating correctional and community settings*. New York: Wiley.

Moos, R. (1976). Evaluating and changing community settings. *American Journal of Community Psychology, 4*, 313–326.

Murray, H. (1938). *Explorations in personality*. London & New York: Oxford University Press.

Naroll, R. (1983). *The moral order*. Beverly Hills, CA: Sage Publications.

Newton, N. (1979). Cross-cultural perspectives. In A. L. Clark & D. D. Affonson (Eds.), *Childbearing: A nursing perspective* (2nd ed., pp. 148–165). Philadelphia, PA: F. A. Davis.

Polansky, N., Chalmers, M., Buttenwieser, E., & Williams, D. (1981). *Damaged parents*. Chicago, IL: University of Chicago Press.

Potter, D. (1954). *People of plenty: economic abundance and the American character*. Chicago, IL: University of Chicago Press.

Riesman, D. (1950). *The lonely crowd*. New Haven, CT: Yale University Press.

Slater, P. (1970). *The pursuit of loneliness*. Boston, MA: Beacon Press.

Sosa, R., Kennell, J., Klaus, M., Robertson, S., & Urrutia, J. (1980). The effect of a supportive companion as perinatal problems, length of labor, and mother-infant interactions. *New England Journal of Medicine, 303*, 597–600.

Unger, D. G., & Powell, D. R. (1980). Supporting families under stress: The role of social networks. *Family Relations, 29*, 566–574.

Webb, W. (1952). *The great frontier*. Austin: University of Texas Press.

Weiss, H. (1980). *Families and neighborhoods*. Unpublished manuscript, Cornell University, Ithaca, NY.

Whittaker, J. (1979). *Caring for troubled children: Residential treatment in community context*. San Francisco, CA: Jossey-Bass.

Whittaker, J. (1983). Social support networks in child welfare. In J. Whittaker, J. Garbarino, & Associates (Eds.), *Social support networks* (pp. 167–187). Chicago, IL: Aldine.

Wilson, E. (1975). *Sociobiology: The new synthesis*. Cambridge, MA: Harvard University Press.

Wohlwill, J. F., & van Vliet, W. (Eds.). (1984). *Habitats for children: The impact of density*. New York: Academic Press.

14

Actuarial and Automated Assessment Procedures and Approaches

Douglas T. Brown

Introduction

During the past 15 years, assessment procedures for professional mental health practitioners have been gradually undergoing a major revolution. The advent of the minicomputer in the 1970s and the microcomputer in the 1980s has significantly influenced the speed with which psychological and other data can be collected and processed. Advanced statistical programs such as SPSS-X, developed in 1984, have enhanced the ability of practitioners to do relatively complex regression analyses including multiple regression, discriminant analysis, and other procedures which provide multivariate prediction models for human behavior.

During the past 5 years, a rapid development stage has occurred in the microcomputer industry. Relatively inexpensive systems (under $10,000) have been created which offer 16-bit microprocessors, large random access memory (1 million bytes or more), and high-speed fixed storage media. This technology has accelerated the development of highly complex multivariate assessment systems for use with adult, adolescent, and child-oriented data. As this chapter is being written, assessment procedures in psychology and the mental health fields are in the process of undergoing a major transformation. The use of microcomputers for the development, standardization, and administration of assessment techniques and batteries has increased dramatically. This process, however, is very much in the developmental stages, and much of what will be presented is a review of that development. As with other disciplines, the mental health field has found itself unprepared to cope with the speed of this technological revolution. Today's advances in microcomputers appear to have a useful life of approximately 3 years. The development of microcomputer hardware is outdistancing the ability of professionals to develop programs which appropriately utilize its capabilities. Therefore, much of what is reviewed in this chapter constitutes rather rudimentary attempts to apply computerization to personality and social–emotional assessment.

Douglas T. Brown. Department of Psychology, James Madison University, Harrisonburg, Virginia.

This chapter will review, historically, developments in automated cognitive and personality assessment. The major types of instrumentation currently in use will be examined, and specific tests will be discussed together with the output generated by these instruments. Methodological and technical considerations will be discussed and critiqued along with the strengths and limitations of various techniques. Finally, case studies will be presented which illustrate the use of computerized assessment with children and adolescents. Throughout the chapter, an attempt will be made to discriminate between adult, adolescent, and child applications; the majority of the most sophisticated techiques, however, are currently in the adult area.

Historical Perspective

The term "actuarial" assessment, when used in the psychology and mental health fields, refers to the use of multivariate statistical procedures for the prediction of behavioral outcomes. The statistical techniques most often employed include multiple regression, canonical correlation coupled with multiple regression, discriminant analysis, and cluster analysis. Prior to the availability of inexpensive sophisticated computerization, these techniques were generally not used in the field because of the extensive mathematical computations necessary. With the use of computers, the amount of time necessary to perform such computations has decreased markedly since 1970. For example, a large-scale discriminant analysis based on 50 variables and 2,000 subjects would have consumed at least 2 hours of computer time in 1967, costing several thousand dollars. With today's more advanced microcomputers, this procedure can be done in a matter of minutes with negligible costs. It is this development that has fostered modern automated assessment procedures.

Automated assessment involves any procedure that attempts to collect and interpret test data through the use of machines. Modern automated assessment systems use rather complicated mathematical algorithms for making behavioral predictions. An algorithm is simply a set of rules for solving a problem in a finite number of steps. These decision rules are built into the computer, based on regression analyses performed on standardization data, at the time that assessment instruments are standardized.

The first applications of automated actuarial systems were developed in clinical psychology. As early as 1968, Fowler and Coyle reported computerized classifications of college students with the Minnesota Multiphasic Personality Inventory (MMPI). Using a UNIVAC 1107 computer (which is not as powerful as today's Apple II) to arrange MMPI scaled scores into Atlas codes, they concluded that the computer more accurately analyzed these three-part codes than did psychologists and counselors who applied their clinical judgments. Thus, with computer technology, the reliability of clinical interpretation was increased.

In 1973, one of the first attempts to develop a psychological battery was described by Paitich (1973). This system, called the Comprehensive Automated Psychological Examination and Report (CAPER), integrated a number of published and unpublished instruments, including the MMPI, 16 PF, Raven, WAIS Vocabulary, Clarke Parent Child Relations Questionnaire, and Clarke Sexual History Questionnaire. The client answered test questions on standard IBM answer sheets and these, in turn, were keypunched and processed on an IBM 370 computer. The computer, utilizing FORTRAN 4 as a program language, scored all of the tests using the raw data and provided printed profiles for each of the tests. The program also provided a number of short verbal descriptive statements about the client based on the test data. Paitich concluded that CAPER provides more reliable scoring and interpretation of personality and cognitive assessment instruments than would be possible through other means.

Another early attempt at computerized assessment is described by Johnson and Williams (1975). A prototypical admissions system was developed whereby incoming clients were given psychological, social, and medical assessments through a computerized screening process on a CRT terminal. This system essentially performed some functions, typically completed by social workers, by providing structured interviews in each of the above areas and compiling a verbal and quantitative report for each client. Furthermore, the system was used to assemble patient data bases over time. In a later study, Johnson, Giannetti, Klingler, and Williams (1980) compared on-line intake procedures with traditional intake procedures, concluding that the computer produced results which were as reliable as conventional methodologies *and* much more cost effective and time efficient. Similar results have been reported by Lyons and Brown (1981).

Perhaps the first assessment instrument adapted to computerization was the MMPI. Miller, Johnson, Klingler, Williams, and Giannetti developed an on-line MMPI interpretative program in 1977, suggesting that previous attempts to computerize the MMPI had resulted in a significant number of misclassifications. Their program employed a scatter analysis to determine if the profile, obtained from a given client, could be matched to known profiles for various psychiatric classifications. The algorithm used for diagnosis employed a 5-point scatter analysis after determining the validity of a given test protocol. Those protocols that could not be matched to a particular diagnostic category were analyzed on a scale-by-scale basis. Reports generated by this technique were both statistical and verbal in nature.

Using a derivative of the above system, Labeck, Johnson, and Harris (1983) compared MMPI diagnosis and interpretation performed by trained clinicians with that of the computer assessment system. Results indicated that the accuracy of computerized MMPI interpretation was equal to or better than that of the clinicians. In addition, the narratives generated by the computer were judged to be significantly better than blind interpretation of similar profiles done by clinicians. Finally, DSM-III diagnostic categories were also identified by the computer, with significant accuracy. Labeck *et al.* concluded that the algorithms employed in their analysis system could not be duplicated by a traditional MMPI analysis using manual scoring. Thus, the computer was found to provide a level of analysis that was not otherwise evident in the professional repertoire of the clinicians. These researchers also concluded that the diagnostic accuracy of their algorithms was at least as good as that provided by a psychologist.

Several computerized models for the interpretation of the Rorschach have been devised. The first of these models, developed by Piotrowski (1974), required a highly reliable coding system for scoring Rorschach responses. More recently, Exner (1974) has revised Piotrowski's system and quantified it for use with children, adolescents, and adults. Finally, Harris, Niedner, Feldman, Fink, and Johnson (1981) describe the development of an on-line Rorschach interpretation method using Exner's Comprehensive System. Using a computer algorithm for Rorschach scoring and interpretation, but not administration, their validity study showed a scoring correlation of $r = .79$ when compared with trained clinicians. Further, the interpretive reports generated by the computer algorithm were judged to be useful and valid, but lacking in adaptive behavior analysis. The computer program's inability to make clinical judgments based on behavioral observations during the administration of the Rorschach was noted as a considerable limitation; clearly, this is an obvious weakness of any computer program used to administer and/or interpret a personality assessment instrument.

As is evident from the studies above, the computer's use in personality assessment has focused primarily on collecting demographic information and administering, scoring, or analyzing specific personality instruments. With few exceptions, most instruments administered and/or interpreted through automated methods have been adapted and/or extrapolated from existing paper and pencil techniques. Notably absent from most of the early computer research, however, is the adaptation of cognitive assessment devices to computer administration and interpretation. Nonetheless, the computer has been used as a very sophisticated "psychometrician."

Space (1981) has provided an excellent review on the breadth of the computer as a psychometrician. These include the use of the computer (*a*) to analyze anxiety and to function as a biofeedback mechanism; (*b*) to provide DSM-III and other kinds of diagnostic categories, (*c*) to collect interview, demographic, case history, and medical history information through CRT terminals, (*d*) to administer and analyze cognitive and personality assessment tools and data, respectively, and (*e*) to produce quantitative and verbal summaries of test information using sophisticated regression techniques. Space cites a number of reasons for the probable future acceptance of the computer as psychometrician. These include the following:

1. There is an increasing demand for psychological and mental health services and a common concern that the time frame between referral, testing, and preparation of reports is too long. Computerized assessment could reduce this turnaround time substantially, for example, by decreasing the need for long waiting lists and/or many hours of test interpretation and report writing.

2. The administration of psychological tests by computer requires only a trained technician rather than a psychologist (or mental health practitioner). This has the advantage of freeing the psychologist to perform other activities.

3. The computerization of psychological instruments provides the potential for performing research and standardizations which were previously not possible. The speed of the standardization process in the future may be enhanced considerably by the ability of computers to rapidly collect and analyze data from discrepant populations.

4. The computerization of psychological instruments should increase the reliability of tests by reducing the amount of administration and scoring error. While this requires proof through further research (see discussion below), computer administration of tests, at the very least, should be identical from administration to administration. To the extent that this is true, computerized reports will be absolutely reliable in the sense that a particular set of responses will result in the same report every time. This contrasts sharply with the literature on inter-report reliability by psychologists.

5. The use of computerized assessment allows for the development of instruments which are very complex in their administration and interpretation (i.e., Rorschach, MMPI, Kelly Role Construct Repertoire Test) and for their wider use because the time-consuming nature of their administrations and scorings have been substantially decreased.

6. Computers allow for the programming of a wide variety of diagnostic responses to a given set of behaviors. This means that rare or unusual diagnostic events can be easily identified by the computer using the best data or procedures available from the profession at a given point in time. Thus, the data base from which a computer works can be infinitely larger than that contained in the average practitioner's repertoire. This suggests that automated assessment could drastically increase the knowledge available for any agency or school setting.

7. The collection of social, medical, and demographic information is often a haphazard procedure in many schools and clinics. The use of computerized data collection for these areas would make this information data base more standard, reliable, and complete. As will be seen from research presented below, the probability of gaining more accurate information could be enhanced by the use of computerized data collection.

Historically, computerized assessment systems have generated considerable criticism from the profession. While more detailed discussion of these criticisms can be found below, the central concerns have been summarized by Space (1981), Sampson (1983), and Brown (1984):

1. Computers are impersonal and therefore insensitive to the feelings of the client being evaluated (this is the most common criticism). Some critics question the quality of data collected under computer conditions.

2. Interfaces between the person being assessed and the computer are poorly designed in that the computer program is often not ergonomically (user friendly) designed.

3. Current computer programs are not interactive in nature for the most part and work on linear models of branching. Thus, some computer programs are not adaptive in their testing style.

4. Computer approaches cannot be easily used with certain populations such as the retarded or severely mentally ill.

5. Since computers cannot make behavioral observations, they often miss extremely "pathological" responses. Thus, behavioral observations cannot be readily factored into the development of a computerized report.

6. Computer-collected information may not be confidential. The collection of large computerized psychological data bases could lead to access by groups or persons not authorized and/or competent to use them.

It is clear from the information already discussed that many of the potential strengths and weaknesses of automated assessment cannot be properly evaluated without further research. The relative recency and availability of automated assessment place this technology in its infancy. As will be evident, much of the hullabaloo currently being expressed by mental health practitioners about automated assessment can be traced to the paucity of research on its efficacy. This, coupled with a lack of understanding of the dynamics of the computer revolution, has created a sense of reactive urgency in the minds of many professionals.

Methodological and Technical Considerations and Limitations of Automated Assessment

Pertinent methodological considerations surrounding automated assessment can be divided into several areas, including (*a*) computer hardware considerations, (*b*) software development considerations, (*c*) the quality of the human/machine interface, and (*d*) ethical considerations. Each of these areas will be discussed and related to relevant literature.

Hardware Considerations

Prior to the introduction of the Apple II computer in 1978, the majority of automated assessment systems had been developed either on mainframe computers (such as the IBM 360 series) or on minicomputers which emerged during the 1970s. While the IBM 360 series was never adequate for the task of regression analyses and report generation, the minicomputers developed by IBM and the Digital Equipment Corporation in the late 1970s did permit the generation of personality assessment reports as described elsewhere in this chapter. Beyond the minicomputers, however, three major events in computer hardware development have provided the current opportunity for advanced psychological assessment. These include the development of the high-speed microprocessor chip, the high-speed random access memory chip, and high-speed high-density data storage media such as that provided by Winchester technology. These advances have allowed modern microcomputer systems to become miniature versions of their mainframe and mini predecessors; in many cases, however, they also have much higher processing speeds. Thus, these machines require less space, less energy, and less money—their costs are now within a price range that permits ownership by individual practitioners.

Many of the more recent automated assessment systems (e.g., Psych-Systems, NCS) have been developed on minicomputers. Generally, these computers contain 16-bit processors with a minimum of 256,000 bytes of random access memory and from 40 to 160 megabytes of fixed disk storage. Some of the more elaborate systems can be as large as 5 million bytes of random access memory and one gigabyte of fixed disk storage. Historically, the major limitation in developing automated assessment batteries was the ability of the computer to store large amounts of statistical and verbal information and to manipulate it rapidly. With the advent of minicomputers, this obstacle was overcome. During the early 1980s when microcomputers such as the IBM XT, Dec Rainbow 100 Plus, and Altos 586 were introduced, the capabilities formerly associated with minicomputers became available to microcomputer users at a fraction of the price. Thus, the most modern microcomputers now being used in automated assessment contain as much as 4 million bytes of random access memory and 160 megabytes of hard disk storage in an enclosure the size of a file cabinet drawer.

As this chapter is being written, new machines are being introduced with 32-bit microprocessor chips which will allow even higher speed data processing and more elaborate statistical and verbal manipulators. These new developments exemplify the recent history of the computer hardware industry. Indeed, it has been so rapid that it is accurate to state that it has outpaced the ability of software developers by at least 5 years. For example, while machines such as the Apple II are relative "antiques" within the microcomputer industry, programs are just now being developed which allow automated assessment on this system. As most of these programs (see Beaumont, 1981, for a description) are relatively simplistic and linear in their design, it is now clear that in order to take full advantage of the potential sophistication inherent in automated assessment, a minimal hardware requirement would include a 16-bit microprocessor with 1 million bytes of random access memory and 40 megabytes of hard disk storage. This would be especially important if interactive and branching applications to be described below are utilized.

Software Considerations

A number of different software approaches have been taken in developing automated assessment systems. Altemose and Williamson (1981) describe two basic models of software development: the linear and the interactive or adaptive models of programming. In the linear model, all clients receive exactly the same form of a given instrument. The adaptive testing model, meanwhile, uses the ability of the computer program to modify test stimuli based on clients' response patterns; Altemose and Williamson refer to this model as the "Intelligent Computer Model."

Practitioners have often assumed that computer programs are adaptively written; that is, they predominantly follow the intelligent computer model. A review of the literature, however (Angle, 1981; Byers, 1981; Johnson & Williams, 1978; Morf, Alexander, & Fuerth, 1981; Sampson, 1983; Vale, 1981), suggests that this is not the case. In fact, the majority of instruments contained on today's assessment systems are not actuarial in nature, but are simply adaptations of the paper and pencil instruments commonly used in clinical and school psychology. Examples of these instruments include computerized versions of the MMPI, 16 PF, Shipley Hartford Intelligence Scale, various Wechsler intelligence scale analysis programs, and a variety of behavioral checklists. As Sampson (1983) points out, the adaptation of these instruments to computerization leads to questions concerning their generalizability given the fact that computer-based norms may differ from the conventionally derived standardization norms for these instruments. This suggests a need for reliability and validity data based on computer presentations of these tests.

A number of researchers have attempted to develop adaptive computerization approaches. Adaptive approaches emphasize branching programs which modify the presentation of stimulus questions based on various client characteristics or responses. In addition, some programs have been developed where ancillary information is collected by the computer at the time of client assessment. Stout (1981), for example, examined response latencies in connection with the computerized administration of the MMPI and a structured interview technique. The structured interview technique used a branching system based on clients' responses. The computer was programmed to measure clients' response latencies on an item-by-item basis and to compare clusters of latency responses based on the types of structured interview questions. This research tended to indicate that when clients viewed certain clusters of questions as problematic, different latency scores resulted when compared with clusters of questions not viewed as problematic. Johnson and Johnson (1981) reported similar findings with the MMPI in which clients' tendencies to fabricate test responses was related to their response latencies. Johnson and Johnson suggested that by using unobtrusive polygraph measures to relate psychological responding to specific stimulus items on a computerized test, areas of maximum client concern could be isolated. This kind of technology, however, has not yet been developed, and some perceive this procedure as having negative ethical implications.

Vale (1981) has provided an excellent review of the fundamental concepts of adaptive testing systems. He notes that the computer selects a given subset of items for administration to a given client based on algorithms which, in turn, are based on three types of branching systems. The first of these system types involves interitem branching, in which each item in the item pool leads to one or more other items based on the item scores. This system is merely binary, and each successive item presented depends on a binary choice made by the client. Many branching systems currently used in education employ this technique. The second basic type involves intersubtest branching. This technique is similar to interitem branching except that clusters of items are first presented to the client. Branching then takes place based on a composite score from a given cluster of items. Thus, branching moves from cluster to cluster or subtest to subtest rather than from item to item. The third type of branching is termed model based. Vale describes this technique quite succinctly:

> Model-based branching strategies are most often based on item response, or latent trait, theory which assumes that item responses are probabilistically related by a specified function to a continuous underlying trait or ability. In these strategies, the score consists of an estimate of the level of ability on the underlying trait that characterizes the individual. Testing begins with the administration of a generally appropriate item. The trait estimate is updated after each item is administered, and the next item, at each stage, is determined by deciding which item of those available, will best improve the trait estimate. (p. 400)

Vale concludes that the currently available microcomputer technology is capable of handling adaptive systems of the type described above, but that lengthy and complex programming is necessary to accomplish test administration at this level of sophistication.

In the area of school psychology, one major actuarial system has been developed by McDermott and Hale (McDermott, 1980; McDermott & Hale, 1982). This system, known as the Multidimensional Actuarial Classification System (MAC), is designed to apply statistical decision rules, modeled after national standards, to the differential diagnosis and classification of child psychopathology. Through these decision rules, the MAC statistically weights the importance of relationships among several psychological factors (e.g., intellectual functioning, adaptive behavior, academic achievement, and social/behavioral adjustment) while producing differential diagnoses in the areas of mental retardation, specific learning disabilities, emotional disturbance, communication/perceptual motor disorders, and academic under- or overachievement.

In order to utilize the MAC, a practitioner must collect and input the following information: (*a*) chronological age, (*b*) an individually administered intelligence test, (*c*) standard scores for academic achievement in all areas of achievement, (*d*) standard scores for the child's level of social maturity (usually based on the Vineland Social Maturity Scale), (*e*) standardized indices of behavioral and emotional adjustment collected through classroom or other observations, and (*f*) other demographic data such as the child's sex and socioeconomic status. Thus, the MAC does not administer the assessments per se. Rather, it analyzes the test data that have been collected by the practitioner and fed into the computer. The computer transforms the data into a standardized format, referencing each instrument's appropriate norms which are stored in its memory. It then makes a differential diagnosis decision.

In creating the MAC, McDermott (1980) used the criteria specified by the American Association on Mental Deficiency (1977) for his classification of mental retardation. His other decision rules were based on the American Psychiatric Association's (1980) DSM-III guidelines. In total, the MAC contains 20 different actuarial decision rules which can be associated with 37 different diagnoses that yield any one of 241 possible combinations of multidimensional classifications. McDermott reports that the MAC's construct validity has been supported through multivariate pattern analyses of these classifications in actual field testings.

McDermott and Hale (1982) evaluated the utility of MAC in a study of 73 children and adolescents referred for psychological services. All of the children were evaluated by trained child psychologists who rendered their specific diagnoses. In addition, data collected in the areas specified above were fed into the MAC, which produced its own diagnostic decisions. The average agreement between the "expert" child psychologists and the MAC averaged approximately 86%, while agreement among the expert child psychologists averaged 76.5%. McDermott and Hale conclude that these findings support the validity of the MAC's classification system, at least when compared with expert psychologists. Furthermore, the MAC's diagnostic reliability appears somewhat superior to that of the expert child psychologists. McDermott suggests that, unlike clinical methods, actuarial assessment does not depend on "clinical judgment." This, therefore, eliminates a significant source of error which leads to unreliability. Stated succinctly, given a particular set of conditions, the computer—unlike the expert child psychologists—will respond with exactly the same diagnostic decisions every time.

Labeck et al. (1983) have shown similar results when comparing diagnostic decisions which utilized DSM-III categories. Comparing diagnostic conclusions reached by trained clinicians and those of a computerized MMPI program, they found exceptionally high congruence between the two methods of diagnosis. Labeck et al. suggest that computerized diagnosis may be somewhat more reliable than clinical judgments based upon the same test data.

Human Interface and Efficacy Considerations

Since the beginning of computerized testing, a considerable debate has surrounded its efficacy. This debate can be divided into two fundamental issues. The first involves the qualitative differences between assessment undertaken by a mental health practitioner in a one-to-one interaction with a client and that undertaken through a computerized assessment system. Basically, the quality of the human/computer interface versus the quality of human/human interface is in question here. The second major issue involves the efficacy of computerized assessment in terms of its quality of judgments versus the quality of judgments made by professional practitioners. This section will attempt to review the data related to these two issues.

The studies examining the human/computer interface present rather contradictory information. Hedl, O'Neil, and Hansen (1973) investigated the affective reactions of clients to computerized intelligence testing versus standard one-to-one intelligence testing performed by psychologists. Based on measures of state anxiety and attitude, they concluded that computer testing procedures produce significantly higher levels of state anxiety and less favorable attitudes about intelligence testing as compared to the traditional intelligence testing methods. Further, Hedl *et al.* concluded that some specific aspects of computerized testing led to heightened levels of anxiety and poor attitudes. These included the lack of the computer terminal's user friendliness during the administration of test items and the unavailability of supportive feedback by the computer throughout the testing situation.

In a more recent study, Skinner and Allen (1983) compared computerized and face-to-face self-report assessment for alcohol, drug, and tobacco use in adults. They hypothesized that computerized structured interviews involving substance abuse would produce more reliable and honest information in this area. Results of their study indicated, however, that this was not the case; the analyses showed no important differences in reliability across the two techniques. Further, an interesting ancillary finding was that clients generally found the computer interview less friendly than that of the personal interview. However, they did consider the computer interview as more interesting and relaxing than the face-to-face interview.

In another interesting study, Quintanar, Crowell, and Pryor (1982) examined linear versus interactive formats for the quality of their human/computer interactions. The results of their study indicated that subjects perceived the interactive computer format more positively and as exhibiting characteristics associated with humanness. However, these interactive programs were also perceived as less honest than the linear programs. The authors suggested that these results reflect the tendency of humans to associate mechanistic or automatic responding with less bias. Another important finding of this study was that subjects exposed to the human-like computer model performed better on the cognitive tasks being presented.

Katz and Dalby (1981) utilized an automated version of the Fundamental Interpersonal Relations Orientation-BC Scales (FIRO-BC), comparing it with traditional paper and pencil techniques utilizing a gifted sample of children. The results of this study indicated that retest reliabilities for the automated version of this instrument were higher than for the paper and pencil version. Reactions of children to the computer-assisted FIRO-BC were extremely positive and improved from the first to the second test administration. Katz and Dalby concluded that it is possible to transfer a paper and pencil test to an automated media application while maintaining high levels of reliability.

Carr and Ghosh (1983a, 1983b) compared the responses of phobic patients to computerized versus traditional methods of assessment by giving 26 randomly selected referred patients an automated assessment interview using a microcomputer program. Over half of the subjects indicated that they found the computer interview more acceptable and that it was easier to communicate with the computer than with a clinician. The results of the computer interview, when compared with those of conventional clinical assessment techniques, correlated quite closely. Carr and Ghosh concluded that the use of automated assessment to identify phobias for treatment is valid, appropriate, and equal in quality to more traditional clinical analyses. On the other hand, Schmid, Bronish, and von Zerssen (1982) used two computer diagnostic systems to evaluate psychopathology in adults. Their findings suggest an incongruence between computer-generated diagnoses and those generated by psychologists, particularly in the areas of organic psychoses, schizophrenia, and depression.

In summary, while much of the data suggest that computerized assessment is more reliable than traditional assessment, the use of computerized systems to form diagnostic impressions is currently at a rudimentary stage of development. The relative paucity of studies in this area suggests that significant research comparing traditional and automated assessment will have to be performed in order to futher validate this procedure. In the area of child psychology, McDermott and Hale (1982) have provided the most formidable example of differential diagnosis as reliably performed by a computer. As with traditional clinical methods of diagnosis, however, the external criteria on which decision rules are built are often themselves not validated (e.g., the definitive characteristics of learning disabilities). These criteria also need equal attention.

Ethical Considerations

A number of divergent concerns related to computerized assessment have been expressed by professionals in this field. These can be grouped into two basic areas: quality control and future impact on the profession. Space (1981) has summarized many of the quality control issues. Since many computerized assessment systems are nonmathematically based, they tend to disregard the individual characteristics of the client, thus losing a great deal of idiographic information. For example, computerized programs are rarely able to ferret out the underlying structure motivating an individual's behavior (some exceptions to this are discussed below). Since a computerized assessment is a preprogrammed event, the interactive control which can be exercised by a client is also limited compared to a standard clinically administered test. Finally, other concerns about the ability of exceptional children and adults to interact effectively with computers have been expressed. These include such factors as reading level and the ability to manipulate computer terminals; both critical variables in the administration of automated assessment techniques.

Sampson (1983) suggests that other technical factors may also influence the quality of automated assessment. These include inadequate or inappropriate norms, failure by test developers to provide reliability and validity data on computer-assisted systems, the inability to generalize test interpretations, and staff resistance to the use of computer systems. Byrnes and Johnson (1981), addressing this latter factor, concluded that professional and staff resistance may be the most critical problem to overcome in the implementation of computerized assessment procedures.

Other researchers have expressed concern about the impact of automated assessment on overall professional functioning. Altemose and Williamson (1981), for example, believe that automated assessment poses a threat to the job security of school and perhaps clinical psychologists. They feel that computer test developers have misled the profession by asserting that much of their software is adaptive in nature and therefore fits into the "intelligent computer model." Altemose and Williamson assert that this simply is not the case, as the majority of computer instruments are rather simplistic in nature and modeled directly after their paper and pencil counterparts. As such, they conclude that current computer techniques do not threaten the traditional role of the school psychologist, but may enhance it. Of greater concern to them is the movement toward the intelligent computer or adaptive assessment models which they perceive as potentially threatening the role of psychologists who perform assessment.

Other theorists (Erdman, Greist, Klein, Jefferson, & Getto, 1981) feel that the intelligent computer model will best help to humanize automated assessment. Further, they believe that the ability of truly adaptive programs to perform advanced statistical and probabilistic analyses should significantly complement current psychological services. This, then, could result in considerably improved perceptions of credibility by consumers of these services.

Brown (1984) has suggested that research is rapidly moving in the direction of the adaptive or intelligent computer model, and that psychologists should quickly acquire additional training in order to be able to operate and interpret the automated assessment systems of the future. Thus, he suggests that it is not a question of *will* these systems be used, but *how* they will be used and how competent mental health practitioners will be to interpret their output.

Concern has been expressed (Turkington, 1984) about the qualifications of those who use automated assessment systems, particularly the use of automated assessment systems by nonpsychologists. For example, interpretation of the more advanced multivariate system's output requires knowledge of multivariate statistics. In fact, the ability to adequately critique many of the more advanced testing systems requires sophisticated knowledge in statistics *and* programming and test design. While many psychologists have simply not acquired these skills as part of their training, the use of automated assessment systems by nonpsychologists (who presumably have little or no training in psychometrics) is of even greater concern. This is especially true when automated assessment systems are applied to personnel screening and to the criminal justice system and when the companies that develop and distribute these systems fail to validate the credentials of those who purchase these systems. Given the fact that much of the software in existence today is at a rudimentary stage of development, the use of automated assessment as the sole decision-making tool in mental health or educational placement is a highly questionable practice, especially in the hands of nonpsychologists. In fact, the American Psychological Association will soon publish guidelines for the development and use of automated assessment systems. These guidelines or standards are badly needed in order to improve quality control in the development of such systems and to set limits on their ethical use.

Ingram (1985) has suggested a number of areas that can facilitate psychologists' evaluations of automated assessment software. These include the following:

1. Is the software based on a good theoretical orientation and are the sources of expertise who helped to develop the software carefully identified?
2. Does the publisher of the software provide ongoing support and updates for the software? Is the publisher committed to the continuous revision and refinement of the software?
3. Does the publisher set guidelines for the ethical distribution of the software; that is, only to professionals who are qualified to use it?
4. Does the software possess adequate security mechanisms which protect the confidentiality of client data?
5. Does the publisher present comprehensive data on the reliability and validity of the test instruments based on administrations by computers to a variety of populations?

6. Is the software easily transportable to a variety of computer hardware and operating systems?
7. Is the software adaptive in nature and interactive with other software programs produced by the publisher or other publishers?
8. Does the publisher provide sufficient data which allow a formal evaluation of the program structure on which the automated assessment system is based?

Very few systems in existence today can meet the above criteria. Many software publishers, because of concerns regarding the theft of their proprietary programming techniques, do not allow ready access to the structure of their systems. This makes formal evaluation of their software difficult or impossible in many instances.

School and Clinical Applications

The utilization of computers to assess children and adolescents in school and clinical settings is still quite limited. The majority of adaptive applications, in fact, have been produced for use with adults. Nonetheless, McCullough and Wenck (1984) have described the types of programs available. These fall into several categories, including (a) those that score and interpret intelligence and adaptive behavior data, (b) programs that generate reports on the basis of intelligence and adaptive behavior data, (c) programs that provide career guidance information, and (d) programs that either produce on-site data bases or allow access to national data bases which are on mainframe computers. Much of the software currently used in school systems is, by necessity, limited by the hardware these systems most often possess (e.g., Apple II, Tandy TRS-80s). These computers are often 8-bit machines which, for the most part, are incapable of supporting adaptive types of testing.

In the area of special education, Okey and McGarity (1982) have described a system for diagnostic testing which acts as an adjunct to a diagnostic teacher by continually assessing the specific objectives delineated on a given student's individual education plan. The program allows the teacher to develop specific items which directly assess the objectives for a particular student, and then it monitors the attainment of these objectives. Bennett (1982) and Williams and Gayeski (1983) have described other uses of microcomputer programs in special education. These include programs that develop individual education plans based on assessment data (e.g., ADEPT, 1982) and programs that perform diagnostic assessment in specific instructional areas such as reading and mathematics.

In the area of advanced automated techniques assessing emotional disturbances and learning disabilities, few programs have been extensively developed. The remainder of this section will be devoted to a review of the major instruments which have been utilized, primarily on minicomputers, for assessing children and adolescents. These instruments vary from very simple adaptations of existing instruments to the computer, to extremely complex multivariate computer systems. Where applicable, sample output from the computer on specific cases will be provided.

Adaptive Behavior Instruments

Two major adaptive behavior instruments have been computerized, the Minnesota Child Development Inventory (MCDI; Ireton & Thwing, 1974) and the Personality Inventory for Children (PIC; Wirt, Seat, & Broen, 1977). In both cases, the versions of these instruments that have been adapted to the 1985 Psych-Systems (of Baltimore, Maryland) automated assessment system will be described.

The Minnesota Child Development Inventory

The Psych-Systems version of the MCDI, administered to mothers of referred children using a computer terminal, contains 320 items which were selected from a pool of 2,000 items on the basis of their age-discriminating power. The MCDI is appropriate for children from 1 to 6 years of age, and its items are grouped into seven scales including gross motor, fine motor, expressive language, language comprehension, situation comprehension, self-help, and personal social. In addition, a general development scale consisting of the most age-discriminating items from all of the above scales provides an index of overall development. Norms for the test are interpreted as being in the normal range, delayed, or advanced for a child's particular chronological age (CA).

Studies performed by Psych-Systems indicate that the validity of a mother's MCDI report is related directly to her level of education and ability to accurately observe the child's behavior. Its reliability is related to the mother's ability to interact effectively with the computer. The MCDI computer output provides a description of the child's current developmental status in narrative form and in profile form. A sample computer printout is provided below based on a child with a CA of 4 years and 3 months. The child was referred for delayed language development.

```
454-54-5454   John Smith      4 yr old white male   17-Mar-85

Child: John


    ------------------------------------------------------------------
    :                :                                               :
    :    MCDI        :   Minnesota Child Development Inventory        :
    :                :                                               :
    ------------------------------------------------------------------


            Test Authors : H. Ireton, Ph.D.,
                           E. Thwing, Ph.D.


The MCDI is a standardized inventory to be completed by a parent
or guardian who knows the child well.   It is designed to assess
the child's current developmental status.

This clinical report is designed to assist in psychodiagnostic
evaluation.   It is for use only by qualified professionals.   The
report was produced by a computerized analysis of the data given by
the client listed above, and is to be used as part of a profession-
al evaluation.  No decision should be based solely upon the contents
of this report, and it should not be used in a clinical setting
without the approval of a professional who is qualified in the
use of psychological tests.
```

The computer program generating this report was designed by Psych
Systems, Inc. , Baltimore, Maryland 21208.   Copyright (C) 1984
by Psych Systems, Inc.   The interpretive analysis utilized in
the interpretation was designed by Harold R. Ireton, Ph. D.   Copyright
(C) 1981 by Harold R. Ireton.   The Minnesota Child Development
Inventory is reproduced by permission, Copyright (C) 1968, 1970,
1972 by Harold R. Ireton and Edward J. Thwing.   Published by
Behavior Science Systems, Inc. , P. O. Box 1108, Minneapolis, Minnesota
55440.   All rights reserved.

Description

This 4 year and 3 month old boy was described by his mother during the
administration of the MCDI. The mother reports less than an 11th
grade education. This raises a question as to whether or not this
person has sufficient reading skills to adequately understand
the inventory items. Thus, the results should be viewed with caution.
This child is reported to have the following handicap or special
problem: Has difficulty speaking to strangers. The presence of a
handicap or special problem may affect the inventory results in
complex ways that make interpretation more difficult.

Current Developmental Status

General Development

This child is displaying significantly delayed development on the
general development scale, according to the informant's report.
Currently, the child's level of functioning as measured by this
scale is more than 30 percent below age level. This is a strong
indicator of a developmental problem in some area. However, generalized
developmental delay cannot be inferred on the basis of this scale
alone.

Motor Development

The child's gross motor development is in the seriously delayed
range, indicating a major gross motor problem. The Fine Motor
score is in the normal range, although the scale lacks comprehensiveness
in this age range.

Language Development

This child's expressive language is significantly below expectations
for children this age. The child's language comprehension is significantly
below age level. A delay on the language comprehension scale is
a strong indicator of a developmental problem. A low score on
this scale could be related to a hearing or language problem,
or to limited intellectual ability.

Adaptive Comprehension

The child's comprehension of situations by primarily non-verbal
means is delayed. Self-Help skills are below what would be expected
for a child of this age.

Personal-Social Maturity

Personal-Social Maturity is well below age level, which may indicate
a major developmental or behavioral problem.

Intellectual Status

The MCDI profile is ambiguous with regard to the child's intellectual
status.

Summary

The score for the following developmental scales fall in the delayed
range: General Development , Gross Motor , Expressive Language
, Language Comprehension , Situation Comprehension , Self Help
and Personal-Social . There is a need for follow-up that should
include at least these areas of delay indicated by the MCDI.
Intellectual status is ambiguous, from these results.

Developmental Age In Months

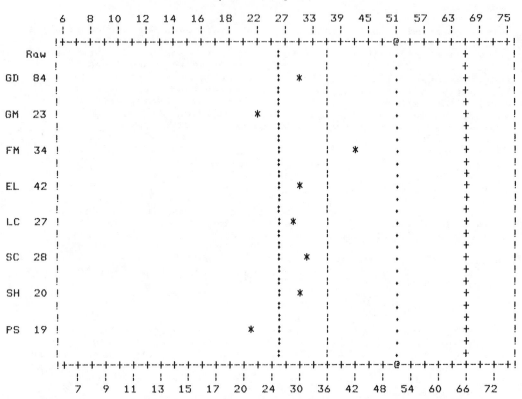

Developmental Age In Months

Graph Key	GD	General Development Scale	Percentage Lines
	GM	Gross Motor Scale	
	FM	Fine Motor Scale	: -> 50% below age
	EL	Expressive Language Scale	
	LC	Language Comprehension Scale	¦ -> 30% below age
	SC	Situation Comprehension Scale	
	SH	Self Help Scale	+ -> 30% above age
	PS	Personal/Social Scale	

Chronological Age Line   @.........@ -> 51 months

NOTE: Graphic representations are based on empirically generated values

Scale Name	Raw Scores	Category
General Development Scale:	84	Delayed
Gross Motor Scale:	23	Seriously Delayed
Fine Motor Scale:	34	Probably Normal
Expressive Language Scale:	42	Delayed
Language Comprehension Scale:	27	Delayed
Situation Comprehension Scale:	28	Delayed
Self Help Scale:	20	Delayed
Personal/Social Scale:	19	Seriously Delayed

```
          Name : John Smith
     Physician : Brown
           Age : 4
           Sex : Male
  Ethnic Group :  1 White
Patient Status :  3 Nonpatient
Education Level :  2 Elementary School
   Occup. Level :  1 Not In Labor Force


              MCDI Raw Data
              -----------------


                 Part One
                 ---------
     1234567890 1234567890 1234567890

  1-   4 1111



                 Part Two
                 ---------
     1234567890 1234567890 1234567890

  1-  30 YYYN**YNNY YYNNYYN*NN NNNYYNNYYN
 31-  60 NYNNN*NNNY NYY*N**Y*N YYNYYN**YY
 61-  90 *N*YNN*YNN YYYNNYNNYY NNNYYNYYYN
 91-120 NYY*NYYNNN NYYY*YNYNY NNY*NNYNNY
121-150 Y*YYY*NNNY *NY*YYNNNY YYY*YNYYYN
151-180 NYYYYYYNYN Y*YNYY*YY* YNYYYY**Y
181-210 NYYNNYNYYN YYNYYYYYYN YY*YNYNN*Y
211-240 YNYNNNYYYY YNNN*Y*NYY NYY*NNYNN*
241-270 NYNY*N*NYY YNYNYNYYYY YNYYNYYY*
271-300 *Y*NNNN**Y *NYNNNYNYY YNYYYNYY*
301-320 YN*YYNYYYN YYYNY*YYNN
```

The MCDI is an example of an instrument that has been adapted for computer without the benefit of renorming. In this case, the computer enhances the test in two ways. First, the reliability of administration is improved, since the test is administered by computer terminal and because a pretest is given to the mother to assess her intellectual ability to respond accurately to the instrument. Second, the scoring and interpretation of the instrument, while not increased in complexity, is accelerated considerably.

The Personality Inventory for Children

The PIC is perhaps the best known and best validated adaptive personality instrument for children (Lachar, Chapter 9 of this volume; Wirt *et al.*, 1977). Designed for use by parents with children from 6 to 16 years of age, the PIC's intent is (*a*) to identify domains that relate to specific behavioral patterns and (*b*) to predict these behaviors and/or patterns by comparing referred children's PIC results with those of numerous other populations with known behavior traits. The instrument contains items which are factored into a number of content areas using the same methodology employed for the MMPI. These content areas include achievement, intellectual screening, development, somatic concern, depression, family relations, lie scale, frequency scale, defensiveness scale, adjustment scale, delinquency scale, withdrawal scale, anxiety scale, psychosis scale, hyperactivity scale, and social skill scale. As can be seen from these scales, multiple validity checks are embedded in the test in order to detect intentional parental misinformation or tendencies to portray the child as more or less pathological in behavior than is truly the case.

An example of a PIC computer analysis for a 13-year-old adolescent referred for emotional disturbance is presented below. The analysis, which was generated with the Psych-Systems minicomputer program, is subdivided into eight sections within the narrative report: (*a*) protocol validity, (*b*) demography, (*c*) family context, (*d*) parental attitude/adjustment, (*e*) child adjustment status, (*f*) cognitive ability and integrity, (*g*) problem areas, and (*h*) personality description.

```
                        13 year old white male     16-Jun-82


             ************************************
             Personality Inventory For Children
             ************************************
Child:
Informant:

This clinical report is designed to aid in psychodiagnostic
evaluation.  It is available only to trained professionals.
This report was produced by a computerized analysis of the
responses provided by the informant listed above.  The report
is to be used in conjunction with professional evaluation.  No
decision should be based solely upon the contents of this report.

The PIC was reproduced by permission.  Copyright (C) 1977 by Western
Psychological Services.  Published by Western Psychological Services,
a division of Manson Western Corporation, Los Angeles, California.

The interpretive logic utilized in this report was designed by
James K. Klinedinst, PHD.  Copyright (C) 1980 by James K. Klinedinst.
All rights reserved.

                    Protocol Validity
This is a valid protocol.


                        Demography
This 13 year old white adolescent boy has been described by his
father.  He has lived in one residence within the past five year
period.

                      Family Context
The information in this section was reported by the father during
administration of the PIC, and may contain information which has
not been shared with the boy.  The family consists of a mother,
father, and three children.  This child is the oldest of three children.
According to the father this child was planned.  The child has
been with the father since birth.  This family functions with reasonable
cohesion and harmony.  Although family functioning is adequate,
there appears to be more than a desirable degree of tension between
members.  The father reports the parents adequately discuss important
matters.

                  Parental Attitudes/Adjustment
This father feels concern about being unable to understand the child's
behavior.  A failure to carry through when control is called for
is suggested.  The relationship between this father and child is
too distant, too disengaged.


Copyright (C) 1980, Psych Systems Inc., Baltimore, Maryland.
```

Present Problem Areas

Problematic behavior, when it occurs, most frequently takes the form of disordered conduct. Areas of behavior clearly suggested for further psychological observation are: activity level, acceptance by peers, managing angry feelings and intelligence and learning ability.

Child's Adjustment Status

Most clinicians would agree that this child is showing clear signs of emotional disturbance and recommend some 'outpatient' form of psychological intervention. Both home and school performance are impaired by this condition.

General Ability/Cognitive Integrity

This boy appears to be less than average in functional intellectual level. An individual intellectual assessment will be required if a more definitive measurement is needed. Given his level of intellectual functioning, he is not achieving academically as well as could be expected. School learning difficulties are present. Reading ability is the most commonly encountered deficiency.

Personality Description

His current interests and attitudes favor active play and physical skill development. He is likely to be seen as noisy, lively, and rough. The respondent is complaining of various social, and moral failures on the part of the child. The themes of conformity and rebellion, responsibility, and acquiring moral values will be an important part of the clinical picture. Such behaviors as disobedience and irritability are expectable.

This child has not yet developed an appropriate degree of self-regulation. The respondent is describing a variety of undercontrolled, excited, socially very undesirable conduct by the child. Temper tantrums are a common complaint. Fighting and cruelty are more likely to appear in the behavior of this child than in that of most.

The adequacy of this child's general abilities and skills is being called into question by the respondent. The clinician should be alert for disturbances in attentional processes. An increased likelihood of encountering distractibility, too much daydreaming, inability to manage complexity, and poor schoolwork is associated with this test pattern.

Obvious internal discomfort and unhappiness are present. The respondent is too closely identified with the child's fears and worries, pessimistic mood and low self-esteem to promote growth-producing activities. The child's behavior is being fostered by the high level of sympathetic or grudging recognition given it by the respondent.

Insufficiently controlled motor activity is being reported. In clinical settings children with similarly elevated profiles are descriptively overactive. The mother may report any of a variety of specific excited behaviors such as 'showing off', talking too much, acting without thinking, performing silly actions, being loud, boisterous, restless, or overactive.

Critical Items

-- DEPRESSION & POOR SELF-CONCEPT --

My child tends to pity him (her) self. (T)
My child has little self confidence. (T)
My child speaks of him (her) self as stupid or dumb. (T)

-- WORRY & ANXIETY --

My child often gets up at night. (T)
Often my child is afraid of little things. (T)
My child sometimes chews on his (her) lips until they are sore. (T)
Sometimes my child gets so nervous his (her) hands shake. (T)

-- REALITY DISTORTION --

My child gets confused easily. (T)

-- PEER RELATIONS --

Most of my child's friends are younger than he (she) is. (T)
My child never takes the lead in things. (T)
My child is very jealous of others. (T)
My child would rather be with adults than with children his(her) own age.
Other children make fun of my child's different ideas. (T)

-- UNSOCIALIZED AGGRESSION --

Often my child smashes things when angry. (T)
Many times my child has become violent. (T)
My child has a terrible temper. (T)

-- CONSCIENCE DEVELOPMENT --

My child is good at lying his (her) way out of trouble. (T)
My child often disobeys me. (T)
I always worry about my child having an accident when he(she) is out. (T)

Critical Items

-- ATYPICAL DEVELOPMENT --

My child has had convulsions. (T)
My child refused or couldn't suck as an infant. (T)

-- DISTRACTIBILITY, ACTIVITY LEVEL & COORDINATION --

As a younger child, it was impossible to get my child to take a nap. (T)
My child seldom gets a restful sleep. (T)
My child has difficulty doing things with his (her) hands. (T)
My child can't seem to keep attention on anything. (T)
My child can't seem to wait for things like other children do. (T)

-- SPEECH & LANGUAGE --

At one time my child had speech difficulties. (T)
My child first talked before he (she) was two years old. (F)

-- SOMATIC COMPLAINTS/CURRENT HEALTH --

Several times my child had complaints, but the doctor could find
nothing wrong. (T)
My child frequently complains of being hot even on cold days. (T)
Skin rash has been a problem with my child. (T)

-- SCHOOL ADJUSTMENT --

Starting school was very difficult for my child. (T)
My child can't sit still in school because of nervousness. (T)
Reading has been a problem for my child. (T)

-- FAMILY DISCORD --

My child seems unhappy about our home life. (T)
We often argue about who is the boss at our house. (T)
The child's father is hardly ever home. (T)
There is a lot of tension in our home. (T)

```
Case #              Ch:

         L   F   DEF ADJ ACH  IS DVL SOM  D  FAM DLQ WDL ANX PSY HPR SSK
120-             +                                                        -120
  -              +                                                         -
  -              +                                                         -
  -              +                                                         -
  -              +                                                         -
110-             +                                                        -110
  -              +                                                         -
  -              +                                                         -
  -              +                                                         -
  -              +                                                         -
100-             +                                                        -100
  -              +                                                         -
  -              +                                                         -
  -              +                                                         -
  -              +                                                         -
 90-             +                                                         - 90
  -              +                                                         -
  -              +                                                         -
  -              +  *           *                                          -
  -              +                                                         -
 80-             +                                                         - 80
  -              +                                                         -
  -              +                                             *        * -
  -              +                                 *                       -
  -     *        +                     *                                   -
 70- --- --- ---+--- -*- --- --- --- --- --- --- --- --- --- --- ----  70
  -              +                                                         -
  -              +             *                                           -
  -              +                                     *                   -
  -              +                                                         -
 60-             +                                                         - 60
  -              +                 *             *                         -
  -              +                                                         -
  -              +                         *                               -
  -              +                                                         -
 50- --- --- ---+--- --- --- --- --- --- --- --- --- --- --- --- ----  50
  -              +                                                         -
  -              +                                                         -
  -              +                                         *               -
  - *            +                                                         -
 40-             +                                                         - 40
  -              +                                                         -
  -              +                                                         -
  -              +                                                         -
  -              +                                                         -
 30-             +                                                         - 30
  -              +                                                         -
  -          *   +                                                         -
  -              +                                                         - 20
 20-             +

         L   F   DEF ADJ ACH  IS DVL SOM  D  FAM DLQ WDL ANX PSY HPR SSK
     R   3   8    5  41  18  18  11   8  18   8  20   6  10  10  14  21
     T  42  71   24  83  69  83  65  58  71  53  73  58  63  76  43  76
```

Case   Ch:

```
          SOM  FAM  ASO  AGN  DVL  WDL  ANX  RDS   EXC  SSK  INT  EXT
 120-                                              +                  -120
   -                                               +                  -
   -                                               +                  -
   -                                               +                  -
 110-                                              +                  -110
   -                                               +                  -
   -                                               +                  -
   -                                               +                  -
 100-                                              +                  -100
   -                                               +                  -
   -                                               +                  -
   -                                               +                  -
  90-                                              +                  - 90
   -                                               +                  -
   -                                               +                  -
   -                                               +                  -
  80-                                              +         *        - 80
   -                                          *    +                  -
   -                                               +    *             -
   -                   *                           +                  -
  70- --- --- --- --- --- --- --- --- --- + --- --- -*- - 70
   -                                               +                  -
   -                        *                      +                  -
   -           *                     *             +                  -
  60-                                              +                  - 60
   -  *                         *                  +                  -
   -     *                                         +                  -
   -                                               +                  -
  50- --- --- --- --- --- --- --- -*- --- + --- --- --- - 50
   -                                               +                  -
   -                                               +                  -
   -                                               +                  -
  40-                                              +                  - 40
   -                                               +                  -
   -                                               +                  -
   -                                               +                  -
  30-                                              +                  - 30
   -                                               +                  -
   -                                               +                  -
   -                                               +                  -
   -                                               +                  -
  20-                                              +                  - 20
          SOM  FAM  ASO  AGN  DVL  WDL  ANX  RDS   EXC  SSK  INT  EXT
    R      8    8   10    8   11    6   10    3    12   21   18   17
    T     58   53   63   73   65   58   63   50    77   76   80   70
```

```
**************************************
Personality Inventory For Children
**************************************

            Supplementary Scales
            --------------------


                Respondent Description Scales
        R    T  0   10   20   30   40   50   60   70  80   90  100
DSM    41   77  !                        !             !    *        !
K      12   26  !              *         !             !            !

                    Prediction Scales
        R    T  0   10   20   30   40   50   60   70  80   90  100
LDP    39   84  !                        !             !        *    !
DP     20   36  !                   *    !             !            !

                Empirical Personality Scales
        R    T  0   10   20   30   40   50   60   70  80   90  100
ES     37   74  !                        !             !*           !
SR     16   35  !                   *    !             !            !
I-E    19   44  !                      * !             !            !

                    Auxilliary Scales
        R    T  0   10   20   30   40   50   60   70  80   90  100
CDY    25   54  !                        ! *           !            !
INF     0   45  !                     *  !             !            !
SD     15   21  !         *              !             !            !
SM     11   57  !                        !    *        !            !
AGM    29   80  !                        !             !      *      !
```

The computerized PIC provides an excellent example of how specific narrative descriptions about a referred child can be generated from a personality instrument which employs multivariate cluster analyses. Unlike the MCDI, the PIC has been standardized on a very large and well-stratified sample. Futher, on-going provisions have been made to collect additional data through computer administration, thus upgrading this standardization. The PIC program also demonstrates quite clearly several of the major advantages that occur when multifactored instruments are administered by computer. First, the speed and reliability of response to the PIC items are increased two-fold. This is critically important for an instrument of 600 items. Next, the scoring and analysis of the instrument are significantly quicker. Results from the test are available virtually within seconds after its administration. Finally, the narrative report produced is based on a cluster analysis of the primary scales. This report would be difficult, if not impossible, to produce manually.

While neither of the instruments described above are adaptive or interactive (during the administration phase), they both illustrate the ease with which personality data can be processed by computer. While the PIC does not produce a differential diagnosis as described by McDermott (1980), the necessary ingredients in terms of discriminant analyses are present to potentially derive such diagnoses. Psych-Systems has announced its intention to develop a program structure which will provide suggested DSM-III child behavior disorder categories. The development of this program would, of course, require careful validation studies, using computer diagnostics versus traditional child clinical diagnostics to determine its accuracy of prediction.

Intelligence Assessment

At this time, no comprehensive intelligence instruments which provide for computer administration have been developed for children. One instrument, the Multidimensional Aptitude Battery (Psych-Systems, 1985e), has been developed for older adolescents and adults. This test is divided into verbal and performance sections similar to the Wechsler scales, with the verbal sections of the test administered by computer and the performance sections administered by a psychologist. Reported concurrent validity coefficients for the instrument range in the low .90s (Psych-Systems, 1985e).

Most of the other instruments developed for computerized intellectual assessment require the psychologist first to administer and score the intelligence test. The most commonly used test, the Wechsler Intelligence Scale for Children-Revised (WISC-R), has a number of analysis programs available which provide quantitative and narrative output. Some of these include systems developed by Southern Microsystems for Educators (Nicholson, 1982), ADEPT Systems (ADEPT, 1982), and Psych-Systems (1985b). All of these programs can run on microcomputers with fixed disks, and they provide a variety of output—some with recommendations for individual education plans. A report generated by the Psych-Systems WISC-R (Honaker, 1982) is provided below. To generate this report, the practitioner must administer and score the WISC-R, produce its scaled scores and Verbal, Performance, and Full-Scale IQs, and provide the computer with these data as well as behavioral observation and/or adaptive behavior data. All of this information is then factored into the final report.

```
858-58-5858  Mary Smith    11 yr old black female  17-Mar-85
```

```
--------------------------------------------------------------------------
:          :                                                             :
:  WISC-R  :  Wechsler Intelligence Scale for Children-Revised           :
:          :                                                             :
--------------------------------------------------------------------------
```

```
            Interpretation : L. Micheal Honaker, Ph.D.
```

```
This clinical report provides a computer analysis and interpretation
of scores obtained from the standard administration of the WISC-R by
a qualified clinician.  The report is designed to assist in
psychodiagnostic evaluation.  It is available only to qualified
professionals.  The techniques utilized in the analysis of the
data and in generation of this report were designed by experienced
behavioral scientists utilizing well validated clinical research.
However this report is to be used in conjunction with professional
evaluation.  No decision should be based solely upon the contents
of this report.
```

The computer program generating this report was designed by Psych
Systems, Inc., Baltimore, Maryland 21208. Copyright (C) 1984 by
Psych Systems, Inc. The interpretive logic utilized in the
generation of the report was designed by L. Michael Honaker, Ph.D.
Copyright (C) 1982 by L. Michael Honaker. Reproduced by
permission and under license from Psychologistics, Inc.,
Indiatlantic, Florida 32903. All rights reserved.

858-58-5858 Mary Smith   11 yr old black female   17-Mar-85

        Name: Mary Smith   Date of Test: 17-Mar-85
         Sex: Female   Date of Birth: 23-Jan-74
      School: Maple Elementary   Race: Black
       Grade: 5
                        Examiner: Brown

                 Current Placement: Emotionally Handicapped
                 Reason for Referral: Emotional Problems

The scores listed below were used for computations in this report. These
age-corrected scaled scores should be checked carefully for errors. If
discrepencies are found, the entire report should be reprocessed.

                  Age Corrected Scaled Scores

        Information   7   Picture Completion   10
        Similarities   11   Picture Arrangement   13
        Arithmetic   7   Block Design   7
        Vocabulary   11   Object Assembly   6
        Comprehension   11   Coding   8
        Digit Span   4

      *** Mary Smith's test age is 11 years, 1 month, 25 days ***

Verbal   Scaled
Subtests: Score   Range

Information   7   Low Average   !---------*
Similarities   11   Average   !-----------*
Arithmetic   7   Low Average   !---------*
Vocabulary   11   Average   !-----------*
Comprehension   11   Average   !-----------*
Digit Span   4   Mental Retardation   !---*
                                                  !
             Average Verbal   8.50   !
----
                                     0   10   19

Performance   Scaled
Subtests: Score   Range

Picture Completion   10   Average   !---------*
Picture Arrangement   13   High Average   !-----------*
Block Design   7   Low Average   !-------*
Object Assembly   6   Borderline   !------*
Coding   8   Low Average   !--------*
Mazes   0   !
                                                  !
             Average Performance   8.80   !
----
                                     0   10   19

```
        Verbal Scale IQ Score            96  39 Percentile
        Performance Scale IQ Score      91  27 Percentile
        Full Scale IQ Score             92  30 Percentile
```

```
   95% Confidence interval for Full Scale IQ Score =  86 to  98
```

```
      Verbal IQ Score - Performance IQ Score =   5  (NS)
```

```
                        Factor Scores:
```

```
   Verbal Comprehension           (VCQ)  100  50 Percentile
   Perceptual Organization        (POQ)   94  34 Percentile
   Freedom from Distractibility   (FDQ)   82  12 Percentile
```

```
                      Factor Differences:
```

```
           VCQ - POQ =    6  (NS)
           VCQ - FDQ =   18  p>.01
           POQ - FDQ =   12  (NS)
```

```
                    Subtest Differences:
```

```
         Subtest Score Minus Mean Verbal Score
         -------------------------------------
   Information                      -1.50        (NS)
   Similarities                      2.50        (NS)
   Arithmetic                       -1.50        (NS)
   Vocabulary                        2.50        (NS)
   Comprehension                     2.50        (NS)
   Digit Span                       -4.50        p<.01
```

```
      Subtest Score Minus Mean Performance Score
      ------------------------------------------
   Picture Completion                1.20        (NS)
   Picture Arrangement               4.20        p<.05
   Block Design                     -1.80        (NS)
   Object Assembly                  -2.80        (NS)
   Coding                           -0.80        (NS)
```

```
        Name: Mary Smith                    Date of Test: 17-Mar-85
         Sex: Female                       Date of Birth: 23-Jan-74
      School: Maple Elementary                      Race: Black
       Grade:  5
                          Examiner: Brown

                   Current Placement: Emotionally Handicapped
                   Reason for Referral: Emotional Problems
------------------------------------------------------------------------
                      Age Corrected Scaled Scores
------------------------------------------------------------------------
         Information       7        Picture Completion     10
         Similarities     11        Picture Arrangement    13
         Arithmetic        7        Block Design            7
         Vocabulary       11        Object Assembly         6
         Comprehension    11        Coding                  8
         Digit Span        4
------------------------------------------------------------------------
```

On this administration of the Wechsler Intelligence Scale for
Children, Mary Smith obtained a Verbal Scale IQ score of 96 and a
Performance Scale IQ score of 91. This results in a Full Scale IQ
score of 92 which falls within the average range of intellectual
abilities. The chances are 95 out of 100 that Mary Smith's true IQ
score falls between 86 and 98. The current Full Scale IQ score
corresponds to the 30 percentile which indicates that Mary Smith is
functioning intellectually at a level equal to or better than
approximately 30 percent of children the same age. Overall,
performance on items tapping verbal comprehension skills was about
the same as that shown on tasks reflecting perceptual-organization
abilities.

Examination of Mary Smith's pattern of performance across the
different subtests suggests relative strengths were exhibited on:
        - Items and tasks tapping the ability to differentiate
            essential from nonessential details
        - Subtests tapping social judgement
        - Subtests necessitating the organization of visually
            presented material
        - Subtests tapping planning ability.
A pattern of relative weaknesses was apparent on:
        - Subtests requiring both long and short term memory
        - Tasks requiring attention to and manipulation of
            numerical stimuli
        - Items reflecting mental alertness and short term
            memory of numerical stimuli.

Overall performance on subtests tapping verbal comprehension
abilities falls in the average range and corresponds to the 39
percentile. Performance was inconsistent across the different
subtests and ranged from the mental retardation to average levels.
No significant strengths relative to overall verbal functioning were
exhibited.
Significant relative weaknesses were shown on subtests tapping:
        - Short term auditory memory and the ability to remember
            the order of symbolic material.

General performance on perceptual-organization tasks falls in the
average range and corresponds to the 27 percentile. There was much
variability across the different subtests and performance ranged
between the borderline and high average levels. Relative to overall
functioning on perceptual-organization tasks, significant strength
was exhibited on subtests requiring:

```
     - Anticipation of consequences and temporal sequencing;
          interpretation of social situations and nonverbal
          reasoning.
No significant relative weaknesses were shown.

                          Implications

The following hypotheses concerning treatment and need for further
evaluation are suggested by the present results.  These hypotheses
should be evaluated in light of Mary Smith's current academic
functioning, cultural and racial background, and situational factors
that may have influenced performance.

Present evaluation results suggest that Mary Smith should be able to
perform academically at a level consistent with same-aged peers.  If
academic difficulties are evidenced, further psychological evaluation
is warranted.




                         ------------------------------------------
                         Brown
                         Examiner
```

As can be seen by inspecting this report, (*a*) information is produced on the relative scatter of scaled scores, (*b*) factor scores are derived using the Kaufman (1975) three-factor structure, (*c*) age-corrected scaled scores are provided, (*d*) a narrative report describing the child's relative strengths and weaknesses is generated, and (*e*) a highly generalized implications section is produced. The report format used to generate this WISC-R analysis is known as "boilerplating" in computer parlance. This technique matches scores or clusters of scores with statements about performance which are stored in the computer. The technique is relatively simplistic and simply provides a description of the various standardized scores presented in the first part of the profile. The program does not integrate other information which may have been collected on the child such as achievement and personality data.

The failure of programs of this type to provide an integrated report has often been cited (Brown, 1984; McCullough & Wenck, 1984) as a major disadvantage for their use in constructing school psychological reports. More comprehensive programs need to be developed which will integrate achievement, personality, and cognitive data and which will provide multivariate prediction of specific behavioral outcomes. Ultimately, programs of this type should administer and score intelligence tests along with other areas of measurements. This has essentially been accomplished with the verbal sections of the WAIS-R; however, the performance section requires innovative and unusual programming techniques which allow the computer to replicate what is now done by psychologists (McLeod, Griffiths, Bigelow, & Yingling, 1982). The use of computerized graphics and color capabilities may form the foundation of the first really unique test devices developed for automated assessment. A rudimentary example of an application of these capabilities is the Visual Searching Task (Psych-Systems, 1985f), which was developed to perform neurological screening.

Personality Trait Instruments for Children and Adolescents

Three personality trait instruments developed for children and adolescents will be discussed below: the Eysenck Personality Questionnaire-Junior (EPQ-J; Eysenck & Eysenck, 1975), the Minnesota Multiphasic Personality Inventory for Adolescents (Hathaway & McKinley, 1982), and the Millon Adolescent Personality Inventory (Millon, Green, & Meagher, 1982). Each of these instruments is based on a factor analytic structure which has been derived either empirically or, in the case of the Millon, on the basis of a theoretical structure. The computer analyses are based on factor scores that the individual attains on each of the specified factors.

The Eysenck Personality Questionnaire-Junior

The EPQ-J consists of 81 items which are factored into four scales: Psychoticism, Extroversion, Neuroticism, and a Lie scale. The automated version of the EPQ-J (Psych-Systems, 1985a) is designed to be used in vocational and other interpersonal settings rather than in psychiatric settings. It provides a brief evaluation of normal personality functioning and therefore is a preliminary screening instrument. The results of an automated EPQ-J, based on a 9-year-old male referred for withdrawn behavior, are presented below. From the narrative output, it is evident that the computer attempts to provide a behavioral description of "probable" overt behaviors based on Z-score interpretations for each of the four major scales.

```
143-34-9231  Mark Jones    9 yr old white male  9-Mar-85
```

```
---------------------------------------------------------------
 :          :                                               :
 :  EPQJR   :  Eysenck Personality Questionnaire, Junior    :
 :          :                                               :
---------------------------------------------------------------
```

```
            Test Authors : H.J. Eysenck,
                           Sybil B.G. Eysenck

        Interpretation : James Wakefield, Ph.D.
```

```
The EPQJr is a brief self-reporting personality inventory appropriate
for boys and girls seven to fifteen.

This clinical report is designed to assist in psychodiagnostic
evaluation.  It is for use only by qualified professionals.  The
report was produced by a computerized analysis of the data given
by the client listed above, and is to be used as part of a
professional evaluation.  No decision should be based solely upon
the contents of this report, and it should not be used in a clinical
setting without the approval of a professional who is qualified
in the use of psychological tests.
```

Mark Jones is socially withdrawn and inhibits his responses. He
tends to avoid others and prefers to work alone rather than in
groups.

He will respond to negative criticism of mistakes more effectively
than praise for good work. He may be able to study for longer
periods of time than other students with similar ability. Learning
should occur best when details are presented before broad principles.
It is important that the teacher give feedback to him in private
whether the feedback is positive or negative. He should also be
allowed to work alone as much as possible. Serious-looking material
should be used rather than highly colored, overly stimulating, or
"entertaining" material. He should have the highest achievement when
classroom tests generally allow him to answer 70 to 75 percent of the
items correctly. It may be necessary to encourage him to work faster
if his concern for accuracy impedes his progress.

Mark Jones is emotional and overreactive. He has difficulty
returning to a normal state after emotional experiences.

He should be reassured and given emotional support prior to beginning
a new or difficult task. Emotional experiences, stress, or the
threat of failure during a task, or associated with the task, will
usually result in lower performance. These experiences should be
avoided as much as possible. A subdued, personal approach combined
with a structured schedule and environment will usually improve
performance. Tests are likely to be threatening for him and should
be deemphasized to avoid extreme emotional reactions. One way to
deemphasize tests is to give more tests that are less important
rather than a few highly important tests. After a test, he will
respond best to private feedback concerning incorrect answers or a
poor performance. When specific fears (e.g. of school, teachers,
peers, etc.) are identified, relaxation techniques and
desensitization are recommended. Supportive counseling will also be
helpful. Individual, rather than group, counseling is recommended.

Summary of Scores

Scale	Raw	Z-Score
P	3	-0.46
E	5	-4.01
N	16	1.14
L	4	-1.40

```
            Name : Mark Jones
       Physician : Brown
             Age : 9
             Sex : Male
    Ethnic Group : 1 White
  Patient Status : 3 Nonpatient
 Education Level : 2 Elementary School
     Occup. Level : 1 Not In Labor Force


              EPQJr Raw Data
              ---------------
        1234567890 1234567890 1234567890

  1- 30 YYNYYYNNYY YYYYNYNYNY NNYNYYNNYY
 31- 60 NNYYNNNYNY NNNNYNNYNN YNYNNNYNYN
 61- 81 NNYYNYNYNN YYYNYYYNNN N
```

The EPQ-J is another example of an assessment instrument which was developed for a paper and pencil format and transported to the computer. Unlike the MCDI, however, the original standardization procedure employed was quite comprehensive. The actual computerization of the EPQ-J is rather simplistic and again uses a technique called "boilerplating" to generate the narrative statements. The EPQ-J is one of the techniques that can easily run on a computer such as the Apple II.

The Minnesota Multiphasic Personality Inventory for Adolescents

The MMPI is perhaps the most thoroughly researched and validated personality instrument using factor analytic techniques. Specifically developed to detect levels of "abnormal" behavior, the MMPI provides pattern analyses of individuals' scores across its factorial scales and compares these patterns with known psychiatric populations. Since the test was originally designed to be multivariate in this respect, it lends itself well to such computer analyses.

The MMPI contains 566 items which are factored into 10 primary scales:

1. Scale 1 (HS)—Hypochondriasis
2. Scale 2 (D)—Depression
3. Scale 3 (HY)—Conversion Hysteria
4. Scale 4 (PD)—Psychopathic Deviate
5. Scale 5 (MF)—Masculinity/Femininity
6. Scale 6 (PA)—Paranoia
7. Scale 7 (PT)—Psychasthenia
8. Scale 8 (SC)—Schizophrenia
9. Scale 9 (MA)—Hypomania
10. Scale 10 (SI)—Social Introversion

In addition, the instrument has three validity scales: the L or Lie scale, the F or Frequency scale, and the K or Correction scale. Numerous other scales have been factored from the MMPI, and at least 100 additional subscales are known to exist in the literature. For proper administration, the MMPI requires a reading level at or above the ninth grade. However, it can be administered verbally by a trained technician. Proper administration and scoring of the MMPI requires a relatively sophisticated computer of the type described earlier.

One of the more sophisticated programs for the interpretation of the MMPI is provided below (Psych-Systems, 1985d). This MMPI was administered by a computer to a 17-year-old adolescent white female referred for delinquent and acting-out behavior. The decision matrix and interpretative scheme utilized by this program is presented in Figure 14-1.

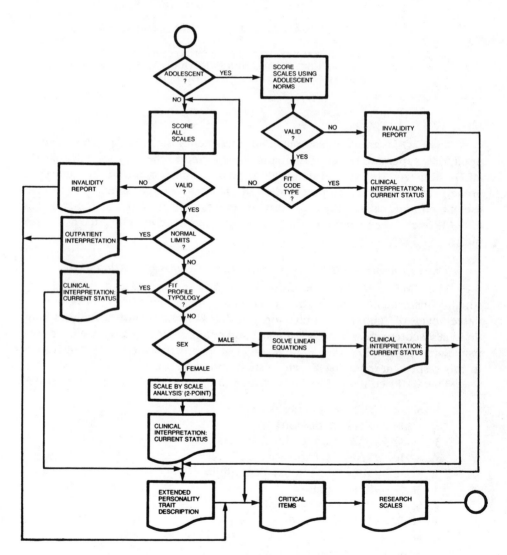

Figure 14-1. MMPI Interpretive Scheme.

003-06-1985 Name Withheld   17 yr old white female 6-Mar-85

```
-------------------------------------------------------------------
:          :                                                      :
:   MMPI   :  Minnesota Multiphasic Personality Inventory         :
:          :                                                      :
-------------------------------------------------------------------
```

TEST AUTHORS: Starke R. Hathaway
J. Charnley McKinley

This clinical report is designed to assist in psychodiagnostic
evaluation. It is available only to qualified professionals.
This report was produced by a computerized analysis of the data
given by the client listed above. The techniques utilized in the
analysis of the data and in generation of this report were designed
by several psychologists, psychiatrists, and other professionals
utilizing highly validated clinical research. However, this report
is to be used in conjunction with professional evaluation. No
decision should be based solely upon the contents of this report.

The computer program generating this report was designed by Psych
Systems, Inc., Baltimore, Maryland 21208. Copyright (C) 1984 by
Psych Systems, Inc. Portions of this report may have been
reproduced or derived from the MINNESOTA MULTIPHASIC PERSONALITY
INVENTORY (MMPI), such being done by permission of and under
copyrights held by THE UNIVERSITY OF MINNESOTA dated 1943, renewed
1970. Rights to the MMPI are licensed through National Computer
Systems, Inc., Interpretive Scoring Systems Division, Minneapolis, MN.

MINNESOTA MULTIPHASIC PERSONALITY INVENTORY
CLINICAL REPORT: ADOLESCENT

Individuals with this profile type appear to be mildly depressed.
Their affect level may be shallow. Referral for treatment most often
occurs because of difficulty concentrating and thinking.

These adolescents resent authority figures and tend to derogate them.
They are argumentative, but also vulnerable to threat and have inner
conflicts about emotional dependency. While they are socially
active, they have troubles with close relationships and extended
personal involvements. Others see them as demanding. Their two
primary defense mechanisms are displacement and acting out.
Histories including trouble with the law, drug abuse, truancy, sexual
promis- cuity, and suicide are common.

MMPI PROFILE: ADOLESCENT

				1	2	3	4	5	6	7	8	9	0
L	F	K		HS	D	HY	PD	MF	PA	PT	SC	MA	SI

	L	F	K		HS	D	HY	PD	MF	PA	PT	SC	MA	SI
R	5	9	12		6	37	24	27	37	17	27	25	13	41
T	49	54	49		45	84	55	70	42	70	65	58	43	62

Welsh Code: 2'46'70-83/195 F/LK
Goldberg N-P Index: 62P

MINNESOTA MULTIPHASIC PERSONALITY INVENTORY
CLINICAL REPORT: ADULT

CURRENT CLINICAL STATUS

This is a valid profile.

This profile suggests the presence of moderate emotional distress
(anxiety, depression, and nervousness), which is accentuated by this
person's tendency to be self-dramatic. Such individuals are
chronically hostile and resentful. Much of their hostility appears
based in their excessive demandingness of others. They are
emotionally dependent and expect others to supply much sympathy,
support and attention. Despite this, they tend to have inner
conflicts about their emotional dependency. They are uncomfortable
with other people, lack poise and self-assurance, and tend to
withdraw from social contacts. With regard to work, they are
apathetic and lack interest and involvement.

Projection and acting-out are preferred defense mechanisms. Impulse
control is deficient. These persons are pervasively self-indulgent
and self-pitying. Serious sexual and marital adjustment difficulties
are relatively common. The prognosis is fair for some improvement
with psychotherapy.

DIAGNOSTIC IMPRESSION

Although a formal diagnosis must be based on demographic, interview
and case history data, psychological test results can sometimes be of
assistance to the clinician in making the diagnostic decision. The
DSM-III diagnostic categories most frequently associated with various
MMPI profile types were identified and subsequently confirmed by a
panel of experienced clinicians. The following, while not presented
as a diagnosis, is a diagnostic possibility based on that consensus.

Impression: Axis I   V71.09 None

                 Axis II 301.84 Passive-Aggressive Personality
                                  Disorder with Depressed Mood

EXTENDED PERSONALITY TRAIT INFORMATION

This person has the capacity to exert substantial control over her
behavior. However, she harbors antisocial attitudes and acting-out
behavior may be the result. She is probably well-controlled
emotionally even to the point of lacking emotional expressiveness.
This person becomes disconcerted when complex situations arise and do
not fit her habitual mode of thinking.

Although currently suffering emotional distress, this person gives
some indication of psychological resiliency. When not distressed she
will be more verbal and relatively at ease in social situations.
Others may see her as usually cheerful and not overly difficult to
approach. She is able to deal with adverse circumstances if given
sufficient support.

She is currently experiencing a good deal of unhappiness and guilt.
She feels that life is a burden that may not be worthwhile, and she
is pessimistic about hopes of improvement. She may also feel that
she is not worthwhile and deserves punishment for her sins, real or
imagined. She thinks of herself as somewhat lacking in
self-confidence. Moreover, she is often overly concerned about the
opinions of others around her.

She views other people as being generally trustworthy, honest, and fair-minded. She may be somewhat lacking in assertiveness and aggressiveness.

She is somewhat lacking in energy and may have difficulty mobilizing her personal resources to meet problems and situations.

She suffers from tendencies toward excessive self-blame, self-pity, worry, demandingness and resentment for real or imagined harms. Preferred defense mechanisms are repression, rationalization and projection.

SPECIAL MEDICAL SYMPTOMS

Results suggest that this individual's predisposition to somatic complaints and concern about health and physical functioning is no greater than average.

ATTITUDES TOWARD WORK

She appears to be normally ambitious in improving her career. She may be viewed as submissive, unassertive, and easily influenced by others. This person may lack the capacity to gain substantial pleasure from her work. She will show innovative approaches to work situations. She is likely to make important decisions impulsively and without sufficient deliberation. Generally, she does not have trust and confidence in her capacity to perform her own work successfully. She lacks a high degree of self-sufficiency. Such individuals tend to have average work attitudes but may lack sufficient self-control for effective job performance. She prefers to work alone and is not empathetic to the needs of others.

MMPI PROFILE: ADULT

```
                              1     2     3     4     5     6     7     8     9     0
        L     F     K        HS     D    HY    PD    MF    PA    PT    SC    MA    SI

100-  ---   ---   ---    +  ---   ---   ---   ---   ---   ---   ---   ---   ---   ---   -100
  -                      +                                                               --
  -                      +                                                               --
  -                      +                                                               --
  -                      +                                                               --
 90-                     +                                                               - 90
  -                      +                                                               --
  -                      +                                                               --
  -                      +          *                                                    --
  -                      +                                                               --
 80-                     +                *                                              -- 80
  -                      +                                                               --
  -                      +                      *                                        --
  -                      +                                                               --
  -                      +                            *     *                            --
 70-  ---   ---   ---    +  ---   ---   ---   ---   ---   ---   ---   ---   ---           - 70
  -                      +                                                   *           --
  -                      +                                                               --
  -            *         +                                                               --
  -                      +                                                               --
 60-                     +                                                               - 60
  -                      +          *                                                    --
  -                      +                                                               --
  -                      +                                                               --
  --  *                  +                                                               --
 50-  ---   ---   ---    +  ---   ---   ---   ---   ---   ---   ---   ---   ---   ---   - 50
  -                *     +  *                                                            --
  -                      +                                                               --
  -                      +                                               *               --
 40-                     +                                                               - 40
  -                      +                      *                                        --
  -                      +                                                               --
  -                      +                                                               --
 30-  ---   ---   ---    +  ---   ---   ---   ---   ---   ---   ---   ---   ---   ---   - 30
  -                      +                                                               --
  -                      +                                                               --
  -                      +                                                               --
  -                      +                                                               --
 20-  ---   ---   ---    +  ---   ---   ---   ---   ---   ---   ---   ---   ---   ---   - 20
        L     F     K        HS     D    HY    PD    MF    PA    PT    SC    MA    SI
  R     5     9    12         6    37    24    27    42    17    27    25    13    41
  K                           6           5                12    12     2
K+R     5     9    12        12    37    24    32    42    17    39    37    15    41
  T    53    64    49        48    84    59    81    39    76    73    72    45    68
```

Welsh Code: 24*678'0-3/19:5   F-L/K
Goldberg N-P Index: 80P

CRITICAL ITEMS (EXTENDED LIST)

These MMPI test items, which were answered in the direction indicated,
may require further investigation by the clinician. The clinician is
cautioned, however, against overinterpretation of isolated responses.

** Unusual Thoughts and Experiences **

I am afraid of losing my mind. (t)

** Depression, Guilt and Self-destructive Feelings **

I have not lived the right kind of life. (t)
I wish I could be as happy as others seem to be. (t)
Most of the time I feel blue. (t)
I do many things which I regret afterwards (I regret things more or
more often than others seem to). (t)
I certainly feel useless at times. (t)
I have difficulty in starting to do things. (t)
At times I think I am no good at all. (t)
I worry quite a bit over possible misfortunes. (t)
I usually feel that life is worth while. (f)
Most nights I go to sleep without thoughts or ideas bothering me. (f)

** Health and Bodily Concerns **

I am in just as good physical health as most of my friends. (f)
I do not tire quickly. (f)

** Sexual Concerns and Problems **

My sex life is satisfactory. (f)
I have never been in trouble because of my sex behavior. (f)

RESEARCH SCALES

                                                    Standard Scores

Special Scales		R	T						
A First Factor	(A)	24	61	¦		¦		*	¦
R Second Factor	(R)	22	60	¦		¦		*	¦
Ego strength (Barron)	(ES)	40	50	¦		*			¦
Caudality (Williams)	(CA)	19	63	¦		¦		*	¦
Social status (Gough)	(ST)	17	49	¦		*¦			¦
Dominance (Gough)	(DO)	8	31	*		¦			¦
Social resp (Gough)	(RE)	15	33	¦*		¦			¦
Manifest anxiety (Taylor)	(MAS)	26	66	¦		¦		*	¦
Dependency (Navran)	(DY)	32	58	¦		¦		*	¦
Prejudice (Gough)	(PR)	7	41	¦	*	¦			¦
Control (Cuadra)	(CN)	29	58	¦		¦		*	¦
Alcoholism (MacAndrew)	(ALC)	20	**	¦		¦			¦
				30	40	50	60	70	

** - Low Addiction Proneness

```
Content Scales (Wiggins)
------------------------------
Social maladjustment         (SOC)  18  65  !              !          *  !
Depression                   (DEP)  19  70  !              !             !*
Feminine interests           (FEM)  19  48  !          *!             !
Poor morale                  (MOR)  14  58  !              !    *      !
Religious fundamentalism     (REL)   1  27 *!              !             !
Authority conflict           (AUT)   6  45  !       *  !             !
Psychoticism                 (PSY)   8  51  !             *             !
Organic symptoms             (ORG)   7  50  !             *             !
Family problems              (FAM)   5  54  !              ! *           !
Manifest hostility           (HOS)   8  49  !          *!             !
Phobias                      (PHO)   5  41  !    *     !             !
Hypomania                    (HYP)   7  37  ! *        !             !
Poor health                  (HEA)   6  50  !             *             !
                                           30    40    50    60    70

Item Factors
(Tryon, Stein & Chu)
---------------------
TSC-I   Social introversion  (I)   16  62  !              !       *  !
TSC-II  Bodily concern       (B)    7  53  !              !*             !
TSC-III Suspicion            (S)    9  55  !              !  *           !
TSC-IV  Depression           (D)   18  77  !              !             !*
TSC-V   Resentment           (R)   10  60  !              !    *      !
TSC-VI  Autism               (A)   10  63  !              !        *  !
TSC-VII Tension              (T)   16  62  !              !        *  !
                                           30    40    50    60    70
```

Standard scores are based on statistics derived according to the
procedures described in Dahlstrom, W.G., Welsh, G.S., & Dahlstrom, L.E.
An MMPI Handbook, Vol. II. Minneapolis, University of Minnesota Press, 1975.

ADDITIONAL SCALES

                                        Standard Scores

```
Factor Scales
(Johnson, Butcher, Null & Johnson)     R   T
------------------------------------   -   -
Neuroticism-Gen'l Anx. & Worry (N)    48  53  !             !*            !
Psychotism-Peculiar Thinking   (P)     1  41  !       *  !             !
Cynicism-Normal Paranoia       (C)     9  45  !          *  !             !
Denial of Somatic Problems    (DSP)   21  60  !             !       *      !
Social Extroversion           (SE)     6  35  ! *        !             !
Stereotypic Femininity        (SF)     8  46  !          *  !             !
Psychotic Paranoia            (PP)     1  41  !       *  !             !
Delinquency                   (DL)     5  54  !             ! *           !
Stereotypic Masculinity       (SM)     2  38  !    *     !             !
Neurasthenic Somatization     (NS)     0  41  !    *     !             !
Phobias                       (PH)     0  33  !*         !             !
Family Attachment             (FA)     9  55  !             ! *           !
Intellectual Interests        (II)     5  47  !       *  !             !
Religious Fundamentalism      (RF)     0  25 *!          !             !
                                             30    40    50    60    70
```

Harris & Lingoes SubScales

```
Subjective Depression           (D1)    22  84  :            :           :*
Psychomotor Retardation         (D2)     8  61  :            :      *    :
Physical Malfunctioning         (D3)     4  55  :            :  *        :
Mental Dullness                 (D4)    12  96  :            :           :*
Brooding                        (D5)     9  83  :            :           :*
Denial of Social Anxiety        (Hy1)    3  48  :          *:            :
Need for Affection              (Hy2)    6  56  :            :   *       :
Lassitude-malaise               (Hy3)    9  74  :            :           :*
Somatic Complaints              (Hy4)    3  46  :          *  :          :
Inhibition of Aggression        (Hy5)    1  34  : *          :           :
Familial Discord                (Pd1)    3  57  :            :    *      :
Authority Problems              (Pd2)    6  69  :            :           *:
Social Imperturbability         (Pd3)    4  39  :     *      :           :
Social Alienation               (Pd4A)  11  70  :            :           *
Self-Alienation                 (Pd4B)   9  70  :            :           *
Persecutory Ideas               (Pa1)    3  5?  :            :    *      :
Poignancy                       (Pa2)    3  55  :            :   *       :
Naivete                         (Pa3)    8  73  :            :           :*
Social Alienation               (Sc1A)   6  60  :            :      *    :
Emotional Alienation            (Sc1B)   4  67  :            :        *  :
Lack of Ego Mastery, Cognitive  (Sc2A)   5  72  :            :           :*
Lack of Ego Mastery, Conative   (Sc2B)  10  90  :            :           :*
Lack Ego Mast., Defect. Inhib.  (Sc2C)   2  52  :          :*            :
Bizarre Sensory Experiences     (Sc3)    2  47  :        *  :            :
Amorality                       (Ma1)    1  47  :        *  :            :
Psychomotor Acceleration        (Ma2)    3  47  :        *  :            :
Imperturbability                (Ma3)    2  45  :       *    :           :
Ego Inflation                   (Ma4)    2  46  :        *   :           :
                                                30    40    50    60    70
```

```
          Name : Name Withheld
     Physician :
           Age : 17
           Sex : Female
  Ethnic Group : 1 White
Patient Status : 3 Nonpatient
Education Level : 2 Elementary School
   Occup. Level : 1 Not In Labor Force
```

MMPI Raw Data

```
        1234567890 1234567890 1234567890

  1- 30 FTFFFTFFTF FTFFTTTTFF TTFTFTFFFT
 31- 60 FTFFFFFFTT TFFFTFFFFF FFFTTFTFTT
 61- 90 TFTTTFTTFF TFFTTTTTFF TTTFFTFFTT
 91-120 FFFTFFFFFF TTFTFFFFFF TFTFFFFFTF
121-150 FFFTFTTTTT FTTTFFTFFF FTFFFFTFFT
151-180 FFTTTFFTFF FFFTTFFFTF TFTTTTTFFT
181-210 FTFFFFTTFT FTTFFTFFTF TFFTFFFTFF
211-240 FFFTFFTFFT FFFTTFFTFT FFFTTTTTTF
241-270 TTTTFFFFFF FFFFFFFFTF FFFFFFTFFF
271-300 FFFFFTFFFF TFFFTTFFFF FFFFTFFFFF
301-330 FFFTFTTTFF FTFTFFFFFF TFFFFFFTFT
331-360 FFFFTTFFFF FFTFFFTFFF FFFFFTFFTF
361-390 FFFFFFTFTT FTFTFTFFFT FFFTFFFFFF
391-420 FFFTTTTTTT TFTTTTFTFT FTFFFTFTFF
421-450 FFFFTFFFFT TFFFFTFFTF FTTTFFTFFT
451-480 TFTTTFFFFT FTTTFTFTFF TTFFFFTTTF
481-510 TFFFFTTFTF FFFFFFTTTF FFFTFFFTFF
511-540 FFFFTTTFFF FTFTFFTFTF TFFFFTFFTT
541-566 FTFTTTTFFF FFFFTFFTFF TTFTFT
```

SPECIAL INSTRUCTIONS FOR USING THE FOWLER CORRECTIONAL REPORT

The Fowler Correctional Report is an MMPI interpretation system for use with law offenders who are eighteen or older. The Correctional Report is not appropriate for use with younger subjects or for individuals not currently in the criminal justice system.

The print-out consists of the following sections:

1. The Narrative Correctional Report. This report is based on the interpretation of the standard MMPI validity and clinical scales. The report is similar in structure to a clinical report, but includes information about management, treatment and rehabilitation issues.

2. The Critical Items. A selection of items which indicate specific areas of concern and might require further investigation by the clinician.

3. The MMPI Profile.

4. Offender Profile and Recommendations. This is a classification system based on research by Dr. Edwin Megaree at Florida State University. Each test subject is placed in one of ten categories or types on the basis of the MMPI profile. A brief report provides a psychological description and treatment recommendations appropriate for the type. Occasionally, an individual will meet the criteria for classification into more than one type. In those cases, the choice of which category to use is a clinical decision. If the clinical information is lacking, it is usually better to choose the type printed first.

5. Content Scales. These are special scales based upon the content of the subject's responses. They indicate how individuals perceive themselves and how they wish others to perceive them. Contradictions between content scale interpretations and the narrative report may suggest efforts on the individuals part to present a distorted picture.

6. Law Offender Scales. Brief interpretations of scales which have particular implications for law offenders.

7. Research Scales and MMPI raw data. A selection of some of the more frequently used research scales, and a grid containing the true-false responses which can be used for future reference or for reproducing the report.

IMPORTANT NOTE: Involvement with the criminal justice system, especially incarceration, may result in severe distress and disorganization in some individuals. When test results are extremely deviant, it is important to re-test the individual several weeks later. In many cases, the re-test will present a less deviant and more accurate picture of the individual's usual functioning level.

```
-----------------------------------------------------------------
:             :                                                  :
:   MMPI      :   Minnesota Multiphasic Personality Inventory    :
:             :                                                  :
-----------------------------------------------------------------
```

FOWLER CORRECTIONAL REPORT

The Minnesota Multiphasic Personality Inventory has been widely used
with law offender clients. This report was produced by a
computerized analysis of the responses of the client listed above.
The interpretation system was developed by Raymond D. Fowler, Ph.D.
It was designed for use in a number of criminal justice applications
including pre-sentencing evaluation, competency determination,
prison classification, rehabilitation planning and probation and
parole assignment. However, it should not be used as the sole basis
for decisions, and recommendations based on this test information should
be supported by other indices. This report should be regarded as
confidential, and only persons with appropriate professional qualifications should have access to it.

The computer program generating this report was designed by Psych
Systems, Inc., Baltimore, Maryland 21208. Copyright (C) 1984 by
Psych Systems, Inc. Portions of this report may have been
reproduced or derived from the MINNESOTA MULTIPHASIC PERSONALITY
INVENTORY (MMPI), such being done by permission of and under
copyrights held by THE UNIVERSITY OF MINNESOTA dated 1943, renewed
1970. Rights to the MMPI are licensed through National Computer
Systems, Inc., Interpretive Scoring Systems Division, Minneapolis, MN.

                  MINNESOTA MULTIPHASIC PERSONALITY INVENTORY
                         FOWLER CORRECTIONAL REPORT

The test results of this person appear to be valid. She seems to
have made an effort to answer the items truthfully and to follow the
instructions accurately. To some extent, this may be regarded as a
favorable prognostic sign since it indicates that she is capable of
following instructions and able to respond relevantly and truthfully
to personal inquiry.

She seems to be a person who experiences recurrent difficulty in
maintaining control over her impulses. When she behaves in a
socially unacceptable manner, she may seem to feel genuine guilt, but
the distress may be more a result of situational difficulties than
internal conflicts. She may exhibit a cyclic pattern characterized
by antisocial behavior, which is followed by distress and superficial
guilt and then by further acting out. This may be associated with a
pattern of excessive drinking. Her behavior seems to show a
self-defeating and self-punitive tendency. She is pessimistic about
the future and distressed about her failure to achieve her goals.
Conflict, for such a person, frequently centers around
dependency-independency needs. She would benefit from an opportunity
```
```

to establish relationships which satisfy her needs for acceptance and support while also permitting experiences in competition and self-expression, thus allowing her to achieve some confidence in her independence and judgment.

She appears to be a hypersensitive person who is overly responsive to criticism and quick to project the blame for her difficulties on others. Although she may be energetic and industrious, with a readiness to become involved in a variety of activities, her tendency to misunderstand and misinterpret the actions of others often leads to difficulties in her social interactions.

She is a rigid person who may react to anxiety producing circumstances with unrealistic fears and compulsive behavior. Chronic tension and excessive worry are common.

There are some unusual qualities in this person's thinking which may represent an original or inventive orientation, or perhaps some thinking disturbance. It should be noted that some temporary disorganization of thought and behavior may be an initial response to incarceration. Further information may be required to make a determination of her mental status.

MMPI PROFILE: ADULT

```
                      1     2     3     4     5     6     7     8     9     0
         L    F    K   HS    D    HY    PD    MF    PA    PT    SC    MA    SI
```

```
          L    F    K   HS    D    HY   PD    MF    PA    PT    SC    MA    SI
R         5    9   12    6    37    24   27    42    17    27    25    13    41
K                         6                5                12    12     2
K+R       5    9   12   12    37    24   32    42    17    39    37    15    41
T        53   64   49   48    84    59   81    39    76    73    72    45    68
```

Welsh Code: 24"678'0-3/19:5   F-L/K
Goldberg N-P Index: 80P

OFFENDER PROFILE AND RECOMMENDATIONS

Type II

This individual is classified as type II on the basis of her MMPI.
The following report describes behavior and experiences which are
typical of type II inmates. It should be kept in mind that this is a
general picture and not all type II characteristics will apply to
every group member.

Psychological description:

-- Group tends to be higher than other offender groups in
   intellectual ability and academic level.
-- Tend to be underachievers. Don't use ability effectively.
-- Relatively mild criminal history is characteristic.
-- Least aggressive and violent of inmate groups.
-- Generally have good relations with authorities and others.

Treatment and management considerations:

-- Should adapt easily to community placement. If placed in prison,
   brief incarceration followed by community supervision is advisable.
-- Separate from more aggressive and predatory groups.
-- Low anxiety, little desire for treatment.
-- Need to be energized to make constructive use of their abilities.
-- Good candidates for educational programs.
-- Could profit from insight-oriented psychothrapy.

Level: Low

Type V

This individual is classified as type V on the basis of her MMPI.
The following report describes behavior and experiences which are
typical of type V inmates. It should be kept in mind that this is a
general picture and not all type V characteristics will apply to
every group member.

Psychological description:

-- One of the better adjusted offender groups.
-- Not psychologically disturbed or excessively impulsive.
-- Most are very low in aggressive or violent behavior.
-- Low in authority conflict; good institutional adjustment.
-- Average in interpersonal relations.

Treatment and management considerations:

-- May be treated in community setting or closed setting.
-- If institutionalized, need help with initial stress.
-- Could profit from stable, supportive relationships with staff
   member.

Level: Low

Type X

This individual is classified as type X on the basis of her MMPI.
The following report describes behavior and experiences which are
typical of type X inmates. It should be kept in mind that this is a
general picture and not all type X characteristics will apply to
every group member.

Psychological description:

-- Aggresive, isolated, poor interpersonal relationships.
-- Psychologically disturbed: severe pathology likely.
-- Conflicts with authorities and poor institutional adjustment
   are common.
-- Extremely anxious, confused, irrational.
-- Expect extreme anxiety, confusion, some irrational thinking.

Treatment and management considerations:

-- Thorough psychiatric evaluation.
-- May require chemotherapy.
-- Consider transfer to forensic unit or mental hospital.
-- Observation period of 60-90 days before developing plan for
   treatment or rehabilitation.

Level: Low

CONTENT SCALES

The following statements are based upon an analysis of the content of
the subject's responses to the MMPI items. The content scales may be
regarded as a measure of how the subject views herself or wishes to
present herself in these areas, and thus may differ from the
descriptions found in the narrative report or from the clinical
impression.

Above each statement is an indication of whether the subject's
professed tendency toward the characteristics described is high, (t
score 70 or higher), moderate, (60-69), or low (40 or lower). Scale
scores between 40 and 60 are noted as average.

Depression (DEP)   HIGH   T= 70
She appears to be deeply depressed. She is overwhelmed by guilt
feelings and she blames herself for her troubles. Life holds little
enjoyment for her and she has difficulty maintaining interest and
involvement in her day to day responsibilities. She feels isolated
from others, sensitive to slights and unworthy of happiness. She
expects punishment and feels that she deserves it.

Poor Morale (MOR)   AVERAGE   T= 58

Psychoticism (PSY)   AVERAGE   T= 51

Phobias (PHO)   AVERAGE   T= 41

Organic Symptoms (ORG)   AVERAGE   T= 50

Authority Conflict (AUT)   AVERAGE   T= 45

Manifest Hostility (HOS)   AVERAGE   T= 49

Family Problems (FAM)   AVERAGE   T= 54

Hypomania (HYP)   LOW   T= 37

LAW OFFENDER SCALES

The following scales were developed with groups of law offenders.
Because they lack extensive validation and clinical use, they should
be cautiously interpreted. It should be kept in mind that while a
high score on a particular scale suggests an increased probability of
the behavior being measured, it is not evidence that the behavior
will occur in any specific individual.

Habitual Criminalism (HC)   HIGH   T= 79
This person has a high score on the habitual criminalism scale.
Offenders with this pattern have a high tendency to continue their
life style with little or no change and to resume old behavior
patterns after incarceration unless constructive intervention takes
place. Elevated scores are more frequent among individuals with
multiple offenses than of first offenders.

Parole Violater (PV)   AVERAGE   T= 52

Overcontrolled Hostility (OH)   AVERAGE   T= 57

Addiction Proneness (AM)   AVERAGE   T= 57

RESEARCH SCALES

                                                    Standard Scores

Special Scales   R   T
-----------------------   --   --
A   First Factor   (A)   24   61   !   !   *   !
R   Second Factor   (R)   22   60   !   !   *   !
Ego strength (Barron)   (ES)   40   50   !   *   !
Caudality (Williams)   (CA)   19   63   !   !   *   !
Social status (Gough)   (ST)   17   49   !   *!   !
Dominance (Gough)   (DO)   8   31   *   !   !
Social resp (Gough)   (RE)   15   33   !*   !   !
Manifest anxiety (Taylor)   (MAS) 26   66   !   !   *   !
Dependency (Navran)   (DY)   32   58   !   !   *   !
Prejudice (Gough)   (PR)   7   41   !   *   !   !
Control (Cuadra)   (CN)   29   58   !   !   *   !
Alcoholism (MacAndrew)   (ALC) 20   **   !   !   !
                                            30   40   50   60   70

** - Low Addiction Proneness

Content Scales (Wiggins)

Social maladjustment   (SOC) 18   65   !   !   *   !
Depression   (DEP) 19   70   !   !   !*
Feminine interests   (FEM) 19   48   !   *!   !
Poor morale   (MOR) 14   58   !   !   *   !
Religious fundamentalism   (REL)   1   27 *!   !   !
Authority conflict   (AUT)   6   45   !   * !   !
Psychoticism   (PSY)   8   51   !   *   !
Organic symptoms   (ORG)   7   50   !   *   !
Family problems   (FAM)   5   54   !   ! *   !
Manifest hostility   (HOS)   8   49   !   *!   !
Phobias   (PHO)   5   41   !   *   !   !
Hypomania   (HYP)   7   37   !   *   !   !
Poor health   (HEA)   6   50   !   *   !
                                            30   40   50   60   70

```
Item Factors
(Tryon, Stein & Chu)
----------------------------
TSC-I Social introversion    (I)    16    62  !              !        *    !
TSC-II Bodily concern        (B)     7    53  !              !*            !
TSC-III Suspicion            (S)     9    55  !              !   *         !
TSC-IV Depression            (D)    18    77  !              !            !*
TSC-V Resentment             (R)    10    60  !              !      *      !
TSC-VI Autism                (A)    10    63  !              !       *     !
TSC-VII Tension              (T)    16    62  !              !       *     !
                                                 30    40    50    60    70
```

Standard scores are based on statistics derived according to the
procedures described in Dahlstrom, W.G., Welsh, G.S., & Dahlstrom, L.E.
An MMPI Handbook, Vol. II. Minneapolis, University of Minnesota Press, 1975.

As is evident in the computer output, a standard score profile is presented utilizing the MMPI's adolescent norms; an adult profile is also generated. The MMPI program requires that a great deal of information be stored in the computer for reference. For example, the computer program (*a*) goes through the process of inspecting the MMPI's validity scales to determine if the entire profile is valid, then (*b*) produces a general personality description together with an analysis of various defense mechanisms. The computer also generates (*c*) a diagnostic impression of the adolescent based on a comparison of the pattern analysis of his or her standard scores with those of known populations in various DSM-III diagnostic categories. Finally, the computer program produces (*d*) extended personality trait information designed to aid in counseling and therapy, while noting (*e*) special medical ramifications along with (*f*) an analysis of vocational and work attitudes. The second section of the report contains (*g*) further factor analytic data based on other research scales which have been factor analyzed in the literature, and (*h*) counseling scales, which represent additional factor analyses, for the purpose of designing counseling and therapeutic intervention.

Two further enhancements are available to the above report. These include the Fowler Correctional Report (Psych-Systems, 1985c) and the ability of the computer to integrate MMPI information with other measures contained on the computer. The Fowler Correctional Report is an extensive analysis of MMPI responses based on known characteristics of correctional populations.

The MMPI analysis system described above is perhaps one of the most sophisticated automated assessment devices in existence today. As can be seen from Figure 14-1, the computer performs a 5-point pattern analysis on the major MMPI scales in order to identify possible DSM-III diagnoses and to produce narrative output. The narrative output contained in this report is much more sophisticated than in other reports described in this chapter. The decision matrix necessary to generate each sentence of the report is extremely complex and based on thousands of possible decision choices. Clearly, the data presented here would be outside of the scope of human potential in the absence of the computer. Indeed, this program is so complex that numerous programmers worked over 10 years to develop it. Further, the program's continual refinements ensure and increase the accuracy of the decision rules it uses.

The Millon Adolescent Personality Inventory

The Millon Adolescent Personality Inventory was developed "for the purpose of identifying, predicting, and understanding a wide range of psychological attributes characteristic of adolescents." It is available for use with adolescents from age 13 and up, is administered by paper and pencil using standard NCS answer sheets, and then is scored and interpreted by computer. The test protocols must be mailed to NCS for scoring and interpretation, and the output is provided in either a clinical or guidance report format. Information is provided on the validity of the particular administration, standard scores are presented for each of the scales along with verbal descriptions of the behavior predicted by these scores, and a paragraph is provided which reviews treatment implications.

The Millon's intent appears to be to provide a system of diagnostic classification for adolescents while also supplying information for counseling and therapy use. The test has three basic dimensions: Personality Style, Expressed Concerns, and Behavioral Correlates. The Personality Styles dimension contains the following subscales: Scale 1, Introversive; Scale 2, Inhibited; Scale 3, Cooperative; Scale 4, Sociable; Scale 5, Confidence; Scale 6, Forceful; Scale 7, Respectful; and Scale 8, Sensitive. These subscales represent the eight basic personality styles evident from adolescents' perceptions of sources of reinforcement and from the coping mechanisms they use to deal with various types of reinforcement.

The Expressed Concerns dimension contains the following: Scale A, Self-Concept; Scale B, Personal Esteem; Scale C, Body Comfort; Scale D, Sexual Acceptance; Scale E, Peer Security; Scale F, Social Tolerance; Scale G, Family Rapport; and Scale H, Academic Confidence. These subscales are derived from many of the developmental tasks suggested by Havighurst and Erickson.

The Behavioral Correlates dimension contains the following: Scale S, Impulse Control; Scale TT, Societal Conformity; Scale UU, Scholastic Achievement; and Scale WW, Attendance Consistency. These subscales have been derived empirically through factor analytic techniques similar to those used with the MMPI.

Several aspects of the Millon make it a rather unusual instrument. First, the test was written in language most adolescents can readily understand; this appears to add significantly to its reliability and credibility with this population. Second, the test was developed not on a model of pathology, but on a model of personality development. The factor analytic data presented in the manual are highly supportive of this model, and the procedures used to standardize this test were unusually rigorous. The computerized report produced by the Millon, however, is not as sophisticated as that for the adolescent MMPI (see above). For the most part, the Millon report is generated using a scale-by-scale analysis rather than a multifactor regression analysis. No data are presented on the interpretative scheme or algorithms used to produce the computerized report. A further analysis of this difficulty is discussed by Brown (1986).

Interpretation

```
                              FIGURE III:1
            Clinical Interpretive Report (Reduced from 8-1/2" x 11")
                                                                    001 0001
                  MILLON ADOLESCENT PERSONALITY INVENTORY
                                CLINICAL REPORT
                  CONFIDENTIAL INFORMATION FOR PROFESSIONAL USE ONLY

            REPORT FOR:                          SEX: MALE     AGE:  16

ID NUMBER:  0123467890        VALID AND RELIABLE REPORT  DATE:  07/06/82

CODE;

6 **4 5 * 8 + 1 + 3 2 7  //F G **-* 8 + H A E + C D  //SS**TTUU* //
                         ----


**************************************************************************
SCALES      * SCORE *         PROFILE OF BP SCORES           *
            *RAW BR*      35   60        75         85      100  DIMENSIONS
********+**+***+***+--------+---+---------+---------+-------+******************
        1   14  47 XXXXXXXX                                      INTROVERSIVE
        +--+---+---+--------+---+---------+---------+-------+------------------
        2    6  27 XXXXX                                         INHIBITED
        +--+---+---+--------+---+---------+---------+-------+------------------
        3   14  31 XXXXXX                                        COOPERATIVE
        +--+---+---+--------+---+---------+---------+-------+------------------
PERSNLTY 4  22  81 XXXXXXXXXXXXXXXXXXXXXXXXXXXXX                  SOCIABLE
        +--+---+---+--------+---+---------+---------+-------+------------------
 STYLES 5   32  75 XXXXXXXXXXXXXXXXXXXXX                          CONFIDENT
        +--+---+---+--------+---+---------+---------+-------+------------------
        6   23  87 XXXXXXXXXXXXXXXXXXXXXXXXXXXXXXXXX              FORCEFUL
        +--+---+---+--------+---+---------+---------+-------+------------------
        7   13  22 XXXX                                          RESPECTFUL
        +--+---+---+--------+---+---------+---------+-------+------------------
        8   18  63 XXXXXXXXXXXXX                                 SENSITIVE
********+**+***+***+--------+---+---------+---------+-------+------------------
        A    9  54 XXXXXXXXXX                                    SELF-CONCEPT
        +--+---+---+--------+---+---------+---------+-------+------------------
        B   10  61 XXXXXXXXXXX                                   PERSONAL ESTEEM
        +--+---+---+--------+---+---------+---------+-------+------------------
        C    3  24 XXXXX                                         BODY COMFORT
        +--+---+---+--------+---+---------+---------+-------+------------------
EXPRESSD D   3  18 XXXX                                          SEXUAL ACCEPTANCE
        +--+---+---+--------+---+---------+---------+-------+------------------
CONCERNS E   6  39 XXXXXXX                                       PEER SECURITY
        +--+---+---+--------+---+---------+---------+-------+------------------
        F   13  91 XXXXXXXXXXXXXXXXXXXXXXXXXXXXXXXXXXXXX          SOCIAL TOLERANCE
        +--+---+---+--------+---+---------+---------+-------+------------------
        G    8  88 XXXXXXXXXXXXXXXXXXXXXXXXXXXXXXXXXXX            FAMILY RAPPORT
        +--+---+---+--------+---+---------+---------+-------+------------------
        H    6  55 XXXXXXXXXX                                    ACADEMIC CONFDNCE
********+**+***+***+--------+---+---------+---------+-------+******************
        SS  27  97 XXXXXXXXXXXXXXXXXXXXXXXXXXXXXXXXXXXXXXXX       IMPULSE CONTROL
        +--+---+---+--------+---+---------+---------+-------+------------------
BEHAVIOR TT 19  81 XXXXXXXXXXXXXXXXXXXXXXXXXXXX                   SOCIAL CONFORMITY
        +--+---+---+--------+---+---------+---------+-------+------------------
CORRE-  UU  18  77 XXXXXXXXXXXXXXXXXXXXXXXX                       SCHOLAST ACHVMNT
        +--+---+---+--------+---+---------+---------+-------+------------------
LATES   WW  15  62 XXXXXXXXXXX                                   ATTNDNCE CNSTNCY
********+**+***+***+--------+---+---------+---------+-------+******************
```

Interpretation

MAPI CLINICAL REPORT NARRATIVES HAVE BEEN NORMED ON ADOLESCENT
PATIENTS SEEN IN PROFESSIONAL TREATMENT SETTINGS FOR EITHER GENUINE
EMOTIONAL DISCOMFORTS OR SOCIAL DIFFICULTIES AND ARE APPLICABLE
PRIMARILY DURING THE EARLY PHASES OF ASSESSMENT OR PSYCHOTHERAPY,
DISTORTIONS SUCH AS GREATER SEVERITY MAY OCCUR AMONG RESPONDENTS WHO
HAVE INAPPROPRIATELY TAKEN THE MAPI FOR ESSENTIALLY EDUCATIONAL OR
SELF-EXPLORATORY PURPOSES; IN AN ACADEMIC COUNSELING SETTING, THE
MAPI GUIDANCE REPORT IS LIKELY TO BE MORE RELEVANT AND PROVIDE A MORE
SUITABLE PICTURE OF THE PSYCHOLOGICAL AND VOCATIONAL TRAITS OF THIS
TEENAGER. INFERENTIAL AND PROBABILISTIC, THIS REPORT MUST BE VIEWED AS
ONLY ONE ASPECT OF A THOROUGH DIAGNOSTIC STUDY. MOREOVER, THESE
INFERENCES SHOULD BE REEVALUATED PERIODICALLY IN LIGHT OF THE PATTERN
OF ATTITUDE CHANGE AND EMOTIONAL GROWTH THAT TYPIFIES THE ADOLESCENT
PERIOD. FOR THESE REASONS, IT SHOULD NOT BE SHOWN TO PATIENTS OR THEIR
RELATIVES.

THIS YOUNGSTER SHOWED NO UNUSUAL CHARACTEROLOGICAL OR TEST-TAKING
ATTITUDES THAT MAY HAVE DISTORTED THE MAPI RESULTS.

PERSONALITY PATTERNS

THE FOLLOWING PERTAINS TO THOSE ENDURING AND PERVASIVE CHARACTERO--
LOGICAL TRAITS THAT UNDERLIE THE PERSONAL AND INTERPERSONAL DIFFICULTIES
OF THIS YOUNGSTER. RATHER THAN FOCUS ON SPECIFIC PROBLEM AREAS AND
COMPLAINTS, TO BE DISCUSSED IN LATER PARAGRAPHS, THIS SECTION CONCENTRATES
ON THE MORE HABITUAL, MALADAPTIVE METHODS OF RELATING, BEHAVING, THINKING
AND FEELING.

THIS YOUNGSTER IS TYPICALLY GREGARIOUS AND FRIENDLY UPON INITIAL CONTACT,
OFTEN MAKING A GOOD FIRST IMPRESSION BECAUSE OF HIS EASY-GOING AFFABILITY.
THIS SOCIABILITY MAY EXPRESS ITSELF AT TIMES IN SELF-DRAMATIZING BEHAVIORS
AND AN IMPULSIVE NEED TO SEEK OUT STIMULATION AND EXCITEMENT. THE OVERALL
STYLE OF SOCIAL LIVELINESS MAY BE SHORT-LIVED SINCE THIS YOUNGSTER IS DISPOSED
TO LOSE HIS TEMPER, BECOME IRRITABLE, IMPATIENT OR BORED WHEN THINGS FAIL TO
GO WELL. IF CROSSED, SUBJECT TO EXTERNAL PRESSURES, OR FACED WITH POTENTIAL
EMBARRASSMENTS, THIS TEENAGER MAY QUICKLY BECOME ILL-HUMORED, QUARRELSOME AND
TOUCHY. THUS, THE CHARACTERISTIC INITIAL IMPRESSION OF SELF-CONFIDENCE AND
AFFABILITY MAY BE QUITE PRECARIOUS, OVERLYING A DEEPER INSECURITY AND DISCON-
TENT AND, HENCE, MAY GIVE WAY READILY TO DEFIANCE, TROUBLES WITH THE LAW AND
FRACTIOUSNESS WITHIN THE FAMILY.

ALTHOUGH THIS YOUNG MAN MAY INITIALLY REACT TO DIFFICULTIES SUCH AS THE
ABOVE BY APPEARING COOL AND INDIFFERENT, BENEATH THIS SURFACE IMPRESSION
THERE ARE APT TO BE STRONG FEARS AND TENSIONS. SHOULD PRESSURE BE PERSISTENT,
HE WILL BE PRONE TO LYING, BECOMING TRUANT AND RUNNING AWAY FROM HOME. SHORT-
TEMPERED, INTOLERANT OF FRUSTRATION AND CRITICISM, HE WILL READILY BECOME
EXCITABLE AND DISOBEDIENT. WHEN MATTERS ARE MORE RELAXED, HE IS LIKELY TO
BEHAVE IN A SAUCY, IF NOT CHARMING MANNER, WITH OBVIOUS EFFORTS TO ATTRACT
ATTENTION AND RECOGNITION.

EXPRESSED CONCERNS

THE SCALES COMPRISING THIS SECTION PERTAIN TO THE PERSONAL PERCEPTIONS
OF THIS YOUNGSTER CONCERNING SEVERAL ISSUES OF PSYCHOLOGICAL DEVELOPMENT,
ACTUALIZATION AND CONCERN. BECAUSE EXPERIENCES DURING THIS AGE PERIOD
ARE NOTABLY SUBJECTIVE, IT IS IMPORTANT TO RECORD HOW THIS TEENAGER SEES
EVENTS AND REPORTS FEELINGS, AND NOT ONLY HOW OTHERS MAY OBJECTIVELY
REPORT THEM TO BE. FOR COMPARATIVE PURPOSES, THESE SELF-ATTITUDES REGARDING
A WIDE RANGE OF PERSONAL, SOCIAL, FAMILIAL AND SCHOLASTIC MATTERS ARE
CONTRASTED WITH THOSE EXPRESSED BY A BROAD CROSS-SECTION OF TEENAGERS
OF THE SAME SEX AND AGE.

EVEN THOUGH OTHER PROBLEMS ARE PRESENT, THIS YOUNG MAN IS WELL INTO THE PROCESS OF DEVELOPING A CLEAR SELF-CONCEPT AND A SERIES OF DIRECTIONS AS TO WHAT HE MAY BECOME. ALTHOUGH NOT FULLY SETTLED IN THIS REGARD, HE DEMONSTRATES A GROWING SENSE OF VALUES AND GOALS FOR HIS FUTURE.

THIS YOUNG MAN REPORTS MODEST SATISFACTION WITH THE PERSON HE IS BECOMING. HE FEELS THAT HE CAN EXPRESS HIMSELF AS AN INDIVIDUAL AND THAT HE IS DEVELOPING A SENSE OF PERSONAL WELL-BEING. THIS COMFORT WITH HIMSELF SHOULD ENHANCE HIS ABILITY TO COPE WITH THE MORE TROUBLESOME ASPECTS OF HIS CURRENT LIFE.

HAVING PROGRESSED THROUGH EARLY ADOLESCENT CONCERNS REGARDING PHYSICAL GROWTH AND APPEARANCE, THIS YOUNG MAN IS UNUSUALLY SATISFIED WITH BOTH HIS LOOKS AND MATURATION, FEELINGS THAT CAN ONLY ENHANCE HIS SELF-ESTEEM AND FACILITATE HIS RELATING COMFORTABLY TO OTHERS.

SEXUALITY IS EXPERIENCED AS COMFORTABLE FOR THIS YOUNGSTER. HE DESCRIBES CONSIDERABLE SATISFACTION WITH THE INTENSITY OF HIS IMPULSES AND THE ROLES THEY REQUIRE OF HIM.

SOCIAL RELATIONSHIPS ARE PERCEIVED AS SATISFACTORY. THERE IS A SENSE OF BELONGING AND IDENTIFICATION WITH HIS PEER GROUP. NEVERTHELESS, SOME CONCERNS ARE EXPRESSED IN THIS SPHERE.

COOL AND DISTANT, THIS YOUTH DEMONSTRATES LITTLE OR NO COMPASSION FOR OTHERS, VIEWING THEIR DIFFICULTIES AS THE PRODUCT OF THEIR OWN WEAKNESSES. HE IS LIKELY TO FEEL NO COMPUNCTION ABOUT IGNORING THEIR NEEDS AND SENSITIVITIES. THIS LACK OF EMPATHY MAY LEAD THIS YOUNGSTER TO SERVE ONLY HIMSELF REGARDLESS OF THE CONSEQUENCES FOR THOSE AROUND HIM.

IN ADDITION TO ANY OTHER DIFFICULTIES, THIS YOUNG MAN DESCRIBES SERIOUS PROBLEMS IN THE FAMILY SETTING. TENSION AND A LACK OF SUPPORT ARE TYPICAL. DEPENDING ON THE PERSONALITY STYLE NOTED ELSEWHERE IN THIS REPORT, THESE DIFFICULTIES MAY REFLECT EITHER SEVERE PARENTAL REJECTION OR, CONVERSELY, A SHARP BREAK ON THE PART OF THIS YOUNGSTER AS HE ASSERTS INDEPENDENCE FROM TRADITIONAL SOCIETAL VALUES.

AS IS QUITE COMMON AMONG TEENAGERS, SCHOOL AND ACHIEVEMENT ARE REGARDED IN BOTH POSITIVE AND NEGATIVE LIGHTS. ALTHOUGH NOT UNIFORMLY SATISFIED WITH HIS LEVEL OF ACADEMIC PERFORMANCE, THIS YOUNG MAN EXPRESSES SOME MODEST GOALS IN REGARD TO ACHIEVEMENT AND A REASONABLE LEVEL OF CONFIDENCE IN HIS ABILITY TO ATTAIN THEM.

Interpretation
BEHAVIORAL CORRELATES

THE SCALES COMPRISING THIS SECTION FOCUS ON PROBLEMS THAT FREQUENTLY COME TO THE ATTENTION OF SCHOOL COUNSELORS, FAMILY AND OTHER AGENCIES, AS WELL AS THERAPEUTIC CLINICIANS. IT SHOULD BE NOTED THAT THESE SCALES DO NOT PROVIDE DIRECT EVIDENCE THAT THE YOUNGSTER HAS OR IS LIKELY TO EXHIBIT THE DIFFICULTIES REFERRED TO. RATHER, THEY GAUGE THE EXTENT TO WHICH THE RESPONSES OF THIS TEENAGER ARE SIMILAR TO THOSE WHO HAVE BEEN IDENTIFIED BY COUNSELORS AND CLINICIANS AS EVIDENCING TROUBLESOME BEHAVIORS SUCH AS IMPULSIVITY, SOCIAL NONCOMPLIANCE, UNDERACHIEVEMENT AND NONATTENDANCE.

EXTREMELY INCAUTIOUS, THIS YOUTH RESPONDS TO MAPI ITEMS IN A MANNER THAT INDICATES A MARKED DISINCLINATION TO RESTRAIN HIS IMPULSES AND TO REFLECT ON THEIR PROBABLE CONSEQUENCES. REPEATEDLY RESPONDING TO MOMENTARY FEELINGS, HE MAY BE CAUGHT IN A VICIOUS CIRCLE OF HIS OWN ACTIONS AND THE NEGATIVE REACTIONS OF OTHERS.

THERE ARE INDICATIONS FROM HIS RESPONSES TO THE MAPI THAT THIS TEEN IS SIMILAR TO YOUNGSTERS DESCRIBED AS SOMEWHAT REBELLIOUS AND SOCIALLY NONCOMPLIANT, A STANCE WHICH MAY BRING HIM TO THE ATTENTION OF AUTHORITIES.

THE RESPONSES OF THIS YOUNG MAN ARE SIMILAR TO THOSE WHO HAVE ESTABLISHED A PATTERN OF UNDERACHIEVEMENT IN ACADEMIC SETTINGS. WHETHER OWING TO A LACK OF MOTIVATION OR A LACK IN BASIC SKILLS, THIS YOUNGSTER IS LIKELY TO HAVE PROBLEMS IN ACHIEVING HIS ACADEMIC POTENTIALS. EFFORTS SHOULD BE DIRECTED TO REDUCE THE PROBABILITY OF FURTHER EXACERBATION.

ALTHOUGH LIKELY TO DEMONSTRATE GOOD SCHOOL ATTENDANCE, THE RESPONSES OF THIS YOUNG MAN INDICATE A MODEST TENDENCY TO BE ABSENT FROM SCHOOL FOR PSYCHOSOCIAL OR EMOTIONAL REASONS.

NOTEWORTHY RESPONSES

THE FOLLOWING STATEMENTS WERE ANSWERED BY THIS YOUNGSTER IN THE DIRECTION NOTED IN THE PARENTHESES. THESE ITEMS SUGGEST SPECIFIC PROBLEM AREAS THAT MAY DESERVE FURTHER INQUIRY ON THE PART OF THE CLINICIAN.

SOCIAL ALIENATION: NO ITEMS

BEHAVIORAL PROBLEMS:

17. WHEN I GET ANGRY, I USUALLY COOL DOWN AND LET MY FEELINGS PASS. (F)
20. I LIKE TO FOLLOW INSTRUCTIONS AND DO WHAT OTHERS EXPECT OF ME. (F)
30. RATHER THAN DEMAND THINGS, PEOPLE CAN GET WHAT THEY WANT BY BEING GENTLE AND THOUGHTFUL. (F)
33. IT IS EASY FOR ME TO TAKE ADVANTAGE OF PEOPLE. (T)
47. WHEN I DO NOT GET MY WAY, I USUALLY LOSE MY TEMPER. (T)
76. MY PARENTS OFTEN TELL ME I AM NO GOOD. (T)
87. PUNISHMENT NEVER STOPPED ME FROM DOING WHATEVER I WANTED. (T)
96. I HAVE A PRETTY HOT TEMPER. (T)
100. I LIKE IT AT HOME. (F)
135. I MAKE NASTY REMARKS TO PEOPLE IF THEY DESERVE IT. (T)

EMOTIONAL DIFFICULTIES:

91. I OFTEN FEEL SO ANGRY I WANT TO THROW AND BREAK THINGS. (T)
113. I AM JEALOUS OF THE SPECIAL ATTENTION THAT THE OTHER CHILDREN IN THE FAMILY GET. (T)
133. SO LITTLE OF WHAT I HAVE DONE HAS BEEN APPRECIATED BY OTHERS. (T)
150. I CAN CONTROL MY FEELINGS EASILY. (F)

THERAPEUTIC IMPLICATIONS

THE FOLLOWING CONSIDERATIONS ARE LIKELY TO BE OF GREATER UTILITY AND ACCURACY DURING EARLY TREATMENT PLANNING THAN IN LATER MANAGEMENT PHASES.

THIS YOUNGSTER IS NOT LIKELY TO BE A WILLING PARTICIPANT IN THERAPY, MO PROBABLY AGREEING UNDER THE PRESSURE OF FAMILY, LEGAL OR DRUG DIFFICULTIES. A TENDENCY TO ATTRIBUTE PAST PROBLEMS TO OTHERS WILL BE EVIDENT AND, EVEN WH ACCEPTING SOME MEASURE OF RESPONSIBILITY, RESENTMENT MAY BE FELT TOWARD THE THERAPIST FOR TRYING TO POINT THESE OUT. THIS TEENAGER MAY SEEK TO BLUFF OR OUTWIT THE CLINICIAN, AN ACTION THAT WILL REQUIRE THE THERAPIST TO RESTRAIN THE IMPULSE TO REACT WITH DISAPPROVAL AND CRITICISM. AN IMPORTANT STEP IN BUILDING RAPPORT IS SEEING THINGS FROM THE VIEWPOINT OF THIS YOUNGSTER. THE THERAPIST MUST CONVEY A SENSE OF TRUST AND A WILLINGNESS TO DEVELOP A CONSTRUCTIVE TREATMENT ALLIANCE. A BALANCE OF PROFESSIONAL AUTHORITY AND TOLERANCE WILL BE NECESSARY TO DIMINISH THE PROBABILITY THAT THE PATIENT WIL IMPULSIVELY WITHDRAW FROM TREATMENT.

Current Limitations and Future Developments

A number of clear limitations exist in the automated software currently available to the profession. For example, very few programs have been developed specifically for use with young children, and those that are available, with the exception of the EPQ-J, collect their data using parents as observers. The need for a relatively high level of reading (sixth grade or above) further restricts the use of many instruments with lower functioning children and adolescents. This is certainly the case with tests like the MMPI which require a relatively high level of vocabulary comprehension.

While many of the studies cited above indicate a relatively positive reaction to computer-administered tests, many clients, in the author's experience, are unable to adequately provide data through this method. Such clients include extremely depressed individuals, individuals with perceptual and motor-learning disabilities, the retarded, and some individuals who exhibit extreme computer phobia. The extent to which computer software has been made user friendly and more human-like has led to improved performances by some in the above groups.

Intelligence testing has not yet been well adapted to the computer. The majority of computer applications fall into systems that measure only verbal and quantitative intelligence through direct practitioner administration, and systems that measure aspects of intelligence through direct computer administration. To date, no attempt has been made to directly measure the perceptual-motor or performance aspects of intelligence using the latter format. The majority of software available in this broad area is geared toward analyzing intelligence data after it has been collected by a practitioner. This, in and of itself, is useful to the extent that the quantitative analyses provided are valid. Most of the programs have been developed for 8-bit microcomputers and are therefore relatively simplistic in their analyses. This is especially true of the verbal reports such programs are able to provide.

Another area of concern involves the profession's ability to evaluate the algorithms which are being employed to generate computer output. Because of concerns about proprietary copyright infringement, many software publishers are reluctant to divulge the mathematical decision rules being used in their report generations. This makes the scientific scrutiny of these techniques difficult and tends to impede research on their validities. Further, the lack of data provided, for example, by NCS on its interpretation of the Millon Adolescent Personality Inventory, makes it difficult for practitioners using this instrument to fully understand the nature of its interpretative scheme. As has been suggested (Brown, 1986), one must simply trust NCS to machine score and interpret the instrument without being able to review the statistical procedures and decision rules used by the computer for making various determinations. If automated assessment is to have future credibility, the techniques used for the collection of data and interpretation must be open to professional scrutiny.

Many practitioners have resisted computerized assessment because of the rapidity of its introduction into the profession. In fact, many of the articles reviewed in this chapter view automated assessment as an impending danger to the profession rather than a potentially helpful tool. This may result from the relative unfamiliarity of practitioners with computers and their use. More fundamentally, some practitioners are concerned that computers may replace them, especially within the domain and function of assessment. In the view of the author, it is critically important that more practitioners obtain training in computer programming and multivariate statistical techniques because a rudimentary knowledge of multivariate analysis will be fundamental to test design and analysis in the future. In the next 5 to 10 years, it is reasonable to assume that highly integrated test batteries will be developed for computers requiring relatively advanced mathematical understandings of their properties. Professional mental health practitioners should not permit themselves to be passive resistors to the development of automated assessment. This could result in their displacement by other professional groups who are more than willing to use automated assessment. For example, the use of automated assessment techniques by psychiatrists who are relatively untrained in psychometrics has been expressed as an emerging concern (Turkington, 1984).

Automated assessment has shown itself to consistently have a number of major advantages. For example, the way items are presented by computer can promote greater individual attention and motivation from those being assessed. Further, there is no question that computers present test items in exactly the same manner given the same conditions every time; this is not the case with human administration. All of these factors reduce inadvertent error and increase reliability. Improved reliability coupled with shorter testing times make automated assessment a more cost-effective means, then, for collecting information. Indeed, the information necessary to produce the MMPI protocol presented earlier was collected in under 1 hour by computer, while the analysis and report printout required 10 minutes. This contrasts with the several hours of administration and scoring time normally required for the MMPI. Much of the data contained in the computerized report are simply not economically obtainable without the use of the computer.

Additionally, the computer offers the advantages of being able to time items and response latencies and to adjust the flow of items contingent on these temporal variables. These capabilities and the quality whereby stimulus items are presented will be enhanced in the future as videodisk technology is employed to vary the format of items and to invent new formats. With this technology, the assessment of many visual-perceptual skills will be possible with the computer.

Without question, in the next 10 years we will see a revolution in the nature of psychological assessment as we know it today. In all probability, more truly useful personality assessment systems will be developed during that short period than in the previous 50 years.

References

ADEPT. (1982). *WISC-R Analysis Program*. Beaumont, TX: Author.

Altemose, J. R., & Williamson, K. B. (1981). Clinical judgment vs. the computer: Can the school psychologist be replaced by a machine? *Psychology in the Schools, 18*, 356–363.

American Association on Mental Deficiency. (1977). *Manual on terminology and classification in mental retardation* (Special Publication No. 2) Washington, DC: Author.

American Psychiatric Association. (1980). *Diagnostic and statistical manual of mental disorders* (3rd ed.). Washington, DC: Author.

Angle, H. V. (1981). The interviewing computer: A technology for gathering comprehensive treatment information. *Behavior Research Methods and Instrumentation, 13*, 607–612.

Beaumont, J. G. (1981). Microcomputer-aided assessment using standard psychometric procedures. *Behavioral Research Methods and Instrumentation, 13*, 430–433.

Bennett, R. E. (1982). Applications of microcomputer technology to special education. *Exceptional Children, 49*, 106–112.

Brown, D. T. (1984). Automated assessment systems in school and clinical psychology: Present status and future directions. *School Psychology Review, 13*, 455–460.

Brown, D. T. (1986). Review of the Millon Adolescent Personality Inventory. *The ninth mental measurements yearbook*. Lincoln: Buros Institute, University of Nebraska.

Byers, A. P. (1981). Psychological evaluation by means of an on-line computer. *Behavior Research Methods and Instrumentation, 13*, 585–587.

Byrnes, E., & Johnson, J. H. (1981). Change technology and the implementation of automation in mental health care settings. *Behavior Research Methods and Instrumentation, 13*, 573–580.

Carr, A. C., & Ghosh, A. (1983a). Response of phobic patients to direct computer assessment. *British Journal of Psychiatry, 142*, 60–65.

Carr, A. C., & Ghosh, A. (1983b). Accuracy of behavioral assessment by computer. *British Journal of Psychiatry, 142*, 66–70.

Erdman, H. P., Greist, J. H., Klein, M. H., Jefferson, J. W., & Getto, C. (1981). The computer psychiatrist: How far have we come? Where are we heading? How far dare we go? *Behavior Research Methods and Instrumentation, 13*, 393–398.

Exner, J. E., Jr. (1974). *The Rorschach: A comprehensive system* (Vol. 1). New York: Wiley.

Eysenck, H. J., & Eysenck, S. B. G. (1975). *Eysenck Personality Questionnaire*. San Diego, CA: Edits/Educational and Industrial Testing Service.

Fowler, R. D., Jr., & Coyle, F. A., Jr. (1968). Computer application of MMPI actuarial systems with a college population. *Journal of Psychology, 69*, 233–236.

Harris, W. G., Niedner, D., Feldman, X. X., Fink, A., & Johnson, J. H. (1981). An on-line interpretive Rorschach approach: Using Exner's Comprehensive System. *Behavior Research Methods and Instrumentation, 13*, 588–591.

Hathaway, S. R., & McKinley, J. C. (1982). *Minnesota Multiphasic Personality Inventory*. Minneapolis: University of Minnesota.

Hedl, J. J., Jr., O'Neil, H. F., Jr., & Hansen, D. N. (1973). Affective reactions toward computer-based intelligence testing. *Journal of Counseling and Clinical Psychology, 40*, 217–222.

Honaker, L. M. (1982). *Wechsler Intelligence Scale for Children-Revised (WISC-R)*. Baltimore, MD: Psych-Systems.

Ingram, R. (1985). *Evaluating psychoeducational software*. Unpublished manuscript.

Ireton, H., & Thwing, E. (1974). *Minnesota Child Development Inventory*. Minneapolis, MN: Behavior Science Systems, Inc.

Johnson, J. H., Giannetti, R. A., Klingler, D. E., & Williams, T. A. (1980). The reliability of diagnoses by technician, computer, and algorithm. *Journal of Clinical Psychology, 36*, 447–450.

Johnson, J. H., & Johnson, K. N. (1981). Psychological considerations related to the development of computerized testing stations. *Behavior Research Methods and Instrumentation, 13*, 421–424.

Johnson, J. H., & Williams, T. A. (1975). The use of on-line computer technology in a mental health admitting system. *American Psychologist, 30*, 388–390.

Johnson, J. H., & Williams, T. A. (1978). Clinical testing and assessment: Using a microcomputer for on-line psychiatric assessment. *Behavior Research Methods and Instrumentation, 10*, 576–578.

Katz, L., & Dalby, J. T. (1981). Computer-assisted and traditional psychological assessment of elementary-school-aged children. *Contemporary Educational Psychology, 6*, 314–322.

Kaufman, A. S. (1975). Factor analysis of the WISC-R at eleven age levels between 6-½ and 16-½ years. *Journal of Consulting and Clinical Psychology, 43*, 135–147.

Labeck, L. J., Johnson, J. H., & Harris, W. G. (1983). Validity of a computerized on-line MMPI interpretive system. *Journal of Clinical Psychology, 39*, 412–416.

Lyons, J. P., & Brown, J. (1981). Reduction in clinical assessment time using computer algorithms. *Behavioral Research Methods and Instrumentation, 13*, 407–412.

McCullough, C. S., & Wenck, L. S. (1984). Computers in school psychology. *School Psychology Review, 13*, 421.

McDermott, P. A. (1980). A computerized system for the classification of developmental, learning, and adjustment disorders in school children. *Educational and Psychological Measurement, 40*, 761–768.

McDermott, P. A., & Hale, R. L. (1982). Validation of a systems-actuarial computer process for multidimensional classification of child psychopathology. *Journal of Clinical Psychology, 38*, 477–486.

McLeod, D. R., Griffiths, R. R., Bigelow, G. E., & Yingling, J. (1982). Computer technology: An automated version of the Digit Symbol Substitution Test (DSST). *Behavior Research Methods and Instrumentation, 14*, 463–466.

Miller, D. A., Johnson, J. H., Klingler, D. E., Williams, T. A., & Giannetti, R. A. (1977). Design for an on-line computerized system for MMPI interpretation. *Behavior Research Methods and Instrumentation, 9*, 117–122.

Millon, T., Green, C. J., & Meagher, R. B., Jr. (1982). *Millon Adolescent Personality Inventory*. Minneapolis, MN: National Computer Systems, Inc.

Morf, M., Alexander, P., & Fuerth, T. (1981). Fully automated psychiatric diagnosis: Some new possibilities. *Behavior Research Methods and Instrumentation, 13*, 413–416.

Nicholson, C. L. (1982). *WISC-R computer report: Southern MicroSystems Educational Software*. New York: Psychological Corporation.

Okey, J. R., & McGarity, J. (1982). Classroom diagnostic testing with microcomputers. *Science Education, 66*, 571–579.

Paitich, D. (1973). Computers in behavioral science: A Comprehensive Automated Psychological Examination and Report (CAPER). *Behavioral Science, 18*, 131–136.

Piotrowski, Z. A. (1974). *Perceptanalysis*. Philadelphia, PA: Ex Libris.

Psych-Systems. (1985a). *The Eysenck Personality Questionnaire-Junior*. Baltimore, MD: Author.

Psych-Systems. (1985b). *Fasttest Automated Assessment System*. Baltimore, MD: Author.

Psych-Systems. (1985c). *The Fowler Correctional Report*. Baltimore, MD: Author.

Psych-Systems. (1985d). *The Minnesota Multiphasic Personality Inventory*. Baltimore, MD: Author.

Psych-Systems. (1985e). *The Multidimensional Aptitude Battery*. Baltimore, MD: Author.

Psych-Systems. (1985f). *Visual Searching Task*. Baltimore, MD: Author.

Quintanar, L. R., Crowell, C. R., & Pryor, J. B. (1982). Human-computer interaction: A preliminary social psychological analysis. *Behavior Research Methods and Instrumentation, 14*, 210–220.

Sampson, J. P., Jr. (1983). Measurement Forum. Computer-assisted testing and assessment: Current status and implications for the future. *Measurement and Evaluation in Guidance, 15*, 293–299.

Schmid, W., Bronisch, T., & von Zerssen, D. (1982). A comparative study of PSE/CATEGO and DiaSika: Two psychiatric computer diagnostic systems. *British Journal of Psychiatry, 141*, 292–295.

Skinner, H. A., & Allen, B. A. (1983). Does the computer make a difference? Computerized versus face-to-face versus self-report assessment of alcohol, drug, and tobacco use. *Journal of Consulting and Clinical Psychology, 51*, 267–275.

Space, L. G. (1981). The computer as psychometrician. *Behavior Research Methods and Instrumentation, 13*, 595–606.

Stout, R. L. (1981). New approaches to the design of computerized interviewing and testing systems. *Behavior Research Methods and Instrumentation, 13*, 436–442.

Turkington, C. (1984, January). The growing use, and abuse, of computer testing. *APA Monitor, 15*(1), 7.

Vale, C. D. (1981). Design and implementation of a microcomputer-based adaptive testing system. *Behavior Research Methods and Instrumentation, 13*, 399–406.

Williams, D. V., & Gayeski, D. M. (1983, February). Interactive assessment. *Instructional Innovator*, 21–22.

Wirt, R. D., Seat, P. D., & Broen, W. E., Jr. (1977). *Personality Inventory for Children*. Los Angeles, CA: Western Psychological Services.

III

Moving from Personality Assessment to Intervention

Intervention programs for referred children and adolescents should follow logically from the previous steps, assessments, and procedures in the personality assessment process. The three chapters in this section discuss how this logical progression can occur. First, the process of writing the personality assessment report and providing feedback to referral sources and the referred child or adolescent is discussed. Then, in Chapter 16, direct and indirect intervention and change procedures are presented, completing the conceptualization of the problem-solving process. Finally, a pragmatic, therapeutic approach to personality and individual intervention is reviewed, once again emphasizing the multimodal, multimethod process.

The Personality Assessment Report and the Feedback and Planning Conference

Howard M. Knoff

The formal, written report, which describes and interprets assessment procedures and results, and the feedback conference, which plans specific intervention directions, often determine the ultimate success of the personality assessment process. Unless the practitioner can concisely and coherently communicate the critical issues and information relevant to a referred child or adolescent, even the most brilliant assessment style, technique, and analysis will be useless or overshadowed. Ultimately, the psychological report and feedback conference have five goals: (*a*) to answer and discuss the initial referral's questions and concerns; (*b*) to analyze the intrapersonal and interpersonal issues and circumstances which cause, support, or maintain the identified referral behaviors or affects; (*c*) to communicate this analysis clearly and effectively to relevant and/or concerned parties such that (*d*) these parties are motivated and able to work cooperatively on a comprehensive intervention program; and (*e*) to provide an additional component to the lasting and documented history of the referred child. This chapter will review the important research specific to psychological reports and feedback conferences and provide practical suggestions toward their most effective formats and presentations.

The Psychological Report

Given its importance to the assessment process, the psychological report has received relatively little conceptual or empirical attention. Generally, most books devoted to the subject provide an underlying philosophy to psychological report writing, a generic model or approach toward organizing the report, and specific adaptations given individual report emphases (e.g., psychoeducational reports, behavioral reports, consultation reports) (Hollis & Donn, 1979; Huber, 1961; Tallent, 1976). Others, however, have addressed these latter, individually tailored

Howard M. Knoff. Department of Psychological and Social Foundations of Education, School Psychology Program, University of South Florida, Tampa, Florida.

reports along with their unique issues and contents. For example, recent articles analyzing reports for children and adolescents have reflected many different perspectives and orientations: special education (Bagnato, 1980; Isett & Roszkowski, 1979; Ownby, Wallbrown, & Brown, 1982), pediatric psychology (Seagull, 1979), parents (Tidwell & Wetter, 1978), and school psychology (Sattler, 1982; Shellenberger, 1982; Teglasi, 1983; Zins & Barnett, 1983). Of the various types of reports, the personality assessment report is perhaps the most criticized (Isett & Roszkowski, 1979; Shellenberger, 1982), yet the most difficult to effectively write and present.

Goals of the Personality Assessment Report

Goal 1: Answering Referral Questions

Paralleling the five goals in the introduction above, the personality assessment report should answer and discuss the referral questions and concerns which initiated the assessment process. To accomplish this completely, the practitioner needs to (*a*) be clear about the purpose of the assessment, and (*b*) keep the reader of the report in mind (Seagull, 1979).

The purpose of the assessment should be fully clarified during the problem identification stage of the four-stage problem-solving process (problem identification, problem analysis, intervention, and evaluation; see Knoff, Chapter 3 of this volume). While the referral source and characteristics (individual vs. group referral, parents vs. school vs. community agency referral sources, collaborative vs. contested referral) may influence the procedures necessary to delineate the assessment purpose(s), all referring parties ultimately should be satisfied with the practitioner's choice of assessment goals. The practitioner should reach a final consensus with the referring parties prior to the problem analysis stage. This consensus process ensures (*a*) that the practitioner and referral source(s) are perceiving the referral similarly, (*b*) that the practitioner's assessments will be geared to the correct concerns, and (*c*) that the assessment report can explicitly address the assessment purposes both when analyzing the collected data and when recommending specific intervention directions. In the final analysis, the congruence between the agreed-upon assessment goals and their discussion in the assessment report will significantly influence the referral sources' satisfaction with the report and the overall assessment process (Knoff, 1982a).

Sometimes the practitioner needs to adapt the assessment goals after the problem identification stage because the initial referral information was incomplete or biased or has since changed. This frequently occurs with personality assessment referrals when the referral sources perceive only the referred child's behavior as contributing to the referred problem. While this is their perception and should be respected, it may not reflect reality as determined by the objective practitioner. This "reality" will be formulated as the practitioner individually assesses the child *and* evaluates the environments and ecological systems which interact with the referred child and the referred situation during problem analysis.

Within the assessment report, the initial and adapted assessment goals both need to be discussed such that the referring parties are exposed to the broader context of the problem. This is a precarious job, because the referring parties are often "implicated" or included within the problem's ecology, when initially they perceived the referral as completely child-specific. This job is not always successfully accomplished; some referring individuals will *never* accept even tangential responsibility for the designated problem. Nonetheless, when it is successful, it is often because the report (and feedback conference) respectfully (*a*) discusses the referring parties' initial perceptions and the original assessment goals; (*b*) attempts to frame those perceptions into a larger problem context identified by the practitioner (see Knoff, Chapter 16 of this volume; Watzlawick, Weakland, & Fisch, 1974); (*c*) provides the referred child's perspective of the problem situation and environment (a perception that often radically differs from those of the referring individuals); and (*d*) suggests interventions which are motivated by everyone's willingness to resolve the referred and larger problems or behaviors.

This immediate discussion began with the first goal (that the assessment report should answer and discuss the referral concerns) and has included a discussion of the diagnostic problem-solving process, especially the fundamental actions which facilitate change during the intervention stage. This demonstrates the interdependent nature of the complete personality assessment process despite attempts to break it down into mutually exclusive activities and component parts. The second characteristic relevant to this immediate discussion is the importance of a writing style directed and sensitive to various consumers of the report.

The primary consumers of the personality assessment report are those individuals who initiated the referral and agreed upon certain assessment goals. These primary consumers might include the child study team in a school setting, the clinical or agency team in a community-based or hospital/institutional setting, and/or the parents or legal guardians (if the referred individual is younger than 18 or the state's specific age of independence). Even if the parents did not initiate the referral but agreed to the formal assessment process (by signing a consent form as mandated, e.g., in the schools by Public Law 94-142), they should still be considered as primary consumers. This is because they have the ultimate responsibility for and the most enduring relationship with their child interpersonally, legally, and practically.

For the primary consumers, the psychological report must be geared to the specific assessment goals outlined and should review only information that is pertinent and necessary to understand the referred situation/environment/individual and to guide a comprehensive intervention. For example, a report written for a school's child study team about an adolescent who is continually truant should not discuss the father's disappointment with his own vocational and financial situation or the adolescent's sexual fantasies and attitudes toward girls. The practitioner's report should address only that information relevant to the truant behavior and its interaction with the educational process and to the goals entrusted to the child study team's professionals. If the adolescent's parents want to understand the noneducational issues which may be affecting the family's dynamics, the practitioner can write a separate report and/or hold separate feedback conferences.

In the private agency or community mental health center, the boundaries which guide the report are less clear. The adolescent's sexual fantasies may be seen as important to a larger problem that the truant behavior only symbolizes. Here, the psychological report still must be tempered by the assessment goals and the interventions that the agency can realistically provide. Further, if the school and agency are working together (given the parents' written release), the agency report may need to be rewritten to address the school's specific concerns and to protect the parents' and adolescent's rights to confidentiality.

The practitioner must also consider secondary consumers when writing the psychological report. Secondary consumers are agencies or individuals who were not involved in the assessment process, yet who will see the report because they have been asked to provide support services or interventions recommended by the report or the feedback conference. Secondary consumers may also be practitioners or agencies who see the report a number of years after it was written as they, for example, try to understand the history behind a long-standing psychological problem. Most psychological assessment reports will be filed in a child's special education file (in school settings) and/or an agency file (in private settings). Legally or ethically, these files should be purged within a specific number of years (set by law or the agency) after contact with the case has ended. However, in the meantime, the reports may be accessible to secondary consumers who improperly use them to create inappropriate biases or prejudices against the child or family. In writing the report, the practitioner can control these abuses by (*a*) designating the report "Confidential—Not to be Reviewed Without a Mental Health Practitioner Present"; (*b*) identifying and writing the report specific to the assessment goals and deleting other irrelevant, confidential data; (*c*) discussing the personality assessment in a state-related (as opposed to trait-related) context emphasizing individual assessment results as applicable only to a certain time, environment, and ecology; and (*d*) ensuring that reports are released only with the parents' or child's (if over 18) written permission.

All of these report writing suggestions and safeguards are provided to protect the confidentiality and future well-being of the referred child or adolescent. As noted throughout this book, there are many variables and interactions which cause, support, or maintain atypical behavior—some in the child's immediate "control," and others beyond that control. These circumstances can change, and the referred child can cease to become a referral concern. The practitioner must write the assessment report assuming a successful resolution of the referral concern and a "closing" of the case's files. The psychological report must protect at all costs the referred individual.

Goal 2: The Report's Contents

The personality assessment report goes far beyond a discussion of the initial referral concerns; it provides an in-depth analysis of the intrapersonal and interpersonal issues and circumstances which cause, support, or maintain the identified and related referral behaviors and/or affects. While there is no style, content, or format that has been empirically identified as "the best" approach to report writing, the literature in this area can be summarized to create a composite or prototypical report (see Sattler, 1982; Shellenberger, 1982; Tallent, 1976; Teglasi, 1983).

Report Heading. As noted above, the top of any psychological report should bear a conspicuous heading: "Confidential—Not to be Reviewed Without a Mental Health Practitioner Present." Below that, generally in block or outline form, are the identifying data on the referred child. This may include the child's name, birthdate, chronological age, address, phone number, parents, school, grade, and some assessment-related data such as date(s) of testing, date of report, and the examiner(s), his or her degree, title, and certification/licensure status. Other important information might include the dates of previous evaluations (especially if done in the same agency or school district) and the presence of any cultural, handicapping, or medical conditions (e.g., English as a second language, hearing impaired, Down's syndrome involved).

Tests Administered/Assessment Procedures. Here, the practitioner should list the tests administered during formal assessment with the referred child, behavior rating scales or other information sources (e.g., checklists, adaptive behavior scales) completed with someone other than the referred child, and relevant conferences, interviews, or reviews of past records (including psychological interviews with child, parents, and/or family). The names of all formal assessment tools should be written out in full with abbreviations in parentheses and any copyright dates, forms, or special scoring systems used. For example, a Rorschach evaluation could be listed as "Rorschach (Exner Comprehensive Scoring System)."

Reason for Referral. This section documents the initial reasons that triggered the referral to the practitioner or agency, and the assessment goals identified during the problem identification stage. If, for example, the child's parents and another referral source disagree on some of the referral reasons, this could be discussed in this section and the different concerns outlined separately.

Background Information. After the practitioner has thoroughly reviewed all the background data (previous assessments, reports, observations, clinical and conference notes, psychological, educational, medical, developmental, and social histories and impressions) and completed the necessary interviews or conferences (e.g., with the agency or child study team, parents, child, and family, and specialized professionals—doctors, teachers, therapists), he or she must clearly and concisely integrate this material into the report. Governed by the assessment goals and the report's consumers, the practitioner includes only that information relevant to an understanding of the referral behaviors, environments, and/or ecology, and to a generation of intervention recommendations and plans. Thus, there is no standard length or format of the Background Information section. It should be as long or as short as is necessary to provide a context to the referral, the assessments chosen, and the comprehensive analyses and conclusions. This context may include previous disagreements about the child's behaviors, therapeutic progress, or treatment plans, as well as descriptions of the child's strengths and weaknesses. Finally, a good Background section can summarize pertinent information, thereby making an extensive review at the feedback conference less necessary, and it can be used later to set the tone of the report, providing an introduction for comparison or clarification.

Assessment Observations. During the personality assessment process, the practitioner generally can observe the referred child in three separate ways: in a common or typical environment known to the child, using formal behavior observation techniques (e.g., at home or in the classroom); during the individual assessment process where the practitioner and child are engaged in a one-on-one interaction; and/or during other assessment procedures where the practitioner–child interactions are more unplanned and open-ended (e.g., individual or family interviews, play interviews, informal conversations). Regardless of the format, all observations are samples of specific behavioral reactions and interactions at specific points in time. The practitioner must look for a generalized picture of the child's behavior based on a cross section of all observations and reports of observations. Deviant or atypical behavior should be noted if it is consistently present across many or all observed environments and situations, or if it recurs predictably in one type of environment or situation.

Previous chapters have comprehensively discussed naturalistic, *in situ*, contrived, and uncontrived observation formats and analyses (see the following chapters in this volume: Garbarino & Kapadia, Chapter 13; Ivey & Nuttall, Chapter

4; Keller, Chapter 11). Observations during individual assessment sessions will be described here.

As with any observation format, the amount of accurate, diagnostic information will be dependent on the practitioner's training, skill, and experience. The individual one-on-one assessment session does not lend itself to structured frequency or time-sampling approaches; securing the child's responses to the chosen test or techniques (e.g., an IQ test, an Incomplete Sentence Blank) is the primary goal. Observational data, then, often are based on significant events or behaviors that occur during testing which are recalled by the practitioner either through clinical notes taken during the session or by memory or impression after the session. The observed behaviors and recollections eventually become diagnostic hypotheses which are compared with referral information, data from other observation formats, and other hypotheses to form a broader picture of the referred child.

To date, there is no empirically sound observational system available for completion by the practitioner during or immediately after the individual assessment session; nor are there procedures to control the potential bias when data (observed or recalled) are generalized into diagnostic hypotheses (Fogel & Nelson, 1983). Thus, the following recommendations are suggested: practitioners (*a*) should recognize that individual assessment observations are based on a relatively narrow, artificial situation and may not represent the child's behavior in "real-life" situations; (*b*) should emphasize observed and documented behavior over recollections or inferences; (*c*) should utilize observers behind one-way mirrors (if available) and determine interrater reliabilities for observations and interpretations; (*d*) should receive supervision in this area when their training, skill, or experience is limited; and (*e*) should evaluate all data within the context of the entire situation or environment by considering consistencies across the entire assessment process, discounting inconsistencies that may be situation-specific and "chance fluctuations."

During the individual assessment session(s), the practitioner can complete four broad categories of observations: descriptive, interpersonal, situational, and intrapersonal. Descriptive observations focus on the referred child's physical or developmental characteristics (appearance, speech quality and vocabulary level, overt nervousness or physical reactions). Interpersonal observations involve the child's behaviors and attitudes toward the practitioner (spontaneous conversation, cooperation, overt anger, level of acceptance and trust). Situational observations analyze the child's attitudes and reactions to the test situation based primarily on the test materials and demands (work style and tempo, reaction to materials, reaction to failure or praise). Finally, intrapersonal observations evaluate the referred child's observed attitude toward him- or herself (self-deprecating statements, self-confidence and poise). Naturally, these categories overlap and are interdependent. Nonetheless, they represent one way to systematically organize assessment observations more meaningfully. These categories are expanded in Table 15-1 which provides a quantitative approach toward observation and diagnostic inference (adapted from Sattler, 1982).

When the Assessment Observations section is written in the personality assessment report, the practitioner must specify the number of observations; who, where, and under what conditions the observations were made; and their relationships to the referral problem or situation (Teglasi, 1983). Only reliable observations should be included in the report, and these observations should be neces-

Table 15-1
Descriptive, Interpersonal, Situational, and Intrapersonal Observations to Assess during Individual Assessment[a]

NAME: _____ BIRTHDATE: _____

GRADE: _____ CHRONOLOGICAL AGE: _____

SCHOOL: _____

DATE(S) OF TESTING: _____

DATE OF REPORT: _____

EXAMINER: _____

TEST(S) ADMINISTERED: _____

Instructions: Place an "X" on the appropriate line for each scale.

I. Descriptive Observations

  A. Behavior or Physical Reactions during Test Session or Performance

    1. Well-groomed   — — — — — — —   Disheveled

    2. Age-appropriate Dress   — — — — — — —   Inappropriate-aged Dress

  B. Behavior or Physical Reactions during Test Session or Performance

    1. Normal Activity Level   — — — — — — —   Hyperactive

    2. Appropriate Affects   — — — — — — —   Depressed/Excitable

    3. Initiates Activity   — — — — — — —   Waits to Be Told

    4. Relaxed   — — — — — — —   Overtly Anxious

  C. Speech and Language

    1. Age-appropriate Language Expression   — — — — — — —   Inappropriate-aged Language Expression

    2. Age-appropriate Articulation   — — — — — — —   Inappropriate-aged Articulation

    3. Age-appropriate Inflection   — — — — — — —   Inappropriate-aged Inflection

    4. Age-appropriate Language Quality   — — — — — — —   Inappropriate-aged Quality

    5. Quiet Volume   — — — — — — —   Loud Volume

    6. Spontaneous Conversation   — — — — — — —   Speaks Only When Spoken To

    7. Reality-Oriented Language   — — — — — — —   Bizarre Language

II. Interpersonal Observations

  A. Attitude toward Examiner

    1. Cooperative   — — — — — — —   Uncooperative

    2. Passive   — — — — — — —   Aggressive

    3. Friendly   — — — — — — —   Unfriendly

    4. Trusting   — — — — — — —   Untrusting

  B. Reaction to Examiner Style/Comments

    1. Comfortable in Examiner's Company   — — — — — — —   Ill at Ease

    2. Needs Little Praise and Encouragement   — — — — — — —   Needs Constant Praise and Encouragement

    3. Accepts Praise Gracefully   — — — — — — —   Accepts Praise Awkwardly

    4. Works Harder after Praise   — — — — — — —   Decreases Efforts after Praise

(*continued*)

Table 15-1
Continued

---

    5. Responds Directly to Examiner — — — — — — Responds Vaguely to Examiner

    6. Responds Quickly to Examiner — — — — — — Responds Only after Urged

III. Situational, Test-Related Observations

  A. Reaction to Test Situation

    1. Absorbed by Tasks — — — — — — Easily Distracted

    2. Persists until Finished — — — — — — Gives Up Easily

    3. Not Aware of Failure — — — — — — Aware of Success/Failure

    4. Works Harder after Success/ — — — — — — Gives Up Easily after Success/
       Failure   Failure

    5. Does Not Accept Failure Easily — — — — — — Accepts Failure Easily

  B. Problem-Solving Behavior/Work Style

    1. Fast — — — — — — Slow

    2. Deliberate — — — — — — Impulsive

    3. Thinks Verbally — — — — — — Thinks Silently

    4. Coordinated — — — — — — Clumsy

    5. Careful — — — — — — Careless

    6. Motivated — — — — — — Not Motivated

    7. Persistent — — — — — — Gives Up Easily or
                                                       Perseverates

    8. Eager to Continue — — — — — — Avoids New Tasks

    9. Challenged by Hard Tasks — — — — — — Prefers Only Easy Tasks

IV. Intrapersonal Observations

  A. Attitude toward Self

    1. Confident — — — — — — Shy, Reserved, Not Confident

    2. Realistic — — — — — — Unrealistic (either over- or
                                                   underrealistic)

    3. Self-Assured about Abilities — — — — — — Unsure of Abilities

    4. Accepts Abilities and Dis- — — — — — — Critical of Abilities and
       abilities   Disabilities

    5. Able to Reinforce/Encourage — — — — — — Self-Deprecating
       Him-/Herself

"Adapted from Sattler (1982) and the Stanford-Binet Intelligence Scale Record Booklet.

sary to a later discussion in the report which crystallizes a major assessment result or conclusion; that is, random or isolated observations should not be reported; the observations reported should relate to the clear, organized analysis and understanding of the child or situation. Finally, the individual assessment observations should provide a statement on the validity of the individual assessment results. When the child's test behaviors or attitudes are inappropriate and interfere with the assessment process, the practitioner should report this, discuss the validity of the present results, and comment on the diagnostic importance of the inappropriate behavior. The practitioner should never be afraid to invalidate a child's assessment results because of poor rapport, motivation, or participation. In fact, it is ethically necessary to do so.

Test Results and Interpretation. This section of the personality assessment report is generally the longest and certainly the most important. Conceptually, the practitioner should review the assessment goals agreed upon with the referring parties in this section as well as assessment goals which surfaced during the interview, observation, and assessment process. Pragmatically, the discussion should describe the child's and ecosystem's strengths and weaknesses along with potential other resources which may be applied during intervention(s). The data, analyses, and discussion should be clear and concise and should contribute directly to an understanding of the referred child and the referral environment and situation.

Most personality or behaviorally oriented referrals will ask related or additional questions which may involve other assessment domains: cognitive or intellectual functioning, academic aptitude and achievement, community and survival skill adaptive behavior and socialization, and vocational aspirations and capabilities. These assessment domains must be integrated into the Test Results and Interpretation section in a logical, organized fashion. Often, this integration involves discussions of domain-specific results and implications (e.g., the referred child's IQ and cognitive style), the referred child's relative strengths and weaknesses within that domain, and results which provide information or clarification of the personality-related referral or issues. A suggested breakdown of this section, integrating personality and other assessment domains, is outlined in Table 15-2.

Within the suggested breakdown for the Test Results and Interpretation section, the practitioner should strategically use test data and descriptions of individual child responses and reactions. The practitioner, however, should avoid a blow-by-blow, test-by-test analysis in lieu of an integrated "case-focused" approach (Tallent, 1976). The practitioner's goal, to convey an understanding and analysis of the referral situation, should not become lost in a technical morass of numbers, norms, and scoring systems. These technical data should be used only to clarify and strengthen the discussion and the reader's understanding. The case-focused approach, therefore, discusses the pertinent assessment results, identified issues, and observed behaviors which support, cause, maintain, or interact with the referred child, situation, or environment. Thus, the Test Results and Interpretation section is best organized by specific case-related issues or analysis conclusions, *not* by the specific assessment procedures or techniques.

Currently, the practitioner must decide which procedures or techniques and which issues or conclusions to discuss and emphasize in the report. As yet, no pervasive decision-making (actuarial) model exists to guide the practitioner's analysis or report writing. The practitioner, however, should focus on data generated through the most reliable and valid assessment procedures and consider data and observations which are seen most consistently across numerous tests or techniques and observational or interview formats (Gresham, 1983; Nay, 1979). Ultimately, the practitioner must use the tests and data which best communicate his or her message; the data should be reported to describe and analyze the referral problem and to accomplish the assessment goals.

The part of the Test Results and Interpretation section that is devoted specifically to personality assessment and the personality or behavioral concerns of the referral can be approached in two ways: an issues approach and/or a perceptions approach. The issues approach clearly defines the specific issues which significantly relate to the referred child or situation, organizing the section's discussion with these issues. These issues may be descriptive (organized by a DSM-III classification with its specific symptoms), interpersonal (organized by specific con-

Table 15-2
Outline of the Test Results and Interpretation Section
of the Personality Assessment Report

I. Cognitive Functioning
   A. Strengths and weaknesses
   B. Relationship to personality or behaviorally based referral problem and identified issues
   C. Assessment of reality testing or coherence of thinking

II. Academic Achievement
   A. Test results vs. Classroom achievement grades
   B. Relationship to personality referral and identified issues

III. Vocational Skills
   A. Strengths and weaknesses
   B. Relationship to personality referral and identified issues

IV. Adaptive and Community Behavior
   A. Strengths and weaknesses
   B. Relationship to personality referral and identified issues

V. Individual Talents
   A. Description and analysis
   B. Relationship to personality referral and identified issues

VI. Personality/Ecosystem Issues
   A. Issues approach (these topics may organize this subsection; as adapted from Tallent, 1976)

Aggressiveness	Goals
Antisocial Tendencies	Hostility
Anxieties	Identity
Attitudes	Intellectual Controls
Aversions	Interests
Awarenesses	Interpersonal Relations and Skills
Background/Socioeconomic Factors	Needs
Cognitive Style/Locus of Control	Outlook and Optimism
Competence and Perceptions of Competence	Perception of Self, Others, Environment
Conflicts	Personal and Social Consequences of
Content of Consciousness	Behavior
Defenses	Psychopathology or DSM-III Classification
Deficits	Rehabilitation Potential, Need, and Prospects
Developmental Factors	Sexual Role, Identity, Behavior, and Desire
Drives	Significant Others (peers, family, adults)
Emotional Controls and Situational Reac-	Social Role, Structure, and Identity
tivity Fixations	Subjective Emotional/Affective States
Flexibility	Symptoms—Physiological and Psychological
Frustrations	Value System and Perspective

   B. Perceptions Approach

Perception of:		
Self	Past	
Peers	Present	
Family	Future	
School	Others	
Community		

---

flicts with significant others), situational (organized by developmental or socio-economic factors), and/or intrapersonal (organized by the individual's needs, drives, perceptions, or behavioral reactions and tendencies). All assessment data and results are integrated into the issue-oriented discussion; there is no need to include data to explain or rationalize an issue's presence unless those data strengthen or clarify the reader's understanding.

The perceptions approach is testimony to the fact that the practitioner often reports the referred child's perceptions of him- or herself and significant others, and not necessarily the reality of these persons or the referral situation. Sometimes the practitioner will find a marked discrepancy between the referred child's perceptions and those of significant others interviewed or observed during data collection. At other times, neither the child's nor significant others' perceptions are congruent with the practitioner's view of the situation or environment. These incongruences are significant, should be documented, and may constitute major issues underlying the referral. Further, successful intervention will be very difficult if all referring parties and significant others cannot understand the child's and each other's perspectives, regardless of their feelings of their accuracy. To this end, the perceptions approach in the psychological report describes the referred child's perceptions of self, peers, family, school, community, past, present, future, and other significant areas. Again, this discussion is based on all the data collection procedures and individual assessments and techniques. The discussion outlines and describes these areas using specific techniques, data, and results only when greater clarity and understanding are needed.

To summarize, the Test Results and Interpretation section is written to describe, analyze, and discuss the significant strengths and weaknesses of the referred child; the characteristics, dynamics, and resources intrapersonally, interpersonally, and situationally within the child, significant others, and the specific ecosystem; and the issues and/or variables which support, cause, maintain, or otherwise interact with the referred child, situation, or environment. This section provides much of the foundation for the recommendations which follow and for the intervention plan discussed during the feedback conference.

Summary and Recommendations. The summary often is the most read section of the psychological report, thus it should be carefully written to emphasize the major aspects of the report. The summary should review the referral concerns and assessment goals which prompted the evaluation and any additional concerns which surfaced during or from parts of the assessment process. The major issues and conclusions discussed in the Test Results and Interpretation section should be reemphasized, especially noting their importance to and clarification of the referral and additional related concerns. No new diagnostic data or impressions are discussed in this section. The summary section is an organized, integrated paragraph or two which encapsulates the entire assessment process and findings.

The recommendations presented in the personality assessment report should be tailored to previous intervention and remedial attempts, the resources and organizational constraints of the intervention settings or environments, and the commitment and ability of the referring parties or significant others to implement them. The practitioner, while collecting background data and impressions, should have identified all previous successful and unsuccessful interventions attempted with the referred child and analyzed the variables and characteristics that made them successful or not. Obviously, the practitioner in the personality assessment report is not going to recommend an intervention that has previously failed unless he or she can demonstrate why it failed, why it will not fail again, and/or how it can be adapted so that it will now succeed.

During the data collection, the practitioner also should have analyzed any possible intervention sites (home, school, community mental health services) to assess the presence of resources (personnel, financial, material, organizational) which will be necessary to the recommended program(s). Recommendations must be specific and realistic. The absence of any necessary resources diminishes the chances that the recommendation will be attempted and erodes confidence in the assessment report and the potential for successful change. This lowered confidence level will also occur when recommendations call for skills that the referred child or significant others do not have, may not be able to learn, or will not learn due to poor commitment and cooperation.

When writing recommendations into the personality assessment report, the practitioner should aim for clarity, specificity, and flexibility. If possible, the recommendations should clearly relate to an issue, dynamic, and situation presented earlier in the report. Recommendations should be specific enough that an intervention program can be developed from the report (or its references) and accurately contain the necessary "therapeutic" components, yet flexible enough to provide those implementing the program room to integrate their own styles and personal approaches (Sattler, 1982; Schellenberger, 1982; Teglasi, 1983).

There are times when it may be advantageous *not* to include recommendations in the personality assessment report until after the feedback conference: when the practitioner is uncomfortable with the commitment of the referred child or significant others or is pessimistic about the potential agreement and cooperation of two separate referring parties (home vs. school); when a comprehensive investigation of previous interventions and ecosystem resources was impossible to accomplish; when the practitioner wants the conference participants to generate ideas with his or her facilitation (as a strategic technique); and when social service or other agencies who have significant (financial and other) control over the final intervention program will be present and have not yet met with the practitioner. In these cases, the practitioner should write a statement in the psychological report noting the reasons for withholding specific recommendations and should still prepare recommendations for discussion at the feedback conference. He or she should write a formal recommendations section after the conference as an addendum to the personality assessment report.

The recommendations section of the report may differ based on where the practitioner is employed and to whom his or her responsibilities are allied. The private or community-based practitioner may provide individual *and* joint recommendations for the community agency, school, and parents, depending on the referral source, those participating during the assessment process, the referred child's age, and where the remedial services are needed or will be delivered from. If, for example, this practitioner is working as an independent evaluator, separate recommendations specific to the home and school or agency participants, respectively, and joint recommendations to be considered by both parties cooperatively may be best—therapeutically, organizationally, and ethically. Similarly, the school practitioner also may provide individual and joint recommendations to home and school individuals, but the school recommendations probably will better reflect the school's resources and organizational dynamics due to the practitioner's "insider" role. Finally, it must be recognized that the school practitioner often is the first to recommend a community-based agency or private practitioner as an intervention component. Thus, at times, the recommendation section may need to be individualized for the private practitioner who will receive the personality assessment report.

When addended recommendations are necessary, both types of practitioners, when they are fully cognizant of the available resources and the personal commitments and abilities of the referring (or participating) parties to change the referral situation or environment, may ultimately write them in one of three ways: (*a*) to reflect the actual intervention programs agreed upon by the conference participants and the specific referral concerns and issues that they will address; (*b*) to reflect the ideal intervention programs necessary for the referral situation, knowing that the conference participants are not psychologically or developmentally ready to provide or commit to these programs or that there are insufficient resources to support these programs; or (*c*) to reflect the agreed-upon intervention programs and how they may be adapted or extended to approximate the ideal intervention programs considered necessary by the practitioner.

To summarize, the report summary reviews the major aspects of the assessment process: the assessment goals, analyses, and conclusions. The recommendations provide individually tailored interventions which are integrated into a comprehensive plan. The recommendations will reflect and be individualized given the practitioner's employment setting (community/agency or school), the referring parties (parents, agency, or school officials), and the age and circumstances of the referred child or adolescent.

Goal 3: The Report's Characteristics

The third goal of the psychological report is to communicate its information clearly and effectively to the relevant and/or concerned parties. Characteristics of good reports, including "pitfalls" to avoid, can be summarized by describing their contents and the practitioner's approach toward interpretation, psychological style and orientation, and communication or writing style. These characteristics will be summarized below (see Sattler, 1982, and Tallent, 1976, for additional commentary); Schellenberger (1982) presents an excellent review of the literature which validates these characteristics and comments.

Initially, the psychological report discusses the specific referral concerns, relating them to the assessment and potential intervention process. In this area, characteristics of a good report include the following:

1. The report clearly identifies the referral's questions and concerns in the Reason for Referral section, discriminates those referral questions which emanated from different referring parties (if present), and responds directly to those concerns by the end of the report. All data and discussion are directly relevant to the referral concerns or additional practitioner concerns identified as a result of the assessment process.

2. The report discusses the most reliable behaviors and conclusions which have been sampled (or described) consistently across the case's interviews, conferences, and observations and across the individual assessments with the referred child. As much as possible, this information should be described behaviorally, and all abstract constructs should be defined with behavioral or clarifying examples.

3. When used, raw data clarify or ensure the understanding of a specific point relative to the analysis or referral concerns. Raw data are not presented indiscriminantly or out of context; it also is not left in the report for the reader's self-interpretation or conclusion.

4. The report describes the unique strengths and weaknesses of the referred child and/or situation such that the individuality of the child and the ecosystem are captured. As much as possible, the child should be viewed in a positive light, and the report written with positive expectations for change (Mason, 1973; Mason & Larimore, 1974).

5. The report does not omit essential information due to a practitioner oversight or bias and does not include minor or irrelevant information or redundancy of information; that is, the presentation is straightforward and objective, and the report is concise.

6. Recommendations are explicit, specific, realistic, implementable, and oriented to curriculum (including social and behavioral) objectives that may be written into the student's individual educational and/or therapeutic plan (Bagnato, 1980). Recommendations are described such that they can be implemented (eventually) without the daily supervision of a mental health practitioner, and are realistic given the resources of the implementing parties.

The practitioner's approach toward data interpretation can sometimes leave the psychological report misleading, inappropriate, or worse—incorrect. Data interpretation, broadly defined, involves the practitioner's choice of appropriate and technically sound assessment procedures and techniques (given the referral and assessment goals), his or her skill in utilizing the collected data effectively, and his or her ability to speculate when necessary beyond the data proper. In this area, characteristics of a good report include the following:

1. Assessment procedures and techniques are presented with a brief description of their administration procedures and the skills, variables, or characteristics that they are purported to evaluate. Special limitations and conditions of the procedures and techniques are discussed if they directly relate to the referral concerns or assessment goals, and rationales or procedures used to overcome these limitations are discussed.

2. The practitioner should responsibly interpret all assessment data, and the psychological report should reflect this through its stylistic and professional tone and format. Interpretations or conclusions are based on the assessment data and on a consistent pattern of behaviors and results taken from the various assessment procedures which adequately sampled significant dimensions and characteristics of the referred child or situation. The practitioner does not overgeneralize from limited data or base his or her interpretations on personal ideas, bias, arbitrariness, or lack of objectivity.

3. Further, the practitioner does not assume a causal relationship between assessment data or results and diagnostic or interpretive characteristics unless there is clear support. Correlational effects do not necessarily indicate causal effects; the practitioner should distinguish these relationships when necessary in the psychological report.

4. When certain conclusions and predictions are necessary or important to the referral and report and it is impossible or unrealistic to collect these data (e.g., can we expect this child to become openly violent again in this situation?), the practitioner should feel free to speculate in the report if he or she is comfortable with that speculation. However, this speculation should occur only to answer specific referral questions or concerns and should be labeled in the report as speculative.

The practitioner's psychological style and theoretical orientation provide the foundation that some feel is mandatory to personality assessment and evaluation (Holzberg, 1968). However, this theoretical orientation sometimes must be tempered during the assessment process and personality assessment report so that a comprehensible interpretation of the data and discussion of the case is available, and so that realistic and pragmatic recommendations and interventions are offered. To that end, the psychological report (*a*) is written for the practical use of the reader, not for the practitioner as a means to "show off" his or her knowledge or theory, to proselytize, or to present an authoritative or dogmatic perspective; (*b*) emphasizes and integrates data and information specifically as they relate to the referred child and/or situation, eschewing a test-by-test analysis or report outline; (*c*) presents information using understandable language, concepts, and examples—thus avoiding discussions that are too theoretical and/or abstract.

Finally, the practitioner's general communication or writing style can influence the effectiveness of the psychological report and the reader's satisfaction with it.

1. Reports should be written in a clear, concise, precise, and straightforward manner. Sentences and sentence structure should be unambiguous and grammatically correct; the reader should understand the report exactly as intended by the practitioner. Further, writing style should be simple and parsimonious, not complex and wordy.

2. Reports use a minimum amount of jargon and technical terminology. When jargon or terminology must be used, they are practically defined and explained, and related to the discussion or conclusion at hand (see Rafoth & Richmond, 1983).

3. Practitioners do not apologize or make excuses for the assessment procedures chosen or the child's assessment results within the report, nor does he or she hedge when the data clearly implicate a certain conclusion or recommendation.

4. Psychological reports are as long as they need to be in order to fully address the referral concerns and the assessment goals. While this may become a personal decision, the practitioner also should gear the report's length (and style) to potential consumers, their perceived motivation and need for detailed information and explanation, and their perceived ability to handle specific amounts of information.

5. Psychological reports are proofread by the practitioner before their distribution to catch style, presentation, and typographical errors.

6. Psychological reports are written, distributed, and discussed in a formal feedback conference in a timely fashion. Reports and data need to have as much relevance as possible so that recommendations and interventions are appropriate, valid, and maximized.

The characteristics and components of a good psychological report, as discussed above in Goals 2 and 3, are exemplified in the psychological reports present in Appendix I of this chapter.

Goal 4: Evaluating the Report

The fourth goal of the psychological report is to motivate referring parties to work cooperatively on a comprehensive intervention program. Obviously, this is the goal of the entire psychological assessment, consultation, and feedback process, and its accomplishment may not be due only to the psychological report or any other single part of the process. Nonetheless, the psychological report should be evaluated, along with other components of the assessment process, to identify its strengths and weaknesses, its ability to motivate and facilitate change, and its needs for adaptation and alteration.

This chapter has used the psychological literature and research to specifically describe the most effective characteristics and components of the psychological report. Research and literature related to evaluating the psychological report can be found in Gilberg and Scholwinski (1983), Hudgins and Schultz (1978), Ownby and Wallbrown (1983), and Shellenberger (1982). Evaluation formats of the psychological report within the entire assessment process are available in Conti and Bardon (1974) and Knoff (1982b).

Because the psychological report's efficacy may not be distinguished from the other assessment item process components, a summative evaluation is indicated. A summative evaluation would occur after the referred child and significant others have implemented an intervention plan and the practitioner is no longer functioning in an "assessment" role. Thus, the practitioner now may be delivering services (counseling, consultation) or may be totally removed from the case. While many evaluative formats are possible and available, only one will be described.

Using the characteristics and components of a good psychological report outlined above, the practitioner can develop an evaluation packet with the following introduction and directions:

> The psychological report describes and analyzes information and assessment results related to a referred child, situation, or environment. In fact, the psychological report may be the most tangible result of the entire assessment and evaluation process. Thus, the effectiveness of the psychological report is critical and should be periodically evaluated.
>
> **Below, different characteristics and components of most psychological reports are outlined. Please evaluate each characteristic/component along the following 5-point scale (circle your evaluation):**
>
> *1.* Characteristic or component's treatment in the psychological report is extremely ineffective; this significantly diminishes the overall utility of the psychological report;
> *2.* Characteristic or component's treatment in the psychological report is ineffective; this diminishes the overall utility of the psychological report;
> *3.* Characteristic or component's treatment in the psychological report is minimally effective; this neither adds nor detracts from the overall utility of the psychological report;
> *4.* Characteristic or component's treatment in the psychological report is effective; this enhances the overall utility of the psychological report;
> *5.* Characteristic or component's treatment in the psychological report is extremely effective; this signficantly enhances the overall utility of the psychological report;
>
> *No Data (ND).* Insufficient data to evaluate this characteristic or component at this time;
>
> *Not Present (NP).* Characteristic or component is absent in the psychological report and cannot be evaluated, *but should have been present in the report.*
>
> **The practitioner then lists the various characteristics and components for an item-by-item evaluation. For example:**
>
> The psychological report describes the referred child using behavioral variables or characteristics .. 1   2   3   4   5   ND   NP
>
> The Test Results and Interpretation section discusses the referred child's significant strengths and weaknesses 1   2   3   4   5   ND   NP

Technical terms and/or jargon in the psychological
report have been minimized or eliminated, and ful-
ly explained where present .... 1 2 3 4 5 ND NP

The psychological report integrates all data and results and does not utilize a test-by-test description
and analysis .... 1 2 3 4 5 ND NP

This evaluation packet can be filled out by all consumers of the psychological report. The evaluation also should ask specific questions which causally relate the
effectiveness of the psychological report with the consumers' success, commitment to, and cooperation with each other and the intervention program.

Goal 5: Protecting the Report

This final goal emphasizes the psychological report's place among other reports and documents which comprise the developmental and chronological, psychological, and/or educational history of the referred child. This history, however, must be controlled by the practitioner so that the confidentiality and privacy
of the referred child, his or her parents, and significant others are maintained.
Further, the practitioner's agency—whether private, public, or governmental—
must have an organized procedure for maintaining confidentiality and privacy in
the storage and disposal of all psychological reports and records (as by The Privacy
Act of 1974).

Confidentiality. While the maintenance of confidentiality between a practitioner and a client in a counseling or therapeutic relationship is unquestioned,
confidentiality during the psychological assessment and report-writing process
is less clear. In this context, the practitioner decides what to include or exclude
from the psychological report based on his or her knowledge of the case and its
intervention direction(s).

Principle 5 (Confidentiality) of the *Ethical Principles of Psychologists* (American Psychological Association, 1981) provides guidelines that the practitioner
should understand and practice. This principle's introduction notes that psychologists are obliged to practice the various principles of confidentiality and should
inform referring parties (*and* referred children if they can comprehend them) of
their right to and the practical limitations of confidentiality. Part *d* of this principle states that the psychologist should "take special care to protect" the best interests of minors or other persons who are unable to give voluntary informed consent or unable to understand their confidentiality rights. Again, this demonstrates
the relatively unspecified guidelines available to the practitioner who must rely
on his or her personal ethics and professionalism.

Part *a* of Principle 5 emphasizes that all information obtained during psychological data collection or assessment (including written) is discussed or dissem-
inated only with individuals "clearly concerned with the case." This section continues, "Written and oral reports present only data germane to the purposes of
the evaluation and every effort is made to avoid undue invasion of privacy." Thus,
the practitioner must weigh the documentation of assessment data and interpretation versus the potential breech of confidentiality and invasion of privacy at all
times. (If a breech or invasion does occur, the parents/guardians of the referred
child have certain privacy and due process rights—see below.)

Finally, Part *c* of Principle 5 reinforces the practitioner's responsibility for
maintaining the confidentiality of reports and records, including their storage and

disposal. As noted above, psychological reports are confidential and are available only to those who are or may be directly involved with a case. Only on rare occasions will the practitioner release the psychological report to another (professional) without the expressed, written permission of the parent or guardian. Principle 5 defines these exceptions as "those unusual circumstances in which not to do so would result in clear danger to the person or others." Characteristics of a written release include the date of the request, the anticipated date of the report's release, who will release and who will receive the released information, exactly what material/documents will be released, the reason for the release, a statement informing the parent/guardian of his or her right to refuse the release process, a statement noting that the signed permission will be restricted to only this one release and report recipient, and a statement outlining how the information recipient will secure the confidentiality and privacy of the released reports or data.

To summarize, Hollis and Donn (1979) provide some general confidentiality and procedural guidelines for the practitioner as follows:

1. Any information is confidential if release would invade the privacy of the individual.
2. Information is confidential if, in the judgment of the practitioner, its release would be detrimental to the client's reputation or mental health.
3. Information that gives only a partial picture of some aspect of a case should be treated as confidential, or used only with extreme care.
4. Information is confidential if obtained in a therapeutic (as opposed to assessment) relationship by means of clinical, subjective, or projective means. (p. 73)

Privacy Rights. Federal law (The Family Educational Rights and Privacy Act of 1974, PL 93-380; The Privacy Act of 1974, PL 93-579) allows parents/guardians or individuals of legal age to review any official files or documents which directly relate to their children (or themselves). This includes files that contain psychological tests and their reported results. These rights are available so that parents can ensure the privacy of information relating to themselves and their child(ren), and to restrict the random accumulation of information about individuals that may be potentially damaging or misconstrued.

While the right to privacy obviously relates to the discussion of confidential information in the psychological report, it also extends to data-gathering methods by the practitioner (Hollis & Donn, 1979). For example, the practitioner has invaded a client's privacy if he or she has represented an assessment procedure or technique's domain in one way and used it in another (e.g., using the Incomplete Sentence Blank projectively, but telling the child it assesses creativity). Another example might involve completing a parent interview—telling the parents that the information is only for choosing an appropriate intervention—and then using the information for a court-requested report.

One gray area of the law is the definition of an "official file or document." For example, is the practitioner's private and personal file of protocols, analyses, and clinical impressions and notes an "official" file? This question remains unanswered, will likely be resolved through litigation and due process hearings, and will likely become specific to certain individual situations and circumstances.

For the record, The Family Educational Rights and Privacy Act of 1974 talks about educational records, not educational or psychological reports, and states that "'educational records' does not include: . . . records . . . created or maintained by a . . . psychologist . . . acting in his or her professional . . . capacity, or assisting in that capacity." The vagueness of this statement explains why this is such a gray area of the law.

If we assume a psychological report may be included in a child's educational records (e.g., through an evaluation based on PL 94-142—The Education of All Handicapped Children's Act of 1975), a parent/guardian would have access and the potential power to change that report. Both the Privacy Act and PL 94-142 permit parents to request an amendment of any information contained in the educational records which they feel is inaccurate, misleading, or which violates their privacy. The educational agency or institution could immediately comply with this request or could deny the request and force the parents to a due process hearing for resolution.

The fifth goal of the psychological report emphasizes the report's place within the documented history of a referred child. Issues of the confidentiality and privacy of the psychological report have been presented. The reader should note that the application of these regulations includes the rights of adolescents of legal age to act on their own behalves. Usually state law will specify this legal age. The reader should be aware of other state laws or regulations which affect the psychological report and the confidentiality and privacy rights of referred children, their parents or guardians, and significant others.

Conferencing and the Personality Assessment Process

The personality assessment process is not a series of isolated contacts between the practitioner and a referred child, his or her parents, or another referral source. This process entails an integrated, interdependent series of contacts and procedures which are organized, premeditated, and goal oriented. Throughout the process, the practitioner must utilize sound observation, interview, consultation, and conferencing procedures. Underlying these procedures are a number of common skills which often are identified as the predominant skills of a competent psychologist or mental health professional; for example, genuineness, listening skills, empathy, the ability to paraphrase, confront, and reflect feelings and thoughts, objectivity, and the ability to encourage and increase communication and collaboration (Benjamin, 1974; Conoley & Conoley, 1982; Losen & Diament, 1978; Sandoval & Davis, 1984).

The conference is an ongoing event which occurs throughout the assessment process, from the origination of the referral to the follow-up conferences which evaluate the success of an implemented intervention program. With most personality or behaviorally oriented referrals, there will be four major conferences: the preassessment, feedback/planning, referred child, and follow-up conferences. Depending on the practitioner's workplace (agency vs. school), his or her style, and the complexity or issues within the referral situation, however, a larger number of smaller conferences may be necessary to accomplish the goals of these four major conferences.

The Preassessment Conference

The preassessment conference generally occurs before the practitioner has formally assessed a referred child, and should involve those individuals that have direct relevance to the referral and the entire assessment process (e.g., parents, teachers, therapists, other specialists, administrators, community or agency representatives). Often, only one individual perceives the need to refer a child. Thus, a referral should be discussed at a preassessment conference to validate the need for the referral and the formal assessment process. If an assessment is appropriate, the conference discussion should allow the various participants to describe their perceptions of the referred child and the referral situation, and their goals for the assessment process. Ultimately, as discussed above, a consensus should be reached as to the primary assessment goals and the assessment responsibilities of the various participating professionals and others who may need to be included (Knoff, 1982a). This consensus hopefully will maximize all of the participants' understanding of the assessment process and their satisfaction, participation, and commitment to future conferences and intervention plans (Knoff, 1983a).

The Feedback/Planning Conference

The feedback/planning conference occurs after all of the assessments, interviews, and observations have been completed. It generally includes all of the professionals and individuals present at the preassessment conference as well as any additional people who may be concerned about or potentially involved in the intervention program(s). During this conference, the mental health practitioner should assert control over the content and depth of the personality assessment and psychological analysis discussion. The personality assessment process has the potential to uncover many personal, intimate details about the referred child, his or her parents, even his or her teachers or peers. This information may not be relevant to the conference's goals or to many participants at the feedback/planning conference and *should not be discussed.* Again, as in the psychological report, the practitioner must protect the confidentiality and right to privacy of the referred child and significant others. For this reason, a series of small meetings prior to the larger feedback/planning conference may be necessary (Knoff, 1983b). For example, the practitioner might set up a separate meeting with the referred child's parents (and the referred child if possible) to discuss the diagnostic findings and the family- or child-oriented recommendations, and to discuss and prepare them for the larger conference. Then, at the main conference, the practitioner can discuss the general results of the assessment process, the specific educationally and therapeutically related results, and the general intervention directions that are necessary or recommended in the personality assessment report. Naturally, this content will substantially differ when the conference is primarily for school versus institution versus agency personnel.

The small feedback conference with the referred child's parents can significantly facilitate the intervention process and its success (Conti, 1983). This conference can be separated into five parts: conference preparation, initial conference analysis, problem discussion, recommendations and intervention planning, and summary. While the initial part occurs before the actual conference, the latter four parts occur sequentially during the conference.

Conference Preparation. The practitioner generally has a wealth of experience and information with the referred child's parents by the time he or she prepares for the small feedback/planning conference. He or she understands their interpersonal styles, their motivations for the referral (if applicable) and/or participation in the assessment process, their assessment objectives and expectations, and their place in the developmental history of the referred child. In addition, the practitioner should understand the emotional status of the parents—individually, with respect to the referred child, and with respect to the referral situation. He or she uses this experience and information to plan the most effective communication style and presentation for the conference and to prepare responses to clarify and respond to the parents' anticipated reactions or concerns. For example, the practitioner might anticipate parental anger, frustration, and resistance based on previous contacts, and should be prepared with responses and conflict resolution procedures (Losen & Diament, 1978).

While preparing for the conference, the practitioner also should analyze the occasion. Often, these feedback conferences initiate a comprehensive, public analysis of the referred child (and parents) and intervention programs which change, if not disrupt, the entire family's life-style and perspective (e.g., a special education placement, institutionalization). Parents are likely to feel anxious about these potentials and about the possibility that they may be blamed for their child's behavior or problems. Further, parents may manifest this anxiety in very different ways: by being passive, aggressive, resistant, sarcastic. Therefore, the practitioner must understand the meaning and potential implications of the conference occasion for its participants and be prepared to react to their emotional reactions and strategies with empathy and his or her own strategic approaches. In this way, the meeting can remain focused on the best interests of the child by ensuring that important issues from the referral situation are addressed.

A third task prior to the conference is to prepare the physical environment or characteristics where the conference will take place. Organizational psychology has consistently demonstrated that environmental factors and their control can influence the success of a conference by influencing communication and interactional processes (Caplow, 1976). These factors include the physical arrangement of the conference room and table, where certain individuals sit during the meeting, where the meeting is held (i.e., at whose "homesite"), how many people participate in the meeting and from which "side" (parents vs. school officials). Depending on the issues relevant to the case, the parents' concerns and styles, and the referred student's best interests, the practitioner must decide where to hold the conference, whom to include (advocates? the school social worker? agency liaisons?), how to arrange the conference room and seating, and how to organize the meeting. All of these factors should be considered prior to the conference, and the practitioner should be able to adapt to unforeseen actions or events. Further, the practitioner should have the conference organized conceptually and procedurally, entering with a written chronological outline. This is especially appropriate for the small parent feedback conference where the practitioner will provide the majority of the factual presentation.

Finally, the practitioner must be aware of him- or herself and his or her role, expectations, and goals for the parent conference. The practitioner should analyze his or her biases in the case, his or her personal attitudes toward the case and conference participants, and his or her personal styles and reactions when angered, frustrated, or confused about the case or conference. With this analysis and self-insight, the practitioner hopefully will maintain his or her professionalism and objectivity during the conference, will demonstrate honesty and empathy, and will be able to resolve any major or minor conflicts or questions all in the best interests of the referred child, parents, and the referral situation.

Initial Conference Analysis. As noted above, after the conference preparation, the remaining four conference components actually occur during the conference. During the initial conference analysis, the practitioner tries to identify and uncover any hidden agenda or feelings that the parents may enter with or experience early on in the meeting. Initially, the practitioner reintroduces him- or herself and others who may be present, reviews the referral concerns and assessment goals, presents a prospective outline of the conference, and asks the parents for their impressions of this introduction and direction (Rockowitz & Davidson, 1979). Then the practitioner takes the first step toward identifying and defusing any hidden agenda or feelings: He or she asks the parents for their observations of the referred child during the assessment process and if they have any concerns at all about the entire process that they would like addressed during the conference. Often, parents with a hidden agenda have it uppermost in their minds, plan to disclose it sometime during the meeting, are emotionally primed in a specific direction (e.g., anger, helplessness), and are oriented toward a specific goal (an apology, making the practitioner feel uncomfortable, revenge). The practitioner's invitation often is too good to pass up; the parents disclose their agenda and/or feelings in no uncertain terms. At this point, and throughout the initial conference analysis, the practitioner focuses on listening to the parents, but also observing their affect, body language, and vocabulary or emotional intonation. In this way, the practitioner validates the parents' agenda, assesses its seriousness, and plans for the best strategic response.

The early disclosure and resolution of the parental agenda or negative feelings have several advantages: (*a*) The practitioner maintains control of the meeting, yet appears to give control to the parents (a significant issue with many parents in this situation); (*b*) the practitioner identifies significant issues early in the conference before the parents become disruptive through aggressive or passive-aggressive comments or behaviors; (*c*) the parents can vent their anger and realize that the practitioner really wants to listen to and help them; (*d*) the parents can resolve their agenda early in the conference, thus leaving the rest of the conference to really listen to the assessment results and proposed interventions. Naturally, not all parents will enter the feedback/planning conference with a hidden agenda or hidden feelings, nor will this strategy uncover and resolve all hidden agendas. Nonetheless, the practitioner can be aware of their possible presence early in the conference by using this technique early in the initial analysis.

Problem Discussion. This part of the conference is for the formal presentation of the assessment results and a discussion of their implications. This presentation can follow the exact organization and format of the psychological report (see above), providing an integrated identification of the specific issues relevant to the referred child and situation and a description of the referred child's various perceptions (e.g., of self, family, school, peers). Throughout the presentation, the practitioner should emphasize that these perceptions and issues are from the child's perspective—they may not reflect reality as the parents know it, but they are important for the parents to understand (Conti, 1983; see Knoff, Chapter 16 of this volume). This emphasis helps to counteract parents' defensiveness, their rejection of assessment results, and their resistance to any recommendations. A discussion of the assessment results' implications allows the parents to react to the presentation and the practitioner to clarify confusing or misinterpreted points.

Recommendations and Intervention Planning. During this part of the conference, the practitioner presents his or her family- or child-oriented recommendations one by one, allowing time after each recommendation for parental reaction. These family-oriented recommendations are discussed in detail as they will only be mentioned briefly (if at all) at the large feedback/planning conference involving all the relevant home, school, and agency participants. Hopefully, the practitioner can successfully "frame" the recommendations in such a way that the parents accept and will implement them (Conti, 1975; Watzlawick *et al.*, 1974). Later in this part of the conference, the practitioner can brief the parents on his or her school, agency, or community-related recommendations and prepare them for the content and process of the larger conference to come.

Summary. During the conference summary, the practitioner briefly reviews the major concerns that initiated the referral, the primary assessment findings, and the specific recommendations and intervention directions. Again, the parents should be asked for their reactions and comments and whether specific issues or concerns have been ignored or overlooked. In this way, the practitioner minimizes any negative (and potentially lasting) feelings that the parents may have from the conference which may affect their behavior/attitudes toward the larger conference or their later commitment to the stated recommendations. Lastly, the practitioner should set a date for the next conference with the parents or discuss and plan for future contacts.

While the characteristics and organization of the small feedback/planning conference with the referred child's parents have been discussed in detail, the same five parts and general considerations are applicable to the larger (or any) conference. Processwise, the larger conference may be more complex and may require more organization and leadership from the chairperson—there are more people in attendance, more varieties of viewpoints, more potential hidden agenda, and more communication patterns to monitor. Nonetheless, the approach, preparation, theory, and practice behind the parent and larger feedback/planning conference are similar (Losen & Diament, 1978).

The Referred Child Conference

At some point after the assessment process and near the feedback/planning conference time, the practitioner should sit down individually with the referred child. Too often, the referred child is the focus of all the assessments and concerns, but is virtually ignored during feedback and planning—he or she becomes an "object" to probe and manipulate rather than a critical, participating partner throughout the assessment and intervention processes. Indeed, the child often holds the ultimate power over an intervention's success: He or she can be resistant, rejecting, mildly cooperative, or well committed to the program and its components. The referred child is often lonely, scared, and isolated during this entire process. Feeling powerless, the child perceives little or no involvement in his or her future. By meeting individually with the child, the practitioner validates the child as an involved partner in the process and provides general assessment feedback, an overview of likely recommendations and changes, and an opportunity to talk about this information and their implications. Often, this conference uncovers some of the child's incorrect perceptions (e.g., my parents are going to send me away, I'm retarded, I'm the one that caused all this trouble and I'm going to be punished) and permits their discussion and correction. If necessary, this conference can be extended to include the child's parents for greater clarification and family relations building. Unfortunately, the practitioner–child conference is the most forgotten in the entire assessment/feedback process. It may be the most important.

The Follow-Up Conference

Once the participants in the feedback/planning conference have agreed on an intervention program, they should next decide how and when to evaluate its effectiveness (see Knoff, Chapter 18 of this volume). Periodically, the intervention team (those conference participants and relevant others who actually implement the intervention) should meet to review the progress of the referred child, the resolution of the referral issues and concerns, and the relationship between the intervention program and these changes. Follow-up conferences should be planned regularly, regardless of the apparent success of the interventions. Obviously, it can be convened before its officially scheduled time if a crisis or pressing need is evident. Overall, in the follow-up conference, the participants (*a*) validate each other's perceptions of the current status of the intervention program; (*b*) analyze the components of the program that are most successful (unsuccessful) or most related to the case's progress (stagnation); (*c*) document overt and subtle changes (positive and negative) in the referred child or situation; (*d*) decide what parts of the program to maintain, change, fine tune, or drop; and (*e*) assess the future progress of the case and plan for the systematic decrease of direct services and the increase of preventive safeguards.

Summary

The present chapter has discussed the psychological and personality assessment report and the various conferences that occur throughout the assessment process which help to structure the report as well as disseminate it. The personality assessment report and the final feedback/planning conference are the most overt results of the entire personality assessment process, and the practitioner must learn to effectively present his or her data, conclusions, and recommendations in both so that the process is considered meaningful and helpful. Supervision and feedback are two effective ways of strengthening one's report writing and conferencing skills. These skills are not necessarily natural or easy; they take training, practice, attention, experience, and hard work.

APPENDIX I: SAMPLE PSYCHOLOGICAL REPORTS INTEGRATING THE PERSONALITY ASSESSMENT PROCESS FOR A REFERRED STUDENT

Below are four psychological reports which describe and integrate the personality assessment process for the respective referred student. These were actual cases (the names have been changed) and the actual reports. The cases briefly are as follows:

Case	Age	Referral Problem
Kelly	10–0	Academic difficulties, emotional reactions to a series of family crises.
Jason	16–10	Extensive history of academic and behavioral problems, diagnosed as attention-deficit disordered with hyperactivity.

| Robert | 13–4 | Received counseling for a number of years, emotional reactions to a series of family losses. |
| Al | 15–3 | Conduct disorder problems in school and at home, close to being suspended from school. |

These reports are presented to demonstrate some characteristics of "good" psychological reports and to exemplify different report styles and organizations. They also demonstrate a progression of report-writing maturity and conceptual skill: Kelly's report was written early in my practitioner experience (1980), Jason's a year later, and Robert's and Al's 2 years later. All of the cases were referred and assessed under the auspices of PL 94-142 and the corresponding State Special Education Law by a child study team. In the first case, I was a District School Psychologist; in the latter cases, I was a private, licensed psychologist working outside of the school district.

PSYCHOLOGICAL REPORT

Name: Kelly *Birthdate:* 9/23
Grade: 5 *Chronological Age:* 10–0
Central Elementary School
Dates of Testing: October 2, 9
Date of Report: October 10

Tests Administered

Classroom Observation
Devereaux Behavior Rating Scale
Wechsler Intelligence Test for Children-Revised (WISC-R)
Bender Visual-Motor Gestalt Test
Kinetic Family Drawing
House–Tree–Person
Incomplete Sentence Blanks
Rorschach
Test for Emotional Development (TED)
Psychological Interview

Referral, Background, and Assessment Observations

Kelly is an attractive, yet self-conscious fifth grader who was referred for evaluation by her mother. Kelly had difficulty passing her academic courses in the fourth grade and is continuing her poorer-than-expected performance in fifth grade. Kelly's family experienced many "life crises" last year with numerous relatives hospitalized, including Kelly's father for a heart attack, and the death of a grandparent. Academic testing was performed to assess Kelly's psychoeducational potential, and personality assessments explored her social–emotional reactions to these life stresses, their relationship to her academic performance, and her current status.

Kelly was initially quiet and hesitant in formal testing sessions and time was spent developing rapport and putting her at ease. She gradually was more spontaneous and was able to talk about her family and herself relatively openly. Personality assessment was very successful with Kelly; she enjoyed the tasks and exhibited little withholding of answers. Kelly has a good sense of humor, but reacted negatively and self-consciously when complimented. Kelly worked capably and with good motivation during psychoeducational testing. She enjoyed many of the tasks and was aware of her successes and weaknesses. Overall, acceptable motivation and rapport were observed during test sessions, and the results appear to validly reflect Kelly's current psychological functioning.

Results

On the Bender Visual–Motor Gestalt Test, a test requiring the reproduction of nine geometric designs, Kelly made two developmental errors (both distortions of angles). Kelly's visual perception and motoric ability, when compared to standardized norms, is appropriate for her age group. Stylistically, Kelly showed some disorganization in planning the designs on the paper; they were out of sequence and a few designs were crowded together. Kelly thought that she "did terrible—messy" and appears somewhat self-critical, however this does not approach rigid perfectionism.

On the WISC-R, Kelly was assigned a Full Scale IQ in the High Average/Average range of intelligence, with a Verbal Scale IQ in the Average range and a Performance Scale IQ in the High Average range. There was a 14-point discrepancy between Kelly's performance and verbal ability, a result which has more educational than diagnostic significance. Overall, Kelly scored at the 84th percentile when compared to same-aged peers.

Kelly's higher performance ability indicates greater comfort and ability in this area. Kelly is more visually oriented, and may prefer nonverbal responses. Kelly showed above-average ability in visual analysis and abstract problem-solving (Block Design), and in anticipating part–whole spatial relationships (Object Assembly). While very competent in this area, she does sometimes need encouragement and consistency in her problem-solving approaches. She does, however, have the capacity to analyze tasks and situations herself and to develop strategies and enact them.

While Kelly's verbal abilities are weaker when compared to her performance skills, they still are average for her chronological age. Kelly demonstrated above-average verbal conceptual thinking and ability in relating things to each other (Similarities). She is aware and able to interact with her environment and possesses a good expressive vocabulary. Kelly shows relative weakness in general information, with a general reluctance to guess at things, and in arithmetic ability where she used her fingers (competently) to count and solve oral word problems. This is somewhat inconsistent with her overall conceptual potential, thus she may require a more visual, concrete approach. Kelly's recall for digit sequences (Digit Span) was below average, showing a need to strengthen her auditory short-term memory or to provide her with techniques to help her processing.

Overall, Kelly has the potential to be an above-average student, to learn and develop competent compensatory and problem-solving strategies, and to experience academic success.

Social–Emotional Status

Personality assessments with Kelly again revealed her above-average intelligence, good creativity, and the potential for appropriate academic achievement. There are indicators of anxiety, especially around issues of homework and interpersonal relationships. Kelly perceives a greater affinity with her father, aunt, and uncle, and manifests some worries about family members' recent hospitalizations.

Self

Kelly has a realistic sense of her abilities and seems comfortable with herself. She is happiest in nonacademic settings, such as riding her aunt's/uncle's horse, but desperately wants a close friend. Kelly can see things positively and shows a desire to compete and win (e.g., when we played *The Game of Life*). She'd rather avoid or deny discussions about her academic record. Kelly has some concerns about her family's health, but these are not overwhelming fears—she wants to be included in the knowledge of life and death situations at home. She appears to have handled her grandfather's death well, because I think she was able to prepare herself. Currently, she appears to identify mostly with her father—this appears to be a long-standing close relationship, but may be accentuated due to his recent heart attack and fears of a reoccurrence.

Peers

Kelly wants a close friend, and this perceived gap is filled through fantasy. Kelly feels lonely and isolated from peers, and this appears real given where she lives. She feels somewhat inferior and inadequate at school (given her poor grades), and this makes her unsure of her social acceptance by peers. She is capable of relating and initiating relationships appropriately, but sometimes tends to withdraw. Her own positive self-concept does not generalize fully into peer interactions.

Family and School

These two systems appear to interact closely for Kelly. She feels intense pressure at home to be successful in school. The pivotal issue appears to be homework. Kelly identifies her mother as most dominant within the family and feels the constant pressure from her to complete homework and perform academically. The result has been a power struggle between mother and daughter, with Kelly withdrawing emotionally and creating psychological barriers. The predominant barriers, a tendency to regress into immature behavior and passive-aggressiveness toward mother, give Kelly control of the situation and counteract her feelings of powerlessness. Another issue here is Kelly's anger with mother about withholding information about family illnesses and hospitalizations.

Kelly's need for more satisfying peer relationships may now be further explained: (1) Here, Kelly can feel good about herself, forget the power struggles at home, and fulfill some of her emotional needs; and (2) Kelly wants a support system in case she loses more relatives, including her father.

Conclusions and Recommendations

Kelly does have the intellectual potential to succeed in school. Her academic performance, however, may be below par because she is using it to assert her own power and self-determination over her mother's academic pressure.

Kelly (and her family) may benefit from counseling to deal specifically with issues of death and potential loss. Individual counseling for Kelly may address her perceptions of family (maternal) pressure to achieve, but this must be coordinated with home. Ultimately, a socialization/counseling group would be appropriate for Kelly to address her needs for peer interactions and acceptance.

Other recommendations will be discussed at the child study team meeting after hearing the other professional reports.

Howard M. Knoff, Ph.D.
School Psychologist

PSYCHOLOGICAL REPORT

Name: Jason
Grade: 11
Central Memorial High School
Dates of Testing: 12/5
Date of Report: 12/15

Birthdate: 1/30
Chronological Age: 16–10

Test Administered

Devereaux Behavior Rating Scale
Wechsler Intelligence Scale for Children-Revised
Rorschach
The Hand Test
Incomplete Sentence Blanks

House–Tree–Person
Kinetic Family Drawing
Minnesota Multiphasic Personality Inventory
Psychological Interview

Referral, Background, and Assessment Observations

Jason has had an extensive history of academic and behavioral difficulties. Last year, his parents enrolled Jason in a private Catholic school because of continuing problems at Central High School. Jason was later seen by a neurologist, who diagnosed him as an attention-deficit disordered child with hyperactivity. His prescribed drug interventions significantly decreased Jason's maladaptive behaviors. Jason and his parents also began to work with a psychiatrist at this time. These sessions were discontinued during this past summer.

Jason's parents desired psychological testing to further clarify Jason's behavioral and personality style. In an interview prior to testing Jason, his father noted that both parents are frustrated with Jason's passivity at home, his lack of enthusiasm and drive, and his relative lack of friends and interpersonal contacts. Jason and his older sister (now attending college) were both adopted (they are not blood relations), and their adoptions were never hidden from them.

Jason was not told about his appointment with me until the previous day. He was somewhat angry at spending a Saturday morning in testing. His school year back at Central High School has been fairly successful so far, and Jason wants to call as little attention to himself as possible. Jason's primary attitudes were, "Why do I need more testing, I'm doing O.K." and "I don't want my teachers involved, they may start perceiving me differently now." Jason's father noted his son's tendency to converse as little as possible. Initially, Jason did talk minimally, but over time he conversed spontaneously and more comfortably. Jason did show appropriate motivation and attention during my assessments, and demonstrated little overt resistance. This evaluation does validly reflect Jason's current intellectual and psychosocial abilities and feelings.

Results

Intellectual Profile

On the Wechsler Intelligence Scale for Children-Revised (WISC-R), Jason, with a chronological age of 16–10, was assigned a Full-Scale IQ of 100 ± 6 with a Verbal scale IQ of 100 and a Performance scale IQ of 100. This places him in the Average classification of intelligence and at the 50th percentile rank of those same-aged peers in the standardization sample.

Jason demonstrated fairly consistent skills across the six verbal subtests. His arithmetic ability was quite good; he quickly answered many of the auditorially given word problems. Jason was also very adept at repeating sequences of numbers both forwards and backwards. There is every indication on this test that Jason has good ability to attend and concentrate on specific memory and academic tasks. Jason demonstrated above-average ability in social comprehension and judgment, the knowledge of societal expectations for good behavior.

Jason's performance subtests were somewhat more scattered, but still within at least average skill levels. Jason scored significantly below his other subtests in the Block Design subtest, a test of abstract, visual-motor skill necessitating good part–whole analysis and visual perception. This was simply a hard test for Jason where he needed more time to complete the designs—one design was completed correctly, but after the permitted time limit. Jason did demonstrate good "stick-to-it-ness" here, and his weakness appears task-specific. He scored significantly high in Picture Arrangement, a test requiring verbal logic, visual discrimination, and anticipation of events.

Overall, Jason has the intellectual potential to achieve academically at an average pace and level. His achievement may be affected by emotionality, motivation, self-concept and self-expectations, his medication, or other environmental influences (teacher attitudes and/or expectations, peer influences, etc.).

Social–Emotional Profile

Clearly, some of Jason's behaviors were relevant to the attention-deficit disorder and the concomitant academic frustration and behavioral impulsivity. Some of Jason's personality style reflects memories and reactions to his premedication behavior. Other parts of his psychological profile reflect other long-standing emotional issues. Some of these issues were undefined by the personality assessment; they may have more meaning to those who have knowledge of Jason's childhood, his reactions to being an adopted child, and the interrelationships among his family.

Jason is feeling a significant amount of frustration and anxiety. Consciously, he will not admit these feelings, nor does he have insight into some of their origins. Jason is repressing—sometimes unsuccessfully—a number of psychological issues. He tries to maintain an excessive self-control, hoping to disregard the issues, but there are too many things/people around him which trigger his emotions. The psychological issues most important/prevalent for Jason are:

1. His adoption and issues around his acceptance/rejection by both his biological and adopted parents;
2. A childhood trauma which significantly influenced his life—perhaps the events surrounding his bicycle accident when he was unconscious for approximately 10 minutes—a trauma which elicits fears of death or concerns about his mind;
3. Concerns about his (in)ability to control himself—this is evident in his sleepwalking and enuresis (until age 9), and in his behavioral outbursts which occur(red) due to both his attention syndrome and his emotional tension;
4. The social and parental results of his medication—not being allowed to get his license or allowed to drink with his friends due to a potential physiological reaction with the medicine;
5. A general fear of being considered different or special, or being singled-out by teacher, or treated specially by peers.

While Jason tries to maintain emotional control, he finds it easiest to withdraw from social and family interactions. Ultimately, however, one of the issues is unchecked and Jason reacts in rebellious, aggressive, and emotional ways. For example, Jason constantly lives with the desire to be tall enough (*like his adoptive father*) to play basketball. Subconsciously, this reminds him that were he a natural son, he would be tall; that he is adopted; and that he was rejected for some reason by his natural parents. His parental rejection just triggers his own negative self-statements, and he eventually projects his anger and frustration outward. The anger is often childish, immature, demanding, unstable, and projected toward authority figures.

Because of his adoption and perceived rejection, Jason has difficulty trusting his current home environment. His affectional needs are disproportionately important; he wants to be assured of his acceptance and love. His needs, however, are unrealistically high and his self-fulfilling prophecy of rejection comes true (in his perception) when his parents can't respond. It is even more difficult because he expects others to understand and "read" his mind and provide him emotional nurturance without his active participation. Later, he can blame others for their "uncaring and unempathetic reactions."

Another dynamic in the family is Jason's relationship with his mother. He perceives her, from his childhood, as overprotective and overdominant. It may be that he was over-indulged (as a reaction to his accident, headaches, and school behavior?) This relationship is particularly important now, as mother is perceived as blocking Jason's move toward independence (symbolized in his driver's license).

Finally, Jason is scared of losing control. He does not feel that he has ever controlled his life, from his adoption, to his accident, to his syndrome and need for medication. His social withdrawal is a defense to maintain control. When he does lose control, he feels guilty and self-defeated. Physically, he feels inferior and impotent. Unfortunately, he may use his antisocial behavior as a way to control others—to make up for his lack of control—or simply as a way to call for help. Regardless, his behavior *is* inappropriate.

Conclusions and Recommendations

Jason has a very complex psychological profile which includes a number of interacting issues. Counseling is a logical recommendation, in fact long-term counseling—individual and family—appears called for. Unfortunately, I do not believe Jason is motivated for counseling, and would reject it in a passive-aggressive way—again, he would not be in control of the decision or the counseling process. Somehow, the counseling idea must be elicited and accepted by Jason. He should know what options are available and be left with the decision where and when. Jason's parents may benefit from counseling support even without Jason.

Academically, Jason seems to be more successful this year. I do not have any specific recommendations at this time. Intellectually he has the potential to be successful; any academic difficulties may indicate a need to check the level of his medication.

Ultimately, Jason may choose to get some support, or he may work things out independently. I hope his conflicts don't become too intense, or if they do, that he heeds their message.

Howard M. Knoff, Ph.D.

PSYCHOLOGICAL REPORT

Name: Robert   *Birthdate:* 1/30
Grade: 6   *Chronological Age:* 13–4
Central High School
Dates of Testing: May 29
Date of Report: June 1

Test Administered

Classroom Observation
Devereaux Behavior Rating Scale
Wechsler Intelligence Scale for Children-Revised (WISC-R)
The Hand Test
Incomplete Sentence Blanks
House–Tree–Person Drawing
Kinetic Family Drawing
Parent and Child Interview

Referral, Background, and Assessment Observations

Robert was referred for an intellectual assessment as part of his 3-year special education review. Social–emotional/personality assessment was requested to clarify some of the significant issues currently in Robert's life/environment in the resource room and counseling support with the school adjustment counselor for the past number of years.

Robert's home situation contains a number of significant stresses: Robert's mother divorced his father when he was approximately 2 years old, remarried him when Robert was about 8, and divorced him again 2 months later. Robert's mother then married another gentleman, who Robert especially liked, who unfortunately died of an infection when Robert was 10. Robert now lives with his mother and half-brother Aaron (aged 3) in a trailer park. Robert's mother worries about his school grades, i.e., whether he'll be retained, but is generally supportive of his counseling and resource room help.

With me, Robert was somewhat tentative and interacted with little eye contact. He was polite, answered my questions quite completely, but admitted he was thinking about not coming for the evaluation. A reasonably good rapport was developed, and Robert appeared to take the tests seriously with appropriate motivation and consideration. This evaluation, therefore, does appear valid and to reflect Robert's current intellectual and social–emotional status.

Results

On the Wechsler Intelligence Scale for Children-Revised (WISC-R), Robert with a chronological age of 13–4 was assigned a Full-Scale IQ of 79 ± 6 with a Verbal scale IQ of 79 and a Performance scale IQ of 82. This places him in the Borderline/Low Average classification of intelligence and at the 8th percentile rank of those same-aged peers in the standardization sample.

Robert's verbal subtests scored fairly consistently in the borderline intellectual range (approximately 4 years below his chronological age). He demonstrated relative strengths in verbal concepts (Similarities) and expressive vocabulary, and relative weaknesses in general academic information and arithmetic. Given the personality testing (below), I feel that Robert's intellectual potential is somewhat higher than revealed here, and that it is depressed due to both emotional reasons and a number of years of poor attention in school due to this emotionality. This is evident in the higher conceptual skills (e.g., Similarities subtest), yet the lower practical day-to-day academic skills.

On the performance subtests, Robert scored fairly consistently in the low average ability range. Robert was relatively strong in the Picture Arrangement subtest (at an age-appropriate level), a test of sequencing picture stories into logical orders. Here, Robert was able to analyze a number of stories and receive bonus points for speed, but as the stories became harder he did not adapt his speed, began to make errors, and did not review his work. This style was also evident in the Block Design subtest where Robert made two consecutive errors (the criterion to stop the test) due to poor analysis and review procedures. I continued the Block Design subtest to test the limits, and Robert correctly reproduced the *next four designs* (including all three 9-block designs)!! If I were allowed to use these test results, Robert's Block Design performance would be age-appropriate, and his Full-Scale IQ 87 ± 6. Thus, Robert's learning/problem-solving seemed to interfere with his WISC-R performance, and may be affecting his academic progress.

Social–Emotional Status

Robert is reacting to and concerned with a number of social and emotional issues. These issues are significantly affecting his attitudes toward himself and his environment and have created a very anxious, depressed child.

Robert has a great need for both affection and security. His affective needs are almost infantile cravings for contact which may relate to significant frustrations during his early childhood. These affective needs are poorly integrated into and dominating his personality. Robert is still (emotionally) very much a child who is dependent on his mother's love and support. His security needs also relate to the family unit—Robert is afraid not only of losing his mother (she was recently hospitalized for emotional reasons), but even for the security of his home (one of his greatest worries is that a truck will run into his trailer home). Both these affective and security needs are out of Robert's control (he could not control his parents' divorces, his stepfather's death), thus he feels helpless in the face of these environmental realities.

These realities have resulted in a number of other social–emotional reactions; Robert tends to withdraw from social interactions with both peers and adults and tends to use fantasy to escape his pressures. Unfortunately, even his fantasy takes on a depressed tone; Robert's person drawing was an old, lonely man who lived in the alleys, was constantly drunk, and had walked the streets for 40 years. Interestingly, Robert enjoys science fiction books.

Robert's self-concept is very low indeed (he noted that sometimes he hates himself). Robert feels lonely, inferior, and socially rejected. He is very sensitive to being slightly overweight, and feels that his peers make fun of and abuse him physically. It was not surprising that school rarely came up during the personality assessment; Robert is dealing with so many other emotional issues that school is (has been) secondary to him. These issues were so strong that I feel they depressed his intellectual evaluation. Clearly, some of these issues need to be resolved before Robert can approach school *and his coming adolescence* in a free, unburdened way.

To summarize, Robert appears to be a depressed child who needs to work through some significant childhood issues. He is psychosexually immature, socially isolated, and has a *very* low self-concept.

Recommendations

Robert needs substantial emotional support. This requires counseling both in the school and through a community agency, and may include both individual and family involvement. Academically, Robert needs continued resource room support. It is not known to what extent Robert's emotionality is depressing his intellectual and academic progress—given counseling support, perhaps this can be addressed in the future. Nonetheless, Robert is missing academic work and exposure; a supportive learning environment is critical to maximize these losses.

Howard M. Knoff, Ph.D.

PSYCHOLOGICAL REPORT

Name: Al   *Birthdate:* 8-11
Grade: 9   *Chronological Age:* 15–3
Central High School
Dates of Testing: 11-13
Date of Report: 11-16

Tests Administered

> Devereaux Behavior Rating Scale
> Wechsler Intelligence Scale for Children-Revised
> Developmental Test of Visual–Motor Integration
> Rorschach
> Incomplete Sentence Blanks
> House–Tree–Person
> Kinetic Family Drawing
> The Hand Test
> Psychological Interview with Child
> Interview with Mother

Referral, Background, and Assessment Observations

Al was referred to investigate his reasons and motivations for not participating in his classes this year and to evaluate some critical behavioral incidents which include bringing liquor to school, a number of detentions, and numerous in-school suspensions which are bringing him close to a suspension. Al entered Central School in the middle of last year and failed his math and science classes for the remainder of the year. A preevaluation conference at Central last year determined that there were no academic reasons for assessments. This year, questions of Al's social–emotional status and whether it is possible for him to function in the regular classroom prompted a formal referral.

An interview with Al's mother revealed that Al had had previous academic difficulties in late elementary school years, and that he went to parochial school in the sixth grade to provide him more structure. While Al didn't like the rigidity of the parochial school, he did do better academically, although he appeared to be an average C student. Al's family moved to Central City because "they were ready for a move." Al's father is self-employed, the move was not financially motivated, and the family discussed the move (in fact, Al was looking forward to the move, according to his mother).

Since the move, Al's mother reports that he has picked up the wrong type of friends, has had trouble with the police, talks about graduating from high school and returning to his first hometown, and has had increasing conflicts with both parents and brothers. Al has increased his requests to sleep over at friends' houses, but on a few occasions he has left the house in anger and stayed out the entire night. Academically, Al's mother feels that he can do the work when he studies, but is unsure of how motivated he is for grades. Last year, he did not appear "visibly" upset about his failures. In fact, he decided not to go to summer school to make these failures up.

An interview with Al revealed that he didn't want to move, and that he does hope to graduate from high school. Many of Al's detentions, according to him, are due to being late for class and fooling around in the hall. This quarter, Al failed four subjects and gym, where he doesn't like to change into gym clothes and forgets them. Al doesn't really know why he failed his subjects last year, and seemed to understand the consequences of bringing liquor into school this year. Socially, Al doesn't see himself in one peer group, but does feel he has friends. Out of school, he does admit to some liquor and drug involvement.

During the formal testing, Al seemed to work to his capacity with appropriate motivation. He understood directions well, took his time in answering questions, and generally reviewed his work. On many of the verbal subtests, Al would repeat the question or problem aloud before answering. This may have been a compensation device when material needed to be accessed from his long-term memory. At times, Al would say that he didn't know answers. This appeared to be an evasive technique—that he didn't want to take the trouble to formulate an answer—and he would usually try when encouraged. Overall, Al did appear to develop an acceptable rapport with me, and thus, these assessments do appear to validly reflect his current intellectual and social/emotional status.

Results

On the Developmental Test of Visual-Motor Integrations, a test requiring the reproduction of geometric designs with paper and pencil, Al correctly drew 22 out of the 24 designs. He demonstrated acceptable visual perceptions, attention to detail, organization, and motor facility. There did not seem to be any visual-motor perceptual problems as assessed by this tool.

On the Wechsler Intelligence Scale for Children-Revised (WISC-R), Al with a chronological age of 15–3 was assigned a Full-Scale IQ of 82 ± 6 with a Verbal scale IQ of 78 and a Performance scale IQ of 90. Al's Full-Scale IQ places him in the Low Average classification of intelligence, and at the 12th percentile rank of those same-aged peers in the standardization sample. There was, however, a significant 12-point difference between the Verbal and Performance scale IQs which may have educational implications. The chances that Al's true IQ falls within the range of scores between 76 and 88 are 95%.

Al's verbal subtests scored consistently in the low average ranges of ability. Al had difficulty recalling general information which is typically learned and memorized in school and had most success with concrete as opposed to abstract material. This was true both given the concreteness vs. abstractness of the questions, as well as with his answers. Overall, the WISC-R's Verbal IQ appears to indicate that Al may have difficulties with some academic classwork. These difficulties become significant given his poor motivation and responsibility for achievement, and his apathy. I do not feel that the Verbal IQ and the significant Verbal/Performance discrepancy reflect Al's more emotional difficulties to a larger extent. The consistency of the verbal subtests points to a more academic/achievement-oriented interpretation.

Al's Performance subtests were also very consistent, scoring in the average to low average ranges. Al appeared to use very capable problem-solving strategies, he took his time, and he reviewed his work. When he did fail the visual-motor tasks in the Performance area, it was because they were above his ability level.

Social/Emotional Status

The personality assessments did indicate a number of significant issues that are affecting Al's social/emotional life and may give some insights into some of his behaviors. Many of these issues revolve around his feelings of powerlessness. Al is currently overreacting to a fairly typical adolescent concern that everyone in his life, except himself, is controlling his every move. This concern seems to have been present for a number of years, however (e.g., Al was placed in parochial school when he was unable to academically achieve and structure himself). At this time, Al is focusing on his "forced" move to Central City. Every bad thing that he does now can be blamed on that; Al is absolving himself of any and all responsibility. Meanwhile, he is fighting this powerlessness in a passive-aggressive manner. His anger is not expressed overtly as much as in a passive way; by not working to his capacity in school, by bringing alcohol to school, troubles with the police, drug involvement. These passive-aggressive behaviors allow Al to control his environment; no one can force him to change them if he doesn't want to.

Al's academic difficulties pose another area of powerlessness. I believe that he *does* need academic support, and I think Al realizes that he doesn't achieve like his peers. But, Al doesn't have control of either the way that he learns or the ways to get the help that he may need. Al's reaction is to not try academically, to passively say that he doesn't know why he failed, and to state that he could achieve if he wanted to. (Incidentally, his decision not to go to summer school was probably a good one; Al most likely escaped another failure experience.)

Much of Al's anger is more actively focused at home. When asked to draw his family doing something together, Al said, "Huh? I don't want to do *that* ." Al is currently rejecting his family as a supportive unit. He rejects his parents as authority figures, expecting them to dominate and control his comings and goings. When too much pressure exists at home, Al either asks to spend nights over at friends or takes control of his life by just leaving without permission.

Many of the family/parental conflicts probably focus on things that Al wants—whether tangible items or privileges. Al has a distinct need to attain goals and privileges that *he* wants. This reflects his significant emotional immaturity and sometimes a lack of understanding and contact with his environment. While he wants these goals, Al either does not know how to appropriately and/or independently attain them, or he does not want to invest the physical and/or psychological energy necessary. Thus, Al expects his environment to give him what he wants.

While he rejects his family as a support system, Al has turned to peers to take up the slack. Unfortunately, this support system is less an interpersonal support system and more of an escape mechanism through near-delinquent acts and drugs. Al is currently using fantasy and drugs to not only escape from his perceived pressures, but again as a way that he can control his life. (He has not yet seen that drugs and peers control his life as much as parents and school.) Adult support systems are also rejected by Al. He appears very suspicious of his environment; he is not willing to enter into another relationship that may require either an emotional investment or another possible loss of control.

Al has no real plans or goals at this time. He is very caught up in the social–emotional issues that he perceives and spends much of his time passively resisting his environment and its demands. He is not currently able to proactively make decisions on how to work with his environment or take responsibility—on a reality level—for changing and moving ahead.

Conclusions and Recommenda.ions

Al does appear to have some significant intellectual/academic weaknesses which are likely to affect his progress in school. While my findings need to be correlated with the academic assessments at the evaluation conference, it appears likely that some change in Al's schedule to include academic support is warranted.

Al also has some significant social–emotional issues which are affecting his perceptions of his environment and his behavior. Individual and family counseling are both recommended. Al needs to deal with his issues of control in the context of the family which he feels is controlling many of his actions/desires. Only after recognizing the reality that the parents need to provide some structure and control and that he is blaming his parents more pervasively for his difficulties can Al begin to deal with his more individual, personal issues.

In school (and in the community), Al must hear the expectations and limitations on his (negative) behavior. This may not currently change his behavior, given his current social–emotional status, but he needs to hear them and get some support to assume his own responsibility over his behavior.

Howard M. Knoff, Ph.D.

References

American Psychological Association. (1981). *Ethical principles of psychologists* (rev. ed.). Washington, DC: Author.

Bagnato, S. J. (1980). The efficacy of diagnostic reports as individualized guides to prescriptive goal planning. *Exceptional Children, 46*, 554–557.

Benjamin, A. (1974). *The helping interview* (2nd ed.). Boston, MA: Houghton-Mifflin.

Caplow, T. (1976). *How to run any organization*. Hinsdale, IL: Dryden Press.

Conoley, J. C., & Conoley, C. W. (1982). *School consultation: A guide to practice and training*. Oxford: Pergamon Press.

Conti, A. P. (1975). Variables related to contacting/not contacting counseling services recommended by school psychologists. *Journal of School Psychology, 13*, 41–50.

Conti, A. P. (1983). Implementing interventions from projective findings: Suggestions for school psychologists. *School Psychology Review, 12*, 435–439.

Conti, A. P., & Bardon, J. I. (1974). A proposal for evaluating the effectiveness of psychologists in the schools. *Psychology in the Schools, 11*, 32–39.

Fogel, L. S., & Nelson, R. O. (1983). The effects of special education labels on teachers' behavioral observations, checklist scores, and grading of academic work. *Journal of School Psychology, 21*, 241–252.

Gilberg, J. A., & Scholwinski, E. (1983). Improving the utility of school psychological reports through evaluation using Stufflebeam's CIPP model. *School Psychology Review, 12*, 346–350.

Gresham, F. (1983). Multitrait-multimethod approach to multifactored assessment: Theoretical rationale and practical applications. *School Psychology Review, 12*, 26–34.

Hollis, J. W., & Donn, P. A. (1979). *Psychological report writing: Theory and practice* (2nd ed.). Muncie, IN: Accelerated Development.

Holzberg, J. D. (1968). Psychological theory and projective techniques. In A. I. Rabin (Ed.), *Projective techniques in personality assessment* (pp. 18–63). New York: Springer.

Huber, J. T. (1961). *Report writing in psychology and psychiatry*. New York: Harper & Row.

Hudgins, A. L., & Schultz, J. L. (1978). On observing: The use of the Carkloff HRD model in writing psychological reports. *Journal of School Psychology, 16*, 56–63.

Isett, R., & Roszkowski, M. (1979). Consumer preferences for psychological report contents in a residential school and center for the mentally retarded. *Psychology in the Schools, 16*, 402–407.

Knoff, H. M. (1982a). Evaluating consultation service-delivery at an independent psychodiagnostic clinic. *Professional Psychology, 13*, 699–705.

Knoff, H. M. (1982b). The independent psychoeducational clinic: Maintaining accountability through program evaluation. *Psychology in the Schools, 19*, 346–353.

Knoff, H. M. (1983a). Investigating disproportionate influence and status in multidisciplinary child study teams. *Exceptional Children, 49*, 367–370.

Knoff, H. M. (1983b). Personality assessment in the schools: Issues and procedures for school psychologists. *School Psychology Review, 12*, 391–398.

Losen, S. M., & Diament, B. (1978). *Parent conferences in the schools*. Boston, MA: Allyn & Bacon.

Mason, E. J. (1973). Teachers' observations and expectations of boys and girls as influenced by biased psychological reports and knowledge of the effects of bias. *Journal of Educational Psychology, 65*, 238–243.

Mason, E. J., & Larimore, D. L. (1974). Effects of biased psychological reports on two types of teachers' ratings. *Journal of School Psychology, 12*, 46–50.

Nay, W. R. (1979). *Multimethod clinical assessment*. New York: Gardner Press.

Ownby, R. L., & Wallbrown, F. H. (1983). Evaluating school psychological reports. Part I: A procedure for systematic feedback. *Psychology in the Schools, 20*, 41–45.

Ownby, R. L., Wallbrown, F. H., & Brown, D. Y. (1982). Special education teachers' perceptions of reports written by school psychologists. *Perceptual and Motor Skills, 55*, 955–961.

Rafoth, M. A., & Richmond, B. O. (1983). Useful terms in psychoeducational reports: A survey of students, teachers, and psychologists. *Psychology in the Schools, 20*, 346–350.

Rockowitz, R. J., & Davidson, P. W. (1979). Discussing diagnostic findings with parents. *Journal of Learning Disabilities, 12*, 11–16.

Sandoval, J., & Davis, J. M. (1984). A school-based mental health consultation curriculum. *Journal of School Psychology, 22*, 31–42.

Sattler, J. M. (1982). *Assessment of children's intelligence and special abilities* (2nd ed.). Boston, MA: Allyn & Bacon.

Seagull, E. A. W. (1979). Writing the report of a psychological assessment of a child. *Journal of Clinical Child Psychology, 8*, 39–42.

Shellenberger, S. (1982). Presentation and interpretation of psychological data in educational settings. In C. R. Reynolds, & T. B. Gutkin (Eds.), *The handbook of school psychology* (pp. 51–81). New York: Wiley.

Tallent, N. (1976). *Psychological report writing*. Englewood Cliffs, NJ: Prentice-Hall.

Teglasi, H. (1983). Report of a psychological assessment in a school setting. *Psychology in the Schools, 20*, 466–479.

Tidwell, R., & Wetter, J. (1978). Parental evaluations of psychoeducational reports: A case study. *Psychology in the Schools, 15*, 209–215.

Watzlawick, P., Weakland, C. E., & Fisch, R. (1974). *Change: Principles of problem formation and problem resolution*. New York: Norton.

Zins, J. E., & Barnett, D. W. (1983). Report writing: Legislative, ethical, and professional challenges. *Journal of School Psychology, 21*, 219–228.

Intervention and the Change Process: Using the Theoretical Assessment Models and Consultation Processes

Howard M. Knoff

Thus far in this book, various authors have focused primarily on the problem identification and problem analysis aspects of the personality assessment process. This process has emphasized (*a*) that effective intervention can only occur when rigorous and individualized problem identification and analysis procedures are completed, and (*b*) that intervention should be related to, indeed directly suggested by, these procedures (see Knoff, Chapter 3 of this volume). This and the next chapter will focus on this problem identification and analysis to intervention transition by reviewing both theoretical and applied intervention perspectives and procedures. More specifically, the theoretical models discussed in Chapters 1 and 3 will be expanded into the intervention domain, while some of the assessment procedures and techniques discussed in Chapters 4–13, which more atheoretically provide practical data and insight into referred children or situations, will be similarly integrated. Finally, this chapter will address *indirect* change processes by applying consultation processes to sociological, systems, and individual change.

Integrating the Theoretical Assessment Models toward Intervention

In Chapter 3 of this volume, Bandura's reciprocal determinism model (1978) was discussed as a conceptual model which integrates behavior, person, and environment characteristics toward a better understanding of child and adolescent personality development. Seven theoretical approaches (the neurobiological, psychoanalytic, humanistic, cognitive-developmental, behavioral, psychoeducational, and ecological approaches) then were described and operationalized to conceptually guide (individually or in combination) the problem analysis process and to assess the different interactions between the reciprocal determinism model's three

Howard M. Knoff. Department of Psychological and Social Foundations of Education, School Psychology Program, University of South Florida, Tampa, Florida.

components. As the problem-solving process moves toward the generation of direct therapeutic intervention strategies and techniques, one additional model must be added: Lazarus's multimodal therapy model (1981).

The Multimodal Model

Lazarus developed multimodal therapy as a comprehensive system which helps to assess individuals' significant distresses and disturbances and to suggest multidimensional treatment directions. Thus, consistent with the philosophy of this book, intervention is inextricably tied to problem identification and analysis procedures. Further, multimodal therapy is founded on the notion that individuals' developmentally atypical or clinically disturbed behavior and personality do *not* have one theoretical or practical explanation or one therapy or treatment approach.

As alluded to in Chapter 3, Lazarus recommends two related practices, systematic eclecticism and technical eclecticism, to mental health practitioners as they attempt to answer the predominant intervention question: "Who or what is best for this particular individual?" Systematic eclecticism suggests that practitioners utilize those theories, assessments, and interventions from the wide assortment available which can be specifically and appropriately applied to referral situations. Indeed, Lazarus states, "A therapist who wishes to be effective with a wide range of problems and different personalities has to be flexible, versatile, and *technically* eclectic" (1981, pp. 4–5). Technical eclectics have the technical knowledge and skill to apply specific strategies to a referred problem even though they may disagree with the theoretical tenets behind the strategies' applications or successes. Lazarus concludes, "Whereas a rigorous scientist cannot afford to be eclectic, an effective therapist will not withhold seemingly helpful techniques, regardless of their point of origin" (1981, p. 5).

Multimodal therapy uses seven interacting modalities or processes to explain the continual development of personality functioning: *B*ehaviors, *A*ffective processes, *S*ensations, *I*mages, *C*ognitions, *I*nterpersonal relationships, and *D*rugs and biological functions. These processes have been combined into an acronym, the BASIC ID, which should remind practitioners that any one or combination of these modalities could be used to explain referred children's primary difficulties and to recommend possible intervention approaches or directions. Naturally, while every modality is present in an individual, each one's impact on personality is unique, unequal, and influenced by the behavioral, personal, and environmental conditions and characteristics of the referred child or adolescent. Thus, the analysis of personality remains individualistic and continues to be tied to ecological and multidimensional variables and events. Below, a brief explanation of each BASIC ID modality is presented.

Behavior

Specific to a personality assessment referral, the behavior modality identifies children's specific inappropriate behaviors and how those behaviors interfere with individual (i.e., child), subsystem (e.g., school or family), or ecological maturation or progress. Naturally, children's behavioral strengths are also analyzed to obtain a more complete sense of their developmental statuses and to identify potential skills and/or resources on which to build intervention programs. All of these behaviors are generally overt and observable, and their frequencies, intensities, and/or durations may be quantified during problem analysis so that a baseline which can later evaluate specific interventions is available. Ultimately, the practitioner needs to decide what to do for specific targeted behaviors; that is, should they be stopped, newly trained, increased, or decreased?

Affective Process

This modality involves children or adolescents' feelings; that is, how does the individual feel? Is he or she happy, sad, angry, altruistic, or what? Further, how do these emotions affect his or her behavior or reactions to certain environments or events? The interactive nature of these modalities is clearly evident in this last question. Generally, none of the modalities will stand alone as the *only* reason for a specific problem; a modality's interaction with other modalities will often best characterize or analyze a referral problem. A child's affective reactions and processes therefore will be most notable for their relationships with and implications for the other modalities in the BASIC ID paradigm.

Sensation

The sensation modality acknowledges a fundamental contrast historically present in psychology between sensation and perception. Sensation is the physiological process (e.g., seeing, hearing, smelling) related to environmental stimulation as opposed to the awareness (i.e., the perception) of that process. Thus, this modality evaluates children's reactions to stimuli which trigger positive and negative sensations. For example, what does he or she like to see or hear, or not like to smell or touch? Do certain behaviors cause feelings of sensory stimulation or certain environments trigger sensations or remembrances of pain or other sensory discomforts? Finally, how do these relate to the referral problem and the other BASIC ID modalities?

Image

The image modality relates to children and adolescents' self-images and their past, present, and future perceptions of themselves. This modality could also relate to self-perceptions of one's physique (e.g., fat, thin, ugly); social, cognitive, or other developmental status; or ethnic, religious, socioeconomic, or family status (e.g., from a broken home, from the "other side of the tracks"). Minimally, this modality is assessed by considering the six different perceptions that children have about themselves. These six "selves" include the following:

1. the person as he or she really is;
2. the person that he or she thinks he or she is;
3. the person that others think he or she is;
4. the person that he or she thinks that others think he or she is;
5. the person that he or she wants to be; and
6. the person that he or she thinks that others want him or her to be.

As with the modalities, any one or combination of these selves could significantly influence a child's image modality. This modality could then be a major determinant of the child's behavioral, person-related, and environmental characteristics and interactions.

Cognition

This modality involves self-beliefs, values, and statements that children and adolescents consciously or subconsciously, overtly or covertly, repeat to themselves which then affect their behavior and attitudes, for example, toward specific people or settings. The rational and irrational self-statements and self-expectations in the rational-emotive therapy approach of Albert Ellis (e.g., "everyone must love and respect me," "I must be kind to all persons"; Ellis & Greiger, 1977) exemplify cognitions which may contribute to children's unhappiness, frustration, or disturbance. Beyond these statements, other important cognitions include children's goals, intellectual interests, and short- and long-term needs.

Interpersonal Relationships

This modality looks at the significant, nonsignificant, and/or potentially significant people in children or adolescents' lives, or, stated another way, the positive, neutral, negative, or nonexistent people who interact directly or indirectly with aspects of children's lives. Implicit in this modality is the interactive nature of children's behaviors, thoughts, and beliefs with the environment. Certainly, from one's biological conception this interactive relationship is a reality of life. Other aspects of interpersonal relationships involve children's expectations of people, things, and events in their environments *and* the expectations of those in the environment for the child. Similarly, how does the child relate to the environment?; that is, is he or she trusting, open, able to freely relate and interact, suspicious, paranoid?

Drugs

This modality involves more than just the drug, medication, or pharmacological involvement of children; it also includes "nutrition, hygiene, exercise, and the panoply of medical diagnoses and interventions that affect personality" (Lazarus, 1981, p. 13). Here, it is important to ascertain children's real or imagined medical concerns; their neurological, biochemical, and physiological statuses (if relevant); and/or their needs for medication or other medically specific interventions (e.g., a wheelchair, a special diet). Again, the relationships between this modality and those in the reciprocal determinism model are apparent. Further, this modality can be a primary factor, all by itself, in those personality and behavioral syndromes that are causally related to physiological or biological states or involvements. Clearly, this modality should be well evaluated or considered during a BASIC ID and/or personality assessment. At the very least, its assessment results could help *to discount* many possible hypotheses or conclusions.

Using the BASIC ID to Guide Comprehensive Personality Assessment

While Lazarus fashioned multimodal therapy as a comprehensive problem identification, analysis, intervention, and evaluation system which can stand alone in its ability to address and resolve multifaceted problems, its full potential as a conceptual model which guides personality assessment and clinical problem solving is not realized without an expansion to include the reciprocal determinism model. This can occur in two ways: (*a*) a categorization of the seven BASIC ID modalities into the behavior, person, and environment components of the reciprocal determinism model; and (*b*) a categorization of each of the seven theoretical problem analysis approaches across the seven BASIC ID modalities.

The BASIC ID and the Reciprocal Determinism Model

Bandura (1978), through his reciprocal determinism model, posits that personality is best explained through the unique, interdependent interactions between one's behavioral, person, and environmental characteristics and experiences. Lazarus (1981), meanwhile, uses the BASIC ID modalities to comprehensively analyze and understand personality. If the reciprocal determinism model were to overlap with the BASIC ID modalities, an even more operationalized and comprehensive model might result. Such a combined model, however, would still have to represent the interactive nature of personality development; that is, the somewhat artificial process of organizing and categorizing components of these models would have to be overcome by flexible, pragmatic use when applied to an actual referred problem.

The behavior component's inclusion in the reciprocal determinism model suggests that children or adolescents' behaviors are related to their personalities and personality developments. Indeed, in some cases, overt behavior and covert or cognitive behavior (e.g., "internalized" self-statements) are the most direct and obvious manifestations of personality and, when observed over time, personality maturation and/or change. Given this perspective, Lazarus's behavior and cognition modalities most logically fit in to operationalize this reciprocal determinism component. Beyond logic, this modality match is conceptually consistent given both Bandura and Lazarus's backgrounds in behavioral theory and practice.

The person component of reciprocal determinism represents the intrapersonal attitudes, beliefs, and characteristics that comprise personality. The modalities specific to this component include the affective processes, sensation, images, and drugs/biological functioning modalities. When fully investigated and analyzed, these modalities facilitate an understanding not only of the person component, but also of its interactions with the other two components of the model. For example, the images modality reveals a child's self-concept and thus reasons why he or she *behaves* self-consciously among peers. Sensation explains a child's reaction to a test when in or near the testing *environment*. Finally, affective processes clarify a child's depressed emotionality and his or her behavioral avoidance of those specific environments that relate to the onset of depression.

The interpersonal relationships modality is most related to the environmental component of the reciprocal determinism model. Here, the interactive nature of the model is especially evident. Clearly, children must interact with those in the environment in order to build relationships which then can influence personality development. As personality further develops, the more mature behavior can then qualitatively affect interpersonal relationships in turn. This modality is the only person-related characteristic to relate dynamically to the environment. This is not to say, however, that other aspects of the environment (e.g., architecture, population density, the presence of crime) do not influence personality development or maturation.

The BASIC ID × Reciprocal Determinism combined model focuses primarily on the personality assessment of referred children, although the environmental component does potentially introduce some ecological considerations into the analysis. As noted in Chapter 3 of this volume, however, the reciprocal determinism model in the context of the problem-solving process can also be differentially operationalized for each of the seven theoretical problem analysis approaches. Thus, another conceptual interaction is possible: the BASIC ID with the theoretical models from the problem analysis process. These combined analyses have the best potential to comprehensively evaluate referred problems *and* to recommend logical and meaningful interventions.

The BASIC ID and the Seven Theoretical
Problem Analysis Approaches

In Chapter 3, the theoretical histories and characteristics of each of the seven problem analysis approaches were presented along with examples of some practical analysis procedures used by each approach. While that discussion will not be repeated, these practical analysis procedures are organized in Table 16-1 into the BASIC ID modalities which they best assess. Practitioners will then have a resource which (*a*) suggests different theoretically based procedures to assess the specific BASIC ID modalities necessary to understand a referred problem and (*b*) organizes a specific theory's analysis procedures across the BASIC ID modalities. Note that some procedures can investigate more than one modality, and that the interactive nature of personality assessment makes any organizational resource like this appear somewhat rigid. In reality, diagnostic flexibility and individualization is always used by the mental health practitioner.

Intervention Possibilities Using the
BASIC ID × Theoretical Approaches Interaction

Now that the various theoretical problem analysis approaches have been organized using Lazarus's BASIC ID modalities, intervention suggestions which consistently follow the analysis procedures can be listed. As noted in Chapter 3, intervention should be based on a probability model; that is, while a great many theoretically and practically based interventions addressing the multifaceted components of a complex referral problem exist, only the high-probability-of-success interventions should be used. These are chosen based on the fact that (*a*) individuals and systems can cope with only a limited number of concurrently implemented interventions at any one time, (*b*) one intervention applied to a strategic point in a system or at a particular point in time may eliminate the need for a host of other interventions, and (*c*) the resources available to actually implement specifically chosen interventions may be limited.

Examples of possible interventions, organized by theoretical approach and BASIC ID modalities, are presented in Table 16-2. Note that an eighth approach, the interactionalist approaches, has been added. As noted in Chapter 1 of this volume, these approaches do have theoretical perspectives of personality development and definite ideas on intervention techniques and strategies. They do not, however, utilize analysis approaches which significanlty differ from the seven approaches outlined above and described in Chapter 3.

Summarizing the Direct Interventions Conceptual Models

This book, especially in Chapters 1, 3, and the present one, has introduced and integrated a number of conceptual models which together guide the personality assessment process. These models will be summarized briefly so that a final integration is available for review.

Table 16-1
Specific Problem Analysis Procedures Organized by the BASIC ID
across the Seven Theoretical Approaches

Approach	BASIC ID modality	Problem analysis procedures
Neurobiological	Behavior:	Behavioral observations in the examining office and in specific other environmental settings; behavior rating scales and reports (including interviews and self-reports) of behavioral symptoms or incidents; behavioral changes and reactions to neurobiological (e.g., physical development and maturation) changes
	Sensation:	Self- or other report of physiological sensations such as aches, pains, dizziness, or tremors, along with when and where they occur and how they seem to go away
	Drugs/Biological functioning:	Comprehensive physiological assessments of growth, neurology, biochemical status, hormonal status, nutrition, hygiene, exercise, allergies, drug involvement; medical and developmental history-taking procedures; other specialized assessment and diagnostic procedures
Psychoanalytic	Behavior:	Behavioral observations or self- and other reports of symptomatic behavior (e.g., obsessive or compulsive behaviors), interviewing
	Affective processes Imagery Cognition Interpersonal relationships:	Projective assessments, psychoanalysis, family history assessment, dream and wish analyses, assessment of psychosexual development and fixations Behavioral observations or self- and other reports, projective assessment, analyses of play and social development, assessment of transference processes in therapeutic environments
Humanistic	Behavior:	Behavioral observations or self- and other reports of unacceptable intrapersonal and interpersonal behavior, interviewing
	Affective processes Imagery Cognition Interpersonal relationships:	Humanistic or supportive counseling/therapy, unconditional positive regard interactions, Q-sort assessment, analyses of wishes or future aspirations, self-concept assessments Behavioral observations or self- and other reports, analyses of play and social interactions/development, assessment of therapy interactions
Cognitive-developmental	Behavior:	Behavioral observations or self- and other reports, developmental scales (primarily norm- or criterion-referenced) assessing current status against developmental expectations, Piagetian behavioral tasks or assessment perspectives looking especially at cognitive development and its effects on other developmental processes, interviewing
	Cognition:	Piagetian tasks that analyze the assimilation and accommodation processes of thinking and interpretation of one's world; assessment using, for example, Kohlberg's "moral dilemmas" to identify one's morals, values, and ethical standings

(continued)

**Table 16-1
(Continued)**

Approach	BASIC ID modality	Problem analysis procedures
	Interpersonal relationships:	Behavioral observations or self- and other reports, analyses of play and social interactions/development with comparisons to normative development at a specific mental or chronological age, use of role play situations to assess children's cognitive understanding of social situations and their resulting interpersonal behavior
	Affective processes Sensation Imagery Cognition Interpersonal relationships	This approach will use any appropriate assessment strategy to develop a normative baseline or set of expectations such that assessed children may be compared to determine their conformity or discrepancy with these expectations. Most assessment here is also based on children's norm- and criterion-referenced levels of intellectual and cognitive status
Behavioral	*Behavior:*	Behavioral observation techniques (see Keller, Chapter 11); behavior rating scale approaches (see Martin, Chapter 10); analyses of children's behavior related to the operant, classical, social learning, and cognitive-behavioral paradigms, interviewing
	Cognition:	Analyses of cognitive behavior, especially through the cognitive-behavioral and rational-emotive paradigms. Assessment of cognitive self-statements, contingencies, reinforcements, and aversive conditions
	Interpersonal relationships:	Similar to assessments of the behavior modality above, with an emphasis on social learning paradigms and techniques; assessments could be in naturalistic, contrived, free-play, or variable-controlled conditions
	Affective processes Sensation Imagery Cognition Interpersonal relationships Drugs/Biological functioning	These may all be behaviorally assessed to the extent that the target behaviors are defined and operationalized in ways that are discrete, reliable to observe, and validly attributed to a specific modality characteristic
Psychoeducational	*Behavior:*	Behavioral observations and behavior rating scale assessments, particularly of school and academic behavior as it relates to acting-out and emotionally disturbed behavior; intellectual and psychoeducational assessment and criterion-referenced and task analyses tied to academic and curricular expectations, interviewing
	Imagery Cognitions	Assessments of self-concept primarily through self-concept scales and self-statements and behavioral manifestations; assessments of cognitive thoughts through *in vivo* statements and social interactions or milieu responses

(continued)

Table 16-1
(Continued)

Approach	BASIC ID modality	Problem analysis procedures
	Interpersonal relationships:	Assessments of social interactions in the environments where they occur; conscious comparisons/analyses of psychoeducational achievement, accomplishments, and desires and their relationships with peer, adult, and significant other interactions
Ecological	*Behavior:*	Analyzed using any appropriate assessment approach, but interpreted in a system's context of the microsystem, exosystem, mesosystem, and macrosystem; behavioral observation of positive, negative, neutral, and nonexistent behavioral interactions, interviewing
	Interpersonal relationships:	Again, analyzed as systems interactions; these interactions include all those relevant and influential to the referred child, even if the referred child is not a direct participant in the interaction; development of ecomaps, use of surveys and observations (see Brassard, Chapter 12, and Garbarino, Chapter 13)
	Affective processes Sensation Imagery Cognition Drugs/Biological functioning	Assessed only to the extent that the referred child interacts with a relevant subsystem individual (e.g., a psychologist or pediatrician) and that the results are applied to an ecosystem understanding and analysis

1. The entire personality assessment process is guided foremost by the problem-solving steps of problem identification, problem analysis, intervention, and evaluation.

2. Within the problem identification step, two major perspectives are used: the developmental perspective and the normative perspective.

3. Within the problem analysis step, three major conceptual models are used and integrated. The reciprocal determinism model analyzes behavioral, person-related, and environmental characteristics of referral problems. Lazarus's BASIC ID modalities also analyze aspects of referral problems focusing primarily on the referred child or adolescent. These modalities, however, fit into the reciprocal determinism model, with the behavior and cognition modalities organized into the behavioral component of the model; the affective processes, sensation, images, and drugs/biological functions modalities organized into the person component; and the interpersonal relationships modality organized into the environmental component.

The last of the three conceptual problem analysis models involves the seven theoretical approaches which lend different perspectives and assessment procedures into this step: the neurobiological, psychoanalytic, humanistic, cognitive-developmental, behavioral, psychoeducational, and ecological approaches. These approaches interact with the BASIC ID modalities—each assessing many of the modalities in theoretically determined ways.

Table 16-2
Specific Intervention Techniques and Strategies Organized by the BASIC ID across the Eight Theoretical Approaches

Approach	BASIC ID modality	Intervention technique
Neurobiological interventions	Behavior:	Physical therapy
		Occupational therapy
		Biofeedback
		Hypnosis
		Drug intervention
		Dietary adaptations
	Sensation:	Hypnosis
		Drug intervention
		Biofeedback
		Physical therapy
	Drugs/Biological functioning:	Drug intervention
		Hypnosis
		Biofeedback
		Specialized physiological/therapeutic treatments
		Dietary adaptations
		Hormonal/biochemical treatment
		Electroconvulsive shock treatment
		Neurosurgery and other surgical operations/techniques
Psychoanalytic interventions	Behavior Affective processes Imagery Cognition Interpersonal relationships	Psychoanalysis Free association Hypnosis Dream analysis Cathartic experiences Insight therapy Transference resolution
Humanistic interventions	Behavior Affective process Images Cognition Interpersonal relationships	Client-centered therapy Self-actualization therapy and/or experiences Insight therapy Self-consistency and congruence activities and experiences Unconditional positive regard experiences
Cognitive-developmental interventions	Behavior:	Social skills and problem-solving training
		Psychoeducational/academic tutoring or special education
		Trial teaching and criterion-referenced teaching
		Mediated learning experiences
		Piagetian-based learning and behavioral curricula
	Cognition:	Values clarification exercises
		Social skills and problem-solving training
	Interpersonal relationships:	Social skills and problem-solving training
		Role playing
		Values clarification exercises
		Play therapy
Behavioral interventions (adapted from Lazarus, 1981)	Behavior:	Behavior rehearsal
		Modeling
		Use of reinforcement paradigms (positive, negative, and aversive)
		Structured learning therapy

(continued)

Table 16-2
(Continued)

Approach	BASIC ID modality	Intervention Technique
	Affect:	Stimulus control techniques
		Classical conditioning/pairing techniques
		Behavioral shaping and chaining
		Anxiety-management training
		Systematic desensitization
	Sensation:	Biofeedback
		Relaxation training
	Imagery:	Positive and negative imagery
		Goal or behavioral rehearsal
	Cognition:	Bibliotherapy
		Ellis' A-B-C-D-E paradigm
		Behavioral problem solving
		Thought-stopping techniques
	Interpersonal relationships:	Social skills and assertiveness training
		Modeling
		Structured learning therapy
		Contingency contracting
		Communications training
	Drugs/Biological functioning:	Behavioral strategies/interventions toward good health habits (nutrition, exercise, anxiety control)
Psychoeducational interventions	Behavior Imagery Cognitions Interpersonal relationships	Psychoeducational/milieu therapy Self-control therapy Modeling Social skills and problem-solving training
Interactionalist interventions	Behavior Interpersonal relationships	Modeling Natural and logical consequences Behavioral contract or plan Encouragement Time-out Reality therapy In-school suspension School or setting removal Behavioral reinforcement
Ecological interventions	Behavior Interpersonal relationships	Use of any relevant interventions suggested above that are strategic, systems oriented, and coordinated to affect a significant reduction in ecosystem stress

4. The intervention step has been separated into direct or child-focused interventions and indirect or consultation-oriented interventions. Direct interventions follow logically from those problem analysis procedures and approaches which are most relevant to the referred problem or child and are organized across the BASIC ID modalities. Thus, the reciprocal determinism model, the BASIC ID modalities, and the theoretical approaches (now including the interactionalist approaches) are all combined for potential use. Indirect interventions involving consultation processes will be discussed below.

5. Finally, evaluation was discussed in terms of process versus product evaluations and formative versus summative evaluations.

As a final note, although presented as one of seven theoretical approaches, the ecological/systems perspective is favored as the predominant, most logical guide to the personality assessment process. This perspective emphasizes that the interdependent systems that include or affect referred children should be targeted for specific and comprehensive evaluation. The goal, therefore, becomes focused on systems analysis and systems change. This allows both *individual* assessments of referred children and *ecological* assessments of influential people, environments, and events in the child's life. This latter assessment sometimes suggests better explanations of the referred problem and more effective intervention directions than the former assessment.

Indirect Intervention Approaches: Consultation Processes

Consultation is a problem-solving interaction between a professional (called the "consultant") and another professional in the same or a different field (called the "consultee") concerning a work-related or professionally oriented problem. In the context of personality assessment, possible consultees could include peer professionals on a school or agency-based child study or mental health team, teachers or child-care workers, or parents. In the case of parents as consultees, it must be clear that they are receiving consultation services and not individual or family counseling or psychotherapy (see below). In most cases, the consultation process is focused on a targeted or referred child (or group of children) who is considered the "client."

Consultation Goals, Philosophy, and a Contrast with Counseling

Consultation follows a problem-solving process that is similar to the personality assessment process; that is, given a specific problem or referral, consultation proceeds from problem identification to problem analysis to intervention to evaluation (Bergan, 1977; Meyers, Parsons, & Martin, 1979). For the purposes of this chapter and book, we shall assume that the multidimensional and multitheoretical problem identification and problem analysis procedures completed as part of a personality assessment are comparable to the same steps when used in a consultation problem-solving process. Thus, we will focus on consultation as an intervention strategy. In context, however, given the procedural philosophy of multisetting, multisource, and multi-instrument assessment and multidimensional intervention (which involves individual therapy for referred children, family therapy, environmental or setting-specific intervention, and organizational or systems intervention where relevant), consultation as an intervention strategy comprises only one part of a comprehensive intervention program. Nonetheless, consultation is a very powerful intervention approach and change process mechanism.

Consultation has two ultimate goals and a number of philosophical tenets. Its first goal is to address problems or children referred by consultees in the most effective manner possible. In achieving this goal, consultation significantly differs from most therapeutic intervention procedures: Consultation occurs as a supportive, problem-solving process for the consultee, often without the consultant's need to directly see or interact with the client (i.e., the referred child). Thus, in consultation, the consultee is wholly responsible for implementing the intervention program for and with the client; the consultant acts as a professional resource and support system. To concretize this with an example, a community mental health practitioner's work with the school staff and parents of a referred child to help them agree on and implement a complementary intervention addressing the child's school phobia demonstrates a consultation intervention. Or, a school psychologist might work as a consultant to the parents of a child to help them decrease the child's resistance toward completing homework.

The second major goal of consultation is to increase consultees' levels of skill, competence, and objectivity such that they are able to intervene with future referred children in more effective ways and with less or no need for consultation services. Thus, consultation as a problem-solving process hopefully "teaches" the consultees how to think about, to evaluate, and to choose appropriate intervention directions such that these skills are generalizable to new and/or different referral problems. In this way, consultation becomes a process which decreases consultees' dependence on other professionals and increases their capacities for independent effectiveness.

The philosophical tenets of the consultation process relate primarily to the relationship between the consultant and the consultee. Obviously, philosophy is often far easier to describe than to implement pragmatically in an imperfect world. Nonetheless, the consultation relationship is a nonhierarchical, peer professional relationship where the consultant has no administrative authority, responsibility, or power over the consultee. The consultant also has no predetermined agenda, theory, or perspective that he or she wishes to impart to the consultee; instead, the consultant tries to work coordinately with the consultee to identify intervention directions or techniques for the troublesome problem(s) of concern. The consultee maintains full responsibility for the referred child and has the right to accept or reject any of the consultant's recommendations and to terminate the consultation relationship at any time (Caplan, 1970). When the consultee is the consultant's mental health practitioner-colleague, the philosophical tenets of consultation appear workable and logical. Further explanation when the consultees are the parents of the referred child, however, is necessary.

Working with parents of referred children presents a significant dilemma for the practitioner, requiring the ability to discriminate between consultation and counseling. Indeed, there is a definite difference between the two. When consulting with parents, the consultant works as a collaborator on child-related problems and there is no focus on parents' emotional reactions to the situation or the change process. The consultant makes tentative suggestions and conclusions because the parents have the ultimate responsibility for making intervention decisions, and the consultant attempts to support the parents' skills, resources, and strengths in making those decisions. When counseling with parents, the mental health practitioner (now not labeled "the consultant") works as an expert on the intra- and interpersonal dynamics of the referred problem with a clear focus on parents' emotional reactions to the situation and the need for behavioral and/or emotional change. The practitioner becomes a facilitator toward change—a process which can involve, consciously or subconsciously, confrontative strategies—because he or she has the responsibility to direct the intervention. Further, the practitioner attempts to weaken parents' resistances so that new perspectives and behaviors can be applied toward problem resolution (Conoley & Conoley, 1982).

When working with parents, the consultant, contrary to the philosophical tenets of consultation, *is* oftentimes an expert. But even as an expert, he or she can stay within the consultation role by not abusing the power often given to an expert and by facilitating parents' own problem solving such that they are able to make intervention decisions. Further, the peer professional characteristic *does* still exist in a consultant–parent relationship, because the parents are, in a sense, expert about their referred child and *their* capacity to help the child or situation to change. Thus, even though a bit harder to conceptualize and coordinate, parents can be consultees in a consultation relationship with a mental health practitioner.

To complete this consultation–counseling comparison, it is critical that the practitioner, prior to conceptualizing the intervention plan (thus, prior to the Feedback Conference—see Chapter 3), consciously decide whether (*a*) to use consultation as part of the plan, and (*b*) to use either consultation or counseling with the referred child's parents as part of the plan. Regardless of which is chosen, the practitioner must sit down with the parents, and perhaps the referred child, to discuss this consultation versus counseling intervention decision with them, the relative characteristics and expectations of the two approaches, parent and child rights and options, and general advantages and disadvantages. Parent consultation and parent counseling in the same intervention plan is not recommended; it would be too confounding, confusing, and contradictory for all involved. Once decided, however, practitioners have an ethical responsibility to tell their consultees how the intervention services will be delivered.

The Types of Consultation and Their Interaction with Prevention

Minimally, there are four types of consultation: client-centered case consultation, consultee-centered case consultation, program-centered administrative consultation, and consultee-centered administrative consultation (Caplan, 1970; Meyers, *et al.*, 1979). While originally categorized as such under the mental health consultation model (see the discussion of consultation models below), these four consultation types suggest a conceptual approach to consultation interactions in general and to consultation-based interventions in particular.

Relative to consultation in general, client-centered case consultation involves problem-solving interactions between the consultant and the consultee which focus on resolving the specific difficulties of the referred child (the client). This type of indirect intervention often occurs when the consultee has attempted numerous intervention strategies with little apparent or lasting change. In an attempt to get another, new perspective on the referred child, the consultee works with the consultant. The consultant, who may observe the client in one or more settings but does not necessarily directly interact with the child (e.g., through interviewing or testing), tries to clarify the consultee's perspectives and perceptions of the problem while facilitating problem solving and an effective direction toward change. Here, it is assumed that indirect intervention through consultation with the consultee, rather than direct "therapy" between a referred client and a mental health practitioner, is the most efficacious intervention approach. For example, there are times when a behavior modification program implemented by the consultee and supervised by the consulting practitioner will be far more effective than a client-centered counseling approach which occurs in the practitioner's office far removed from the problem environment.

The consultee-centered case consultation is similar to the case-centered type in that the initial consultant–consultee interaction is motivated by some difficulty with a target client or group of clients. With this type, however, the consultant during the course of the consultation interactions recognizes either (a) that the "problem" is not truly client-specific but is actually consultee-specific, or (b) that the client problem would be more efficiently handled by intervening with the consultee rather than with the client. For both of these possibilities, the consultee may require consultative support in improving his or her skill, objectivity, knowledge, and/or self-confidence. Thus, the consultee-centered consultation is used to improve the consultee's professional or interpersonal weaknesses or limitations which are hindering the relationship with the client and causing or supporting the referred difficulty.

Program-centered administrative consultation focuses on strengthening and improving the programs where referred clients are placed (e.g., in private or public schools and mental health agencies, respectively) because administrative/organizational improvements, not direct-service/client intervention improvements, are necessary for more effective services. Here, the consultant works with all those consultees who have direct or indirect program responsibility and influence, addressing those administrative and organizational weaknesses or gaps which are detracting, directly or by implication, from program participants' progress or problem resolutions. For example, problems with some referred clients may be due more to lack of support staff (i.e., budgetary constraints) or staff coordination than to specific client-related interventions or therapy programs. Problem-centered administrative consultation, therefore, focuses the intervention process on the staffing needs, thereby hoping to indirectly affect the clients' problems as well.

Consultee-centered administrative consultation is the conceptually broadest of the four consultation types. This consultation interaction analyzes entire organizational systems (e.g., school districts, mental health agencies, governmental services, or communities at large) and their effectiveness in dealing with and preventing mental health-oriented problems. The consultant here helps consultees to focus on referred clients from the most removed, yet most critical consultation position. If consultees cannot conceptualize intervention and the administration of intervention from a planned, proactive, and systemic perspective, then intervention will be forever practiced in a reactive, crisis-oriented, situation-specific manner where client change may occur but never truly be prevented. This discussion alludes to the three major levels of preventive services, a discussion of which occurs after the conceptual summary below.

With use of the problem-solving personality assessment process, appropriately referred problems generally require intervention in one or a combination of the following areas: the areas addressing referred children's individual intrapersonal needs; referred children's interpersonal needs; others' needs, perceptions, and interactions with referred children; administrators' or agency directors' staffing and programming needs for these children; and administrators' or agency directors' comprehensive programming needs in order to prevent future referrals of a similar type. If indirect intervention, as defined by the consultation approach, is one facet of the intervention program, the four types of consultation noted above can individually address specific parts of these intervention areas and needs. For example, client-centered case consultation can address referred children's individual intra- and interpersonal needs, consultee-centered case consultation can address the needs of those who interact with referred children, program-centered administrative consultation can address administrators' or agency directors' needs, and consultee-centered administrative consultation can address the comprehensive, preventive planning which focuses on system needs.

Specific to prevention, there are three major levels of preventive services: tertiary, secondary, and primary. In many ways, this entire book has concentrated on tertiary prevention by describing programs that provide assessment and intervention services to individuals who manifest significant personality or behavioral problems at the time at which they are referred. Tertiary prevention programs and consultation emphasize direct service to the consultee and, as noted above, indirect or direct service to the referred client. Further, each component of the tertiary problem-solving process is directed toward resolving the referred problem only and toward preventing its future occurrence and the need for re-referral. While all four types of consultation could be used during tertiary prevention, the two case-centered consultation types are most commonly used because they deal with consultees' direct-service problems.

A practitioner coordinating a secondary prevention program first identifies a school, agency, or community population that has historically exhibited recurrent social–emotional or behavioral problems, and then develops an intervention program to prevent these problems from occurring in other "at-risk" groups who present the precursor characteristics of the original, identified population. A secondary prevention team, for example, might identify problems within an emotionally disturbed/learning-disabled junior high school population comprised of students who originally were labeled learning disabled, but who later exhibited "emotionally disturbed" behavior to avoid their academic failures and frustrations (Knoff, 1983). In such a program, the practitioner and/or team would assess and intervene with elementary school learning-disabled students who are at risk, given an assessment of previously identified precursor characteristics, for the same type of emotionally disturbed behavior when they reach junior high school. Secondary prevention, therefore, emphasizes direct services to consultees as at-risk groups are identified and assessed and then served by preventive programs, but indirect services to the participating children or adolescents. Thus, consultees, not consultants or mental health practitioners, should publicly direct and implement the preventive intervention program. Secondary prevention programs are truly preventive in nature and all four types of consultation could be used—the two administrative-centered consultation types while conceptualizing the program and its potential impact, and the case-centered types as implementation problems arise and are resolved.

Primary prevention programs generally involve an entire system (e.g., a school district or community) which is grappling with complex, multifaceted problems that require coordinated attention and intervention. Rochester, New York's Primary Prevention Project, for example, coordinates Rochester's community mental health networks, school districts, parents, and the university to address and prevent pervasive mental health and behavioral problems in children. Primary prevention, therefore, does not target a specific at-risk population, but attempts to prevent common mental health difficulties within an entire system's population. This involves direct consultation with consultees targeted from the large systems and organizations of interest; the affected population only indirectly is aware of the consultation process. Primary prevention is the most preventive of the three types, the most proactive, and usually the most cost-effective. As noted above, consultee-centered administrative consultation is its cornerstone, although all four consultation types could be involved (Knoff, 1984a).

The Multimodal Consultation Models

So far in this chapter, the underlying characteristics of consultation have been described along with the four general types of consultation and their relationships with preventive services and interventions. One final piece to this indirect intervention puzzle remains. Analogous to the multiple intervention models specific to direct interventions (see the BASIC ID × theoretical approaches interaction above), there are multiple models of consultation intervention. These seven consultation models are combined conceptually, referred to as the "multimodal consultation" models, and are represented with the acronym PROB^{L}EMAPS: the *P*rocess, *O*rganizational development, *B*ehavioral, *M*ental health, *A*dvocacy, *P*sychoeducational, and *S*trategic consultation models, respectively (Knoff, 1984b). These seven models are described briefly below; those models most relevant to the personality assessment, intervention, and problem-solving process are discussed in the greatest detail.

Process Consultation

Process consultation looks primarily at the effects of (*a*) environmental characteristics and events and (*b*) individuals' interpersonal interactions, especially within groups or group formats, on individual and group effectiveness and productivity. From a personality assessment perspective, the process consultant helps consultees to perceive, understand, and accept or adapt these characteristics' and interactions' impacts on referred individuals by addressing, minimally, the following process components: communication, members' roles and functions in relevant groups (e.g., in a school building or treatment team), group problem solving and decision making, group norms and group growth, leadership and authority issues and dynamics, and intergroup cooperation and competition. Thus, process consultants assume that some children are referred for individual personality assessment when their problems actually are symbolic of poor adult-directed group process. Take, for example, the class filled with discipline problems because the school principal and classroom teacher have difficulty implementing their leadership and authority roles. Surely, the students do not require personality assessment or individual therapy; instead, the process consultant needs to intervene directly with the principal and teacher to change the processes interfering with appropriate student discipline. This change procedure ultimately should indirectly alter what was originally presented as the "target" behavior problem. Process consultation is comprehensively discussed and analyzed by Schein (1969).

Organizational Development (OD) Consultation

OD consultation includes a variety of perspectives and intervention techniques used on the assumption that organizational change can influence group and individual behavior both directly and indirectly. The goals of OD consultation are (*a*) to increase the effectiveness of organizations' abilities to set and accomplish their agenda and goals and (*b*) to increase responsiveness to internal and external changes which affect the organization, both while simultaneously maintaining organization members' personal satisfaction and individual growth. In some ways, OD consultation is similar to process consultation except that organizations are far more complex, comprising multiple, interdependent, and interacting groups. OD consultation differs further in that organizations often are influenced by other organizations in their communities or by ecological macrosystem variables (i.e., community values and ideologies). From a personality intervention perspective, an organizational development consultant working with a district superintendent or mental health center director could identify organizational goals toward primary, secondary, and tertiary mental health directions and could resolve a staff's resistance toward working as an interdisciplinary, cohesive team. Again, the OD consultant assumes that some individual child problems actually represent organizational systems problems, and that changes at an organizational level do affect group processes and individual child behavior. Additional reading in OD consultation is available by Jerrell and Jerrell (1981) and Schmuck, Runkel, Arends, and Arends (1977).

Behavioral Consultation

Behavioral consultation uses the behavioral theories, models, and approaches discussed in Chapters 1 and 3 within the problem identification, problem analysis, intervention, and evaluation problem-solving process to help *consultees* to behaviorally understand and change targeted behavior problems or situations. The primary goals of behavioral consultation are to guide the consultee (*a*) to successfully analyze, intervene, and change targeted client behavior(s), (*b*) to develop skills and strategies which can be generalized to similar, future behavioral problems, (*c*) to use behavioral research and theory in pragmatic, applied ways, and (*d*) to help others to see the value of behavioral paradigms and interventions. Thus, behavioral consultation is generally client-specific rather than group- or organization-specific, and the emphasis is on supporting consultees as they implement the intervention and behavior change strategies with children and adolescents. This consultation model, therefore, is very interested in the development of child-specific interventions within the personality assessment model. Further reading on this model is available from Bergan (1977) and Keller (1981).

Mental Health Consultation

Much of the introduction to this section on consultation processes was descriptive of mental health consultation. In the personality assessment process, mental health consultation focuses primarily on consultee-centered case consultation and the four reasons why consultees need this type of consultation: to address deficiencies in knowledge, skill, confidence, and objectivity. Lack of objectivity is particularly emphasized in this model, as some consultees are thought to misperceive children's behavior (e.g., considering it "disturbed") due, for example, to transference or too much emotional involvement. The mental health consultant guides the consultee toward greater objectivity (or knowledge or skill or confidence) such that referred children are perceived more accurately and realistically. This process entails a close, trusting relationship between the consultant and consultee and interventions which are accepted as facilitative and related to problem resolution. Mental health consultation, therefore, is one of the more consultee-focused intervention models. It is discussed more comprehensively by Meyers (1981), Meyers *et al.* (1979), and Caplan (1970).

Advocacy Consultation

Advocacy consultation is both generic to mental health service delivery and specific to identified client populations. In its generic sense, the advocacy consultant tries to change target groups' attitudes and behaviors toward consultees' or clients' legal and human rights through publicity and consciousness-raising activities. Assuming that those in mental health and/or educational service delivery fields are advocates for children and adolescents, advocacy consultants address ways to help others to understand client needs, characteristics, and rights. In its specific sense, advocacy consultation takes place when specific groups (e.g., the emotionally disturbed, the physically handicapped) require help, for example, in ways to publicize their needs for services and more equitable treatment. Overall, then, advocacy consultants (a) target the change process in directions of power equalization, (b) focus on social systems rather than individual clients or overall groups, (c) plan for multifaceted and multidimensional intervention, (d) work with and toward political action, and (e) are generally oriented toward facilitation and cooperation, yet activism if necessary. Advocacy consultation, therefore, is somewhat removed from intervention planning for individually referred children; it looks for interventions that politically and legally affect entire classes or clusters of children. Advocacy consultation is highlighted by Conoley (1981) and Biklen (1974).

Psychoeducational Consultation

Consultants using this model emphasize the need for continuing consultation and support so that recommendations by a child study or agency team, based on the problem analysis results of the personality assessment process, are actually operationalized and implemented. Psychoeducational consultants, therefore, are trying to ensure that assessment results, interpretations, and recommendations are considered and appropriately used by consultees who have the day-to-day responsibility of managing referred clients' programs. In many ways, the psychoeducational consultation process is embodied in the pragmatic personality assessment process described in Chapter 3. This discussion reinforces the critical importance of preassessment conferences, feedback conferences involving all the individuals relevant to a specific referral, the ongoing evaluation of intervention programs, and follow-up consultation initiatives. These are all activities that could utilize the expertise of psychoeducational consultants for the most effective service delivery. Psychoeducational consultation, therefore, directly relates to many aspects of the personality assessment process, specifically the need to actually operationalize and implement relevant, realistic intervention plans for referred clients. Additional support for this model is available from White and Fine (1976).

Strategic Consultation

Strategic consultation involves community-wide change through the identification of pervasive system, group, and individual needs and the development of comprehensive planning and service-delivery programs. This requires an analysis of the community ecosystem and an identification of specific "leverage points" through which the change process can be most effectively attained. Strategic consultation, thus, is systemically more involved than either organizational development or process consultation, yet it most certainly uses some of their specific perspectives and techniques. Related to the personality assessment process, strategic consultation is somewhat far removed from direct client intervention; it is more oriented to the implementation of secondary and primary prevention programs which obviate the need for direct services to individually referred clients. Strategic consultation's primary goal, then, is to motivate and support all facets of the community to identify and commit their resources and organizations toward promoting positive mental health practices and attitudes. Conoley and Conoley (1981) have written more extensively on strategic consultation.

Each of the seven consultation models discussed above brings its own uniqueness to the multimodal approach. While space limitations allow only brief descriptions of the models, it is evident that the behavioral, mental health, and psychoeducational consultation models are more related to the client-centered and consultee-centered case consultation types; the process and organizational development models are related to the program-centered administrative consultation type; and the advocacy and strategic models are related to the consultee-centered administrative consultation type. Specific to developing intervention programs for referred clients within the personality assessment process, the behavioral and psychoeducational consultation models appear to be the most relevant.

Using Multimodal Consultation

Similar to Lazarus's multimodal therapy, which uses whatever BASIC ID modalities seem necessary to effect *direct*, therapeutic change in specific referred children, the multimodal (PROB^LEMAPS) consultation models are used to advance those *indirect* consultee and client changes necessary to intervention success. The multimodal consultant therefore employs a process whereby the seven consultation models are considered individually and then in combinations for their potential contributions to a successful intervention. As described by Knoff (1984b), there are four assumptions inherent in the multimodal consultation process:

> 1. Referral problems, whether client-centered, consultee-centered, program/curriculum-centered, or organization/administration-centered, often require two or more of the PROB^LEMAPS consultation models for effective resolution. While a referral problem may be resolved through one consultation model, it is likely that characteristics of this model overlap with those of another consultation model such that the second model is unnecessary. For example, an administrative problem may suggest the need for both organizational development and process consultations yet be resolved through organizational development consultation alone because its dynamics/interventions resolve the organizational development components of the problem *and* indirectly or vicariously resolve the problem's process components. As noted above, however, most complex referral problems need and must formally use two or more relevant PROB^LEMAPS consultation models for optimal success.
>
> 2. While a number of consultation models might possibly resolve a given referral problem, there is often a preferred consultation model (when one model generalizes enough to make additional models redundant) or combination of models which are most efficacious. While the literature has rarely investigated consultation models' relative efficacy (e.g., Jason, Ferone, & Anderegg, 1979), this heuristically oriented assumption suggests that empirical evidence will ultimately support the use of certain consultation models with certain complexes of referral problems and ecosystems.
>
> 3. The concurrent use of parallel or interacting consultation models for a referral problem, when empirically tested and supported, will produce a more efficient problem resolution than the nonconcurrent, isolated use of the same consultation models. For example, if it has been empirically determined that a referral problem is best resolved through mental health, process, and psychoeducational consultations, the systematic and concurrent implementation of these consultation models should resolve the problem more effectively than the segregated implementation of each

model to its respective conclusion. In effect, this assumption reinforces the notion that referral problems reflect an interaction of interdependent subsystems, not isolated subsystem problems that can be resolved individually. Stated another way, the multimodal (concurrent) implementation of two (or more) consultation models is more effective than the cumulative influence of the same models implemented apart.

4. Multimodal consultation involves both subjective and objective analysis, and the interventions are based on a probability model. While the efficacy of specific consultation models with certain complexes of referral problems should be empirically derived, it must be acknowledged that some consultation models (e.g., mental health, advocacy consultations) rely more on the consultant's subjective impressions and interpretations than on standardized assessment procedures and actuarial decision-making for success. Thus, multimodal consultation assumes a flexible consultation approach which is directed toward efficient change; a process which should be sensitive to both the subjective and objective components of problem-solving and decision-making (Watzlawick, Weakland, & Fisch, 1974). (pp. 85–86)

As noted in the assumptions above, there is a conceptual consistency between multimodal consultation and the personality assessment process described in Chapter 3 (e.g., the need for empirical derivations, the dependence on a probability model). Further, the use of multimodal consultation as part of an intervention program is consistent with these previous discussions. This process should entail a consideration of all potential interventions relevant to the referral situation from each individual consultation model. These interventions should then be synthesized (see Maher, 1981, for a decision-making model) such that an integrated, individualized consultation intervention program has been developed for the specific referral situation and its unique ecological circumstances (see Knoff, 1984b, for a complete discussion of this process). As noted above, this process comprises only the indirect consultation services necessary to an intervention plan; direct interventions for referred children or environments should also be planned and implemented.

To summarize, this chapter has reviewed both the direct (BASIC ID × theoretical approaches) and indirect (multimodal consultation: PROBᴸEMAPS) intervention approaches which are a necessary part of the personality assessment process. To conclude this chapter, some aspects of the change process as a whole will be considered.

The Change Process

Interest in the process of social–emotional and behavioral change has a history that far predates the literature which first addresses formal approaches to personality assessment. Certainly, many of the Greek philosophers (e.g., Plato and Aristotle) debated about the elements of change and the ways that change occurs and/or can be influenced. Given its extensiveness, no attempt will be made to comprehensively present this history. Instead, some of the characteristics that affect change will be presented, and the change process will be related to the personality assessment process.

Relationship Enhancement and Client or Consultee Change

Given the reciprocal determinism model, children and adolescents' behavioral and/or social–emotional changes occur when one or more interactions between the model's components create change; that is, referred problems are most often resolved when there are changes in the referred person, the problem environment, the targeted behavior, the person–environment, person–behavior, environment–behavior interactions, and/or the person–environment–behavior interaction. (This assumes that changes in the referral source's perceptions of the problem occur as part of an environmental change.) Because change, regardless of its location in the reciprocal determinism model, requires interactions between people (e.g., in a multidisciplinary team, among a mental health practitioner and the referral source and referred child, between a consultant and a consultee), the quality of the relationship during the change process often becomes critically important. Indeed, as Goldstein (1980) notes, "There now exists a wide variety of research evidence, from several different types of two-person interactions, to indicate that the quality of the helper–client relationship can serve as a powerful positive influence upon communication, openness, persuasibility and, ultimately, positive change in the client" (pp. 19–20).

Goldstein (1980), summarizing the literature from both empirical and theoretical perspectives, presents a "relationship enhancement" progression which considers the dynamic characteristics that most facilitate client change. While this progression is applicable primarily to direct intervention services and therapeutic change, it can be easily generalized to include indirect services and consultative change. This adapted progression is presented in Table 16-3.

Relationship enhancers involve interpersonal variables and social psychological interactions which improve the quality of the relationships between practitioners and referred children or consultants and consultees. Ten variables and their correlations with positive relationship enhancement are shown in Table 16-3 and discussed below. The first three variables are enhancers which help to attract children (or consultees) to mental health practitioners and their interaction or change process. Next, practitioner characteristics which strengthen these relationships and continue to ensure change are described. Finally, the need to consider the practitioner–child interaction itself is presented.

Table 16-3
The Progression from Relationship Enhancement to Change from the Direct and Indirect Service Perspectives[a]

Relationship enhancers	Relationship components	Relationship consequences	Outcome
Child/adolescent or consultee			
Structuring			
Imitation			
Conformity			
Mental health practitioner			
Expertness	Liking	Communication	
Credibility			Child/adolescent
Empathy	Respect	Openness	or
Warmth			consultee change
Self-disclosure	Trust	Personality	
Physical closeness and posture			
Mental health practitioner–child/adolescent or consultee matching			

[a] Adapted from Goldstein (1980).

1. *Structuring* or preparing children (or consultees) for practitioners and the intervention or change process involves presenting the practitioner as a positive, helpful person whom the child will like and describing what to realistically anticipate from the practitioner and the change process. These activities have demonstrated, in research and practice, their effectiveness in increasing practitioner and child (or consultee) relationships.

2. *Imitation* or modeling a positive relationship with the practitioner also facilitates the relationship-building and change process. For example, peer professionals' respect and friendliness toward a practitioner in parents' or referred children's presence can suggest to those observers that the practitioner is an "OK" person to like and with whom to interact.

3. The pressure to *conformity* may be used when structuring or imitation procedures do not work. Here, having the child state that he or she will like working with the practitioner after others have commented similarly can create a pressure to conform which, with its "public" commitment, can create powerful relationship enhancement attitudes and behaviors.

4. Characteristics of the mental health practitioner known to strengthen the practitioner–child relationship include practitioner expertness, credibility, empathy, warmth, self-disclosure, and physical closeness and posture. While these are all definitionally clear to any mental health practitioner, their use during relationship-building and intervention should be individualized to the specific child or adolescent (or consultee). Often these variables relate to relationship enhancement in an "inversed-U" relationship; that is, for any individual, there will be an optimum level of perceived expertness or credibility or warmth or whatever. Above and below that level, the full benefit of the variable to relationship enhancement will not be realized, and the variable's presence may in fact weaken or destroy the relationship. For example, too little warmth will not allow rapport and trust to develop, whereas too much warmth may scare or smother the child or adolescent.

5. Practitioner–child (or consultee) matching alludes to the need to individualize relationships and interpersonal interactions. Every mental health practitioner is not suited to intervene, therapeutically or otherwise, with every child or adolescent. Practitioners often know who their favorite clients or populations are, that is, with whom they most enjoy working and with whom they get the best results.

While the research literature is generally inconclusive, Goldstein (1980) has summarized some of the tentative conclusions specific to the practitioner–child matching process:

> 1. Helper and client hold congruent expectations of the role each is to play in the relationship. They understand and agree upon their respective rights and obligations regarding what each is expected to do and not to do during their interactions.
> 2. Helper and client are both confident of positive results from their meetings. Each anticipates at least a reasonably high likelihood of client change.
> 3. Helper and client come from similar social, cultural, racial, and economic backgrounds.
> 4. Helper and client are similar in their use of language, conceptual complexity, extroversion-introversion, objectivity-subjectivity, flexibility, and social awareness.
> 5. Helper and client are complementary or reciprocal in their need to offer and receive inclusion, control, and affection. The need for inclusion relates to associating, belonging, and companionship versus isolation, detachment, and aloneness.

Control is a power or influence dimension, and affection refers to emotional close-ness, friendliness, and the like. Helper and client are complementary or reciprocal on these dimensions if the level of inclusion, affection, or control which one member needs to offer approximates the level of that dimension which the other member needs to receive. (p. 47)

According to Goldstein (1980) and as depicted in Table 16-3, the relation-ship enhancers improve the practitioner–child relationship in three areas: liking, respect, and trust. These, in turn, relate to the relationship consequences of im-proved or optimal communication, openness, and persuasibility which are nec-essary for positive and effective change.

Goldstein's relationship enhancement progression and the discussion above presents one way to look at the change process. Certainly, change can be ad-dressed from other theoretical, pragmatic, even paradoxical, perspectives. None-theless, the perspective presented here is one of the more comprehensive, athe-oretical perspectives; that is, it can be applied to many of the other perspectives; indeed, it is fundamental to most of them.

Summary

Change occurs throughout the personality assessment process (Conti, 1983). From the receipt of the referral to the preassessment conference to the assessment to the intervention and follow-up, impressions are being gathered, attitudes are being formed, and interpersonal conclusions are being reached. All of the rela-tionship enhancement variables are active throughout the personality assessment process, and any one variable or interaction can make or break the practition-er/referral source/referred child relationship, and thus, the intervention program. The practitioner must be consciously aware of the dynamics of change throughout the assessment process.

One important dynamic that is often mentioned during any discussion of change is resistance. Indeed, like the change process itself, a discussion of resist-ance is well beyond the scope of this volume (see Haley, 1963, 1973; Lankton, 1980; Watzlawick *et al.*, 1974, for more extensive coverage). However, Conti's (1983) suggestions for overcoming resistance are particularly noteworthy and, in fact, they provide an excellent philosophy to the personality assessment and inter-vention process: "The psychologist can defuse this resistance by re-emphasizing (*a*) that the information reflects the child's perspective of reality which may or may not be accurate; (*b*) the clients are free to accept or reject the analysis, rec-ommendations, and/or consultation; and (*c*) the clients can always approach other professionals for their opinions or recommendations" (p. 438).

To summarize this section and chapter, the change process has been dis-cussed extensively from many different empirical and theoretical perspectives. The mental health practitioner must be aware of the dynamics of change and be prepared to deal with it as a *process*. In some ways, the change desired in the re-ferred child and the technical techniques and strategies used toward change are concrete products. The dynamics of change involve process. Both of these prod-uct and process concerns must be addressed—they are interdependent. Practi-tioners cannot choose to attend to one over the other. If they do, true change will be unlikely, and the entire personality assessment process will not realize its potential to improve the lives of children, adolescents, and those around them.

References

Bandura, A. (1978). The self-system in reciprocal determinism. *American Psychologist, 33*, 344–358.

Bergan, J. R. (1977). *Behavioral consultation*. Columbus, OH: Charles E. Merrill.

Biklen, D. (1974). *Let our children go: An organizing manual for parents and advocates*. Syracuse, NY: Human Policy Press.

Caplan, G. (1970). *The theory and practice of mental health consultation*. New York: Basic Books.

Conoley, J. C. (Ed.). (1981). *Consultation in schools: Theory, research, procedures*. New York: Academic Press.

Conoley, J. C., & Conoley, C. W. (1981). Strategic consultation: Community care givers in the schools. In J. C. Conoley (Ed.), *Consultation in schools: Theory, research, procedures* (pp. 201–222). New York: Academic Press.

Conoley, J. C., & Conoley, C. W. (1982). *School consultation: A guide to practice and training*. Oxford: Pergamon Press.

Conti, A. (1983). Implementing interventions from projective findings: Suggestions for school psychologists. *School Psychology Review, 12*, 435–439.

Ellis, A., & Greiger, R. (1977). *Handbook of rational-emotive therapy*. New York: Springer.

Goldstein, A. P. (1980). Relationship-enhancement methods. In F. H. Kanfer & A. P. Goldstein (Eds.), *Helping people change* (pp. 18–57). Oxford: Pergamon Press.

Haley, J. (1963). *Strategies of psychotherapy*. New York: Grune & Stratton.

Haley, J. (1973). *Uncommon therapy: The psychiatric techniques of Milton H. Erikson, M.D.* New York: Norton.

Jason, L. A., Ferone, L., & Anderegg, T. (1979). Evaluating ecological, behavioral, and process consultation interventions. *Journal of School Psychology, 17*, 103–115.

Jerrell, J. M., & Jerrell, S. L. (1981). Organizational consultation in school systems. In J. C. Conoley (Ed.), *Consultation in schools: Theory, research, procedures* (pp. 133–156). New York: Academic Press.

Keller, H. R. (1981). Behavioral consultation. In J. C. Conoley (Ed.), *Consultation in schools: Theory, research, procedures* (pp. 59–100). New York: Academic Press.

Knoff, H. M. (1983). Learning disabilities in the junior high school: Creating the six-hour emotionally disturbed adolescent? *Adolescence, 18*, 541–550.

Knoff, H. M. (1984a). A conceptual review of discipline in the schools: A consultation service-delivery model. *Journal of School Psychology, 22*, 335–346.

Knoff, H. M. (1984b). The practice of multimodal consultation: An integrating approach for consultation service delivery. *Psychology in the Schools, 21*, 83–91.

Lankton, S. (1980). *Practical magic*. Cupertino, CA: Meta Publications.

Lazarus, A. A. (1981). *The practice of multi-modal therapy*. New York: McGraw-Hill.

Maher, C. A. (1981). Decision analysis: An approach for multidisciplinary teams in planning special service programs. *Journal of School Psychology, 19*, 340–349.

Meyers, J. (1981). Mental health consultation. In J. C. Conoley (Ed.), *Consultation in schools: Theory, research, procedures* (pp. 35–58). New York: Academic Press.

Meyers, J., Parsons, R. D., & Martin, R. (1979). *Mental health consultation in schools*. San Francisco, CA: Jossey-Bass.

Schein, E. H. (1969). *Process consultation: Its role in organization development*. Reading, MA: Addison-Wesley.

Schmuck, R. A., Runkel, P. J., Arends, J. H., & Arends, R. I. (1977). *The second handbook of organization development in schools*. Palo Alto, CA: Mayfield.

Watzlawick, P., Weakland, C. E., & Fisch, R. (1974). *Change: Principles of problem formation and problem resolution*. New York: Norton.

White, P. L., & Fine, M. J. (1976). The effects of three school psychological consultation models on selected teacher and pupil outcomes. *Psychology in the Schools, 13*, 414–420.

17

Personality Assessment and Individual Therapeutic Interventions

H. Thompson Prout

The psychological treatment of children's and adolescents' problems is a challenging task carried out by professionals in a variety of settings. It is, by nature, a task different from counseling and psychotherapy with adults. Children, and particularly adolescents, rarely seek out therapy voluntarily and often have a distorted view of the therapeutic process and its purposes. They are often brought or sent to treatment by an adult in their environment. In fact, children's views of and "motivations" for treatment are often at cross purposes with those who have made the referral. For example, during the problem identification and analysis stages of the personality assessment process, some children may not even acknowledge a problem, much less offer information that can help to clarify the situation.

Children and adolescents also present a more complex clinical picture because of developmental issues. Determining what is "normal" behavior is a difficult task in itself, but may be more confusing with children because developmental and chronological age levels often determine whether a behavior falls within normal or expected limits. Children's more limited verbal and cognitive development also limits the type of therapeutic strategies that can be employed; that is, they may be unable to talk and think through issues in the same manner as adults.

Environmental changes also tend to affect children more. Children and adolescents are usually reactors to situations rather than initiators of change. Children are dependent on the environment and are relatively powerless to effect change. The child is subject to many stressors (e.g., family dissolution and disruption, school stresses, community crises) over which he or she has little control. Yet, these events can have profound emotional impact. In general, child and adolescent therapy can be a vastly different enterprise than adult therapeutic intervention. In many ways, these differences may make assessment even more crucial to to overall process.

A philosophy inherent in this book is that personality assessment and ther-

H. Thompson Prout. School Psychology Program, State University of New York at Albany, Albany, New York.

apeutic interventions with children and adolescents should be guided by "intelligent eclecticism" and should be multimodal in nature (Prout, 1983; Prout & Brown, 1983a). Intelligent eclecticism refers to the perspective that no one theory or therapeutic approach can explain all child/adolescent disorders, problems, or psychopathology, much less offer treatment guidelines that are appropriate for all problems. Prout and Brown (1983b), in their summary and comparison of different therapeutic approaches, noted that various theories differ in the degree to which they deal with certain aspects of intervention. For example, some approaches offer comprehensive parent counseling packages (e.g., Adlerian approaches), some appear well suited for work with adolescents (e.g., reality therapy), and some offer a well-detailed developmental framework (e.g., psychoanalytic theory). The intelligent eclectic approach assumes that mental health practitioners will assess referred problems and select theoretically based strategies that best match the presenting concerns; that is, practitioners should not force referred problems into inappropriate theoretical frameworks. While there are obvious limitations to eclecticism—no practitioner can be conversant and comfortable with all major approaches—it is conceivable that the same practitioner might employ behavioral contracting with an acting-out adolescent, yet use nondirective counseling with a shy, withdrawn younger child. In fact, the combining of strategies and techniques from different theoretical schools is not only seen as acceptable, but desirable.

The multimodal view of treatment has been popularized by Lazarus (1976, 1981) and applied with children by Keat (1979). In the present context, multimodal treatment implies a relatively broad view of what is "psychotherapeutic" for a child or adolescent. Multimodal refers to the many potential interventions that might be used when working with troubled children. For example, traditional individual psychotherapy, a classroom-affective education program, parent counseling, or an alternative school program might all yield psychotherapeutic benefits for children or adolescents. Further, teachers, parents, and other school or agency personnel might be used as therapists or treatment agents. Finally, treatment may be implemented in a variety of settings.

The multimodal view also calls for the combined use of several modalities. A disturbed child would not be seen solely for individual psychotherapy. The mental health practitioner would coordinate a comprehensive package that might include individual therapy and other family, school, and community interventions. This multimodal view, therefore, assumes that the more interventions that can be combined, that is, the more modalities involved, the more likely that therapeutic goals will be realized. Certainly the key to the success of multimodal treatment, as supported by Lazarus and Keat, is the careful assessment of the referred problem and the careful selection of treatment modalities.

At a philosophical and idealistic level, it is clear that assessment should be an integral part of the planning and implementation of treatment programs. Pragmatically, however, it is unclear whether psychological or behavioral assessment actually leads to better treatment. In fact, the more traditional, test-oriented assessment approaches have been particularly criticized on this issue. Keefe, Kopel, and Gordon (1978), in comparing behavioral assessment with traditional assessment, have noted that "[t]he link between traditional assessment and treatment is a weak one. Diagnostic classification often leads to differential treatment only on a gross level (e.g., inpatient versus outpatient treatment). Similar treatment procedures are often used irrespective of assessment information (e.g., Daily, 1953)" (p. 13).

Similarly, Tallent (1976), in discussing the utility of psychological reports in psychotherapy, cites several studies suggesting that assessment is not considered very useful by psychotherapists. Finally, Barrett, Hampe, and Miller (1978), in their review of the outcome research in child psychotherapy, conclude that individuals' responses to treatment clearly seem to be related to the diagnostic categories assigned to them. However, this research and the assessment-intervention relationship are hindered by poor classification systems and inadequate or inappropriate child and adolescent assessment measures.

Behaviorally oriented practitioners have claimed that the close interface of assessment and treatment is a particular strength of their approach (e.g., see Goldfried & Linehan, 1977; Keefe *et al.*, 1978). According to Nelson and Hayes (1981), however, this relationship has not yet been demonstrated: " . . . there is a need to experimentally demonstrate that specific methods of behavioral assessment actually lead to better treatment" (p. 25). To summarize, it appears that the actual utility of assessment (behavioral or traditional) in planning and conducting treatment programs is unclear and has not been empirically demonstrated at this time. Despite this equivocal situation, good clinical practice still dictates that assessment remain an important part of a comprehensive treatment approach.

The purpose of this chapter is to review and discuss the role of assessment in the development of therapeutic interventions for children and adolescents. The purposes of assessment for intervention will be reviewed, an assessment-based model of intervention will be presented, the role of assessment within specific theories of psychotherapy will be discussed, and the use of self-report measures will be considered.

The Purpose of Assessment in Therapeutic Intervention

The general purposes of personality assessment, and assessment in general, have been discussed previously in this book. One of these purposes involves treatment or intervention planning. Palmer (1970), in fact, has stated that this is the primary purpose: " . . . the essential purpose of a psychological assessment is to determine the nature and extent of the disturbance in order to select and formulate the model(s) of behavior change" (p. 5). Within this realm, there are a number of personality assessment activities that relate directly to the development of treatment programs. Practitioners of all theoretical orientations may engage in these general activities, but the specific strategies within each activity will often be dictated by and consistent with the practitioner's personal therapeutic orientation. Below is a discussion of these general intervention planning activities.

1. *Establish a baseline.* As the assessment process proceeds, the extent or severity of the referred problem is determined so that intervention planning can begin. The assessment to intervention transition may initially involve the establishment of a problem's baseline, resulting in its quantitative evaluation (e.g., frequency of hitting), a rating of its intensity or severity (e.g., mild vs. moderate anxiety), or relative presence or absence of some clinical sign or symptom (e.g., signs of depressed mood in a thematic procedure). These baseline figures permit the evaluation of treatment progress by determining how successful treatment has been and whether a change in the treatment approach is necessary.

2. *Pinpoint treatment targets*. This activity involves problem identification and definition resulting in an operationalization of intervention focuses and directions; this allows the practitioner to set goals and/or objectives and to prioritize the most significant of the referred problems. The generality or situational nature of the problems may also be assessed here. Finally, this procedure may reveal themes or content that should be pursued in individual therapy sessions. For example, a behavior therapist might specifically delineate target behaviors related to aggression, while a more dynamically oriented therapist might direct his client toward dealing with affective responses to significant others.

3. *Assess developmental status*. The nature of child and adolescent interventions requires that treatment be appropriate for the developmental level of the child. This includes two aspects, designing treatments that are appropriate (*a*) for children's cognitive and language levels (e.g., using language appropriate for a child with cognitive abilities in the 8-year-old range), and (*b*) consideration of the child's level of social–emotional development (e.g., level of social skill development). This latter aspect may also be a treatment target. Assessing presenting problems within a developmental framework also determines whether they are "true" problems or essentially normal developmental patterns. Certain fears, for example, may be considered normal at one age level and abnormal at another age. Finally, developmental assessment may also identify relative strengths or assets that children can utilize during treatment.

4. *Assess children's views of the problem*. This includes assessing children's perceptions and understanding of the presenting problems. Here, practitioners are concerned with whether children acknowledge that a problem exists, and then with their views of the various factors relating to the problem. Related to this are children's understandings of the treatment process and their willingness (i.e., motivation) to cooperate with treatment. This may involve prognostic assessments of whether children are open to direct intervention.

5. *Assess relevant environmental factors*. This activity involves assessing school, family, peer, and community factors that may influence the treatment plan. This may reveal factors that need to be considered in treatment, yet may not be the target of direct intervention. For example, a resistant, abusive parent may not be accessible for direct intervention along with the referred child, yet may play an important role when planning the content of individual sessions with the child. Conversely, an environmental assessment may indicate intervention directions besides those involving direct work with the child. Certainly, a comprehensive treatment plan might include individual counseling with the child, as well as teacher consultation and parent counseling.

6. *Select appropriate treatment strategy*. As noted above, the intelligent eclecticism approach in selecting treatment approaches is strongly advocated. This approach posits that the assessment process should yield data which help to select the therapeutic approaches that best address children's specific problems; that is, practitioners should not expect that a single treatment approach will be appropriate for all, or even most, problems. The assessment process may also identify behavior patterns that have clearly identified and proved treatment strategies. For example, past research demonstrates that certain anxiety disorders respond well to desensitization techniques (Prout & Harvey, 1978).

7. *Evaluate efficacy*. All of the activities discussed above represent clinical practices that could (and maybe should) be conducted by all practitioners in their professional work. This last activity involves the use of assessment to evaluate intervention program efficacy and/or to conduct more basic research on the outcomes of specific interventions. The use of appropriate outcome measures and methodologies allows the evaluation of specified techniques which are used to resolve specific problems. This activity therefore can potentially address a much debated question in the mental health field, the effectiveness of psychotherapy and other intervention strategies.

A Model of Intervention

Current thinking among theorists in psychotherapy suggests that the therapeutic process should no longer be viewed as magical and directionless. Indeed, most, but not all, theories of psychotherapy ascribe to some relatively standard, albeit individualized, intervention procedure. This usually involves problem identification, problem definition, assessment, intervention goal setting, and various stages of therapeutic change. Behaviorally oriented practitioners are perhaps most identified with this systematic, active, problem-focused approach to psychotherapy.

A systematic, step-by-step view of the intervention process has been advocated by a number of professionals, most notably Gottman and Leiblum (1974) and Brown and Brown (1977). Both sets of authors present flowcharts diagramming their decision-making models of intervention. These models, attempting to demystify the process that leads to change, view the counselor/therapist/mental health practitioner as the manager or agent of change. The therapeutic relationship, while still viewed as important, is not seen as the sole key to the change process. Instead, the activities of and decisions by the practitioner and the client (e.g., referred child or adolescent and/or parents) are deemed to be crucial to the overall process. These two models, as advocated above, also emphasize the use of assessment data throughout the intervention process. While these models are generally compatible with intervention approaches associated with behavior therapy, they are essentially atheoretical in nature, particularly the one developed by Gottman and Leiblum. Thus, while ongoing assessment is dictated in both the problem assessment and evaluation phases, it could involve either direct behavioral observations or repeated administrations of more traditional projective measures, two seemingly disparate approaches to assessment.

An assessment-based model of intervention is presented in Figure 17-1 primarily as a guide for the practitioner. Clearly, it does not outline an absolute procedure; there will undoubtedly be cases that do not fit completely within this model. Nonetheless, this model emphasizes the systematic, data-based planning and implementation of interventions, consistent with the purposes of assessment discussed previously. Further, the role of assessment in designing individually based interventions is implicit in this model; that is, assessment dictates the choice of therapeutic strategy. Finally, assessment is seen as an ongoing process where the practitioner and client(s) receive feedback when goals have been met and when a change in strategy might be necessary. Thus, the "looping" nature of the model is a key element. This feature emphasizes a "let's go back and take another look" attitude when, for example, an initial assessment is not totally accurate and its reevaluation is necessary in order to change a therapeutic direction.

This author is reminded of a case encountered in his first professional posi-

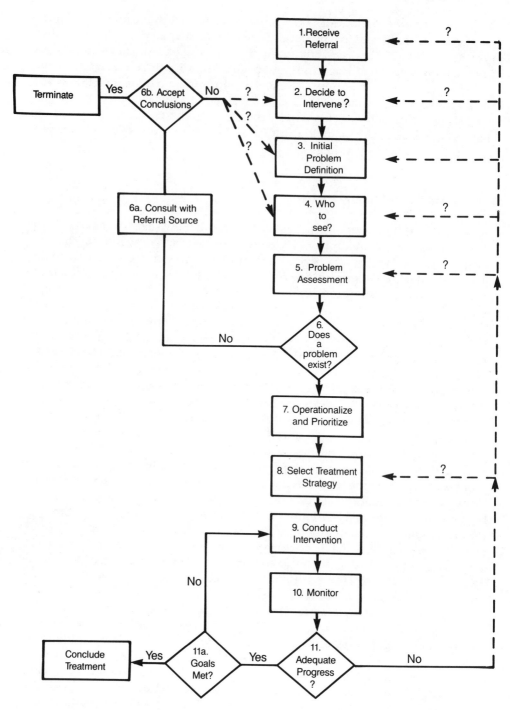

Figure 17-1. An assessment based model of intervention.

tion as a psychologist in a child guidance clinic. A family brought in their 9-year-old son because of school problems largely revolving around poor grades. After the initial assessment, some educational recommendations were formulated and a program of supportive counseling focusing on the school problems was begun. The initial assessment had revealed no major individual psychopathology and no significant family dysfunctions. Within a short period of time, however, an extremely abusive family situation was discovered along with periodic near-psychotic rage episodes by the referred boy where he threatened the rest of the family with knives. Needless to say, it was necessary to "loop back" rather quickly, to reassess the new information presented, and to change directions. To continue solely with the original school focus would have been ridiculous.

Below is a descriptive "walk through" of the flowchart presented in Figure 17-1. Again, this model is presented as a guide, and the steps are not seen as mutually exclusive or chronological; that is, some of the activities may occur concurrently and it may not be necessary to totally complete Step 2 before beginning Step 3. This presentation should be compared with the pragmatic problem-solving process described in Chapter 3 of this volume.

Step 1: Receive Referral. This simple first step is often overlooked in the assessment process. Indeed, information sometimes gathered at later stages in the assessment process could or should be obtained at this stage. For example, contrast the difference between receiving a note from a teacher that says "Please see Johnny Smith for counseling" versus a well-detailed referral form that allows you immediately to begin your problem analysis. Certainly the referral form or procedure should assist in making decisions about the types of information that will be collected during the more in-depth assessment procedures. Further, a special section of the referral form (or a separate form) for or to plan intervention-specific referrals could be useful at this stage.

Step 2: Decide to Intervene. This stage poses the questions: "How was the decision made to refer the child or adolescent for intervention?" and "Who made the decision?" As noted previously, children rarely refer themselves for treatment; usually, some adult in their environment has initiated the referral. Part of the process at this step is to assess the ownership of the "problem," that is, who views or has labeled the child's behavior as problematic? The motivations, expectations, and perceptions of those who might potentially be involved in the intervention are also assessed at this level. In addition to the child's perceptions of the referral and referred problems, the views of parents and teachers are important here. For example, individuals' perceptions of the therapeutic process may limit the interventions available as options. A teacher who expects the practitioner to perform "magic" in once per week counseling sessions with a child may not be open to a consultation approach. Similarly, the stereotypes that clients bring to treatment may influence the practitioner's selection of a strategy. A parent in counseling who expects you to be analytic, supportive, and reflective may respond poorly to attempts to set up a home-based reinforcement program.

The goal at this level, then, is to identify those who acknowledge that a problem exists, analyze perceptions, expectations, and motivations that may either hinder or facilitate treatment, and target attitudes that need modification before beginning the treatment program that focuses on the specific referral problems. This latter goal may involve pretherapy counseling or consultation for referred children, referral sources, or both.

Step 3: Complete Initial Problem Definition. This step represents an initial attempt at problem definition which then generates a direction for more formal problem assessment. The referral information structures the preliminary priorities of the assessment package, and tentative operational definitions of referral concerns are developed. These initial priorities and definitions are the working hypotheses that will be adapted or validated during the problem assessment activities (e.g., Step 5), and they help determine who will participate in the assessment process (i.e., Step 4).

Step 4: Decide Who to See. As mentioned above, children's behavior is often dependent on environmental factors. At this stage, practitioners decide from whom to obtain data during the assessment process (e.g., parents? teachers? peers? siblings? social service personnel? school administrators?) and what settings to evaluate relative to the occurrence of the referral problem(s) (e.g., home? school? specific classes? community?). A major goal here is to design an assessment package that will address the setting-general versus situation-specific aspects of referral concerns, to analyze discrepancies in perceptions of the "problem" among those in the environment, and to begin to identify individuals and behavior settings that might be involved in the intervention. Using the initial priorities and definitions developed in Step 3, the type of information needed from particular individuals can be determined.

Step 5: Complete Problem Assessment. At this point, a formal assessment of the referral concerns begins. Using the priorities developed in Step 3, the practitioner selects assessment techniques that will help to further define problem areas and/or confirm or disconfirm working hypotheses. As noted previously, this model is intended to be atheoretical and compatible with the many assessment approaches discussed in the other chapters of this book. Thus, this step may involve the first significant differences among practitioners of different theoretical persuasions. For example, assume that an initial screening has identified depression as a potential problem area for a child. Certainly depression can be assessed through a variety of modalities and techniques. Self-report inventories (e.g., Children's Depression Inventory, Beck Depression Inventory), behavior rating scales (e.g., Child Behavior Checklist and Child Behavior Profile), structured clinical interviews (see Chapter 4 of this volume), peer ratings (Peer Nomination Inventory for Depression), direct observation, incomplete sentence responses, objective measures from parental reports (e.g., Personality Inventory for Children), thematic analysis of responses to projectives (e.g., Thematic Apperception Test), and DSM-III criteria might all be used, consistent with the more reliable multimethod approaches (Gresham, 1983; Nay, 1979), to assess the clinical concept of depression. Thus, the same clinical question can be addressed in a variety of ways. Problem assessment also serves to establish a baseline that can be used as a reference and comparison point to evaluate the intervention program.

Step 6: Determine if a Problem Exists. This question represents the first major decision point in the assessment process as diagrammed in Figure 17-1. Based on the assessment data, the practitioner decides if a problem exists that warrants intervention. With children, this is often a difficult question because child development data and research indicate that certain problem behaviors reported by parents are actually normative (e.g., MacFarlane, Allen, & Honzik, 1954). If the data suggest that a genuine problem exists, then the planning and implementation of the intervention program (i.e., Step 7) should begin.

If the assessment data indicate that a problem of significant concern is not apparent, then the next step is to "loop back" and consult with the original referral sources (see Substep 6a). This, in effect, is also a therapeutic activity, as reassurances can be very comforting. The referral sources obviously may choose to accept or reject the practitioner's assessment conclusions of the situation (Substep 6b). If they accept the conclusion that a problem does not exist, the assessment process is completed and terminated. If they do not accept the assessment conclusions, it will be necessary (in lieu of a referral to another practitioner) to loop back into the initial assessment sequence. This may involve identifying and/or addressing other issues, involving other individuals in the assessment, reworking the initial priorities and definitions, and/or completing additional assessments. Significantly, the refusal of the referral sources to accept the conclusion of "no real problem" may itself become a treatment target.

Step 7: Operationalize and Prioritize. The decision that a problem exists implicitly leads to the decision to intervene. Thus, at this point, the problem concerns related to a referral and problem assessment are put into an operational framework which is then prioritized. This activity will dictate the focus of intervention strategies, their chronological implementations (if they must be staggered), their interrelationships, and the process of monitoring treatment progress. For example, again using the example of depression, the practitioner may decide that this primary problem needs specific attention during the intervention program. The interventions planned, however, will obviously depend on the practitioner's therapeutic orientation; different orientations will focus on different aspects of this problem. For example, a behavior therapist might focus on increasing prosocial behaviors, a cognitive or rational-emotive therapist might concentrate on irrational self-statements, and a psychodynamically oriented therapist might attempt to resolve some past internal conflict. While it is likely that some aspects of this operationalization were done during the planning of the problem assessment, actual treatment goals or objectives are set at this stage.

Step 8: Select Treatment Strategy. Based on the decisions in the previous steps, the practitioner selects and plans specific interventions to match the specific delineated problems. Again, within the limits of the practitioner's comfort and technical expertise with different approaches, this should be a thoughtful and systematic process. A wide variety of intervention options exist (see Keat, 1979; Prout & Brown, 1983a); if there is blind adherence to one approach, the bulk of the assessment activities are a waste of time. Again, intelligent eclecticism is recommended.

Step 9: Conduct Intervention. At this step, specific intervention strategies are implemented. Thus, there may be several steps in the treatment process involving different behavioral settings and individuals at different points.

Step 10: Monitor. Using the data gathered in Step 5, the practitioner readministers all or part of the problem assessment package, comparing the new results with the baseline data. Monitoring essentially analyzes the progress being made toward the treatment goals. The implications of this data comparison are used for the decisions made at Step 11.

Step 11: Evaluate for Adequate Progress. It is best to conceive of Steps 9–11 within an ongoing and continually looping back process which addresses the efficacy of the intervention program. Thus, the practitioner should be continually evaluating the implemented treatment strategies to assess their progress toward the treatment goals, and ultimately, the successful attainment of those goals. When adequate progress is observed, a decision to continue treatment as originally formulated is usually made. If the treatment goals and objectives have been met (Step 11a) and all parties agree with this evaluation, the assessment and treatment process is concluded. If adequate progress is lagging, the practitioner may loop back to several points in the process. Usually, a return to Step 8 to modify the treatment strategy and select another option is logical and appropriate; however, an entire reassessment and redefinition of the problem may be necessary. In the case cited above, the boy originally referred for school problems, it was essentially necessary to disregard the entire initial assessment and start at the beginning by reframing the referral concerns.

In summary, a systematic approach to therapeutic intervention is advocatd, irrespective of the practitioner's orientation. Further, this approach emphasizes an ongoing interface between assessment and intervention. This interface should allow for better selection of treatment strategies as well as for better monitoring of therapeutic progress.

Assessment and Theories of Psychotherapy

Prout and Brown (1983a) have identified six major theoretical approaches to counseling and psychotherapy with children and adolescents: behavior therapy, reality therapy, person-centered therapy, rational-emotive therapy, Adlerian therapy, and psychoanalytic/psychodynamic therapy. Although these theoretical approaches share a common goal of identifying variables which facilitate a better understanding of children's specific problems or psychopathologies, each one offers a unique view of personality, psychopathology, assessment, and psychotherapeutic intervention, and a particular framework or orientation. As noted above, however, these six therapeutic approaches are not necessarily consistent with the eight models of disturbed behavior presented in Chapters 1 and 3, nor are they necessarily consistent with the specific assessment techniques outlined in Part II of this book.

The multimodal practitioner who is an intelligent eclectic will quickly recognize that (*a*) any psychotherapy approach should be used if it will potentially address some facet of a referral problem—regardless of its consistency with eight models of disturbed behavior and/or the previously reviewed assessment techniques, and (*b*) that the imperfect interaction between the six counseling approaches and the eight theoretical models again is acceptable and expected within the multimodal assessment process approach. Indeed, psychotherapy is only one component of the comprehensive assessment and intervention process which is guided by the eight models of disturbance. And as noted, the six counseling approaches do not always fit into the eight theoretical models in a clear and consistent way. For example, none of the psychotherapy approaches could be categorized within the realm of the neurobiological model. Yet, some individual therapy approaches can be effective with neurologically based problems (e.g., behavioral strategies for hyperactive children; see Prout, 1977). On the other hand, the psychoanalytic and behavioral psychotherapy approaches are generated from and are consistent with the psychoanalytic and behavioral models of disturbed behavior, respectively. Finally, the approaches and models can be selectively used, again if necessary for a therapeutic gain. For example, behavior rating scales (see Chapter 10) and behavior observation techniques (see Chapter 11) are usually associated with the behavioral model, yet they could be used by a nondirective practitioner to monitor increases in the prosocial behavior of a shy, withdrawn child. Similarly, a reinforcement program to increase the on-task classroom behavior of academically low-achieving children might also be evaluated through the assessment of their affective changes.

Below, the six major theoretical approaches to individual counseling and psychotherapy with children and adolescents will be discussed in greater detail.

Behavior Therapy

Of all the theories related to psychotherapy, behavior therapy presents perhaps the most complete and comprehensive system of intervention-based assessment. This comprehensiveness exists due to the variety of different views within behavior therapy to explain behavior, that is, classical conditioning, operant learning, social learning theory, and cognitive-behavioral. These different views, however, are all linked together by a broad learning theory foundation that emphasizes environmental and social influences in the development of psychological disorders.

Kanfer and Saslow's (1969) classic S-O-R-K-C conceptualization of assessment still offers a most useful and broad-based assessment perspective by emphasizing both overt and covert aspects of behavior. "S" or *stimulus* focuses on antecedent events; "O" refers to *organismic* or biological variables; "R" or *response* encompasses a variety of motor, verbal, cognitive, emotional, and physiological behaviors occurring in the situation; "K" or *contingency* describes the probability relationships among variables; and "C" or *consequences* refers to the events that follow targeted responses. Inherent in the model is the identification and analysis of the learning history, variables, and processes that led to the development of the problem behavior, and more specifically, the delineation of learning variables that can be utilized in a change program.

Consistent with the S-O-R-K-C conceptualization, Ross (1980) has offered a behavioral definition of children's psychological disorders: "A psychological disorder is said to be present when a child emits behavior that deviates from an arbitrary and relative social norm in that it occurs with a frequency or intensity that authoritative adults in the environment judge, under the circumstances, to be too high or too low" (p. 9). This definition emphasizes the environmental and social context in viewing behaviors as either excessive or deficient. Rather than utilizing broad labels or global descriptions, the behavior therapist describes and then classifies behavior into one of these categories. An excess behavior occurs at too high a rate, with too much intensity, or for too long. Conversely, a deficit behavior occurs not at all or at too low a rate, with too little intensity, or too slowly. A hyperactive child, for example, may present an excess of motor activity, while a withdrawn child may be deficient in prosocial skills. Thus, the behavioral assessment approach focuses, to a degree, on the quantification of targeted problem behaviors.

The behavioral observation strategies discussed in Chapter 11 of this volume provide good examples of this aspect of behavioral assessment. While quantifying behavior involves objective procedures for the most part, it still requires judgments on whether behavior is excessive or deficient for a specific situation. This judgment may be facilitated through the use of behavior rating scales (see Chapter 10), which usually compare target behaviors to some standard (usually to other students in the class).

The behavior therapist strives for a thorough behavioral description of the referred concern. Data are generated to permit judgments about the appropriateness or inappropriateness of target behavior within the social context, and information gathered to analyze the learning pattern is later used to develop the change program. In addition to the behavioral assessment strategies discussed in this volume, there are a wide variety of other assessment and intervention techniques associated with the behavioral perspective. The reader is referred to Ollendick and Hersen (1984) and Mash and Terdal (1981) for complete discussions of these techniques. Briefly, however, these techniques include the following:

1. *Behavioral interviewing*. Behavioral interviews usually focus on parents, teachers, or other significant adults in the child's environment. These interviews elicit descriptions of antecedent, consequence, and other behavioral variables and characteristics from the adult perspective, and they tend to be relatively structured with the goal of producing specific types of information. Children are also sometimes interviewed within a behavioral format. For example, reinforcement menus, which assess children's preferences for activities and tangible rewards, are sometimes used in an interview form.

2. *Self-report measures*. These will be discussed in the next section of this chapter.

3. *Peer ratings*. These measures are similar to behavior rating scales except that they are completed by children in the target child's environment. Also called sociometric measures, they typically ask a child to rate others in a class on certain variables, or might ask questions like "Who in your class is sad?" or "Who in your class is a bully?"

4. *Role plays*. Role play assessments ask a child to act out how he or she would respond in certain situations. This assessment method is often used in social skills training. A child, for example, might be asked to show how he or she would make friends with another child.

5. *Specific behavior rating scales*. In addition to the general behavior rating scales discussed in Chapter 10, a wide variety of scales exist to assess specific behavior problems. Scales have been developed, for example, addressing hyperactivity, aggression, social skills, fears and anxieties, and various learning patterns.

Reality Therapy

Reality therapy was developed by psychiatrist William Glasser (1965) based largely on his clinical work with juvenile delinquents. Reality therapy espouses the view that identity is the single most basic requirement of all humans, transcending all cultures and existing from birth to death (Glasser & Zunin, 1979). The theory does not advocate individual diagnosis, believing that this actually does a disservice to the client. Instead, the key to understanding behavioral problems, according to reality therapy, rests with the differentiation between a "successful identity" and a "failure identity." Those with successful identities feel loved and cared for, are given recognition for achievements, enjoy themselves, and have a sense of belonging and self-worth. Much of this sense of self-worth comes from maintaining satisfactory standards of behavior and receiving recognition for that.

A failure identity is essentially equivalent to psychopathology within this system. Failure identity children believe that they are no good, worthless, and will be unsuccessful at things they attempt. Further, they see little chance of happiness or success in the future, and consider themselves "losers." Because they have given up, they are often described as apathetic, unmotivated, uninvolved, unconcerned, and indifferent. They tend to be self-critical, irrational, and irresponsible. The clinical problems resulting from this self-view include depression and withdrawal, acting out, thinking disturbances, and sickness (Fuller & Fuller, 1983).

Reality therapy itself does not have a formal assessment process associated with its clinical procedures. Much of its diagnostic and assessment approach occurs within the context of the therapeutic interview. Two underlying philosophies of reality therapy's therapeutic process, however, suggest that using other theories' methodologies is acceptable. First, reality therapy places considerable emphasis on the need to intervene with and change present or existing behaviors. Thus, the need for the behavioral assessment of problem behaviors to assess change is implied in the theory. A reality therapist, then, would be comfortable collecting data to show, for example, an increase in a child's homework completion or a decrease in arguing. In fact, much of the therapeutic process in reality therapy involves the counselor and child making a plan for change. This plan is developed with a built-in evaluative mechanism to determine if change has occurred, and much of the responsibility for assessing the change is left to the child.

The second underlying philosophy involves the assessment of changes in children's self-concept or self-esteem. Although rarely recommended as part of the therapeutic process, the improvement of attitudes toward self, with concomitant changes in behavior, is often a treatment goal. Assessment of self-concept and self-esteem has been a common discussion point in outcome studies of reality therapy. For example, in the outcome studies reviewed by Fuller and Fuller (1983), measures of self-concept were utilized the most to assess change.

To summarize, formal psychological assessment is not an important activity for reality therapists. While this therapeutic model does assess change, it is usually within the context of the therapeutic process. Nevertheless, as discussed above, related assessment models and techniques—notably behavioral approaches and the use of self-report measures—are not inconsistent and can be useful to the reality therapy process.

Person-Centered Therapy

Person-centered counseling/therapy, originally known as client-centered therapy, is a nondirective approach developed by Carl Rogers in the 1940s and 1950s. Developed partially in reaction to the then dominant psychoanalytic approaches and their emphasis on diagnosis, interpretive work, and past experiences, this theory has developed a reputation of being against testing, diagnosis, and formal assessment. In fact, some of Rogers's earlier writings (1951) suggest that diagnosis runs counter to the therapeutic process.

Psychopathology within the person-centered system revolves around the individual's sense of self. The adjusted person has a positive self-concept and accurate perceptions and awareness of self. Maladjustment occurs when incongruence exists between individuals' views of themselves and their reality of experience (Meador & Rogers, 1979; Rogers, 1959). The maladjusted person will also no longer be self-actualizing or engage in activities that promote, maintain, and enhance personal growth. According to this approach, children develop psychopathology when they negatively react to conditional love (Moore, 1983).

In person-centered counseling/therapy and its child counterpart, nondirective play therapy (Axline, 1947), no formal assessment process is recommended. Thus, practitioners who practice within this framework probably will not conduct formal testing or diagnostic interviews. Instead, the *clients* provide the content for the therapy sessions, through either conversation or symbolic play, while the practitioner attempts to empathetically understand their personal experience. In essence, then, "diagnostic" assessment in this system occurs when the practitioner reflects the affective component of the client's statements. There are, however, some exceptions to this assessment perspective.

Rogers and Dymond (1954), despite Rogers's antitest view, did develop a self-report measure of self-concept. This measure has not held a prominent place in the therapeutic process and has been used more within a research context. Coopersmith (1959) reworded the items on this scale and developed a children's Self-Esteem Inventory (see discussion in the next section). Finally, Palmer (1970) also discussed the use of testing as an adjunct to client-centered therapy. He feels that a variety of associative techniques (e.g., TAT, sentence completion techniques) can help to identify children's views of their selves and assist in promoting their affective expression. Palmer does note, however, that "orthodox" client-centered therapists would probably not be comfortable with this. Thus, the typical person-centered perspective puts little emphasis on the rule of psychological assessment in the therapeutic process, choosing to emphasize primarily intervention and dynamic change.

Rational-Emotive Therapy

Rational-emotive therapy, developed by Albert Ellis, has its own detailed description of psychopathology and a well-defined assessment system. The rational-emotive therapist attributes most maladaptive or disturbed emotions, feelings, and/or behaviors to faulty thinking and irrational beliefs. For example, if a person is depressed about a failure situation, the rational-emotive therapist will devote most of his or her efforts toward understanding the client's thoughts and beliefs about the failure. He or she will spend less time assessing the behaviors related to the failure while also deemphasizing the affective reaction of the depression. Thus, the therapist identifies and views the irrational beliefs (e.g., I must be successful in everything I attempt) as the cause of the disturbed emotions; that is, the failure did not cause the person to become depressed; rather, the irrational beliefs about the failure led to the depression.

Rational-emotive therapy's A–B–C format provides the key toward understanding its perspective of psychopathology and its assessment approach (Ellis, 1977). "A" refers to activating experience or activating event. This is something that happens in an individual's life that is followed by "C" or the consequence. Consequences can be both emotional and behavioral, and they are often the presenting problems that bring a person to treatment. In the example above, the failure experience would be "A" and the depression would be "C." Ellis notes that most emotional disturbances stem from the faulty assumption that "A" causes "C" when in reality it is the beliefs ("B") about the activating event that cause the disturbed consequences. Detecting these irrational beliefs and faulty thinking processes are the primary activities in rational-emotive assessment. Grieger and Boyd (1983) have described a variety of childhood emotional problems within this framework, listing both the manifestations of the problems and the likely irrational ideas behind the disturbed behaviors and emotions. For a complete discussion of psychopathology from a rational-emotive perspective, the reader is also directed to Grieger and Grieger (1982).

Grieger and Boyd (1980) describe assessment in this system as "rational-emotive psychodiagnosis," a problem identification and analysis process. This activity is generally conducted within the context of a directed or semistructured interview wherein the therapist has specific areas and types of information that need to be discussed. The general goal is to determine which types of problems the child or adolescent presents, and to conceptualize these problems in A–B–C formats. Again, the emphasis is on eliciting the client's thinking patterns and irrational beliefs by listening for irrational self-statements and beliefs, the client's causal attributions, and distorted perceptions of reality. The therapist will also note the absence of coping self-statements and poor problem-solving and solution-generating skills.

DiGiuseppe and Bernard (1983) describe a variety of assessment techniques for use with children within this approach. These include both rating methods and associative techniques—feeling scales, subjective units of discomfort scale, feeling charts, hand puppets, sentence completion techniques, think aloud approaches, and TAT-like approaches. These techniques promote verbal expression, help to clarify and measure perceived and actual emotional consequences, and elicit information about children's thoughts and beliefs. Similarly, Young (1983) discusses techniques for use with adolescents. Noting that adolescents generally will be open to more verbal assessment and therapeutic approaches and may be able to complete therapy-related homework assignments, therapists might ask them to describe in writing those problems encountered at school or at home in an A–B–C format. Specific forms are available for these homework assignments (Ellis & Grieger, 1977).

In general, rational–emotive therapy puts considerable emphasis on assessment and views assessment as an ongoing part of the therapeutic process. In addition to conducting interviews, the therapist may utilize a variety of rating tasks, written assignments when developmentally appropriate, and associative techniques. The rational–emotive therapist borrows techniques more commonly associated with other theoretical schools (e.g., puppet play, sentence completion, TAT-like approaches), but uses these techniques to elicit information relevant to the rational-emotive conceptualizations of the problem or problem situation.

Adlerian Therapy

The Adlerian theory of personality greatly emphasizes the influence of family and the development of life-style in children's early years. Life-style represents a basic orientation toward life providing a "guiding line" as the base of the personality that includes his or her complexes of prejudices, biased apperceptions, conclusions, and convictions (Dinkmeyer, Pew, & Dinkmeyer, 1979). Family influences are critical, particularly the birth order of the referred child compared to his or her siblings, the family constellation, and the family atmosphere. As the life-style develops, the individual's private logic, life plan, and fictional goals become a more important force in behavior.

According to Adlerian theory, the discrepancy between one's life-style and the reality of one's life experience is a factor in the development of psychopathology. Mental illness is viewed as a combination of mistaken beliefs, extreme discouragement, and a faulty private logic (Dinkmeyer & Dinkmeyer, 1983). "Neurotic" problems result from the condition of failure and discouragement. Neurotics possess basic common sense and are aware of what they should do, yet they avoid certain life tasks and/or choose incorrect paths of action. They may present an image of "really trying," but simply fail to accept the basic responsibilities of life. In this context, children's problems are best understood in terms of the goals of their behavior and misbehavior. Getting attention, showing their power, getting even, or furthering one's disability are the primary goals of children's misbehavior. Adolescent problems are interwoven with the task of value formation.

The role of formal psychological assessment within the therapeutic process is a subject of some debate among many Adlerians. Mosak (1979) states that Adlerians are divided on the issue of psychological testing and notes that most Adlerians avoid nosological diagnosis because it represents a static view of the individual and ignores personality growth and development. Older, European-trained Adlerians are strongly antitesting, but some more recently trained professionals do use some associative assessment techniques.

Adlerian therapists, much like rational-emotive therapists, conduct directed or semistructured interviews to obtain data relevant to understanding referred problems—all within their particular theoretical framework. Further, Adlerian practitioners have developed a number of assessment aids to assess individuals' life-styles including interview guides, life-style inventories, and self-report and rating scales (Dinkmeyer *et al.*, 1979). For example, Dinkmeyer and Dinkmeyer (1977) have developed the Children's Life-Style Guide (CLSG), a modification of a similar adult assessment instrument. The CLSG is a structured questionnaire that provides an outline and format for life-style assessment. First, children are asked to make comparisons between themselves and their siblings. The second section then deals with children's "psychological movement," eliciting information about their goals and beliefs and their attitudes about school, future plans, and social relationships. Children are also asked to describe their perceptions of each parent, how they feel they are treated at home, and to recall early childhood recollections and to specify "three wishes." The total assessment summarizes the child's beliefs about him or herself, the world, and others; describes the child's motivations (goals and intentions); and addresses the child's choices of behaviors to reach life goals. Adlerians place considerable importance on the life-style assessment, yet similar to other theories, they do not use psychological testing in the traditional sense.

Psychoanalytic/Psychodynamic Therapy

Psychoanalytic theory has perhaps the most extensively developed system of psychotherapy along with a well-detailed description of psychopathology. The basic tenets of the theory are described in Chapter 1 of this volume. While the validity of some of its basic assumptions and techniques is arguable, the depth and breadth of psychoanalytic theory for explaining human behavior is impressive. In fact, the extensiveness of the theory precludes a discussion of psychopathology in this brief context.

Psychoanalytic therapists, depending on their particular orientation within the analytic system, focus on a variety of internal person variables. The cornerstone of psychopathology is the model of intrapsychic conflict which occurs when an individual's id, ego, and superego forces are imbalanced (Weisz & Benoit, 1983). Understanding unconscious drives and forces and related defense mechanisms is thus seen as the key to understanding overt behavior. Psychosexual development is also important to the understanding of the child's developmental progress. Early trauma is seen as the basis of pathogenic behavior. The overall goals in assessment, therefore, include the assessment of the id, ego, and superego; determining what defense mechanisms are used by the individual; developing hypotheses about unconscious forces and probable conflicts; and relating these to current and/or fixated levels of psychosexual development.

According to Palmer (1970), most psychoanalytic approaches utilize formal psychological assessment and/or testing prior to the beginning of therapy. Most often, this includes the Rorschach (see Chapter 5) and/or one of a number of thematic assessment approaches (see Chapter 6). The psychoanalytic therapist also uses a variety of other techniques within the interview or therapy context. These include the interpretation of play, free association (generally for the older child or adolescent), and other associative techniques. The diagnostic play session can vary from a relatively nondirective assessment to structured play in a playroom set up with certain materials (e.g., a dollhouse, mother doll, father doll) to elicit specific information.

In general, psychoanalytic therapists conduct relatively formal and thorough diagnostic workups as part of the treatment process; assessment is a major component of this clinical work. This is an interesting contrast to the other theories of psychotherapy discussed above in that the psychodiagnostic and psychopathology aspects of this theory exist almost independently from its intervention techniques; that is, some practitioners consider psychoanalytic diagnostic assessment as an end in itself rather than a means to develop a treatment plan.

Self-Report Measures

Self-report measures, sometimes called objective personality measures, rely on individuals' reports of the problems they are experiencing or individuals' personal perceptions of their personality characteristics. These measures are often used in individual therapy to target clients' problems and to monitor therapeutic progress. Some practitioners, in fact, use brief self-report measures during each session for this latter purpose. Self-report measures are most often paper and pencil measures which require children or adolescents to rate themselves or to respond to the accuracy of statements (e.g., "Yes-No" or "True-False") which attempt to describe them. These measures have been used extensively with adults and increasingly with children and adolescents. The Minnesota Multiphasic Personality Inventory (MMPI) is the most frequently used self-report instrument, and it is seen by many as a prototype of this assessment technique.

Self-report measures generally fall into two categories; multiscale inventories and single scale measures. The typical multiscale measure assesses a number of variables within the same instrument; thus, scores are produced for a number of scales (representing these variables) within the administration of one measure. In addition to the economy of multidimensional assessment with multiscale measures (i.e., it is not necessary to separately assess different personality characteristics), they also allow for the differential assessment of their various characteristics. For example, the MMPI is well known for its use of profiled configurations, or combinations, of scales to more precisely assess personality problems. Further, multiscale measures are less likely to obscure important characteristics that may be related to primary presenting problems.

From a negative perspective, multiscale measures have the disadvantage of being longer and more time consuming, and thus less likely to be used continuously to assess therapeutic change. The single scale measures (although many do have subscales) usually focus on one clinical variable. Depression, anxiety, and self-esteem are among the most common variables to be assessed by single scale measures. The measures tend to be briefer and most useful when the presenting clinical problem is moderately well defined and when data are desired about its intensity or severity. Because of their brevity, they can be used regularly during the therapeutic process to monitor change. However, a significant disadvantage is that they are not comprehensive, and thus, they assess clinical variables individually—isolated from other variables. For example, anxiety and depression often occur together clinically. If only a depression measure is used, some critical aspect of treatment related to anxiety may be overlooked.

The objective measures have been developed through three general test development approaches: factor analysis, criterion-keyed or empirically based approaches, and rational or content-oriented approaches. Item selection during factor analysis is primarily based on a statistical correlational model which determines how well individual items "hang together" in factors. Each factor's label is based on the apparent theme or content shared by the items that correlate together. The criterion-keyed approach bases its item selection on the degree to which an individual item correlates with or is answered by specific clinical groups. For example, if "depressed" individuals tend to consistently respond to an item in a certain way, then that item would be placed on a depression scale.

A criticism of both these approaches is that item selection decisions are primarily statistically based and may make little sense from a clinical standpoint. For example, consider the two items "I like to watch ice hockey" and "I am often sad." If the first item correlated with other items reflecting depression (i.e., factor analysis), or if depressed individuals tended to give a certain response to that item (i.e., criterion-keyed), then that item could be placed on a depression scale even though there is no rational link between ice hockey and depression. Conversely, if the second item reflecting sadness was not statistically reliable or predictive, it could be omitted from a depression scale despite the fact that a report of sadness is viewed as a primary characteristic of depressed clients. While this situation is unlikely to occur, it is possible within the statistically based models. The rational approach, on the other hand, selects items based on practitioners' or researchers' clinical knowledge about the problem or characteristic. Thus, specific items can be included on a measure even if they do not meet statistical criteria. The sadness item, therefore, could be included on a depression scale even if depressed individuals tended to respond to it in a random fashion.

Needless to say, there has been considerable debate among personality test developers about the relative merits of various item selection approaches. Interestingly, the three approaches discussed above tend to produce remarkably similar scales (see Burisch, 1984, for a clear and entertaining discussion of these issues). Further, many tests are constructed using a combination of these approaches. The last section of this chapter will briefly describe some general measures of personality and some self-report measures of depression, anxiety, and self-esteem that can be used with children and/or adolescents.

General Self-Report Measures

As mentioned above, the MMPI is often considered the prototype of the self-report personality inventory. The basic scale is 566 items long, produces 10 clinical scales and 4 validity scales, and was developed using a criterion-keyed approach. This approach is similar to that used to develop the Personality Inventory for Children (see Chapter 9 of this volume).

The MMPI has probably been the subject of more clinical research studies in recent years than any other individual psychological test. As a result, there are literally hundreds of other clinical scales that have been developed using its basic item pool and test construction approach. While the MMPI is primarily used with adults, it has also been appied clinically with adolescents, although the basic norms are likely to yield somewhat distorted interpretations when used with adolescents (French, Graves, & Levitt, 1983). Norms exist for adolescents as young as 14 (Marks, Seeman, & Haller, 1974), and Hathaway and Monachesi (1961) have compiled descriptions of adolescent profiles.

Cattell, Eber, and Tatsuoka (1970) used a factor analytic approach to develop the Sixteen Personality Factor (16 PF) Questionnaire. This instrument is designed to be factorially pure, with each scale assessing a basic aspect of personality structure. This measure tends to relate to more normal personality patterns as opposed to the pathological patterns emphasized by the MMPI. Using the same statistical approach and developmentally appropriate adaptations, Cattell and his colleagues have also developed the High School Personality Questionnaire (ages 12–18), the Children's Personality Questionnaire (ages 8–12), and the Early School Personality Questionnaire (ages 6–8). Included among the traits measured on these scales are intelligence, emotional stability, dominance, conscientiousness, enthusiasm, shrewdness, sensitivity, anxiety, extraversion, independence, and creativity.

Recently, Millon, Green, and Meagher (1983) introduced the Millon Adolescent Personality Inventory with items specifically designed for adolescent populations. Using a combination of test construction procedures, this scale has both a factor analytic and external validation base. The scale produces scores in three areas: personality styles, expressed concerns, and behavior correlates. The dimensions measured include normal personality patterns (e.g., introversive, inhibited, confident, forceful) as well as scales to assess more clinical concerns (e.g., self-concept, peer security, impulse control). The scale, however, is not as clinically oriented as the MMPI; nor is it as oriented toward normal personality patterns as the 16 PF series of instruments.

Measures of Depression

The concept of childhood depression, and its existence, have been controversial until only recently. Historically, much of the clinical literature on depression has hypothesized that children could not experience "true" depression because they were not at sufficient cognitive and/or emotional levels of development. This view has now been abandoned by most researchers and practitioners in the field (Costello, 1981; Lefkowitz & Burton, 1978). Nonetheless, the assessment of depression in children is a relatively recent phenomenon.

Perhaps the best known single measure of depression is the Beck Depression Inventory (Beck, Ward, Mendelsohn, Mock, & Erbaugh, 1961). This is a 21-item scale where the client chooses one of four statements, arranged by the severity of the symptom, to describe each item. The scale is recommended as a way to monitor the treatment of depression, and it has norms available for its use with adolescents (Teri, 1982).

Specific to other measures of depression, Kovacs and Beck (1977) developed a downward extension of the Beck Depression Inventory, the Children's Depression Inventory, for use with children as young as 8. The items on this scale have developmentally appropriate language and use a three-statement format instead of the four statements described above. As with the adult version, a single depression score is produced. Lang and Tisher (1978) have developed the Children's Depression Scale (CDS) where children describe themselves, guided by a series of statements, using a 5-point rating scale which extends from a "very right" to a "very wrong" description. The scale produces two main scores, one for depressive symptoms and one for reports of pleasurable or positive experiences, and hypothesizes that depressed children *will* report their depressive symptoms as well as a few things that they find positive in their lives. The depression scale also yields six subscales: affective response, social problems, self-esteem, preoccupation with own sickness and death, guilt, and pleasure. A unique aspect of the CDS is that it also provides a format that allows adults who know the child to make similar sets of ratings.

Measures of Anxiety

The measurement of anxiety in children has received considerable attention from researchers and practitioners. For example, Barios, Hartman, and Shigetomi (1981) listed 17 self-report measures of anxiety or fear from their extensive review. These measures range from situationally specific instruments to those that assess general anxiety. As an example of the former, Sarason, Davidson, Lighthall, Waite, and Ruebush (1960) developed the Test Anxiety Scale for Children to assess anxieties specifically related to test and school situations.

Currently, two general measures of anxiety are most frequently used with children: the Revised Children's Manifest Anxiety Scale (RCMAS) and the State–Trait Anxiety Inventory for Children (STAIC). Both of these measures are downward extensions of instruments developed originally for use with adults. The RCMAS was developed by Reynolds and Richmond (1978) as a revision of an earlier scale authored by Castenada, McCandless, and Palermo (1956). Given the RCMAS's series of statements, the child decides whether each item applies to him or her, responding appropriately with a "Yes" or "No." In addition to a general anxiety score, the RCMAS has subscales for Physiological Anxiety, Worry and Oversensitivity, and Concentration Anxiety, and a Lie scale. Recent grade-by-grade national norms have been published for elementary and high school students (Reynolds & Paget, 1983).

The STAIC (Spielberger, 1973) is based on Spielberger's well-known work emphasizing two distinct types of anxiety: state anxiety, which is related to situational variables and is subject to varying degrees of stress, and trait anxiety which is viewed as a more stable personality characteristic. The STAIC produces scores for both of these dimensions and asks children to rate themselves on current feelings (how you feel right now) and on more general descriptions of themselves and their affect.

Measures of Self-Esteem

As previously noted in this chapter, the individual's view of self—whether it is called self-concept, self-esteem, self-acceptance, or identity—plays an important role in a variety of the therapeutic approaches and personality theories. Improving self-concept is often a therapeutic goal, and problems with poor self-concept or low self-esteem are frequently viewed as related to other client-specific disorders and problems. In fact, many therapists, particularly those adhering to "humanistic" perspectives, feel that the improvement of clients' self-concepts or self-esteems decreases or eliminates problems like anxiety, depression, or acting out. The measurement of this concept has a long history in applied psychology. Unfortunately, there is some disagreement on specific definitions, and the terms cited above are not necessarily interchangeable (Goodstein & Doller, 1978). Indeed, the accurate perception of oneself can be vastly different from how one values him- or herself.

A variety of self-esteem and self-concept measures have been developed for use with children and/or adolescents. The Tennessee Self-Concept Scale (Fitts, 1964) consists of a series of self-descriptive statements from which an individual chooses one of five responses from "completely true of me" to "completely false of me." The scale produces a variety of subscales (e.g., social self, family self) as well as a total positive self-concept score. This scale may be used with clients over 12 years of age.

Lipsitt (1958) developed the Self-Concept Rating Scale for Children, which has children rate themselves on a series of trait-descriptive adjectives that are each preceded by "I am. . . . " The 5-point rating scale allows children to rate a trait from "not at all" to "all of the time." Lipsitt also developed The Ideal Self-Rating Scale for Children using the same trait adjectives introduced instead with the stem "I would like to be. . . . " Scores are produced on each scale and then combined for a discrepancy score.

Coopersmith (1959) modified a scale originally developed by Rogers and Dymond (1954) to produce a children's Self-Esteem Inventory. Items are checked "like me" or "unlike me" to describe how the child usually feels. The scale assesses the child's perceptions in four areas: peers, parents, school, and family.

The most widely used instrument for assessing children's self-concept is the Piers–Harris Self-Concept Scale (Piers, 1969), which is entitled "The way I feel about myself." This scale can be used with third to twelfth graders and uses a "Yes/No" format for a series of child-appropriate statements. Although the scale statistically shows a number of factors, its single score is considered to be an adequate general measure of self-concept (Goodstein & Doller, 1978).

Summary

This chapter has focused on and advocated the use of personality and behavioral assessment within the context of counseling and psychotherapy with children and adolescents. Personality and behavioral assessment has a number of purposes in planning, selecting, monitoring, and evaluating therapeutic intervention; further, it can serve as the foundation for a systematic approach to intervention. This chapter has also espoused a multimodal and "intelligent eclecticism" view of conducting interventions with children, suggesting that practitioners choose among a variety of intervention strategies and that these interventions be multifaceted.

The major theories of counseling and psychotherapy presented in this chapter all have different views of the role of assessment in their particular therapeutic theories. These views range from considerable emphasis on the therapy/assessment interface to those that place almost no value on assessment as a facilitator of therapeutic change. In addition to the various assessment approaches discussed in this book, self-report objective measures are seen as having particular value for counselors and therapists. Currently, personality assessment and therapeutic intervention are often loosely linked. Future developments hopefully will foster a closer bond between these two clinical activities.

References

Axline, V. (1947). *Play therapy*. Boston: Houghton-Mifflin.

Barios, B. A., Hartman, D. P., & Shigetomi, C. (1981). Fears and anxieties in children. In E. J. Marsh & L. G. Terdal (Eds.), *Behavioral assessment of childhood disorders* (pp. 259–304). New York: Guilford Press.

Barrett, C. L., Hampe, I. E., & Miller, L. (1978). Research on psychotherapy with children. In S. L. Garfield & A. E. Bergin (Eds.), *Handbook of psychotherapy and behavior change* (2nd ed., pp. 411–436). New York: Wiley.

Beck, A. T., Ward, C. H., Mendelson, M., Mock, J., & Erbaugh, J. (1961). An inventory for measuring depression. *Archives of General Psychiatry, 4*, 53–63.

Brown, J. H., & Brown, C. S. (1977). *Systematic counseling*. Champaign, IL: Research Press.

Burisch, M. (1984). Approaches to personality scale construction: A comparison of merits. *American Psychologist, 39*, 214–227.

Castenada, A., McCandless, B. R., & Palermo, D. S. (1956). The children's form of the manifest anxiety scale. *Child Development, 27*, 317–326.

Cattell, R. B., Eber, H. W., & Tatsuoka, M. M. (1970). *Handbook for the Sixteen Personality Factor Questionnaire (16 PF)*. Champaign, IL: Institute for Personality and Ability Testing.

Coopersmith, S. A. (1959). A method for determining types of self-esteem. *Journal of Abnormal and Social Psychology, 59*, 87–94.

Costello, C. G. (1981). Childhood depression. In E. J. Mash & L. G. Terdal, (Eds), *Behavioral assessment of childhood disorders* (pp. 305–346). New York: Guilford Press.

Dailey, C. A. (1953). The practical utility of the psychological report. *Journal of Consulting Psychology, 17*, 297–302.

DiGiuseppe, R., & Bernard, M. E. (1983). Principles of assessment and methods of treatment with children: Special considerations. In A. Ellis & M. E. Bernard (Eds.), *Rational-emotive approaches to the problems of childhood* (pp. 45–88). New York: Plenum Press.

Dinkmeyer, D., & Dinkmeyer, D., Jr. (1977). Concise counseling assessment: The children's life style guide. *Elementary School Guidance and Counseling, 12*, 117–126.

Dinkmeyer, D., & Dinkmeyer, D., Jr. (1983). Adlerian approaches. In H. T. Prout & D. T. Brown (Eds.), *Counseling and psychotherapy with children and adolescents* (pp. 287–328). Tampa, FL: Mariner.

Dinkmeyer, D., Pew, W. L., & Dinkmeyer, D., Jr. (1979). *Adlerian counseling and psychotherapy*. Monterey, CA: Brooks/Cole.

Ellis, A. (1977). The basic clinical theory of rational-emotive theory. In A. Ellis & R. Greiger (Eds.), *Handbook of rational-emotive therapy* (pp. 3–34). New York: Springer.

Ellis, A., & Greiger, R. (Eds.). (1977). *Handbook of rational-emotive therapy*. New York: Springer.

Fitts, W. H. (1964). Tennessee Self-Concept Scale. Nashville, TN: Counselor Recordings and Tests, Department of Mental Health.

French, J., Graves, P. A., & Levitt, E. E. (1983). Objective and projective testing of children. In C. E. Walker & M. C. Roberts (Eds.), *Handbook of clinical child psychology* (pp. 209–243). New York: Wiley.

Fuller, G. B., & Fuller, D. L. (1983). Reality therapy approaches. In H. T. Prout & D. T. Brown (Eds.), *Counseling and psychotherapy with children and adolescents* (pp. 165–222). Tampa, FL: Mariner.

Glasser, W. (1965). *Reality therapy*. New York: Harper & Row.

Glasser, W., & Zunin, I. (1979). Reality therapy. In R. J. Corsini (Ed.), *Current psychotherapies* (pp. 302–339). Itasca, IL: F. E. Peacock.

Goldfried, M. R., & Linehan, M. M. (1977). Basic issues in behavioral assessment. In A. R. Ciminoro, K. S. Calhoun, & H. E. Adams (Eds.), *Handbook of behavioral assessment* (pp. 15–46). New York: Wiley.

Goodstein, L. D., & Doller, D. L. (1978). The measurement of the self-concept. In B. B. Wolman, *Clinical diagnosis of mental disorders* (pp. 445–474). New York: Plenum Press.

Gottman, J. M., & Leiblum, S. R. (1974). *How to do psychotherapy and how to evaluate it*. New York: Holt, Rinehart, & Winston.

Gresham, F. (1983). Multitrait-multimethod approach to multifactoral assessment: Theoretical rationale and application. *School Psychology Review, 12,* 26–34.

Grieger, R. M., & Boyd, J. B. (1980). *Rational-emotive therapy: A skills based approach*. Princeton, NJ: Van Nostrand-Reinhold.

Grieger, R. M., & Boyd, J. B. (1983). Rational-emotive approaches. In H. T. Prout & D. T. Brown (Eds.), *Counseling and psychotherapy with children and adolescents* (pp. 101–164). Tampa, FL: Mariner.

Grieger, R. M., & Grieger, J. (Eds.). (1982). *Cognition and emotional disturbance*. New York: Human Sciences Press.

Hathaway, S. R., & Monachesi, E. D. (1961). *An atlas of juvenile MMPI profiles*. Minneapolis: University of Minnesota Press.

Kanfer, F. H., & Saslow, G. (1969). Behavioral diagnosis. In C. M. Franks (Ed.), *Behavior therapy: An appraisal and status* (pp. 417–444). New York: McGraw-Hill.

Keat, D. B. (1979). *Multimodal therapy with children*. Oxford: Pergamon Press.

Keefe, F. J., Kopel, S. A., & Gordon, S. B. (1978). *A practical guide to behavioral assessment*. New York: Springer.

Kovacs, M., & Beck, A. T. (1977). An empirical-clinical approach toward a definition of childhood depression. In J. G. Shchulterbrandt & A. Raskin (Eds.), *Depression in childhood: Diagnosis, treatment and conceptual models* (pp. 43–57). New York: Raven Press.

Lang, M., & Tisher, M. (1978). *Children's depression scale*. Hawthorn, Victoria, Australia: Australian Council for Education Research Limited.

Lazarus, A. A. (1976). *Multimodal behavior therapy*. New York: Springer.

Lazarus, A. A. (1981). *The practice of multimodal therapy*. New York: McGraw-Hill.

Lefkowitz, M. M., & Burton, W. (1978). Childhood depression: A critique of the concept. *Psychological Bulletin, 85,* 716–726.

Lipsitt, L. P. (1958). A self-concept scale for children and its relationship to the children's form of the Manifest Anxiety Scale. *Child Development, 29,* 463–472.

MacFarlane, J., Allen, L., & Honzik, M. (1954). *A developmental study of the behavior problems of normal children between twenty-one months and fourteen years*. Berkeley: University of California Press.

Marks, P. A., Seeman, W., & Haller, D. L. (1974). *The actuarial use of the MMPI with adolescents and adults*. Baltimore, MD: Williams & Wilkins.

Mash, E. J., & Terdal, L. G. (Eds.). (1981). *Behavioral assessment of childhood disorders*. New York: Guilford Press.

Meador, B. D., & Rogers, C. R. (1979). Person-centered therapy. In R. J. Corsini (Ed.), *Current psychotherapies* (pp. 131–184). Itasca, IL: F. E. Peacock.

Millon, T., Green, C. G., & Meagher, R. B. (1983). *Millon Adolescent Personality Inventory*. Minneapolis; MN: Interpretive Scoring Systems.

Moore, H. B. (1983). Person-centered approaches. In H. T. Prout & D. T. Brown (Eds.), *Counseling and psychotherapy with children and adolescents* (pp. 223–286). Tampa; FL: Mariner.

Mosak, H. H. (1979). Adlerian psychotherapy. In R. J. Corsini (Ed.), *Current psychotherapies* (pp. 44–94). Itasca, IL: F. E. Peacock.

Nay, W. R. (1979). *Multimethod clinical assessment*. New York: Gardner Press.

Nelson, R. O., & Hayes, S. C. (1981). Nature of behavioral assessment. In M. Hersen & A. S. Bellack (Eds.), *Behavioral assessment* (pp. 3–37). Oxford: Pergamon Press.

Ollendick, T. H., & Hersen, M. (1984). *Child behavioral assessment: Principles and procedures*. Oxford: Pergamon Press.

Palmer, J. O. (1970). *The psychological assessment of children*. New York: Wiley.

Piers, E. V. (1969). *Manual for the Piers-Harris Children's Self-Concept Scale (The way I feel about myself)*. Nashville, TN: Counselor Recordings and Tests.

Prout, H. T. (1977). Behavioral intervention with hyperactive children: A review. *Journal of Learning Disabilities, 10*, 141–146.

Prout, H. T. (1983). Counseling and psychotherapy with children and adolescents: An overview. In H. T. Prout & D. T. Brown (Eds.), *Counseling and psychotherapy with children and adolescents* (pp. 1–34). Tampa, FL: Mariner.

Prout, H. T., & Brown, D. T. (Eds.). (1983a). *Counseling and psychotherapy with children and adolescents*. Tampa, FL: Mariner.

Prout, H. T., & Brown, D. T. (1983b). Summary and comparisons of approaches. In H. T. Prout & D. T. Brown & (Eds.), *Counseling and psychotherapy with children and adolescents* (pp. 425–448). Tampa, FL: Mariner.

Prout, H. T., & Harvey, J. R. (1978). Applications of desensitization procedures for school-related problems: A review. *Psychology in the Schools, 15*, 533–541.

Reynolds, C. T., & Paget, K. D. (1983). National normative and reliability data for the Revised Children's Manifest Anxiety Scale. *School Psychology Review, 12*, 324–336.

Reynolds, C. T., & Richmond, B. O. (1978). What I think and feel: A revised measure of children's manifest anxiety. *Journal of Abnormal Child Psychology, 6*, 271–280.

Rogers, C. R. (1951). *Client-centered therapy*. Boston, MA: Houghton-Mifflin.

Rogers, C. R. (1959). A theory of therapy, personality, and interpersonal relationships. In S. Koch (Ed.), *Psychology: A study of a science (Vol. III.): Formulation of the person and the social context* (pp. 119–132). New York: McGraw-Hill.

Rogers, C. R., & Dymond, R. F. (1954). *Psychotherapy and personality change*. Chicago, IL: University of Chicago Press.

Ross, A. O. (1980). *Psychological disorders of children*. New York: McGraw-Hill.

Sarason, S. B., Davidson, K. S., Lighthall, F. F., Waite, R. R., & Ruebush, B. K. (1960). *Anxiety in elementary school children*. New York: Wiley.

Spielberger, C. D. (1973). *Manual for the state-trait anxiety inventory for children*. Palo Alto, CA: Consulting Psychologists Press.

Tallent, N. (1976). *Psychological report writing*. Englewood Cliffs, NJ: Prentice-Hall.

Teri, L. (1982). The use of the Beck Depression Inventory with adolescents. *Journal of Abnormal Child Psychology, 10*, 277–284.

Weisz, F., & Benoit, C. (1983). Psychoanalytic approaches. In H. T. Prout & D. T. Brown (Eds.), *Counseling and psychotherapy with children and adolescents* (pp. 329–388). Tampa, FL: Mariner.

Young, H. S. (1983). Principles of assessment and methods of treatment with adolescents: Special considerations. In A. Ellis & M. E. Bernard (Eds.), *Rational-emotive approaches to the problems of childhood* (pp. 89–108). New York: Plenum Press.

IV
Summation and Integration

A final chapter is used to summarize the major perspectives and recommended practices throughout this book with an eye toward the strengths and weaknesses of the personality assessment process and the future needs in this important research and service-delivery area.

Conclusions and Future Needs in Personality Assessment

Howard M. Knoff

To conclude and summarize this book, a discussion of three predominant dimensions of personality assessment is necessary. These relate to the practice of personality assessment—from the problem identification and analysis to intervention and evaluation steps; the need for ongoing research to further improve individual personality assessment tests and techniques and to evaluate the efficacy of assessment models, procedures, and decisions; and the training of personality assessment processes in preservice, internship, and continuing education domains. This summary chapter will review the major points made throughout this book, organized by these three dimensions, emphasizing future needs in the field of personality assessment.

The Practice of Personality Assessment

1. *Personality assessment is a hypothesis-testing, problem-solving process that works within a probability model.*

The personality assessment process, as discussed consistently throughout this book, involves the steps of problem identification, problem analysis, intervention, and evaluation. Each step builds onto the next such that logical, meaningful, and conceptually planned intervention programs arise from the assessment activities, analyses, and interpretations. These interventions result directly from hypotheses which, based on the assessment data (e.g., from interviews, observations, direct testing), explain the referred or actual problem and suggest problem resolution directions. These hypotheses are refined and tested clinically and/or empirically throughout the assessment process, yet often most consciously during the evaluation of intervention efficacy and client satisfaction.

Despite the logic and organization of the personality assessment process,

Howard M. Knoff. Department of Psychological and Social Foundations of Education, School Psychology Program, University of South Florida, Tampa, Florida.

mental health practitioners still will never be able to predict without error how an individual will behave or emotionally react in all situations or environments. This is because there are too many overt and covert (intrapersonally) and direct and indirect (interpersonally and environmentally) variables which differentially, and sometimes unpredictably, influence and affect children and/or adolescents at any point in time. The vast number of variables and interactions, in addition to the complexity of what we call "personality," preclude the practitioner from assessing every conceivable dimension of a referred child or adolescent. Thus, practitioners, during the personality assessment process, attempt to sample strategic aspects of personality utilizing those assessments that give the best picture of the referred child.

The personality assessment process, therefore, proceeds with the concurrent goals of minimizing the probability of diagnostic and practitioner error while maximizing the probability of a successful intervention program. Implicit in these goals, *and* the hypothesis-testing model and the lack of perfect prediction in personality assessment noted above, is the existence of probability. Indeed, probability is evident throughout the assessment process, for example, in the probability of choosing the correct referral problems, the correct and most effective assessment procedures, the correct interpretations and conclusions, and the correct intervention strategies. Practitioners structure and complete their assessment procedures seeking high probability of success results. Perfection is not expected (indeed, it is impossible), but persistence and the ability to generate new directions and strategies in the face of transient setbacks *is* expected.

2. *Personality assessment is a multitrait, multisetting, multimethod assessment approach which is sensitive to the ecological and reciprocally determined nature of personality.*

Throughout this book, each chapter has added a conceptual and pragmatic building block to what has become a multimodal, multimethod approach to personality assessment. Using Bandura's (1978) reciprocal determinism model which analyzes personality through the interaction of behavioral, person-oriented, and environmental domains, the problem-solving process of personality assessment was systematically expanded to include Nay (1979) and Gresham's (1983) multimethod assessment approaches, Lazarus's (1981) multimodal theoretical approaches, the seven (or eight) theoretical explanations of disturbed behavior, Bronfenbrenner's (1979) ecological approaches, and Knoff's (1984) multimodal consultation approaches. The integration of all of these approaches demonstrates, once again, (*a*) the complexity of personality and the personality assessment process, (*b*) the need for a hypothesis-testing, probability-based perspective toward assessment, and (*c*) the advantage of being "technically eclectic" (Lazarus, 1981), that is, of having the ability to integrate different theoretical and conceptual perspectives into the personality assessment process and to apply different procedures and interventions correctly and appropriately even when they are not consistent with practitioners' personally accepted theoretical orientations or models.

3. *Personality assessment should be practiced morally, ethically, and from an orientation of advocacy and respect for client rights.*

Relatively speaking, personality assessment procedures have not received significant amounts of attention through litigation in state or federal courts of law. Professionally, however, most associations representing the various groups of mental health practitioners have ethical principles and standards which include guidelines addressing the practice of personality assessment. For example, the American Psychological Association has standards addressing the construction and publication of assessment tests and procedures, the professional practice of psychology, and the professional practice of its currently recognized specialty groups in psychology: school, counseling, clinical, and industrial organization. While there are no assurances that adherence to a professional association's ethical standards will prevent litigations focused on the personality assessment process, these standards do provide some protection from individual liability and some demonstration of professional accountability if followed.

More generally, an orientation toward advocacy and respect for client rights is strongly recommended as an on-going practice and philosophy for all practitioners. Practitioners should have children's and adolescents' best interests in their thoughts and actions at all times, even if this requires professional decisions and recommendations that are unpopular with supervisors and/or employing schools or agencies. Practitioners should clearly identify their primary client(s), their biases and conflicting interests, and the skills and special expertises that they have available to address referred problems or concerns. Further, they must be sensitive to the potential implications and consequences to those participating in any facet of a personality assessment, as well as to the potential complications of labels, special remedial placements and programs, and lapses in professional confidentiality.

4. *The implications of school versus clinic or agency referrals, involvements, and intervention programs should be acknowledged and planned for during the personality assessment process involving children and adolescents.*

Personality assessment completed by school practitioners is different from personality assessment completed by clinic or agency practitioners. Similarly, intervention programs implemented by or in school versus agency settings often significantly differ. Generally, mental health services and perspectives in school settings are guided by a psychology × education interaction; that is, disturbed "psychological" behavior is primarily identified (*a*) by its impact on the referred child's educational and developmental progress, and (*b*) by its ability to disrupt others' educational progress. Similarly, school-based interventions are developed not only to resolve social–emotional, behavioral, or self-image problems, but also to facilitate a return to educational progress and learning. Agency-based personality assessment, meanwhile, can look more purely at the child's or adolescent's psychological status and needs. Intervention here is often focused on psychological change, although an agency might consult with school personnel to help them understand the intervention programs and their implications for educational practice.

Clearly, mental health practitioners must be aware of and sensitive to the differences between school and agency referrals, assessments, and intervention programs while making referral sources and, in certain cases, referred individuals aware of their differences and implications. These differences also need more research attention such that service delivery in both of these settings can become more effective and comprehensive.

Research in Personality Assessment

5. *Personality assessment is not yet a science, but should maintain that as an aspiration and goal.*

The entire personality assessment process, from problem identification to evaluation, must continue to be actively researched so that the most effective and empirically based procedures can be identified for use in the field. Practitioners should recognize that many decisions required during the comprehensive personality assessment process currently are based on clinical, not empirical, judgments; that is, (*a*) the empirical research has not addressed many of these process areas, and (*b*) practitioners sometimes rely more on their clinical training and experience than on the results of the available, methodologically sound research evaluating assessment practices and programs. While I do not believe that the need for clinical judgment will ever become unnecessary, especially given the complexity of referred problems noted above, certainly research results can highlight the most significant procedures, variables, or characteristics present and interacting given specific types of referrals and referral situations. This empirical emphasis, therefore, can decrease practitioners' potential for clinical error, for example, when specific decisions are required during the assessment process, by increasing the appropriateness, reliability, and validity of the data available to guide those decisions. Given additional research, especially in the use of the multimethod model, assessment decisions and conclusions can become more empirically and clinically defensible in the field.

Given the discussions in this book, a number of research areas are evident and necessary. These include the need for research:

1. To validate the existence of the seven (or eight) theories explaining emotionally disturbed or disturbing behavior and to investigate their individual contributions to the multimodal, multimethod perspective of personality assessment.

2. To improve current classification systems for emotionally disturbed children and adolescents, based more directly on empirical (e.g., actuarial) data. This can potentially improve interprofessional communication, assessment to intervention efficacy, and generalizations of clinical work with specific disturbed samples.

3. To investigate the effectiveness and to validate and refine the multimodal, multimethod assessment process, its impact on referral children and adolescents across time and settings, and its effects on the social psychological/therapeutic change process across specifically involved ecosystems.

4. To evaluate the psychometric properties of existing personality assessment tests, techniques, and procedures—from diagnostic interviews to behavioral approaches to projective techniques to family and ecological assessments—thereby validating their existences as appropriate tools which produce meaningful and reliable results.

5. To identify personality domains and characteristics not addressed by existing personality assessment tests and procedures, and to remediate those needs by constructing well-standardized tests which have sound psychometric properties and documented clinical utility.

6. To continue the evaluation and development of automated personality assessment procedures and other computer applications directed at the personality assessment process and its resulting services for referred children and adolescents.

7. To further clarify the psychological change process such that intervention programs can be more reliably and validly identified given specific as-

sessment conditions, results, and characteristics, and so that the differential effectiveness of multimodal therapeutic and/or consultation approaches can be demonstrated.

8. To ascertain the overall efficacy of mental health services, from tertiary to secondary to primary prevention approaches, such that professional integrity and accountability are evident and so that our professional practices can be defended as necessary and important to the continuing development of sound mental health in our children, adolescents, communities, and society.

The call for additional research validating the multimodal, multimethod assessment process reinforces a major assumption echoed throughout this book: that this is currently the most defensible personality assessment approach available to mental health practitioners. Briefly, the effectiveness of this approach has been demonstrated using separate models developed by Campbell and Fiske (1959) and Cronbach and Gleser (1957). Campbell and Fiske's multitrait–multimethod model provides an approach to establish the construct validity of different psychological tests or techniques while facilitating a conceptual understanding of the personality assessment process and its classification and intervention components. The multitrait–multimethod can evaluate separate traits (e.g., hyperactivity, conduct disorder, and aggressiveness) measured by different methods (e.g., observation, standardization tests) determining (a) if the methods adequately measure the trait and (b) if the traits are functionally similar or distinct (Gresham, 1983). Thus, this model, through continuing research, can evaluate psychodiagnostic tools in a personality assessment battery and their ability to validly, consistently, and meaningfully assess empirically derived traits.

Cronbach and Gleser's (1957) model also assesses practitioners' use of personality assessment procedures and their contributions toward accurate classification and effective intervention. This model, however, involves decision-making theory and emphasizes the validity of the decision process and results (i.e., placement and programming) as opposed to the independent validities of specific tests and techniques. Each test, therefore, is evaluated on its contribution to the decision process by investigating how recommended and implemented services, based on assessment data, results, and analyses, correlate with therapeutic and functional change. Decision-making theory, according to Rabin and Hayes (1978), clearly points to the need for multimethod assessment batteries.

Both models have received support in the theoretical and research literature (Cascio & Silbey, 1979; Gresham, 1983; Nay, 1979). Additional research, however, is necessary to apply this support to different types of personality-related referral problems and to make these general assessment models more known and routinely used by mental health practitioners.

Training for Effective Personality Assessment

6. *Personality assessment is both a content and a process-oriented skill which requires sound training, supervision, and continuing education.*

Very little research is available documenting the most effective ways to teach personality assessment to graduate-level students or advanced practitioners. Thus, any discussion of training, supervision, and continuing education needs in personality assessment reflects one's personal experiences and biases while, at the same time, identifying potential research hypotheses that need to be empirically validated.

In my opinion, personality assessment is a skill that develops over time with training, supervision, and on-going experience. While there are individual differences among mental health practitioners with regard to their clinical insight and their abilities to conceptualize referral problems and directions and to integrate vast amounts of diverse data, personality assessment training and experience, nonetheless, provide the critical foundations which allow these differences to surface.

Training in personality assessment involves much of the content that practitioners need to deal with the technical aspects of the process: for example, learning what the theories of disturbed and disturbing behavior or personality are; how specific assessment tools are constructed, evaluated, given, scored, and interpreted; and what the research says about specific interventions for specific childhood disturbances or disorders. All practitioners need this theoretical and practical knowledge, usually provided in a classroom setting or through individual research and reading, to put the assessment process and its specific component procedures and activities into a professional context. To simply give a projective or some other assessment technique without any previous training or experience in personality assessment is dangerous (to the referred child when inappropriate recommendations result from poor assessment procedures and/or interpretations) and, in my mind, potentially unethical. Consistent with Lazarus's notion (1981) of the technical eclectic, practitioners must be sure of their technical training and knowledge before attempting personality assessments, even under supervised conditions.

Supervision is critical during practitioners' first years in the field (whether in an internship or actual job setting) as they begin to do more case-related personality assessments. (Note that I refuse to specify how many years are necessary because this is practitioner- and situation-specific and often of a qualitative nature.) Regardless of one's classroom training and knowledge, no instructor or book can adequately simulate the complexities of an actual personality assessment referral and process. Not only must practitioners individualize and apply the specific skills learned during training, but they must do it while individualizing the assessment to the unique ecosystem of the referred child or adolescent and the characteristics of the referred setting (e.g., school or agency). Clearly, every case referred for personality assessment has its own idiosyncrasies, and practitioners benefit from supervised experiences across many cases so that a broad foundation of knowledge and application of skills develops over time. Thus, there is no substitute for clinical experience and supervision because they allow practitioners (*a*) to implement and test their knowledge and training under realistic circumstances and conditions, and (*b*) to learn from these case experiences *and* from the close guidance of a more knowledgeable, experienced colleague, yet (*c*) to be protected from conceptual and technical errors occurring during the personality assessment process due to their inexperience and/or misapplication of knowledge. To expand this latter point, the supervision process protects referred clients from errors made by inexperienced practitioners due to lack of skill, knowledge, confidence, or objectivity. Supervision, therefore, is the process part of personality assessment training. This experiential process is a necessary part of training; the knowledge of assessment theories and techniques is necessary but *not* sufficient to develop effective practitioner skills and expertise.

Continuing education involves both the content and process components of personality assessment skill building. As documented by this book, personality assessment models, theories, and practices continue to flourish. This places a professional burden on practitioners in the field to continually maintain their skills by updating their knowledge (the content) and experience (the process). Continuing education could involve, for example, on-going reading in the field; attending workshops, seminars, or university courses; obtaining new assessment tools for critical use and review; or participating in a colleague study group which discusses innovations in the field. Regardless of the type of involvement, continuing education is a professionally necessary activity—it is recommended by most professional associations and mandated, in fact, by some states for on-going certification or licensure.

Summary

Personality assessment with children and adolescents is a common, on-going activity in mental health practice. This book has been dedicated to the practice, research, and training of personality assessment for all mental health practitioners (e.g., psychologists, social workers, counselors, and therapists). While this is a comprehensive text, in my opinion, this book should not be used as a license attesting to practitioners' expertise in personality assessment. Rather, I hope that it becomes part of one's training, a basis for another's practical experience, and/or a foundation for others' continuing education in what will continue to be a vibrant, changing, and often controversial field.

References

Bandura, A. (1978). The self-system in reciprocal determinism. *American Psychologist, 33*, 344–358.

Bronfenbrenner, U. (1979). *The ecology of human development*. Cambridge, MA: Harvard University Press.

Campbell, D. T., & Fiske, D. W. (1959). Convergent and discriminant validation by the multitrait-multimethod matrix. *Psychological Bulletin, 56*, 81–105.

Cascio, W. F., & Silbey, V. (1979). Utility of the assessment center as a selection device. *Journal of Applied Psychology, 64*, 107–118.

Cronbach, L. E., & Gleser, G. L. (1957). *Psychological tests and personnel decisions*. Urbana: University of Illinois Press.

Gresham, F. (1983). Multitrait-multimethod approach to multifactored assessment: Theoretical rationale and practical application. *School Psychology Review, 12*, 26–34.

Knoff, H. M. (1984). The practice of multimodal consultation: An integrating approach for consultation service delivery. *Psychology in the Schools, 21*, 83–91.

Lazarus, A. A. (1981). *The practice of multi-modal therapy*. New York: McGraw-Hill.

Nay, W. R. (1979). *Multimethod clinical assessment*. New York: Gardner Press.

Rabin, A. I., & Hayes, D. L. (1978). Concerning the rationale of diagnostic testing. In B. B. Wolman (Ed.), *Clinical diagnosis of mental disorders: A handbook* (pp. 579–600). New York: Plenum Press.

Appendix[1]

A Summary of Selected Personality Assessment Tools Available to Mental Health Practitioners

Tests Reviewed

The Achenbach Child Behavior Checklist
Blacky Pictures Test
Children's Apperception Test
Conner's Parent Rating Scales
The Conner's Teacher Rating Scale
The Family Coping Strategies Inventory
Family Inventory of Life Events and Changes
The Family Satisfaction Inventory
The Forer Structured Sentence Completion Test
Goodenough Harris Drawing Test
The Hart Sentence Completion Test for Children
The House–Tree–Person Technique
The Kinetic Drawing System: Family and School
The Make-A-Picture Story Test
The Miale-Holsopple Sentence Completion Test
The Michigan Picture Test-Revised
Missouri Children's Behavior Checklist
Personality Inventory for Children, Revised Format
The Quality of Life Inventory
Quay–Peterson Behavior Problem Checklist-Revised
The Rohde Sentence Completion Method
Roberts Apperception Test for Children
The Rorschach: The Comprehensive System
The Rotter Incomplete Sentence Blank
The Sacks Sentence Completion Test
School Apperception Method
Teacher Version of the Achenbach Child Behavior Checklist
Thematic Apperception Test

[1]The author wishes to acknowledge the assistance of Deborah F. Rous in compiling this Appendix.

The Achenbach Child Behavior Checklist (1983)

Authors: T. M. Achenbach and C. S. Edelbrock

Publisher: Psychiatric Associates
  c/o Department of Psychiatry
  University of Vermont
  Burlington, Vermont 05401

A. Description of Test

  1. Standardization Population
  Clinically referred children from 42 mental health agencies located in the eastern United States formed the basis of the clinical sample. Parents completed the CBCL at the various agencies during intake procedures; 2,300 completed CBCLs were obtained from the mental health facilities. The sample population consisted of 81% white people, 17% black people, and 2% other.

  2. Time to Assess
  15–17 minutes.

  3. What It Assesses
  The test investigates profiles of behavior problem children. The two major areas are: (a) Internalizing Syndromes and (b) Externalizing Syndromes. Additionally, there are up to 15 other scales which describe specific types of behavioral problems (e.g., depression, somatic complaints, social competency). The test gives descriptive statements, not diagnostic entities. It provides information about both behavioral assets and behavioral problems.

B. Scoring/Interpretation
  For the behavior problem areas, the questions are open-ended. For the behavioral asset assessments, there are four response choices for each of the three scales. The parent states what types of social, school, and other activities the child is involved in and the degree of involvement or success based on the 4-point scale ("Don't Know" to "Average" or "Failing" to "Above Average"). All data are entered on the Child Behavior Profile (CBP). The examiner compares the child's profile with typical children of the same age and sex. He or she can also review the specific behavioral syndromes manifested by the child. Percentiles and T scores are available. Clusters of responses offer descriptive statements, not diagnostic entities.

C. Norms
  The test was normed on a population different from the standardization population on which the

645

questions and scales were based. This population consisted of 1,442 children who could not have had mental health services during the previous years. Children's names were randomly selected in the Washington, D.C., Maryland, and northern Virginia areas. Fifty children of each sex, at each age (4–16) having SES and racial distributions consistent with the clinical samples, were selected: 80.5% were white, 18% black, and 1.5% other. The checklist was completed by mothers in 83% of the cases, by fathers in 13.5% of the cases, and other guardians in 3.5% of the cases.

D. Validity and Reliability
   1. Reliability
      Internal Consistency is more than adequate.

      Interclass Correlation Coefficient (obtained by a test–retest procedure where the correlation coefficient is affected by the consistency of the rank ordering of the items of the CBCL over time) is high.

      Temporal Stability is excellent

      Test–Retest: For Hyperactive is excellent; for Schizoid or Anxious factor is very good; for child care workers vs. parents is very good.

      Interparent Agreement is good to excellent.

   2. Validity
      Convergent Validity [with Conners Parent Questionnaire (Conners, 1973) and the Quay–Peterson Revised Behavior Problem Checklist (Quay & Peterson, 1983)] was generally adequate for Somatic, Impulsive–Hyperactive, Social Withdrawal, Aggressive, Internalizing, and Externalizing.

      Discriminate Validity: The test has been able to discriminate between clinical and nonclinical samples. There were 18% misclassifications for the behavioral area and 16% misclassifications in the social competence area.

Blacky Pictures Test (1950)

Author: Gerald S. Blum

Publisher: Psychological Corporation
          757 Third Avenue
          New York, New York 10017

A. Description of Test
   1. Standardization Population
      No norms or standardization population.
   2. Time to Assess
      Approximately 30 minutes.
   3. What It Assesses
      This test assesses the psychosexual development of children ages 5 and over. It is a thematic projective technique which utilizes 11 cards depicting a family of dogs as the major story characters. Thematic areas assessed include such problems as attitudes toward siblings and parents, characteristic defense reactions, negative self-perceptions, and sexual identity processes.

C. Scoring/Interpretation
   The manual recommends that scoring be based on spontaneous stories, answers to inquiry questions, cartoon preferences, and related comments on other cartoons. There are 13 separate psychosexual dimensions through which the interpretations are made. There are several different guides for interpretation and the scoring methods vary accordingly. It has a very good, clear, objective manual.

D. Norms
   None.

E. Validity and Reliability
   1. Reliability
      Test-Retest: Good to fair.

      Interscorer: Adequate for protocols, but not for spontaneous stories, reliable for research but not necessarily for individual clinical assessment.

2. Validity (for the original revised edition)

Construct Validity (factor analysis): Adequate for males only.

When the validity was tested with people who were presumed to possess certain of the traits the test measures, almost all predictions were confirmed.

Children's Apperception Test (1976)

Authors: Leopold Bellak, M.D., & Sonya Sorel Bellak

Publisher: C.P.S., Inc.
P.O. Box 83
Larchmont, New York 10538

A. Description of Test
   1. Standardization Population

   Two hundred records of children between ages 3 and 10 provide normative data which may be used to "appraise the relative degree of discordance between" unconscious tendencies and manifest behavior for diagnostic purposes, and to establish age norms for certain phases of dynamic development. No other data are given.

   2. Time to Assess
   Approximately 30 minutes.

   3. What It Assesses
   It is a thematic projective technique where children are presented with cards portraying animals in typically human situations. They are asked to tell a story about each picture.

   The pictures are designed to evoke fantasies relating to problems of feeding and other oral activity, sibling rivalry, parent–child relations, aggression, toilet training, and other childhood experiences. It investigates individual differences in perception of standard stimuli. It is designed to explore the child's structure and how he or she deals with the problems of growth. It can reveal the dynamics of interpersonal relationships, of drive constellations, and the nature of defenses against them. The basic framework seems to be psychoanalytic and the authors claim it is culture free.

C. Scoring/Interpretation
   Responses are recorded verbatim and are analyzed according to the Interpretation section. The Interpretation section suggests 10 variables which should be studied in the subject's response, i.e., the main hero (self-concept); main needs and drives of the hero—which may correspond to the subject's needs and drives. There is a record sheet which facilitates interpreting responses and a "short form" which c. n place the subject in the Psychotic, Borderline, Neurotic, or Normal range.

D. Norms
   The test is designed for use between ages 3 and 10. The CAT-H (using humans instead of animals) is used with children with an MA beyond 10 years. The sample is small (200). The authors feel the individual case may stand by itself and does not need to be validated. There are no normative data on children's responses at different ages.

E. Validity and Reliability
   The authors claim that they interpreted the samples' responses blindly and then reviewed clinicians' records. Their interpretations matched the diagnoses of the clinicians. The authors hope that eventually quantitative data regarding responses at different ages will be established.

The Conners Parent Rating Scales (1982)

Author: C. K. Conners

A. Description of Test
   1. Standardization Population
   The test is based on a listing of behavior problems compiled by Cytryn, Gilbert, and Eisenberg (1960). Five factors now comprise this new, shortened version of the original Parent Rating

Scale (1969, 1973), which contained eight major factors for 683 children between 6 and 14. The shortened version was devised to simplify scoring and interpretation.

2. Time to Assess
Approximately 15 minutes.

3. What It Assesses
This 48-item instrument assesses five factors: Conduct Problems, Learning Problems, Psychosomatic Problems, Impulsivity-Hyperactivity, and Anxiety. The items lend themselves to screening for other specific child behavior problems. The test has been useful in assessing drug-induced treatments of hyperactive children (Sprague & Sleater, 1973).

C. Scoring/Interpretation
Each item is answered "Not at All," "Just a Little," "Pretty Much," or "Very Much." The number of points assigned to each answer is 0, 1, 2, or 3, respectively. Scores are obtained by adding raw scores on different factors; means for each factor are obtained and transformed into T scores. A T score of 70 is used as a cutoff score for identifying significant behavior problems.

D. Norms
Normative data were obtained from parents of 750 children in Pittsburgh, Pennsylvania. The parents' names were selected from a telephone book, and the parents were asked to complete a questionnaire for each child between 3 and 17. The average age of the children was 9.9, but the number of children sampled at each age is not given. 55% were males and 45% were females. 98% of the sample was white, 1% was black, and 1% other.

E. Validity and Reliability
1. Reliability
Item-Total Correlation: Ranging from $r = .13$ to $r = .65$.

Between Mother and Father: Stable reliability.

Between Teacher and Parent: Adequate, not as good as mother and father.

Test-Retest: Adequate, but it varies among the different factors, different ages, and different versions of the PRS.

2. Validity
Different factor structures have been found to have different validity.

Convergent (with Quay–Peterson Behavior Problem Checklist): Good validity. Hyperactivity has also been found to correlate significantly with the Werry–Weiss–Peters Activity Rating Scale; however, the hyperactivity measure can be unstable across time, and does not correlate with objective measures of activity. Boys are assigned more pathological symptoms than girls. Mothers rate more harshly than fathers.

The Conners Teacher Rating Scale (1982)

Author: C. K. Connors

A. Description of Test
1. Standardization Population
The 39 items on the Teacher Rating Scale are based on the items of the Parent Rating Scale which were based on eight major factors for 683 children between 6 and 14.

2. Time to Assess
Approximately 15 minutes.

3. What It Assesses
This is a short rating scale designed to be used in a school setting. It is mainly used to assess hyperactive children, but it also has scales to potentially assess Conduct Disordered, Emotional-Overindulgent, Anxious-Passive, Asocial, and Daydreaming/Problem Attendance children.

C. Scoring/Interpretation
Each item is answered "Not at All," "Just a Little," "Pretty Much," or "Very Much." The number of points assigned to each answer is 0, 1, 2, or 3, respectively. Scores are obtained by adding raw scores on different factors; means for each factor are obtained and transformed into T scores. A T score of 70 is used as a cutoff score for identifying significant behavior problems.

D. Norms

The TRS has been normed on four different populations in four different cultures yielding somewhat similar factors. Although the sample populations varied from small and inadequate to large and representative, the factors were similar and the test is seen to be valid cross-culturally.

E. Validity and Reliability

1. Reliability

The reliability varies depending on the version used and the different factors.

Internal Consistency [Trites, Blouin, & LaPrade (1979) version]: Fair to good. Generally, the internal consistency of the 39-item TRS appears adequate.

Teacher–Teacher Agreement (Adelaide version): Adequate and stable, with the exception of the Tension-Anxiety factor.

Interscorer: No data available.

Test-Retest (Adelaide version): Over 1 month and 1 year, reliability was good. With certain factors and certain ages the reliability varies from poor to adequate.

2. Validity

Construct Validity: Appears adequate; Trites's (1979) large normative sample appears to provide a firm foundation for six basic factors.

Criterion Related: Adequate

Discriminate: Good for normal vs. hyperactive children; the TRS is sensitive to drug treatment and behavior therapy. Glow *et al.*'s (1982) multimethod factor matrix of the TRS provides good discriminant validity for Hyperactive-Inattentive, Unforthcoming-Unassertive, Socially Regressed, Depressed Mood.

Goyette *et al.*'s (1979) version found that sex and age played a part in diagnoses to a greater extent than Trites *et al.*'s (1979) version.

Convergent Validity: The Hyperactive factor was found to correlate with other behavior rating scales (Quay–Peterson Behavior Problem Checklist, David's Hyperkinetic Rating Scale, Devereaux Elementary School Behavior Scale, Behavior and Temperament Survey, and School Behavior Survey), peer evaluation, direct behavioral observations, standardized achievement scores, and other teacher behavior surveys. In other studies, does not correlate with behavioral measures of activity such as teacher behavioral observations, actometer, stabilimeter, or structured freeplay observations. Some support for validity in diagnosing depression.

The Family Coping Strategies Inventory (F-COPES) (1982)

Author: D. H. Olson, H. I. McCubbin, H. Barnes, A. Larsen, M. Muxen, M. Wilson

Publisher: c/o Dr. David Olson
Family Social Science
290 McNeal Avenue
University of Minnesota
St. Paul, Minnesota 55108

A. Description of Test

1. Standardization Population

Forty-nine coping strategies were compiled from a review of the literature. The items were given to 119 college students, reduced to 30 items, and then were factor analyzed. This 30-item instrument was used with a national sample, cross-validated, and the items were reduced to 29 with five resulting factors.

2. Time to Assess

Approximately 15 minutes.

3. What It Assesses

Designed to assess the problem-solving approaches and behaviors used by families in response to family or family-related problems or difficulties. The five factors include Acquiring Social Support, Reframing, Seeking Spiritual Support, Mobilizing Family To Acquire and Accept Help, and Passive Appraisal.

B. Scoring/Interpretation

Respondents are presented with a statement, and they rate their degree of agreement with it on a 5-point scale. A sum score for each subscale, as well as a total score is obtained. The total score indicates the number and degree of coping strategies that the individual perceives the family using.

C. Norms

Norms appear to be obtained from the national survey, and percentile norms, means, and standard deviations are available.

D. Validity and Reliability

1. Reliability

Scorer: Sufficient for use in research and screening.

2. Validity

Construct: Factor analyses yielded the same five factors in two different studies.

Family Inventory of Life Events and Changes (FILE) (1983)

Authors: H. I. McCubbin and J. M. Patterson

Publisher: c/o Dr. H. I. McCubbin
Family Social Science
290 McNeal Avenue
University of Minnesota
St. Paul, Minnesota 55108

A. Description of Test

1. Normed on a national, stratified, cross-sectional sample of intact couples representing all stages of the family life cycle (independent husband sample, $N = 1,330$; independent wife sample, $N = 1,410$). Sample tended to be more midwestern in region, more Lutheran in religion, more inclusive of first marriages than for the nation as a whole.

2. Time to Assess

Approximately 20 minutes.

3. What It Assesses

It is a self-report inventory to assess normative and nonnormative family stresses. The test assesses families, not individuals. Factor analytic studies yielded nine subscales: conflict between family members, marital conflict, pregnancy and childbearing strains, finance and business strains, work–family transitions and strains, illness and family care strains, family losses, family transitions in or out of the nuclear family, family legal strains.

B. Scoring/Interpretation

Completed by having family members check off whether a particular life event or strain has occurred over the past year. Five FILE scores are possible, depending on the needs of the researcher or clinician: the Family Readjustment score, Family Life Events score, Family–Couple Life Events score, Family–Couple Discrepancy score, and the Family Pile-up score.

C. Norms

Norms based on the national, stratified, cross-sectional sample of intact couples are available for all of the scales noted above.

D. Validity and Reliability

1. Reliability

Scorer: Adequate for research but not for individual diagnoses.

Internal Consistency: Reduced by including rare life events, e.g., deaths. Three of the nine subscales have adequate reliability, while six do not.

Test-Retest: For 4–5 weeks, good.

2. Validity

Construct: Factor analysis in two studies revealed almost identical factors.

The Family Satisfaction Inventory (1982)

Authors: D. H. Olson and M. Wilson

Publisher: Dr. David Olson
Family Social Science
290 McNeal Avenue
University of Minnesota
St. Paul, Minnesota 55108

A. Description of Test
1. Standardization Population
The data from 438 university students were factor analyzed, reducing the Inventory's original 28 items to 14. These items were then standardized on a national stratified cross-sectional sample of intact couples. They were mostly midwestern, religious Lutheran, first marriage couples.
2. Time to Assess
Approximately 15 minutes.

3. What It Assesses
The test assesses one of 14 concepts addressing the family's cohesion (the emotional bonding of individuals in the family) and adaptability (the extent to which a family can change its prior structure, role relationships, and relationship rules when situations require this).

B. Scoring/Interpretation
The individual responds to questions regarding the family, rating his or her degree of satisfaction with the aspect in question. The scale is scored by tallying an unweighted total score of the 14 items. There are percentile norms, means, and standard deviations from the national survey to aid interpretation.

C. Norms
Based on the national, stratified, cross-sectional sample of intact couples.

D. Validity and Reliability
1. Reliability
Interscorer: Very good.

Test-Retest: Over a five week period—adequate.

2. Validity
Construct: A correlation between the family and life satisfaction from the national survey yielded a significant positive correlation. Correlations between this test and other related measures of family satisfaction were positive.

The Forer Structured Sentence Completion Test (1950)

Author: Bertram R. Forer

Publisher: Western Psychological Services
12031 Wilshire Boulevard
Los Angeles, California 90025

A. Description of Test
1. Standardization Population
None.

2. Time to Assess
Approximately 30 minutes.

3. What It Assesses
Through a projective, sentence completion format, this test is designed for use with adolescents aged 10–18 and adults. It assesses dominant needs or drives, causes of various personality trends, reactions to interpersonal relationships, predominant emotional attitudes, direction and amount of aggressive tendencies, and total affective level. There are also guidelines regarding expected response trends for certain personality types.

B. Scoring/Interpretation

There are separate editions for boys, girls, men, and women, each with 100 items. The manual offers a number of guides and hypotheses which may be used to facilitate interpretation of the responses. However, much of the interpretation is based on speculation from comparing and contrasting the responses. Item responses are organized into seven major areas (e.g., affective level, aggressive tendencies) and point out evasiveness, individual differences, and defense mechanisms.

C. Norms

There are no data about norms in the manual.

D. Validity and Reliability

There are no validity or reliability data in the manual. This is a clinical or diagnostic instrument, and the validity and reliability may correlate with the skill and experience of the diagnostician.

Goodenough Harris Drawing Test (1963)

Author: Dale B. Harris

Publisher: Psychological Corporation
757 Third Avenue
New York, New York 10017

A. Description of Test

1. Standardization Population

Three hundred children at each year level between the ages of 5 and 15 were selected to be in the standardization sample. They were selected so as to be representative of the United States population with regard to father's occupation and geographical region (1963).

2. Time to Assess

Approximately 20 minutes.

3. What It Assesses

The test may be administered individually or in groups. It assesses reasoning, spatial aptitude, and perceptual accuracy; emphasis is placed on the child's accuracy of observation and the development of conceptual thinking. Harris claims that the various scores combine to give an estimate of the child's intellectual maturity, but it should not be used for important decisions such as placement. It gives an initial impression of a young child's general ability level.

B. Scoring/Interpretation

There are Draw-A-Man, Draw-A-Woman, and Draw Yourself subtests. The Draw-A-Man and Draw Yourself subtests have 73 scoreable items each, the Draw-A-Woman subtest has 71 scoreable items. There is also a Quality scale where the entire drawing is scored by matching the child's drawing with one of the 12 samples in a graded series that it most closely resembles. There is also a short scoring guide for experienced examiners.

C. Norms

Point scores are changed to standard scores with a mean of 100 and standard deviation of 15; percentile ranks and averaged standard scores are also available.

D. Validity and Reliability

1. Reliability

Test-Retest: After 1 week, adequate.

Split-Half: Good.

Rescoring: Excellent; the examiner effect is negligible for point scores.

Interscorer: Better for the point scale than for the quality scale. However, the quality scale has good interscorer reliability.

2. Validity

Construct Validity: Correlations with other intelligence tests are all over .50. It correlates highest with tests of reasoning, spatial aptitude, and perceptual accuracy. The test may measure somewhat different functions at different ages, the extent of which is not entirely known. Scores tend to be related to the amount of experience with representational art within each culture.

The Hart Sentence Completion Test for Children (HSCT)

Author: Darrell H. Hart

Publisher: c/o Dr. Darrell Hart
Educational Support Systems, Inc.
2828 East 33rd South
Salt Lake City, Utah 84109

A. Description of Test
1. Standardization Population
While norms are currently being compiled, the HSCT has been used in a number of studies with school children, typical and with a range of learning and adjustment difficulties, whose data can be used for comparison purposes.
2. Time to Assess
15–30 minutes.
3. What It Assesses
It is a sentence completion test which is consistent with child development principles instead of general personality theory. It assesses the child's perceptions on four dimensions: (*a*) family environments, (*b*) social environments, (*c*) school environments, and (*d*) interpersonal or internal conditions. It is used for educational or therapeutic interventions.

B. Scoring/Interpretation
There is a scale rating system and an item-by-item rating system. In the former, the examiner makes a "gestalt" summary, his overall impression of the child, along a 5-point continuum from positive to negative. This is a subjective judgment. The item-by-item system provides the examiner with criteria which facilitate the rating of child responses. The items are scored using a template, and the complete ratings may be profiled for interscale comparisons.

C. Norms
Normative data are presently being compiled and are not yet available for various classification groups.

D. Validity and Reliability
Scale Rating System
1. Reliability
Interscorer: Moderate to good.
Interrater: When reflecting specific needs and clinical symptoms or syndromes—not adequate.
2. Validity
Five out of eight scales distinguished between emotionally handicapped and typical children.
Item-by-Item System
1. Reliability
Interscorer: Good.
2. Validity
Differential: Data significantly differed among emotionally handicapped, learning-disabled, and normal subjects.

The House–Tree–Person Technique (1948)

Author: J. N. Buck

Publisher: See various books from
Western Psychological Services
12031 Wilshire Boulevard
Los Angeles, California 90025

A. Description of Test
1. Standardization Population

No specific standardization population covering the technique is comprehensive. A number of studies with different populations are available.

  2. Time to Assess
     Approximately 20 minutes.

  3. What It Assesses
     The child is asked to draw a house, tree, and person on separate pieces of paper with an inquiry process to get more information about each drawing in between. As a projective drawing technique, different clinicians interpret different meanings for the drawings, specific characteristics of the drawing, or certain drawing or response styles. Generally, the house drawing is used to reveal the psychological status, attitudes, or perceptions that the child has about his or her home environment. The tree drawing is said to reveal children's intrapersonal, interpersonal, and environmental adjustment. The person is said to reveal issues and attitudes about self-concept and self-perception.

B. Scoring/Interpretation
   Scoring is generally by evaluating the drawing as a whole, specific characteristics of the drawing, and content of the drawing from the inquiry process. Many studies provide interpretive hypotheses to these areas, best summarized by Ogdon (1977, Western Psychological Services).

C. Norms
   Again, no comprehensive norms are available.

D. Validity and Reliability
   Dependent on specific individual's scoring criteria, experimental samples, and methodological integrity.

The Kinetic Drawing System for Family and School (1985)

Author: H. M. Knoff and H. T. Prout

Publisher: Western Psychological Services
           12031 Wilshire Boulevard
           Los Angeles, California 90025

A. Description of Test

  1. Standardization Population
     No single, comprehensive standardization population for the System has been used. A number of studies and scoring systems for the Family or School Drawing, respectively, have been published. These are summarized in the manual.

  2. Time to Assess
     Approximately 30 minutes.

  3. What It Assesses
     These projective drawing techniques separately assess individual issues, perceptions, attitudes toward, or dynamics relevant to family or school environments or interactions, respectively. Taken together, the drawings can be differentially assessed to note common themes, situation-specific issues or dynamics, or the carry-over of particular themes or issues from one setting into another. The drawings are completed by having the child complete separate drawings of themselves and others doing something together in the two environments.

B. Scoring/Interpretation
   The manual summarizes scoring characteristics and hypotheses generated by others which are in the literature. Scoring generally addresses Actions Between Figures; Figure Characteristics; Position, Distance, and Barriers; Style; and Symbols. A number of objective scoring systems for the two separate drawings are summarized in the manual.

C. Norms
   None developed for the comprehensive System.

D. Validity and Reliability
   None available for the comprehensive System. A number of studies are available for the separate

drawings, indicating adequate scoring reliability depending on the objective scoring system used. Validity data are dependent on the individual characteristics studied, the samples used, and methodological integrity. These are all reviewed in the manual.

The Make-A-Picture Story Test (1952)

Author: E. S. Schneidman

Publisher: Psychological Corporation
757 Third Avenue
New York, New York 10017

A. Description of Test
  1. Standardization Population
     Not available to report; very difficult to develop standardized procedures with the MAPS given the variety and possible combinations of stimuli and pictures.
  2. Time to Assess
     Approximately 60 minutes.
  3. What It Assesses
     Essentially a variation of the TAT for individuals aged 6 through adulthood, the MAPS has individuals make their own pictures by selecting one or more human-like or animal cutouts from a variety of figures and placing them on one of 22 backgrounds, and then having them tell a story about the created picture. Generally assesses the same potential dynamics, themes, and presses of the TAT.

B. Scoring/Interpretation
   While a variety of quantitative schemes are available, they are generally not time-efficient. Qualitative interpretation comparable to the TAT is most used; this, therefore, varies, depending on clinician skill and experience.

C. Norms
   None developed due to stimulus characteristics of the test.

D. Validity and Reliability
   None to report.

The Miale–Holsopple Sentence Completion Test (M-HSCT) (1954)

Authors: J. A. Holsopple and F. Miale (1954)

Publisher: C. C. Thomas
Springfield, Illinois

A. Description of Test
  1. Time to Assess
     Untimed; no approximate time available.
  2. What It Assesses
     This is a projective, sentence completion test which is global, unstructured, and untimed. Based more on psychoanalytic premises, it is designed to elicit information that is less well defended in the individual's personality structure.

B. Scoring/Interpretation
   There is no formal scoring system. A global, qualitative analysis is suggested. "Types of response phrasing" are provided to assist in interpretation.

C. Validity and Reliability
   The validity of the test is highly dependent on the skill and experience of the practitioner.

The Michigan Picture Test-Revised (MPT-R) (1980)

Author: M. L. Hutt

Publisher: Grune and Stratton
111 Fifth Avenue
New York, New York 10003

A. Description of Test
   1. Standardization Population
   Standardized on a representative sample of children from public school populations and children with behavioral and personality problems from child guidance clinics.
   2. Time to Assess
   Approximately 40–50 minutes.
   3. What It Assesses
   A thematic instrument designed for children aged 8–14 or in grades 3–9, the MPT-R's major objective is to differentiate children with emotional maladjustment from those with satisfactory emotional adjustment. The MPT-R has 15 cards, and 5 "core" cards are recommended as the minimal battery, with up to 7 additional cards to "round out" the administration process. Children make up a story with a beginning and an ending for quantitative and qualitative analyses.

B. Scoring/Interpretation
   Scoring criteria are available in the manual. Interpretation is based on the normative sample and a Tension Index, a Direction of Forces Index, a Tense Score, and a Combined Maladjustment Index. Other information scored includes psychosexual levels, interpersonal relations, personal pronouns, and popular objects.

C. Norms
   Available in the manual.

D. Validity and Reliability
   1. Reliability
   Interrater Reliability: Adequate.
   2. Validity
   Discriminate Validity: The scales were able to significantly discriminate adjusted from maladjusted children.

   These are preliminary results and the author notes that additional reliability and validity study is needed.

Missouri Children's Behavior Checklist (MCBC) (1969)

Authors: J. O. Sines, J. D. Parker, L. K. Sines, and D. R. Owen

A. Description of Test
   1. Standardization Population
   Standardization data were collected from a wide array of settings in the United States and Canada, including child psychiatry, pediatric, and mental health clinics. Most children were seen for psychological evaluations. There were 404 boys, 250 girls, ages 5–19. The psychometric properties were constructed from the sample of males. The number of subjects in each age group varied extensively. The effects of age, sex, and SES were not tested.
   2. Time to Assess
   15–20 minutes.
   3. What It Assesses
   The test is a behavior rating scale designed to contribute to the differential diagnosis of behavioral pathology in children 5–16. It yields ratings across six dimensions (Aggression, Inhibition, Activity Level, Sleep Disturbance, Somatization, and Sociability). It has been useful in identifying clusters of behavioral symptomology across different populations.

B. Scoring/Interpretation

The 70 items are rated "yes" or "no," as to whether the child has shown the particular behavior during the past 6 months. All six scales are scored and a Total Pathology score is also given. The scoring system is relatively easy. The child receives one point for each item reported in the pathological direction. The higher a child's score on any factor, the greater the possibility of that child exhibiting the deviant behavior described by the factor. On the Sociability dimension, a higher score indicates more positive behavior.

C. Norms

A number of normative groups are available for comparison purposes; the lack of one accepted normative sample may be a disadvantage. DeFilippis (1979) randomly selected names from public school files of a midwestern community. 302 mothers of children aged 7–9 completed the MCBC. Sex, SES, and IQ were tested for effects on the score. No effects for SES or IQ were obtained. Males differed from females on several factors. A cutoff point of 150 above the mean was suggested for the Total Pathology scale. Kelly and King (1980) provide normative data for 437 black children ages 5–16. Males and females were combined in each age group. Samples ranged from $N = 9$ for the age 5 group to $N = 61$ for age 10. Age and sex effects were found. Again, only males were included in the sample which provided psychometric properties.

D. Validity and Reliability

All validity and reliability data must be viewed in the light of the variable norms.

  1. Reliability

Internal Consistency: Dimensions are relatively inadequate.

Scoring Reliability: No data, but the yes/no format facilitates scoring.

Interrater Reliability: Good between mothers and fathers.

Temporal Stability: No data.

  2. Validity

Discriminate: DeFilippis's (1979) cutoff score correctly identified 89% of children recommended for treatment.

Construct: No formal factor analysis of the MCBC has been published. A factor analysis of the original 95-item version of the MCBC with 120 males, aged 9–11 (McMahon et al., 1979), revealed two reliable factors: Aggression and Social Responsibility (a third factor was dropped due to limited items).

Differential: Adequate for developmentally disabled, psychiatric, and normal populations. In some studies, differences between males and females were found, and in some, no differences were found. There is some evidence for four factors—Aggressive-Action, Inhibited, Mixed Disturbance, and Normal—but the use of these factors in classifying children referred to a guidance clinic resulted in 50% misclassifications. There is some evidence for identifying "at-risk" preschoolers.

Personality Inventory for Children, Revised Format (1982)

Authors: Robert D. Wirt, Philip D. Seat, David Lachar (Manual),
         James K. Klinedinst (Manual) and William E. Broen (Test)

Publisher: Western Psychological Services
           12031 Wilshire Boulevard
           Los Angeles, California 90025

A. Description of Test

  1. Standardization Population

Norms for ages 6–16 years based on a sample of 2,390 children and adolescents, and a sample of nearly 200 normal boys and girls ages 3–5 years. 81.5% of the normative samples were selected from children attending regular classes in the Minneapolis public schools. The remainder of the sample was obtained from mothers of children being seen for nonpsychological programs at a Minneapolis medical center, from cooperating organizations, and from door-to-door canvassing.

2. Time to Assess
   Approximately 45–60 minutes.

3. What It Assesses

   It is an objective, empirically derived questionnaire with 600 true/false questions which are answered by an adult who is knowledgeable about the child (usually the mother). The mother gives information about the child's current problem and case history and a personality profile results. The test can be used for children aged 3–16. The PIC has four validity and screening scales and 12 clinical scales.

   There are three "validity scales": (*a*) L scale (determines whether child is made to appear in an unrealistically favorable light); (*b*) F scale (consisting of rarely endorsed items); and (*c*) Defensiveness scale (designed to assess parental defensiveness about the child's behavior).

   The Adjustment scale is a screening scale used to identify children in need of psychological evaluation.

   The remaining 12 scales are clinical scales designed to assess the child's cognitive development, academic achievement, emotional and interpersonal problems, and the psychological climate of the family. Additionally, there are supplementary scales to clarify diagnoses in individual cases.

B. Scoring/Interpretation
   Scoring is facilitated by a grid for each scale or computerized scoring and interpretation. Each scale is standardized to a *T* score with a mean of 50 and standard deviation of 10 (higher scores indicate greater probability of psychopathology or deficit). Interpretation is based on comparisons to the norms, to identified clinical groups, through actuarial decision models, and through profile classifications.

C. Norms
   Based on the two samples described above, which range from ages 3–16. These have been analyzed by sex, age, occupation of head of household, and education of parents. All scales have been factor analytically derived. Mean profiles of other specialized diagnostic groups are given to aid in profile interpretations.

D. Validity and Reliability
   Extensive reliability and validity data reported in the manual. Construct validity appears especially good.

The Quality of Life Inventory (1982)

Authors: D. H. Olson and H. Barnes

Publisher: c/o Dr. David Olson
            Family Social Science
            290 McNeal Avenue
            University of Minnesota
            St. Paul, Minnesota 55108

A. Description of Test
   1. Standardization Population
      Based on a national, stratified, cross-sectional sample of intact families (husbands and wives) and male and female adolescents.

   2. Time to Assess
      Approximately 15 minutes.

   3. What It Assesses
      Parents and adolescents rate their degree of satisfaction with the family and other aspects of their lives. The family and practitioner can identify areas where support and stress subjectively impact family members. This test utilizes a subjective instead of an objective statistical approach, i.e., instead of utilizing social and economic indicators, the respondents are asked whether they are satisfied with certain aspects of their lives.

B. Scoring/Interpretation
   A total scale unweighted sum score is obtained and is interpreted using percentile norms for husband, wife, and male and female adolescent groups, respectively.

C. Norms

Percentile norms were obtained for husbands, wives, and male and female adolescents.

D. Validity and Reliability

1. Reliability

Scorer: Very good.

2. Validity

Construct: Obtained through factor analysis which gave support for the initial conceptual structure of the scale.

Quay–Peterson Behavior Problem Checklist-Revised (1983)

Authors: H. C. Quay and D. R. Peterson

Publisher: c/o Dr. H. C. Quay
University of Miami
Coral Gables, Florida 33134

A. Description of Test

1. Standardization Population

The original Behavior Problem Checklist (BCP) was derived from factor analytic studies of the presenting problems of children seen in a child guidance clinic and from similar analyses with a sample of typical children from grades K–6. The Revised BCP expanded the scale to 89 final items and factor analyses were completed for four samples: 276 cases (ages 5–22, 72% male/28% female) from two private psychiatric residential facilities; 198 cases (3–21 years old, 64% male/36% female) who were outpatients and inpatients; 114 children (X age = 10 years old, 72% male/28% female) from a private school for learning-disabled children; and 172 children (39 girls, 133 boys) from a community school for the developmentally disabled.

2. Time to Assess

Approximately 30 minutes.

3. What It Assesses

This behavior rating scale uses its 89 items to investigate the behavior traits of children and adolescents. It consists of four major scales (Conduct Disorder, Socialized Aggression, Attention Problems-Immaturity, Anxiety-Withdrawal) and two minor scales (Psychotic Behavior and Motor Excess). The BCP has been used in applied settings for the purposes of screening and assessment and to provide epidemiological data.

B. Scoring/Interpretation

The items are scored on a 3-point system (no problem, mild problem, or severe problem). Items were selected for the scales based on their loadings on one factor only, their consistency of placement across the four standardization samples, and their size of factor loading. Interpretation is based on an individual's profile across the six scales and comparisons with the normal and clinical samples.

C. Norms

Available for the Behavior Problem Checklist (Manual, 1979), and for the normal and clinical samples described above (Manual, 1983).

D1.Validity and Reliability (for the Revised Behavior Problem Checklist, 1983)

1. Reliability

Internal Consistency: For major scales, excellent; for minor scales, adequate.

Interrater: Limited preliminary data appear adequate.

2. Validity

Much of the concurrent, predictive, and construct validity of BCP assumed to generalize to the Revised-BCP.

Discriminant Validity: 77% of a clinical group correctly identified with 23% false positives; 87% of elementary school group correctly classified with 13% false positives—both for males. For females, 91% of the former group correctly identified with 23% false positives; 7% false positives in the latter group.

D2. Validity and Reliability (for the Behavior Problem Checklist, 1979)
1. Reliability
Internal Consistency: Adequate.
Test-Retest: For 1 week, excellent; for 1 year, adequate.
Interrater: (*a*) Parent/parent (moderate to fairly high), (*b*) Parent/teacher (somewhat uneven), (*c*) Parent/counselor and teacher/counselor (adequate but somewhat lower than parent/parent).
2. Validity
Appears adequate regarding developmental changes.
It is sensitive to group differences regarding different family structures.
There is a significant correlation between certain BPC scales for boys and measures of marital hostility or aggression.
There is a significant correlation between the transgressor (those who cheated on a task) and the Conduct Problem scale.
Validity appears adequate when the BPC is correlated with other similar measures.
Construct Validity: Found to be adequate based on factor analysis. Similar factors were obtained with other standardization samples. Where black children are concerned, there is an additional factor reflecting resistance by black children to expectations within white academic settings.

The Rohde Sentence Completion Method (1957)

Author: A. R. Rohde

A. Description of Test
1. Standardization Population
None.
2. What It Assesses
It uses Murray's (1938) conceptual scheme of presses and needs to assess personality dynamics. Diagnostic and personality-related hypotheses are generated based primarily on individuals' psychological motivations.
B. Scoring/Interpretation
There are no formal scoring criteria. Sentence completions are interpreted at the overt content level of attitudes and values, the latent content level of underlying personality dynamics, and the global level of overall functioning. The manual provides descriptive examples and case studies.
C. Norms
None in evidence.
D. Validity and Reliability
No data available.

Roberts Apperception Test For Children (1982)

Authors: Glen E. Roberts, Ph.D., and Dorothea S. McArthur, Ph.D.

Publisher: Western Psychological Services
12031 Wilshire Boulevard
Los Angeles, California 90025

A. Description of Test
1. Standardization Population
Standardized on a sample of 200 "well-adjusted" children of both sexes, with efforts to include representative cross sections of all SES statuses.
2. Time to Assess
Administered in 20–30 minutes and scored in 15–20 minutes.

3. What It Assesses

This is a thematic technique for children aged 6–15 which uses an objective scoring system and norms. Designed to assess children's perceptions of interpersonal situations, including their thoughts, concerns, conflicts, and coping styles, the RATC is made up of 27 stimulus cards (11 with both male and female versions) of which 16 are administered at any one time. The child tells a story about each picture, including what led up to the picture and how the story ends.

B. Scoring/Interpretation

An explicit scoring system yields adaptive scales (reliance on others, support to others, support of the child, limit setting, problem identification, and three resolution scales) and clinical scales (Anxiety, Aggression, Depression, Rejection, Unresolved). In addition, there are other critical indicators and collections of scores, all of which are compiled on an Interpersonal Chart. Scores are compared to the normative data, and the manual provides numerous case examples.

C. Norms

Standardization data are organized into four age groupings (6–7, 8–9, 10–12, 13–15), and raw scores are converted and analyzed through T scores.

D. Validity and Reliability

1. Reliability

Interrater and Split-Half: Acceptable.

2. Validity

Convergent and Discriminate: Initial data appear promising. RATC able to separate clinical from nonclinical groups at a highly significant level.

The Rorschach: The Comprehensive System (1974)

Author: J. E. Exner, Jr.

Publisher: Rorschach Workshops
11 Beaver Drive
Bayville, New York 11709

A. Description of Test

1. Standardization Population

Extensive normative data based on the protocols of 1,870 nonpatient children and adolescents (ages 5–16) tested by 147 examiners across the country in proportions roughly comparable to United States census data across stratified variables.

2. Time to Assess

Varies with the age of the examinee.

3. What It Assesses

The Rorschach operates primarily as a perceptual-cognitive task. Subjects are presented separately with 10 inkblots and asked "What might this be?" An inquiry process deduces how they saw what they saw. Analysis provides insight into how individuals structure their perceptual-cognitive experiences and their characteristic dispositions and current emotional and attitudinal states. Comparisons with norms and clinical groups provide some other diagnostic hypotheses and conclusions.

B. Scoring/Interpretation

Each individual response to a Rorschach card is coded across seven major categories: location determinants, form quality, organizational activity, popularity, contents, and special scores. Interpretation is based on normative comparisons and analysis of these scoring areas, as well as considerations of Rorschach responses at specific age levels, typical patterns of development for children and adolescents, and trends toward the stability of personality dimensions that affect the predictability of behavior from one age to another.

C. Norms

Norms are available for the various scoring categories for 12 age ranges across the 5–16 age span.

D. Validity and Reliability

1. Reliability

Test-Retest: Adequate to very good: dependent on the age of the examinee.

2. Validity

Good discriminate validity across many clinical groups (e.g., schizophrenia, depression, anxiety-withdrawal, conduct disorder).

Extensive validity studies indicate excellent clinical promise diagnostically.

The Rotter Incomplete Sentence Blank (RISB) (1950)

Authors: Julian B. Rotter and Janet E. Rafferty

Publisher: The Psychological Corporation
304 East 45th Street
New York, New York 10017

A. Description of Test

1. Standardization Population
Three forms of this 40-item test are available, with norms published in the manual.

2. Time to Assess
Approximately 15–20 minutes.

3. What It Assesses
This is a projective technique which reflects students' wishes, desires, fears, and attitudes. Available in three forms with a quantitative scoring system, the RISB is designed primarily as a screening device with an overall adjustment index score.

B. Scoring/Interpretation
A scale value is assigned to each response in accord with the general principles stated in the manual by matching responses with various samples (extremely well adjusted to those in need of psychotherapy). There are 10 scoring principles. Interpretations can be made through any theoretical framework or common sense. The manual gives examples. There are no cutoff scores, but one may refer to the table of percentiles to compare the individual to the norm samples. Interpretation is often dependent on practitioner experience and skill.

C. Norms
For the college group, the RISB was given to 299 entering freshmen at Ohio State University. The mean was 127, the standard deviation was 14 for both males and females. Norms and percentiles for the other two forms and groups are available.

D. Validity and Reliability

1. Reliability

Split-Half: Adequate.

Interscorer: Excellent.

These types of reliability are important for this test, which involves judgment.

2. Validity
Differentiation: Significantly differentiated between adjusted and maladjusted males and females.

The Sacks Sentence Completion Test (SSCT) (1950)

Authors: J. M. Sacks and S. Levy

A. Description of Test

1. Standardization Population
Nonobjective scoring and interpretation system.

2. What It Assesses
The Sacks uses sentence stems to assess each of 15 separate attitudes (e.g., toward mother, friends, fears). It is designed to identify areas of disturbance as well as an overview of inter-relationships among various attitudes.

B. Scoring/Interpretation

The responses are grouped and individually rated on 3-point scales using a nonobjective scoring system. This is supposed to determine the degree of disturbance present.

C. Norms

Nonobjective scoring system.

D. Validity and Reliability

None evident.

School Apperception Method (1968)

Authors: Irving L. Solomon, Ph.D., and Bernard D. Starr, Ph.D.

Publisher: Springer Publishing Company, Inc.
200 Park Avenue South
New York, New York 10003

A. Description of Test

1. Standardization Population

There is no formally identified standardization population. The content of the pictures was determined by the authors' varied experiences in school psychology. After using it with children in school and clinic settings, revisions were made and the final series of cards was chosen.

2. Time to Assess

Approximately 40 minutes.

3. What It Assesses

Developed for children in grades K–9, the SAM consists of 22 cards of detailed drawings depicting school-related and classroom scenes. The authors suggest administering 12 cards of this projective, thematic technique to children, requiring the telling of a story with a beginning and an ending for each picture. The SAM is designed to elicit information regarding children's significant emotional and academic adjustment difficulties in school. This may include perceptions of teachers and peers, attitudes toward academic activities, and expectations of interpersonal interactions.

B. Scoring/Interpretation

Children's stories about the stimulus cards are recorded on a protocol. The manual suggests various evaluative systems [especially noting Bellack's (1974) TAT/CAT scoring guidelines] and also provides its own framework with nine categories for interpreting the SAM stories or responses. Additional information is provided with sample responses and interpretations.

C. Norms

Unsubstantiated.

D. Validity and Reliability

Not reported in manual.

Teacher Version of the Achenbach
Child Behavior Checklist (in press)

Authors: C. S. Edelbrock and T. M. Achenbach

Publisher: Psychiatric Associates
c/o Department of Psychiatry
University of Vermont
Burlington, Vermont 05401

A. Description of Test

1. Standardization Population

Teachers completed the checklist for 450 boys referred to 18 mental health agencies in the eastern, midwestern, and southern parts of the country. 80% of the boys were white, 19% were black, and 1%, other. There was an equal number of boys at each age level from 6 to 11. 22% were considered upper SES, 39% were middle SES, and 39%, lower SES.

2. Time to Assess
15 minutes.

3. What It Assesses
This behavior rating scale addresses behavioral symptomology in the school setting consisting of 118 specific behavior problems; it is normed for ages 6–11, with additional norms forthcoming. It yields scores on multidimensional behavior problems, adaptive functioning, and school performance. A factor analysis produced two main factors (Internalizing/Externalizing and a Mixed factor) and eight second-order factors (anxious, social withdrawal, unpopular, self-destructive, obsessive-compulsive, aggressive, nervous-overacting, and inattentive).

B. Scoring/Interpretation
Teachers are asked to respond to some items on a 3-point scale regarding a student's behavior; school performance is rated by identifying the child's grade level of specific academic subjects along a 5-point scale; adaptive functioning is rated on a 7-point scale. Raw scores are plotted on the Teacher Profile and are transformed into T scores and percentile ranks based on the normative sample described below.

C. Norms
Three hundred teachers completed the Teacher Report Form questionnaires. There were 50 boys at each age level from 6 to 11. They had a similar SES breakdown as the referred group of boys in the standardization sample. Other normative data for other age groups are in progress. As yet, the checklist has only been normed with boys.

D. Validity and Reliability
1. Reliability
Internal Consistency: Adequate (based on CBCL).

Interrater and Interscorer: No data.

Test-Retest: For 1 week to 2 months, excellent for disturbed children and children with behavioral or emotional problems. This should be interpreted cautiously because there was a small sample size.

2. Validity
Content: Good based on CBCL.

Discriminative: Effectively discriminates between clinically referred boys and nonreferred boys.

Convergent: The internalizing factor was found to have good correlations with observational ratings. Total behavior was found to correlate positively with observations, negatively with on-task behavior. Adaptive functioning and school performance correlates negatively with problem behavior and positively with on-task ratings of behavior.

Thematic Apperception Test (1938)

Author: Henry A. Murray

Publisher: Harvard University Press
79 Gasden Street
Cambridge, Massachusetts 02138

A. Description of Test
1. Standardization Population
Depends on the scoring approach used. Those most commonly available are Morgan and Murray (1935), Bellak (1947), Eron (1950), and Murstein (1963). The presence of a scoring system does not always suggest a clearly specified standardization population.

2. Time to Assess
Approximately 45 minutes based on 10 cards.

3. What It Assesses

One of the most prevalent projective, thematic techniques, the TAT was developed to reveal individuals' dominant drives, emotions, traits, and conflicts by identifying significant interpersonal needs, presses, and themas. The TAT consists of 31 cards, with some specific to male/female children, adolescent, and adult issues, respectively. Generally, approximately 10 cards are given for a single administration and individuals are asked to tell a story with a beginning and end related to the stimulus card.

B. Scoring/Interpretation

A number of quantitative scoring schemes and rating scales have been developed that yield good scorer reliability (see above). These procedures are seldom used in clinical practice because they are time consuming. Thus, the practitioner's skill and experience are often most necessary for interpretation.

C. Norms

Depends on scoring approach, although norms not readily available.

D. Validity and Reliability

Validity and reliability are hard to establish because of the open-ended, free response nature of the task and the difficulty of finding criteria against which to validate inferences. A variety of formal scoring systems and methods of administration have been developed, and the scoring systems are yielding increasingly more valid and reliable results.

Author Index

667

Subject Index